Metals as Biomaterials

Wiley Series in Biomaterials Science and Engineering

Commissioned in the UK on behalf of John Wiley & Sons, Ltd by Medi-Tech Publications, Storrington, West Sussex RH20 4HH, UK

Series Advisors

Robin N. Stephens
AVE (UK) Limited, Burgess Hill, UK

Julian H. Braybrook
Laboratory of the Government Chemist, London, UK

Patrick M. Maloney
CellPro Inc, Bothell, Washington, USA

Providing readers with comprehensive, authoritative and timely information in this fast-developing area of research and biomedical technological advancement, this series encompasses topics in biomaterials science and engineering including the structure and function of materials and devices, their individual actions and interactions, and practical and clinical applications.

Books in the *Wiley Series in Biomaterials Science and Engineering* are designed to help stimulate further developments in biomaterials science and engineering by disseminating up-to-the-minute, quality information to academic and industrial research and development scientists employed in all areas of the medical, biomedical and bioengineering sciences, whether in medical device R&D, pharmaceutical and pharmacological research or materials science, and to clinical specialists in prosthetics and surgery.

RECENT TITLES IN THE SERIES

Biosensors in the Body; Continuous in vivo *Monitoring*
Edited by David M. Fraser (0 471 96707 6)

Biocompatibility Assessment of Medical Devices and Materials
Edited by Julian H. Braybrook (0 471 96597 9)

Design Engineering of Biomaterials for Medical Devices
David Hill (0 471 96708 4)

Metals as Biomaterials
Edited by J. Helsen and H.J. Breme (0 471 96935 4)

FORTHCOMING TITLES IN THE SERIES

Computer Technology in Biomaterials Science and Engineering
Edited by J. Vander Sloten (0 471 97602 4)

Metals as Biomaterials

Edited by

Jef A. Helsen
Faculty of Metallurgy and Materials Engineering, Catholic University of Leuven, Leuven, Belgium

and

H. Jürgen Breme
Department of Metallic Materials, University of the Saarland, Saarbrücken, Germany

JOHN WILEY & SONS
Chichester · New York · Weinheim · Brisbane · Singapore · Toronto

Copyright © 1998 by John Wiley & Sons Ltd,
Baffins Lane, Chichester,
West Sussex PO19 1UD, England

National 01243 779777
International (+44)1243 779777
e-mail (for orders and customer service enquiries): cs-books@wiley.co.uk
Visit our Home Page on http://www.wiley.co.uk
or http://www.wiley.com

All rights reserved. No part of this publication may be reproduced, stored in a retrieval
system, or transmitted, in any form or by any means, electronic, mechanical, photocopying,
recording, scanning or otherwise, except under the terms of the Copyright, Designs and Patents Act
1988 or under the terms of a licence issued by the Copyright Licensing Agency,
90 Tottenham Court Road, London, W1P 9HE, UK without the prior permission in writing of the
publisher with the exception of any material supplied specifically for the purpose of being
entered and executed on a computer system for the exclusive use by the purchaser of the
publication.

Other Wiley Editorial Offices

John Wiley & Sons, Inc., 605 Third Avenue,
New York, NY 10158-0012, USA

WILEY-VCH Verlag GmbH, Pappelallee 3,
D-69469 Weinheim, Germany

Jacaranda Wiley Ltd, 33 Park Road, Milton,
Queensland 4064, Australia

John Wiley & Sons (Asia) Pte Ltd, 2 Clementi Loop #02-01,
Jin Xing Distripark, Singapore 129809

John Wiley & Sons (Canada) Ltd, 22 Worcester Road,
Rexdale, Ontario M9W 1L1, Canada

Library of Congress Cataloging-in-Publication Data
Metals as biomaterials/edited by J.A. Helsen and H.J. Breme
 p. cm. – (Wiley series in biomaterials science and engineering)
 Includes biographical references and index
 ISBN 0-471-96935-4 (hardcover: alk. paper)
 1. Metals in medicine. I. Helsen, J.A. II. Breme, H.J. III. Series.
R857.M37M48 1998
610′.28–dc21
DNLM/DLC
                                                                          98–9264
                                                                             CIP

British Library Cataloguing in Publication Data
A catalogue record for this book is available from the British Library

ISBN 0 471 96935 4

Produced and typeset in 10/12 pt Times by Gray Publishing, Tunbridge Wells.
Printed and bound in Great Britain by Biddles Ltd, Guildford and King's Lynn.
This book is printed on acid-free paper responsibly manufactured from sustainable
forestry, in which at least two trees are planted for each one used for paper production.

Contents

List of contributors   vii

Foreword   ix

Preface   xi

1. Selection of materials   1
   H.J. Breme and J.A. Helsen

2. Metals and implants   37
   H.J. Breme, V. Biehl and J.A. Helsen

3. Shape memory alloys   73
   J. Van Humbeeck, R. Stalmans and P.A. Besselink

4. Degradation (*in vitro–in vivo* corrosion)   101
   D. Scharnweber

5. Surfaces, surface modification and tailoring   153
   H.J. Breme

6. Special thin organic coatings   177
   H. Worch

7. Adhesion of polymers   197
   W. Possart

8. Adhesion to ceramics   219
   H.J. Breme, M.A. Barbosa and L.A. Rocha

9. Biological response and biocompatibility   265
   H.F. Hildebrand and J.-C. Hornez

10. Tissue–implant interaction   291
    R. Thull

11	Cells and metals *D.B. Jones*	317
12	X-ray photoelectron spectroscopy *J.J Pireaux and J. Riga*	337
13	Atomic force microscopy *U. Hartmann*	359
14	Electrochemical impedance spectroscopy as a surface analytical technique for biomaterials *J. Hubrecht*	405
15	Retrieval analysis *P. Laffargue, H.J. Breme, J.A. Helsen and H.F. Hildebrand*	467
Index		503

Contributors

M.A. BARBOSA — *INEB-Mat, Institute of Biomedical Engineering, 823 Rua do Campo Alegre, 4150 Porto, Portugal*

P.A. BESSELINK — *Memory Metal Holland, Gronausestraat 1220, 7534 AT Enschede, The Netherlands*

V. BIEHL — *Department of Metallic Materials, University of the Saarland, PF 151150, D-66041 Saarbrücken, Germany*

H.J. BREME — *Department of Metallic Materials, University of the Saarland, PF 151150, D-66041 Saarbrücken, Germany*

U. HARTMANN — *Institute of Experimental Physics, University of the Saarland, D-66041 Saarbrücken, Germany*

J.A. HELSEN — *Department of Metals and Materials Engineering, Catholic University of Leuven, W. de Croylaan 2, B-3001 Leuven, Belgium*

H.F. HILDEBRAND — *Biomaterials Research Group, Biophysics Laboratory, Faculty of Medicine, University of Lille, 1 Place de Verdun, F-59045 Lille Cedex, France*

J.-C. HORNEZ — *Biomaterials Research Group, Biophysics Laboratory, Faculty of Medicine, University of Lille, 1 Place de Verdun, F-59045 Lille Cedex, France*

J. HUBRECHT — *Department of Metals and Materials Engineering, Catholic University of Leuven, W. de Croylaan 2, B-3001 Leuven, Belgium*

D.B. Jones	Department of Experimental Orthopaedics, Philipps University, D-35033 Marburg, Germany
P. Laffargue	Service de Traumatologie et de Chirurgie Orthopédique A, CHRU de Lille, Hôpital Roger Salengro, Lille Cedex, France
J.J Pireaux	LISE, University Faculties of Notre-Dame de la Paix, University of Namur, 61 rue de Bruxelles, B-5000 Namur, Belgium
W. Possart	Structural Research, Polymers and Interphases, University of the Saarland, PF 151150, D-66041 Saarbrücken, Germany
J. Riga	LISE, University Faculties of Notre-Dame de la Paix, University of Namur, 61 rue de Bruxelles, B-5000 Namur, Belgium
L.A. Rocha	University of Minho, Campus de Azurien, 4810 Quinarex Codex, Portugal
D. Scharnweber	Institute of Materials Science, Technical University of Dresden, D-01069 Dresden, Germany
R. Stalmans	Department of Metallurgy and Materials Engineering, Catholic University of Leuven, B-3001 Leuven, Belgium
R. Thull	Division of Experimental Dental Medicine, Bavarian Julius-Maximlians University of Würzburg, Pleicherwall 2, D-97070 Würzburg, Germany
J. Van Humbeeck	Department of Metallurgy and Materials Engineering, Catholic University of Leuven, B-3001 Leuven, Belgium
H. Worch	Institute of Materials Science, Technical University of Dresden, D-01069 Dresden, Germany

Foreword

Developments in recent years in bioactive materials, polymers, composite materials and ceramics, as well as present and future trends toward hybrid material systems and tissue engineering, could give the strong – but wrong – impression that there is no longer any future for metals and alloys as biomaterials.

Where alternative materials are proposed to cope with specific shortcomings of metals (such as corrosion), they often show their deficiencies, especially in their mechanical properties. Therefore it remains very important to think in terms of metal-based biomaterial systems, in which the intrinsic strengths of metals are fully exploited while state-of-the-art engineering methods are used to overcome their weaknesses.

Over the last two decades, research and development and innovation in materials engineering have led to considerable improvements in metal and alloy properties as well as to new types of products for a wide area of of medical applications. A special case is the one presented by the shape memory alloys, which have recently led to rather spectacular medical applications.

For these reasons, this up-to-date reference book on metals as biomaterials clearly fills a gap.

It starts with a general chapter on the selection of biomaterials, emphasising mechanical criteria such as strength, stiffness (E-modulus), fracture toughness and fatigue resistance. In the following chapter, a comprehensive knowledge base (including numerical data) on metal implants is provided. A specific chapter is devoted to shape memory alloys.

A second group of chapters deals with the intrinsic shortcomings of metals, i.e. corrosion, wear resistance, tissue response and systemic biocompatibility, and the engineering methods to deal with them: surface treatment and modification, thin organic coatings, ceramic coatings, polymer–metal macrocomposites.

This book on metals as biomaterials comes just in time. It is not meant to pay tribute to the instrumental role that metals and alloys have played in the lives of millions of patients over the last 30 years, although implicitly it does, in a most convincing way. It is a handbook and reference book for professionals in industry, clinics and research, and a fundamental textbook for all biomaterials students.

The expertise of the two editors Jef Helsen and Jürgen Breme and the authors of the different chapters – all widely known experts in their fields – provide this book with a label of outstanding quality.

Georges van der Perre
Department of Mechanics, University of Leuven, Belgium

Preface

Once something has been proven to be good, it may, under certain circumstances, turn out to be an obstacle to the development of something even better, especially when massive economic interests are involved. This fact also holds for the field of implantology, a branch of medical technology that depends, as almost no other field of research, on the interdisciplinary endeavour, for example of surgeons, biologists, engineers, physicists and chemists. Nevertheless, in the last few decades great progress has been made possible due to the fact that medicine has been provided with materials which fulfil at least in part the required functions.

In the 1960s corrosion fatigue was a common material 'disease' in hip stems and osteosynthesis plates but has been generally eliminated by the alloys now used for weight-bearing implants. The effect of the allergen nickel is also almost completely eliminated. The ingrowth of cementless hip stems has been made possible by the use of plasma-sprayed hydroxyapatite coatings. The wear resistance of artificial joint materials is substantially improved. Heart valves have become reliable devices. We now have at our disposal artificial arteries and veins, ligaments, eye lenses, kidney dialysis, cardiovascular and urological stents, artificial limbs and so on – a long list of advances which improve substantially the health and comfort of the human race.

More recently, and consistent with the progress of medical technology, tailor-made products are being used, which due to the complexity of the problem may often no longer be made of a single material, but of a composite in which each of the individual components has its own function to perform, for example structural components with functional coatings. Research now concentrates increasingly on the interface between living and non-living material because very little is as yet understood about the interactions which occur there. The advances in implantology research are documented by a large number of annual international and national conferences with their proceedings and in addition by publications in such relevant journals as *Biomaterials*, *Journal of Biomedical Material Research*, and so on. It is only with great difficulty that the non-scientist is able to absorb and filter this deluge of information with respect to its relevance or the mass of individual results. The present book, the first in a series dealing with the most commonly used materials – metals, ceramics and polymers – is devoted to metals and is intended to serve as a guide to all those engaged in the field of metallic implant materials. The intention of the editors was to offer a concise textbook compiling numerical data on metals and alloys of biomedical relevance on the one hand, and describing the interaction of metals with cells and tissues on the other.

The book opens with a chapter on the philosophy (principles) of materials selection, a basic issue in the development of an implant. Chapter 2 compiles the numerical chemical, physical and mechanical data for all metals and alloys of biomedical relevance now in use or with a potential for use in the future. They include stainless steels, cobalt–chromium alloys, titanium and its alloys, dental restoration and refractory materials. A separate chapter is devoted to shape memory alloys. These alloys are newcomers in the biomedical field with interesting prospects for a bright future. Nothing in nature is inert and metals, too, degrade. The biological environment is particularly aggressive towards metals. The degradation of metals, corrosion, is described in electrochemical terms and this aspect is dealt with in Chapter 4. The materials scientist wants to select a material that best fits the intended application. If it does not exist, he or she has to create it. So the materials scientist is committed to tailoring a material to fulfil the requirements. Chapters 5–8 deal with materials which 'engineer' surface modification, organic coatings, adhesion to polymers and ceramics. We mentioned earlier the lack of an overall scientific picture of the interaction of materials with living matter. The major question here is the study of the interaction of metals and alloys with tissues and with cells. This topic is dealt with in Chapters 9–11. Mention of the instrumentation used to assess properties and interactions should certainly be included in this textbook. However, the arsenal of instruments is so vast that we have limited ourselves (Chapters 12–14) to a few techniques not currently covered by other biomaterials textbooks: X-ray photoelectron spectroscopy, atomic force microscopy and electrochemical impedance spectroscopy.

During the last two decades a vast amount of industrial and academic research has been devoted to the constellation of new materials. Most of the metal alloys we use today cannot be defined as new. The same can be said about ceramics and polymers. Many of these materials were developed decades ago but gradually and by appropriate production techniques promoted to biometals, bioceramics or biopolymers. Attempts to substitute metals by materials of the other generic classes were often not successful. Metals and their alloys exhibit a particularly excellent long-term stability of mechanical loads (tension stresses) and are as such not easily substituted, in particular in weight-bearing implants. This will probably be the situation for the years to come. Moreover, biocompatibility can be improved by appropriate tailoring of the surfaces (e.g. coating) or the bulk (e.g. by making composite materials with a gradient in elasticity modulus). However, a gradual substitution by other high-tech materials will definitely take place in the future until the point is reached where organs will be regenerated and the need for biomaterials will be drastically decreased – but before that happens, this book will long be outdated. In the opinion of the editors, the question whether or not there is a need for a book on metals as biomaterials may be answered by a convincing yes.

1
Selection of materials

H.J. BREME[1] AND J.A. HELSEN[2]
[1]University of the Saarland, Saarbrücken, Germany
[2]Catholic University of Leuven, Leuven, Belgium

1.1 INTRODUCTION

In order to provide a device or facility, certain specific property requirements pertaining to both the material and the product must be fulfilled (Figure 1.1). The material-specific properties, which are listed in Table 1.1, include mechanical, physical, chemical and physicochemical properties. Of additional importance in the case of biomedical devices are the biological properties (biocompatibility and bioadhesion), which are influenced by the physical, chemical and physicochemical behaviour of the material. The relevant properties specified by the product are summarised in Table 1.2. In the following an example is discussed for the evaluation of an implant (hip prosthesis) construction starting from the first concept to the realisation via a hierarchical analysis.

The characteristics of the environment in which an implant has to operate and the function it has to perform set the boundary conditions for the design of a new implant. Based on these conditions a scientist will develop a first concept. The more

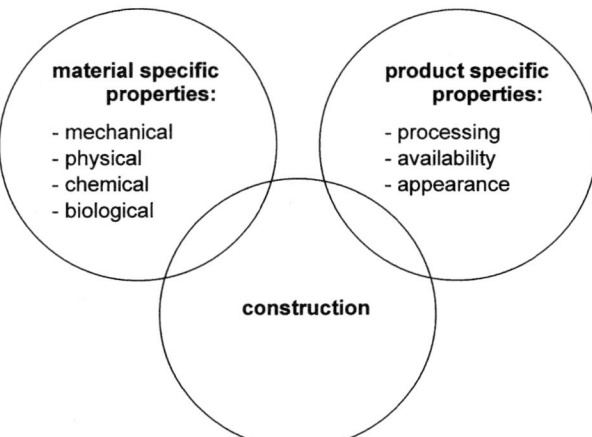

Figure 1.1 Material- and product-specific properties leading to a construction.

Metals as Biomaterials ISBN 0 471 96935 4 Edited by J.A. Helsen and H.J. Breme. © 1998 John Wiley & Sons Ltd

Table 1.1 Material-specific properties with respect to biomedical constructions

Properties	Relevant to biomaterials
Mechanical	According to the loading
Yield, tensile (compression) strength	Important
Ultimate tensile (compression) strength	Important
Elongation at fracture	Important
Reduction in area	Important
Fracture toughness	Important
Fatigue strength	Very important
Young's modulus	Very important
Creep resistance	Important for polymers only
Structure	Important
Wear, abrasion resistance	Very important
Physical	Only for specific applications, e.g.:
Density	orthopaedic implants
Acoustics	ultrasonic monitoring
Electrical resistivity	heart pacemaker leads
Magnetism	probes in NMR spectroscopy
Optical properties	mirrors
Thermal expansion	bone cement and composites (metal/ceramics, etc.)
Chemical (surface)	
Oxidation	Very important (repassivation)
Corrosion and degradation resistance	Very important
Wear, abrasion resistance	Very important
Biological	
Bioadhesion (osteoconductivity, osteointegration)	Very important
Immune response (allergic, toxic, mutogenic, carcinogenic)	Very important

NMR, Nuclear magnetic resonance.

precisely these conditions are determined, the more concrete a concept will be. Subsequently, two routes can be followed. The ideal approach is that the implant is designed in as much detail as possible according to the actual state of the art, followed by either the selection of existing materials meeting the requirements of the design, or the creation of new, dedicated materials. The more materialistic route is to carry out the design in a progressive way, continuously considering what is possible with the available materials. In any case, the designer will conduct a materials selection process, first, among the generic classes and, secondly, within a given generic class. This book starts from the assumption that the designer has selected a metal for a reason which is obvious to the designer. The selection within the generic class of metals will then be discussed.

A new implant will be created to meet the requirements of a surgeon, a professional designer or a scientist as a natural issue of newly acquired knowledge. It always starts as a concept which is translated into a first design and then passes

SELECTION OF MATERIALS

Table 1.2 Product-specific properties with respect to biomedical constructions

	Relevant to biomaterials
Processing	
Melting	Important for metals
Casting	Important for metals
Forming	Important for metals
Welding	Important
Brazing	Important
Machining	Important
Powder technology	Important for special materials (tailored) and devices
Availability	
Price of material	Important
Cost of processing	Important
Appearance	Important only for visible constructions, e.g. crowns and bridges in dental restoration and for subcutaneous implants

consecutively through a number of steps before the design is manufactured and marketed. Each step represents a fairly tight relationship of the design to the material: requirement on the market, cost, availability of new materials or new manufacturing techniques, improvement of the new design with respect to competing and existing products, and many other technical, medical and commercial considerations. The ultimate selection of the materials will be a direct consequence of the functional analysis of the organ to be supported or replaced. Feedback from experimental *in vitro* and *in vivo* tests may correct the selected material.

For any selection process the designer follows a strict hierarchy. Possible hierarchical trees for the analysis of the functions to be performed in a total hip replacement are shown in Figure 1.2. The hip joint is taken as an example of a heavy-duty application where the mechanical properties of the materials used for its production are of major importance for the success of the prosthesis. The concept adopted here as an example is a modular, non-cemented total hip prosthesis consisting of a cup (pelvic part), the head fitted to the tapered neck of the stem (articulating part) and the stem with a Young's modulus gradient (femoral part) (Figure 1.2a). The cup is in contact with the pelvic bone and is made out of a polymer, coated with hydroxyapatite or backed by a coated or non-coated metal cup. The cup may be either all ceramic or all metal. The outer surface is either coated for ingrowth and cementless implantation or non-coated for cemented fixation. Whether the bulk is a polymer, a ceramic or a metal, it should be resistant to wear and, because it is subject to severe loads, resistant to creep (Figure 1.2b). The counterpart of the cup is a ball, typically of a modular design, fitted with a tapered connection to the femoral part. It may be made of a ceramic or a metal with high compressive strength and should be highly resistant to wear and corrosion (Figure 1.2c).

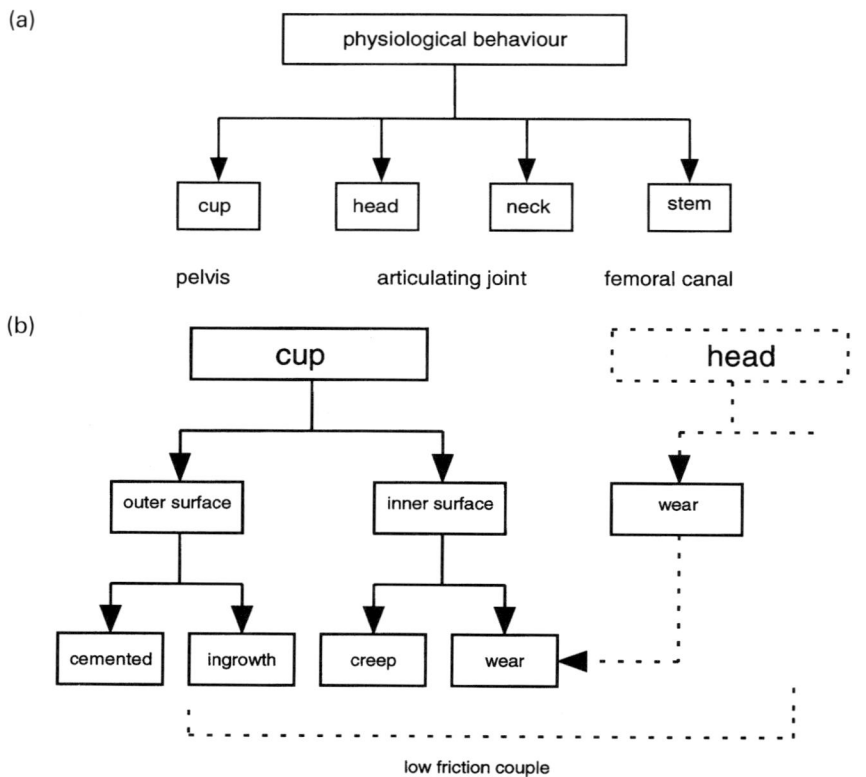

Figure 1.2 (a) Modular hip prosthesis: main components. (b) Pelvic part of the hip prosthesis. The main requirements to be taken into account when designing the cup of a new prosthesis. (c) and (d) opposite.

Moreover, it should form a suitable low-friction couple with the cup material and an acceptable corrosion couple with the metal of the femoral part. The body weight is transmitted to the femur through the contact zone between the stem and the femoral cortex. It is subject to strong bending stresses, micromovements of the stem provoke wear and a bad design may cause considerable stress shielding. Its surface may be the bare metal or it may be coated with hydroxyapatite. The Young's modulus of the materials used may be hypoelastic, hyperelastic or isoelastic with cortical bone. A complex material with a gradient in the Young's modulus, low at the surface (similar to bone) and high near the core (Figure 1.2d), may also be conceived.

The example given illustrates the complexity of the selection of materials, because they must simultaneously meet contradictory requirements. The number of variables already mentioned is high and the list is not exhaustive. The great variety of possible combinations is also reflected in the variety of designs that are commercially available. The selection of materials is, however, only one part of the whole development process of an implant. A flow sheet of the experimental steps to

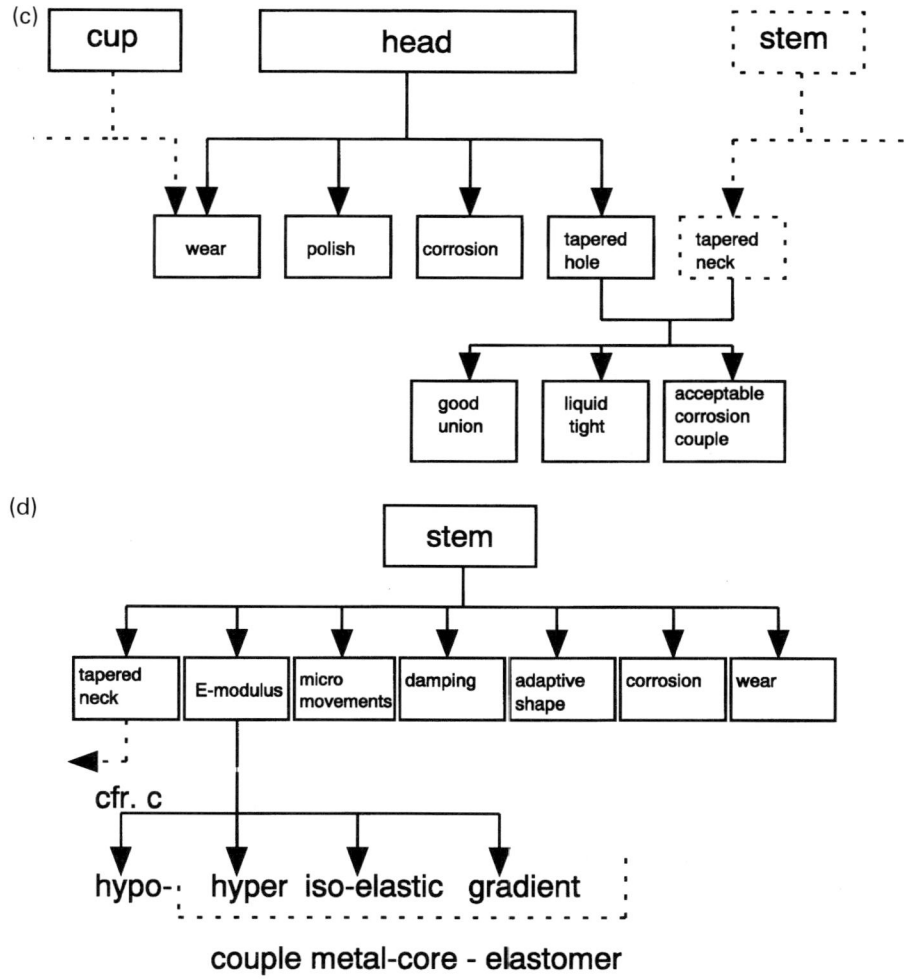

Figure 1.2 (c) Articulating part of the hip and its mechanical and chemical requirements. (d) Femoral part of the hip prosthesis. Four possible configurations are suggested for the mechanical properties to be imposed on the material: hypoelastic, hyperelastic or isoelastic with respect to cortical bone or with a gradient in the E-modulus.

be taken after a functional analysis and selection procedure is shown in Figure 1.3. More details on different experimental items such as premedical tests, toxicity and surface modification are discussed in the following chapters. The flow sheet shows different feedback loops, illustrating that, as the test procedures approach the final design, subparts, if not major parts, of the concept will have to be modified.

A good guide to the preliminary materials selection is the *Elsevier Materials Selector*, edited by Waterman and Ashby (1991). A number of materials selection

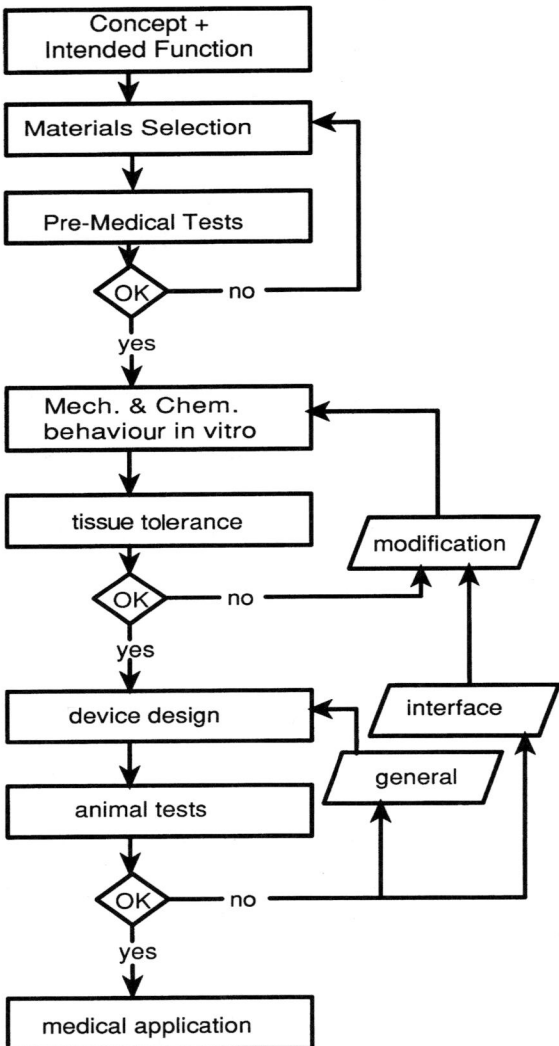

Figure 1.3 Flow sheet of the consecutive steps to be followed during the development of a new prosthesis.

charts shows how to maximise a given property for a minimum of another property. The Young's modulus versus density chart shows at a glance the classes of materials that combine the highest modulus with minimum weight, highest torsion strength with minimum weight, strength with expansion coefficient, loss-coefficient with modulus, strength with cost, etc. There also exists a software version of this system, *The Cambridge Materials Selector* (Version 2.0) (Cebon and Ashby, 1994). The user can thus compose his or her own materials property charts by placing any of the

SELECTION OF MATERIALS

listed properties against any other. Unfortunately, no charts yet exist for selecting materials on the basis of biocompatibility and biofunctionality criteria, e.g. highest strength and minimum immune response. A selection of data sources for metals, books and software is collected in Table 1.3. An attempt is made in Chapter 2 to collect exhaustively most of the engineering properties of the metals and alloys used for biomedical purposes.

1.2 HISTORY OF AN ALL-METAL PROSTHESIS

Good ideas do not necessarily lead to better implants. The use of silicone rubber as an elastic cushioning material in a total hip prosthesis for both the femoral and acetabular components was such an idea in the 1970s. It can be considered as the remote onset for the concept of prostheses made of materials with a gradient in

Table 1.3 Data sources (books and software) for metals: properties and selection

Books
ASM Handbooks No.1 (1990) to No. 19 (1996) (all aspects of metals and ceramics), ASM International, Ohio, USA
ASTM *Annual Book of ASTM Standards*
MRS *Proceedings of Annual Fall Meeting*
Handbook of Corrosion (1995), ASM International, Ohio, USA
Boyer, R., Welsch, G. and Collings, E.W., (1994) *Materials Properties Handbook: Titanium Alloys*, ASM International, Ohio, USA
Guide to Materials Engineering and Data Information (1986), ASM International, Ohio, USA
Pollock, D.D., (1993) *Physical Properties for Engineers*, CRC Blackwell Library Services, Oxford.
Software
TAPP version 3.0 (1996) A materials database of over 30 000 compound phases, solutions and phase diagrams ESM Software, Hamilton, USA
Cuthill, J.R., Gokcan, N.A., and Morral, J.E. (1988) *Computerized Material Databases*, Metallurgical Society, Worchdale, USA
The Materials Property Data Network (1995) STN International, CAS, Columbus, USA
International Metallic Materials Cross-reference Database Software (1996) Genium Publishing Corporation, Schenectady, USA
ASTM Stahlschlüssel with CD-ROM (1996) ASTM and Technical Standard Services, Hitxhin, UK
Materials selection books
Cornish, E.H. (1985) *Materials Selection and Design*, UK Information Sources, Chameleon Press
Waterman, N.A. and Ashby, M.F. (1996) *Elsevier Materials Selector*, Elsevier Applied Science, London
Ashby, M.F. (1994) *Materials Selection Wallchart*, Chapman and Hall
Materials selection software
Cambridge Materials Selector (1995) CMS 2.0 Software, Granta Design, Cambridge, UK

The list is non-exhaustive.

Young's modulus (Esslinger and Rutkowski, 1973; Repo *et al.*, 1986; Newcombe *et al.*, 1987). The practical implementation of the idea failed because the authors neglected to make the appropriate material selection and carry out subsequent testing. In the history of science forgotten ideas are often reinvented a couple of decades later. A few authors are attempting now to exploit the same ideas again, but only with careful selection and extensive testing of the materials before starting implantation (Helsen *et al.*, 1993; Jaecques *et al.*, 1995). Their research philosophy was based on flow sheets, as given in Figures 1.2 and 1.3.

Another example is the all-metal modular hip prosthesis. Hip prostheses will be referred to often not because they are more important than other replacements in hard or soft tissues but, in the discussion of metals, hip and knee prostheses are the examples *par excellence* of heavy-duty applications of metals. The articulating part of the prosthesis is the combination of a ball rotating in a socket, at first glance a simple mechanical part that should be easy to substitute by a mechanical equivalent. The physiological and morphological reference frame of a healthy human hip joint is shown in Figure 1.2a. This joint belongs to the class of synovial joints. The osseous parts are covered by articular cartilage, the composition of which is beyond the interest of this chapter. The cartilaginous surface has a very low coefficient of friction, and is wear resistant, slightly compressible and elastic. It is ideally constructed for easy movement and able to absorb the large forces of compression and shear generated by gravity and muscular power. It is partly enclosed by a fibrous capsule and the sliding is lubricated by the synovial fluid which is a true non-Newtonian fluid (i.e. viscoelastic). The shape of this joint is not spherical but slightly ovoid. Contact between the surfaces of the ball and socket is maximum in only one position. The degree of movement is limited when compared, for example, to the shoulder: flexion of 90–100° from the vertical and around 10–20° beyond the vertical (Williams *et al.*, 1989, pp. 470, 473, 475, 523). So far a (non-exhaustive) qualitative description of the performance of a healthy joint has been given. A normal healthy joint shows zero wear. For many reasons, e.g. osteoarthritis or rheumatic diseases, the joint can become deficient to such an extent that it has to be replaced entirely by a mechanical substitute. After this short description of the physiology of the hip joint, it will be clear that the mechanical constraints for substituting the natural device with an artificial one are far more demanding than they would seem at first glance.

The search for the perfect articulating pair has a history as long as hip arthroplasty itself. Artificial joints are subject to wear, whereby the amount of wear particles released into the capsule is of particular importance for the longevity of the implant fixation (Willert *et al.*, 1993; Streicher *et al.*, 1996). Polymethylmetacrylate (PMMA), teflon and other materials were tried and rejected for different reasons. The most long-standing combination since the early 1960s is the couple between an ultra-high molecular weight polyethene cup (UHMWPE) and a ball of a CoCr alloy. This couple provoked relatively little trouble provided the life expectancy of the (older) patients was not too long and implantation in younger patients was not frequent. Wear debris from polyethene seems to be the major reason for aseptic

SELECTION OF MATERIALS

loosening (Simon, 1994). Modification to the bulk, the surface and the subsurface of the UHMWPE by dispersion hardening or implantation of nitrogen or other atoms is one approach used to tackle wear resistance (Lee *et al.*, 1993, Liao, 1995). Another improvement might be the substitution of metal with ceramic femoral balls, which is reported to be more favourable (Zichner and Willert, 1992). An all-metal design, however, seems to be the most promising and economically feasible alternative. Although a good idea, it was not successful from the beginning (McKee, 1982) but breakthroughs occurred during the 1990s. From 1988 to June 1996 the implantation of about 50 000 metal combinations was reported (Schmidt *et al.*, 1996). The analysis of retrieved prostheses after several years of implantation confirms the very low wear rates predicted by *in vitro* experiments. Two parameters have proved to be of utmost importance in the success of the metal combination (Streicher *et al.*, 1996; Schmidt *et al.*, 1996):

- the use of a CoCr alloy with high carbon content, thermomechanically processed, which gives rise to small interdendritic carbides (e.g. type F75 or ISO 5832–12, see Chapter 2, Table 2.23, with >0.2% C).
- appropriate clearance between cup and ball.

A further improvement was the reduction in the ball diameter to 28 mm. Using this design, together with the high degree of polish of both parts possible for F75-type alloys, friction moments are obtained which are comparable to or even lower than for the same alloy with respect to UHMWPE. Hip simulator experiments gave wear rates of 10–20 µm per year in the initial phase below 10^6 cycles (about 2 years' function *in situ*). The rate slowed down to stationary values of about 6 µm per year or below for longer periods. The wear was similar for both the cup and the ball. All of these results were valid for hip simulator experiments in moist air or Ringer's solution with calf's serum. The *in situ* observations fitted well to those predicted by simulation for the actual *in situ* period of 10–17 years. For at least one of the marketed prostheses, the metal-to-metal articulation was introduced into an existing successful design whereby all components remained unchanged. The metal sliding surface was solidly anchored inside the polyethene cup, which was in itself already a technical challenge. The cup itself was backed by a metal shell. This particular aspect is mentioned here because it demonstrates how economic considerations are one of the many boundary conditions in the design of a prosthesis.

The above discussion focused on the improvement of the tribological properties of a total hip prosthesis. The construction process of the whole prosthesis will now be examined. As an example, the production steps of a cementless hip stem and cup are discussed (data provided by Sulzermedica, The Alloclassic Hip System).

1.2.1 FORGING

A cylinder of commercially pure titanium (ISO 5832–2) is heated to about 900°C and forged into a protoshape of the shell. The material is pressed into the die with a force of approx. 300 tons in one blow (Figure 1.4a, b). The stem forging is considerably more complicated because of its asymmetrical shape and material distribution. The dies and the forging process are thus controlled more frequently. The forging starts from a bar of the forging alloy Ti6Al7Nb (ISO 5832–11) after heating to about 900°C (Figure 1.4c). The first step is to upturn the end which will later be the proximal stem area (Figure 1.4d). After removing the flash, the forging is reheated. The lower part of the forging is then stretched using drawing rolls (Figure 1.4e). After reheating, the CCD angle is formed and the part is prepressed in another die. With one final blow, the part achieves its final form (Figure 1.4f–h). All of these forming steps are necessary in order to meet the final shape tolerances. A small stub is left on the tip of the stem, for holding the part during later machining operations. From the forging flash the forge master can determine the optimum material distribution in the die. The forging flash is sheared off while still warm. Ferritic residue is removed using an abrasive blasting process to permit easy examination of the surface. Subsequently, stem and cup forging are machined down to the precise final shape. Both forgings have a machining allowance, i.e. they are larger than the final product.

1.2.2 STEM MACHINING

The forging of the stem is clamped at the neck and the stub at the distal end. The contour is milled and holes are drilled in the trochanter wing. Following this, the distal tip is rounded and the extraction hole is drilled in the proximal part (Figure 1.4i, j). Most care is taken in the machining of the 12/14 taper spigot because the tolerances for diameter, roundness, straightness and angle are very tight. The taper spigot is machined so that its surface is threaded, 70 µm deep at the small diameter end and becoming gradually flatter towards the larger diameter end (Figure 1.4k). This fine thread deforms plastically when the ball head is impacted on to the stem and thus matches the inside taper. Size and taper angle are engraved on to the end face of the taper spigot. In the next operation all corners are rounded and ground by a robot-controlled machine in order to remove any notch effects.

1.2.3 MACHINING THE CUP SHELL AND BALL HEAD

The forging for the cup (Figure 1.4b) is machined inside and outside on a lathe in several steps (Figure 1.4l). The thread is cut and the kidney-shaped openings in the roof of the cup are made on a milling machine (Figure 1.4m, n). The tooth profile is formed on an automatic grinding machine and sharp edges are carefully removed. The ball head and the articulating metal insert in the cup are made from a forging CoCrMoC alloy. The first step in the manufacturing of the ball head is to turn the inside conical taper, followed by premachining of the articulating surface, with machining allowance (Figure 1.4o, p). In a grinding and polishing machine, the head is given its exact diameter and its special surface quality, which is checked under a microscope (Figure 1.4q). The dimensional inspection, with a tolerance of 1 µm, is

SELECTION OF MATERIALS

carried out on a three-axis measuring machine. In manufacturing the cup articulating surface, the outer form is finish machined first and then the articulating surface is premachined with machining allowance. The articulating surface is then ground and polished in several process steps.

1.2.4 MACHINING THE CUP

The inner and outer form, particularly the recess for the titanium disc and the space for fixing the articulating insert, are machined from bars of medical-quality polythene (polyethylene) (Figure 1.4r–t). Four polyethene stubs to prevent rotation of the insert are anchored in predrilled holes by friction welding. A disc is punched out of commercially pure titanium sheet, coarse blasted and laser marked. It is fixed in the base of the insert, and prevents direct contact between polyethene and bone after implantation (Figure 1.4u). Using a special process of the manufacturer, the articulating surface is bonded in the polyethene part, which is complicated by polyethene having a much greater coefficient of expansion than metal (Figure 1.4v). This was taken into account in the design of the bond.

1.2.5 FINISHING THE STEM AND SHELL

The machined stem and the shell do not yet have, amongst other things, the rough surface necessary for osseointegration. The implant surfaces, which have direct contact with bone, are coarse blasted. These are the body of the stem and the outside of the shell. The remaining areas, the stem neck and the inside of the shell, are fine blasted (Figure 1.4w, x). Compared with applied rough coatings, blasting reduces the strength of the base material only insignificantly. The blasting process leaves a microstructured surface almost completely free of contamination.

The above summary is a partly detailed description of the manufacturing process of an all-metal hip prosthesis. The choice of this system as an example does not imply in any instance pronouncing a preference for one manufacturer or another or advancing an opinion about the medical merits of the design. The motive was only that the description of this device allowed the pinpointing of details of a production process which are cardinal to the success of a complex implant, i.e. the problems relating to joining various materials (discussed in detail in the following chapters), improvements in the structure and thus the mechanical properties of the alloys used (forging and heat treatment), avoiding notches by careful rounding of corners (initiation of cracks, corrosion), surface polishing of articulating surfaces (tribological properties, wear), blasting of surfaces in contact with bone (osseointegration) or preventing bone contact with polythene (titanium backing of the polyethene insert, wear of polyethene), surface structure of the taper spigot, etc. This illustrates the topics that must be dealt with in hierarchical trees, as discussed above.

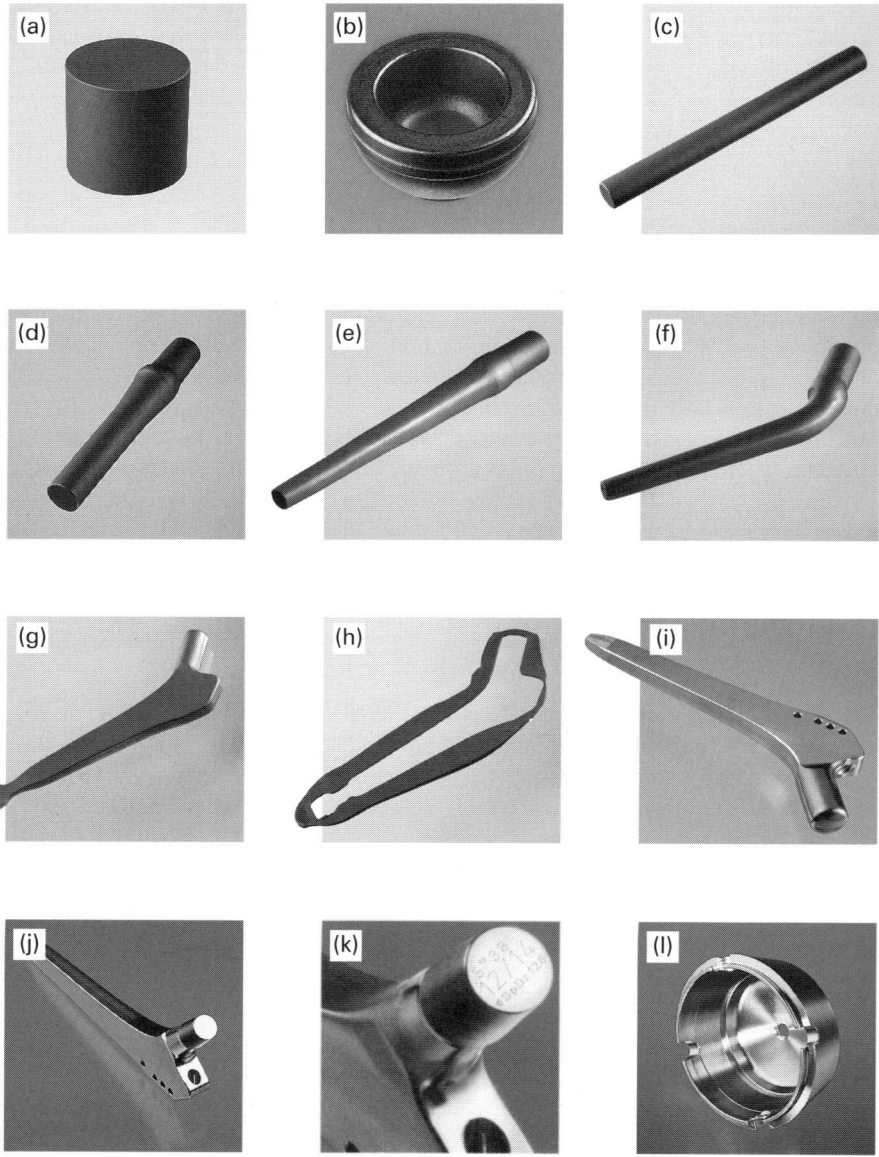

Figure 1.4 Manufacture of an all-metal total hip prosthesis: (a) titanium cylinder for the production of the shell; (b) shell forging after pressing operation; (c) Ti6Al7Nb bar for the production of the stem; (d) upsetting; (e) drawing; (f) bending; (g) final forming operation and dimensional inspection; (h) sheared of flash; (i) machining of the contours and surfaces, drilling holes; (j) machining the taper spigot; (k) rounding the stem corners and dimensional inspection; (l) turning the onside contours of the titanium shell. (m)–(x) opposite.

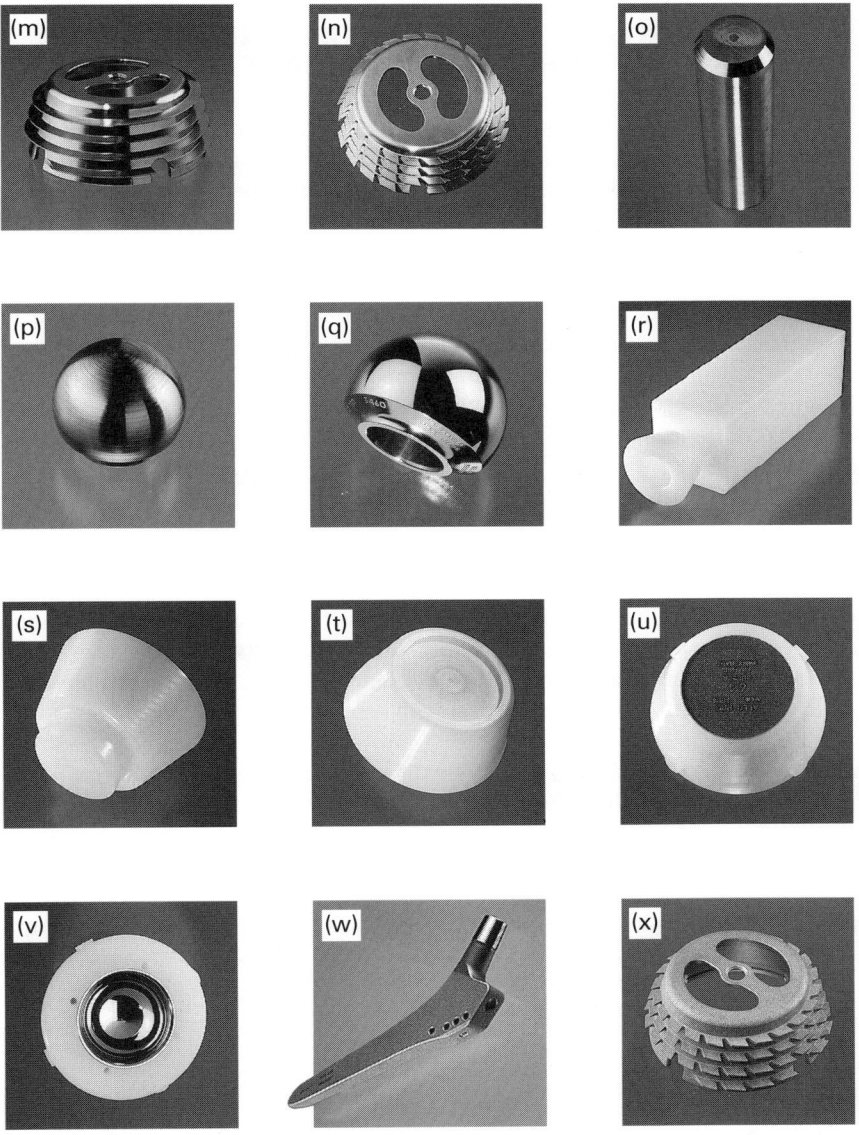

Figure 1.4 (continued) (m) Milling the openings in the roof of the shell and the thread flanks; (n) grinding the tooth form and dimensional inspection; (o) bar of the CoCrMoC alloy for the ball head; (p) machining the ball head; (q) polishing the surface and dimensional inspection; (r) bar of high-purity, medical-quality polyethene, starting material for the cup insert; (s) machining the outer form; (t) machining the recess for the titanium disc; (u) pressing in the titanium disc and friction welding the four stubs; (v) fitting the internal articulating surface and dimensional inspection; (w) coarse blasting the stem surface, fine blasting the neck area, laser marking, cleaning, final inspection and packaging. (Photographs courtesy of Sulzermedica.)

1.3 COMPARISON OF THE VARIOUS BIOMATERIALS WITH REFERENCE TO THE MOST IMPORTANT REQUIREMENTS

In principle, two types of medical devices can be distinguished: structural and functional constructions. Since the functional devices must be produced according to specific physical and/or biological requirements, in most cases tailored materials related to the application (see Chapter 5) must be used for the constructions. Therefore the following discussion of materials selection will be limited to materials for structural devices. For these materials, in addition to processability and availability, mechanical, chemical (surface) and biological properties play a predominant role. In the following, the different groups of biomaterials (metals, ceramics, polymers and carbon) are first compared by means of a discussion of these properties in an overview. Subsequently, the various metallic biomaterials in use are discussed more specifically, including the possibilities of improvements to their properties.

1.3.1 MECHANICAL PROPERTIES

In a discussion of mechanical properties the type of mechanical loading must be indicated. The metallic materials are suited to every kind of loading depending on their specific properties, while ceramics and carbon can be highly loaded only by compression stresses (Table 1.4). Because of defects such as porosity and inclusions, tensile stresses which, under tension, bending and torsion, may occur statically and dynamically, will have an effect. Even grain size and distribution may have an influence. This notch sensitivity caused by the defects is also responsible for the poor fracture toughness of these materials. A great effort has therefore been made to improve these properties. Zirconia has a higher toughness and fatigue strength

Table 1.4 Response of biomaterials to different types of mechanical loading

Type of Loading	Metals	Ceramics and carbon	Polymers
Static			
Tension	Suitable	Not suitable	
Compression	Suitable	Suitable	
Bending	Suitable	Not suitable	Suitable only under low stresses
Torsion	Suitable	Not suitable	
Dynamic			
Tension compression	Suitable	Not suitable	
Pulsating tension	Suitable	Not suitable	
Pulsating compression	Suitable	Suitable	Suitable only under low stresses
Reversed bending	Suitable	Not suitable	
Impact	Suitable	Not suitable	

SELECTION OF MATERIALS

(Table 1.5) than alumina, since the transformation from the tetragonal to the monoclinic phase can be suppressed through stabilisation, for example, by yttrium oxide. In addition, during crack formation and propagation at the crack tip, the transformation from the metastable tetragonal to the monoclinic phase induces compression stresses whereby more energy is required to advance the crack (Christel et al., 1989). The mechanical properties of polymers (examples are given for PMMA and UHMWPE in Table 1.5) are poor under both tensile and compression stresses. In addition to wear, which will be discussed with the chemical (surface) properties, creep in polymers is one of the most critical problems. Considering the limiting facts for ceramics, carbon and polymers for structural biomedical devices, in most cases the use of metallic materials is preferred. Ceramics and polymers are only applicable in special parts of the construction where, for example, extensively high tensile stresses are absent, as in hip prosthesis heads or cups, respectively. Nevertheless, when metallic materials are used, one has to consider their different properties. For example, the fracture toughness, K_{IC}, increases if the ultimate tensile strength decreases. The same behaviour occurs (Figure 1.5) upon observation of the fatigue strength and the deformability of the material, which can be described by the elongation at fracture. With increasing fatigue strength the elongation at fracture is diminished. This fact is important for implants that must be adapted to the environment, such as plates used in maxillofacial surgery. However, the metallic materials offer a wide range of mechanical properties so that a suitable selection according to the mechanical requirements should be possible.

Structural medical devices made of metals can be classified into two groups:

- low-loaded implants (e.g. plates and screws for maxillofacial surgery)
- high-loaded implants (e.g. hip and knee prostheses).

Table 1.5 Typical mechanical properties of different biomaterials

	UTS (MPa)	Fatigue strength[a] (MPa)	K_{IC} (N mm$^{-3/2}$)	A (%)
CrNi–steel (X2CrNiMo18153)	490–690	200–250	2400–2700	>40
CoCr alloy (Co20Cr35Ni10Mo)	800–1200	550–650	1500–1850	8–40
cp-Ti, grade 2	390–540	150–200	2080–2320	22–30
Ti alloy (Ti6Al4V)	930–1140	350–650	1525–1750	8–15
Al$_2$O$_3$	350	0/400[b]	95–180	<1
ZrO$_2$	350–400	0/450[b]	160–250	<1
PMMA	24–48	20–30	30–50	<1
UHMWPE	37–46	16	–	
200–525				
Cortical bone	80–150	–	–	–

See Chapter 2 for further details.
UTS, Ultimate tensile strength; K_{IC}, fracture toughness; A, elongation at fracture.
[a]Rotating/bedding.
[b]Compression/compression.

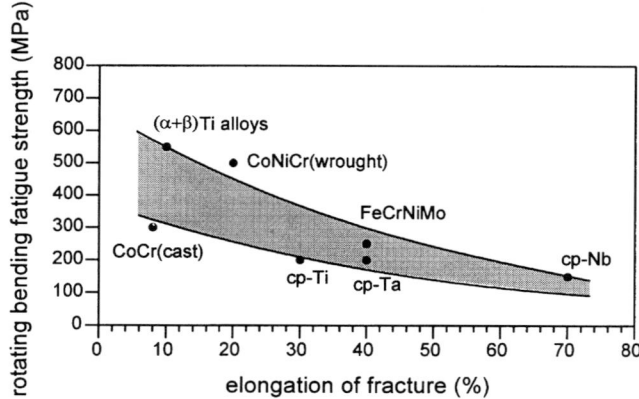

Figure 1.5 Elongation at fracture as a function of the fatigue strength (metallic biomaterials).

For the second group the strength properties, especially the fatigue strength of the material are of foremost importance. In principle, the strength of metallic materials can be improved by the application of the following methods:
- solid-solution hardening by substitution and/or interstitials
- precipitation (dispersion) hardening
- cold deformation
- reduction in the grain size
- texturing.

All of these methods can be used alone and in various combinations. However, an improvement in the strength properties by means of the hardening methods may influence other properties such as the chemical and biological behaviour of the material in a negative, undesirable manner.

The possibilities for applying solid-solution and precipitation hardening can be seen from binary phase diagrams and, with better accuracy, in quasi-binary sections of multielement phase diagrams and temperature–time transition (TTT) diagrams of the various alloys. The most common binary phase diagrams, for example, for titanium in combination with different alloying elements, are shown in Figure 1.6a–d. Figure 1.6b is characteristic of substitution elements such as V, Ta and Nb. This type of diagram is also typical of other base elements, e.g. Fe(Ni) or Cr(Ni). The substitution of the matrix element by elements providing a high solubility causes only a slight hardening effect because a high solution demands similar atom radii of the substitute to the matrix atom, whereby only low residual stresses in the lattice are produced. By comparison, interstitial atoms, e.g. oxygen in titanium or carbon in iron (Figure 1.6d), may lead to higher stresses and therefore can be more effective. Precipitation hardening compared with solid-solution hardening can have an extremely high strengthening effect, depending on the precipitated secondary

SELECTION OF MATERIALS

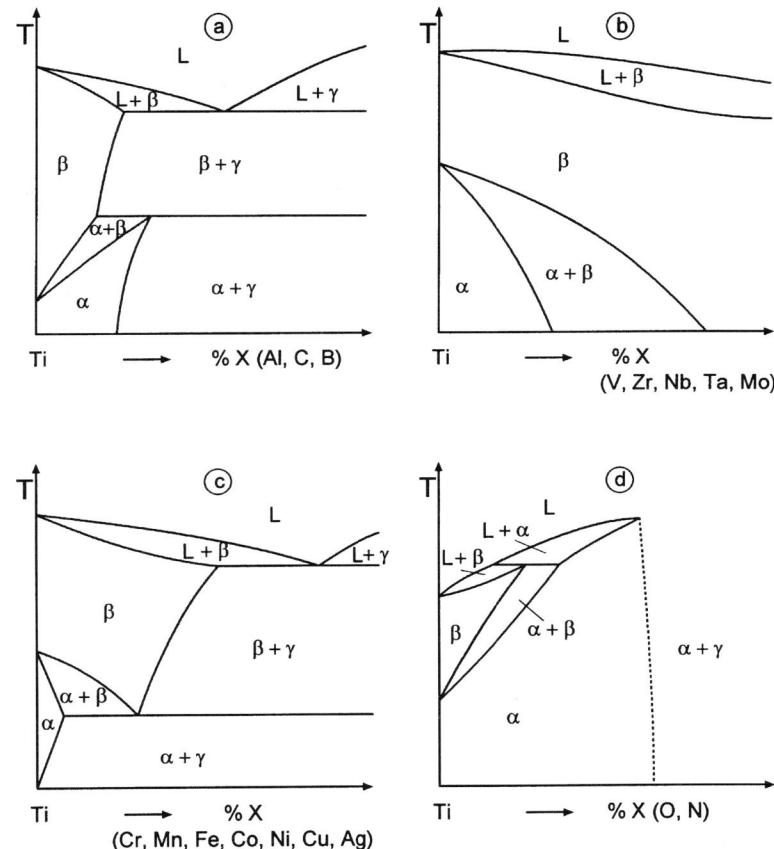

Figure 1.6 Types of linear (Ti–X) phase diagram.

metallic or intermetallic phases (Figures 1.6a, c). In particular, coherent and semicoherent secondary phases can be very effective because they are able to produce long-distance stresses in the lattice. Using an ageing procedure (variation in the annealing temperature and time) the optimum size and distance of the precipitations can be achieved by hindering the dislocation migration. Depending on the alloy, the optimum precipitation of coherent or semicoherent particles can be supported by a preliminary cold deformation because, owing to favourable energetic phenomena, the dislocations are potentially preferred sites for the precipitation of secondary phases.

Stainless steels have corrosion problems, and a single-phase (γ)-microstructure, as shown by the quasi-binary section in the system Fe–Cr–Ni (Figure 1.7) (Schafmeister and Ergang, 1938/39), is sought, so that only a relatively ineffective solid-solution hardening by substitution occurs. Therefore the only method of

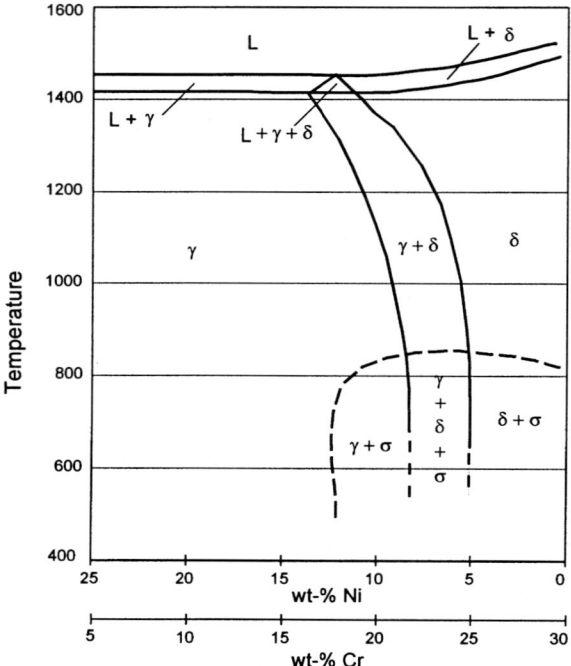

Figure 1.7 Quasi-binary section in the ternary system Fe–Cr–Ni (Schafmeister and Ergang, 1938/39).

increasing the strength properties of stainless steel is cold deformation, in which the migration of dislocations is hindered owing to their multiplication. Because of the increased energy level of the microstructure, the corrosion resistance in a sodium chloride solution will be decreased by cold deformation (Figure 1.8). Also, owing to their fcc lattice, the CoCrNi alloys with a Cr content of about 18–21 wt% and containing Mo or W show a good cold deformability and strengthening which can be further increased by the precipitation of a hexagonal ε-phase in the temperature range of 400–600°C. A quasi-binary section (Smith and Yates, 1968) of the multiphase alloys, of which Co35Ni20Cr10Mo (MP35N) is the most important representative, is shown in Figure 1.9. The precipitation of the hcp platelets is induced by the stress and the mechanical deformation. A further increase in the hardness and strength properties of alloys containing Mo can be achieved by a cold deformation followed by ageing in the temperature range of 500–600°C with an ensuing precipitation of the intermetallic phase Co_3Mo. In addition to the interstitial solid-solution hardening with oxygen, cold deformation for cp-titanium, cp-niobium and cp-tantalum is a useful method for increasing the strength properties, including the fatigue properties. Compared with stainless steels, cold deformation with cp-titanium as well as with cp-niobium and cp-tantalum is not known to produce

SELECTION OF MATERIALS

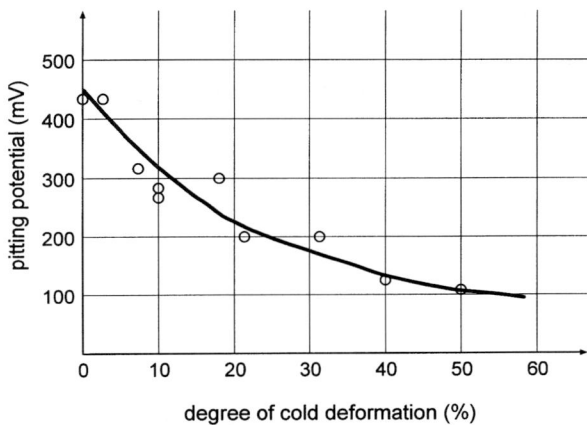

Figure 1.8 Influence of cold deformation on the corrosion behaviour of 316L.

negative effects on the corrosion resistance in a sodium chloride solution. In contrast to stainless steel and cp-titanium, CoCr and Ti alloys show only a poor cold deformability due to the precipitation hardening of secondary phases. Moreover, these secondary phases are able to guarantee a fine-grained microstructure, providing an increase in the strength properties because they are able to impair the grain growth of the matrix phase during hot deformation and/or annealing at higher temperatures.

The CoCr alloys containing carbon are also hardened by the precipitation of carbides. According to the C content the portion of precipitated carbides can be so

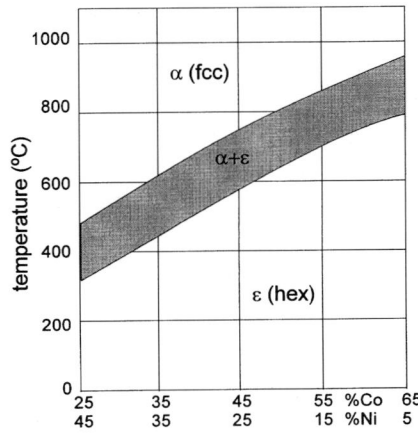

Figure 1.9 Quasi-binary section of CoNi multiphase alloys (Smith and Yates, 1968).

great that a deformation of the material is not possible. Devices consisting of such alloys can be produced only by casting. However, the advantage of CoCr materials containing carbide precipitations is an improved abrasion resistance, thus permitting their application in the manufacture of articulating components, e.g. head balls of hip prostheses. In general, wrought materials are preferred to cast materials because of their lack of such defects as pores, segregations and shrinkage cavities which may arise during solidification of the castings and which, because of the notch effect of these defects, decrease the strength properties, especially fatigue. The skill in optimising the strength properties of wrought materials by precipitation hardening lies in allowing a minimum of deformability (an elongation at fracture of about 10%) in order to avoid the risk of brittle fracture.

A precipitation hardening of titanium alloys is brought about by intermetallic phases which can occur in the α- as well as in the β-phase. Stabilisation by different alloying elements of the α-phase (e.g. Al, O) and the β-phase (e.g. V, Fe, Mn, Nb, Ta) takes place. At a content of more than 5 wt% aluminium the precipitation of Ti_3Al in the α_2-phase begins, as can be seen from the quasi-binary section in the ternary phase diagram of Ti6Al4V (Figure 1.10). This α_2-phase provides an extremely high hardening effect so that the aluminium content in titanium alloys must be limited to a maximum value of 8 wt%. Owing to the large amount of the Ti_3Al-phase, a higher aluminium content would cause an embrittlement of the material so that no deformability of the material would be possible. Alloys

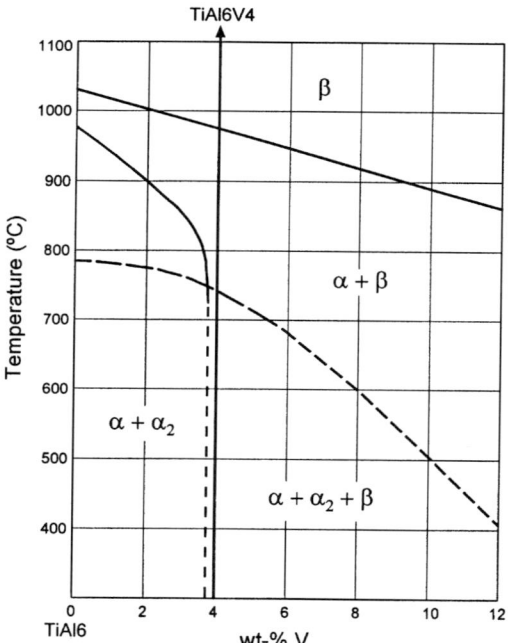

Figure 1.10 Quasi-binary section in the ternary system Ti–AlV.

SELECTION OF MATERIALS

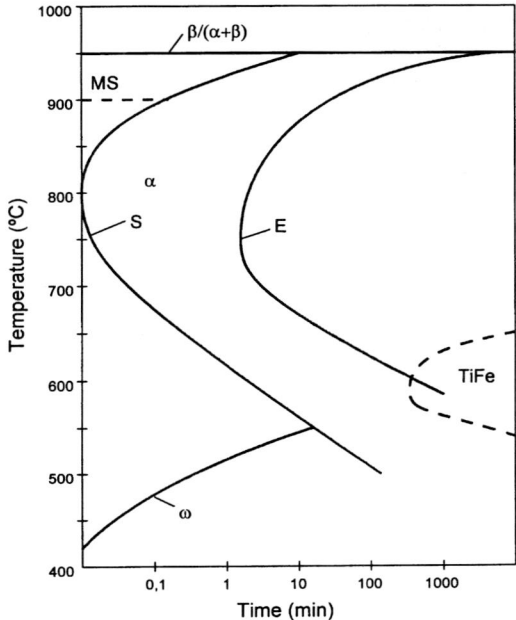

Figure 1.11 TT diagram of Ti5Al2.5Fe (Breme and Schade, 1985).

containing β-stabilising elements are also hardened by the ω-phase, which is precipitated in the β-phase. Figure 1.11 shows the TTT diagram of the alloy Ti5Al2.5Fe (Breme and Schade, 1985). The precipitation of the ω-phase can be brought about by ageing in the temperature range of 400–600°C (isothermal ω-phase). Besides this isothermal precipitation, an athermal precipitation during cooling from higher temperatures is known. Since the ω-phases are composed of titanium and the β-stabilising element, local enrichment of these elements occurs. As related to Ti6Al4V, the vanadium content can locally reach a level of 20–25%. This content must be regarded as critical because of the toxicity of vanadium, which will probably cause a disease to occur. Fortunately, the ω-particles are submicroscopically small. Nevertheless, the development of titanium alloys such as Ti5Al2.5Fe (Zwicker *et al.*, 1980) and Ti6Al7Nb (Semlitsch *et al.*, 1985), which contain no toxic elements, is justified. Of the above-mentioned strengthening methods, grain refining, which acts according to the Hall–Petch relation, is automatically conducted for two-phase or multiphase alloys because the grains of the different phases hinder each other in their grain growth. In contrast to fcc or bcc materials, hexagonal materials such as titanium are predestined for texture strengthening. The effect can be suitable if, for example, the main loading occurs in a rod in the longitudinal direction and a high strength is required in the rod axis. By rolling an (α+β)-titanium alloy in the low (α+β)-phase field the basal planes of the hexagonal cells will be orientated perpendicular to the rod axis so that the strength

Table 1.6 Mechanical properties of Ti5Al2.5Fe rolled at 850°C in different directions

Position of sample	$E \times 10^3$ (MPa)	$R_{p0.2}$ (MPa)	R_m (MPa)	A_5 (%)	Z (%)
Parallel	109	784	967	13	35
45°	116	876	913	12	30
Perpendicular	124	926	1015	12.5	32.5

$R_{p0.2}$, Yield strength; R_m, tensile strength; A_5, elongation at fracture; Z, reduction in area.

properties of the material will be more parallel, rather than perpendicular, to the rod axis. However, a texture with different properties in different directions can have undesirable effects. A sheet of Ti5Al2.5Fe alloy that has been rolled in the low (α+β)-phase region (750–85°C), and from which a ball head of a hip prothesis is to be made, shows a texture. The basal planes of the α-grains have a crystallographic orientation parallel to the surface of the sheet. This fact explains the higher strength properties perpendicular to the sheet compared with those that are parallel to the sheet (Table 1.6). In addition, because of the texture, a difference in Young's modulus was measured in both directions. This effect can cause difficulties under service conditions because the elastic strain differs according to the direction (Figure 1.12). The elastic deformation of the ball consisting of the titanium alloy shows a

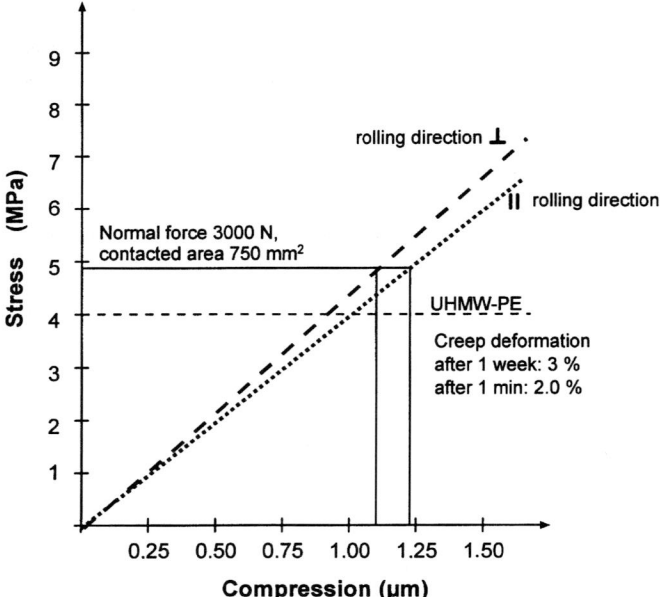

Figure 1.12 Influence of anisotropy on Young's modulus (sheet made of Ti5Al2.5Fe).

SELECTION OF MATERIALS

difference of about 0.2 µm parallel and perpendicular to the rolling direction. Therefore a cup consisting of polyethylene can be locally loaded by compression so that creep deformation will occur if the compression force amounts to 3000 N. Taking into account a contact of 675 mm^2, which was experimentally determined, between the polyethylene cup and the head with a diameter of 32 mm, the calculated stress of 4.8 N mm^{-2} is able to produce creep of the polyethylene of more than 2% in 1 min (Zwicker and Breme, 1984).

Of outstanding importance for a medical device is its stiffness S, which can be defined as the product of the moment of inertia I and of Young's modulus E:

$$\mathrm{BF} = \frac{\sigma_b}{E}. \tag{1.1}$$

A low stiffness as close to that of the natural bone as possible provides a good load transfer whereby the stimulation of new bone formation is realised. While stress shielding (high stiffness) results in bone resorption (Figure 1.13), a low stiffness under static and/or dynamic loading will provide an elastic elongation of the cells in the neighbourhood of the implant whereby the production of calcium, which is the basis for bone formation, is stimulated. In the region of the physiological stress and strain, respectively, bone formation and resorption are balanced. A decrease in the stress in this region causes resorption, which decreases the cross-section of the bone whereby stress and bone formation are increased until equilibrium is again achieved. Using animal bones it has been shown that the physiological stress for the cortical bone amounts to about 25–45 N mm^{-2} (Rubin *et al.*, 1990). Concerning the remodelling, the bone has two reaction possibilities. Besides the change in the cross-section, which requires a considerable amount of time (several months), within a shorter period a change in density may occur owing to the reception (high strain) or release (low strain) of calcium. The release of calcium causes a decrease in both the tensile strength and Young's modulus (Figure 1.14) (Natali and Meroi, 1989), whereby an automatic control system with a closed loop again becomes active, because a decrease in Young's modulus (lower stiffness) causes a higher strain and an increased calcium production. Figure 1.15 shows schematically the closed loop

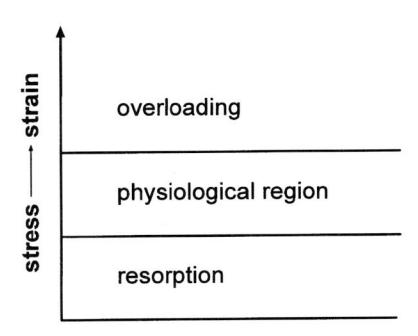

Figure 1.13 Stimulation and resorption of the bone as a function of loading (schematic).

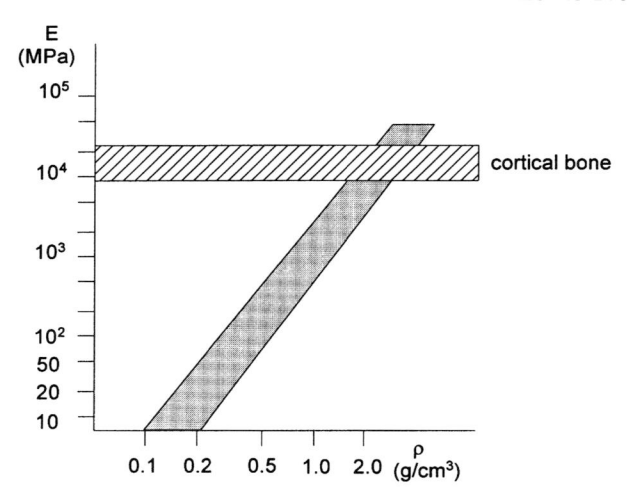

Figure 1.14 Young's modulus of the bone as a function of density (Natali and Meroi, 1989).

that is assumed to govern Wolff's law (Hart et al., 1984; Roesler, 1987). The ability of the bone to adapt and react according to the state of loading and its ability to translate mechanical signals into biomedical signals imply that it must have internal strain sensors and transducers (Kydd and Daly, 1976; Carter et al., 1987). For these considerations one must take into account the fact that the human bone possesses individual properties that depend, for example, on the age of the patient. Considering the fact that the moment of inertia is in most cases given by the geometry of the landscape (biology), Young's modulus should be as close as possible to that of the bone (E = 10 000–20 000 N mm^{-2} for the cortical bone), so that the implant will have isoelastic behaviour corresponding to that of the bone. Considering this dependence, the most important mechanical properties can be summarised by the definition of the biofunctionality BF, which can be described by the quotient of the fatigue strength σ_b (e.g. rotating bending strength) for Young's modulus:

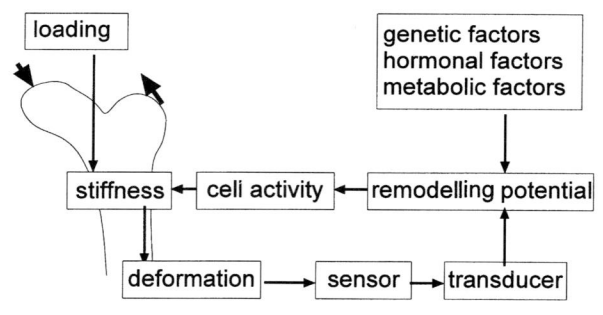

Figure 1.15 Strain adaptive bone remodelling according to Wolff's law (Hart et al., 1984).

SELECTION OF MATERIALS

Table 1.7 Biofunctionality (BF) of different biomaterials

	Fatigue strength[a] (MPa)	$E \times 10^3$ (MPa)	$BF \times 10^{-3}$
Metals			
FeCrNiMo (e.g. 316L)	250	210	1.2
CoCr, cast	300	200	1.5
CoNiCr, wrought	500	220	2.3
Ti alloys ($\alpha+\beta$)	550	105	5.2
cp-Ti	200	100	1.8
cp-Nb	150	120	1.3
cp-Ta	200	200	1.3
Ceramics			
Al_2O_3	0/400[b]	380	0/1.05[b]
ZrO_2	0.450[b]	170	0/.2.6[b]
Polymers			
PMMA	30	25	1.2
UHMWPE	16	1.2	13.3

$$BF = \frac{\text{fatigue strength}}{\text{Young's modulus}}.$$

[a]Rotating/bending.
[b]Compression/compression.

$$BF = \frac{\sigma_b}{E}. \tag{1.2}$$

This relation takes into account the outstanding importance of Young's modulus. The BF values of the various biomaterials are given in Table 1.7 and Figure 1.16, which show the superiority of titanium and its alloys over other metallic materials. The biofunctionality of UHMW polymers is extremely high. Nevertheless, because of their extremely low fatigue strength the application of these materials in highly loaded structural implants is impossible.

In the case of metallic and ceramic materials there exists the possibility of decreasing Young's modulus by porous sintering. Theoretically, Young's modulus can be calculated according to Equation (1.3):

$$E_p = E_0 (1 - 1.21 \, p^{2/3}), \tag{1.3}$$

where E_p is the modulus of the porous sample, E_0 the modulus of the bulk material and p the porosity (Ondracek, 1988). Figure 1.17 presents the influence of porosity on Young's modulus calculated from Equation (1.3) for different biomaterials. Since a high porosity stands for low strength properties, the superiority of titanium materials can be deducted from this diagram. Further details concerning the possibilities of a decrease in Young's modulus, especially of titanium materials, are given in Chapter 5.

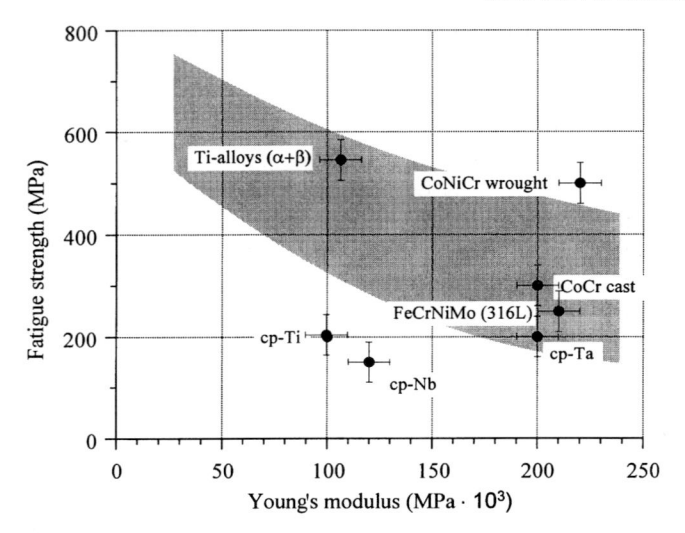

Figure 1.16 Biofunctionality of various metallic materials.

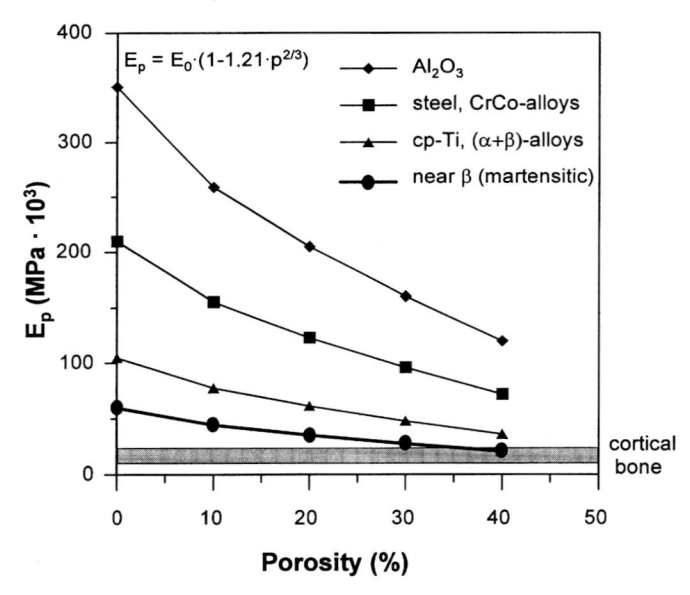

Figure 1.17 Young's modulus of various biomaterials as a function of porosity.

1.3.2 SURFACE (CHEMICAL) PROPERTIES

While the surface properties (oxidation, degradation and abrasion) have a subordinate character for ceramics, they are of great importance for metals and polymers. For metallic materials the presence of an oxide layer is the basis for their

SELECTION OF MATERIALS

corrosion resistance. It is of fundamental importance that following damage to this oxide layer, e.g. by surgical instruments, a repassivation by oxidation takes place. By contrast, oxidation of polymers, e.g. UHMWPE, leads to increased degradation. This oxidation may be caused by loading the material. With knee prostheses, it was shown that in the load-bearing area the molecular weights were reduced and the most damaged areas were heavily oxidised. Therefore, a synergy seems to exist between maximum shear stress and chemical reaction by oxidation. By oxidation, especially of the grain boundaries, the device may be damaged through fatigue or creep (Nagy and Li, 1990). Auto-oxidation is known to take place in polymers in contact with enzymes via the production of hydrogen peroxide and a hydroxyl radical (Williams, 1992). The wear and abrasion properties have a complex character, depending on different factors such as partners of fretting, lubricant, articulating velocity, contact area and temperature. With polyethelene, both adhesive and abrasive wear have been observed (Bartel *et al.*, 1986). The coefficient of friction, frictional torque and therefore the heat generated seem to be lowest for ceramics in contact with an UHMWPE surface. An increased local heat can increase the creep and oxidation of UHMWPE (McKellop *et al.*, 1981). Comparing zirconia with alumina a wear rate with a value five times lower has been observed with zirconia in contact with UHMWPE (Schwartz, 1990).

In order to avoid damaging the surface layer, coatings of hard layers of non-abrasive materials that also show favourable fretting behaviour are recommended, especially for the movable parts of implants consisting of metals with a low abrasive resistance (Zwicker *et al.*, 1984; Higham, 1985; Williams and Buchanan, 1985). Examples illustrating improvements to the friction and abrasive behaviour in metallic materials are given in Chapter 5. Surface layers produced by different methods can also improve the corrosion resistance of metallic materials. In spite of this passive layer the metallic materials exhibit a general corrosion in the body fluid which depends on the basic material itself (Fraker *et al.*, 1983).

The current density of various materials was determined as a function of the potential difference between the anodic and cathodic branches of the current potential curves in 0.9% NaCl with a stable redox system, $Fe(CN)_6^{4-}/Fe(CN)_6^{3-}$. The saline solution containing this redox system had a resting potential closely resembling that of a tissue culture fluid which has a redox potential of 400 mV. Ti and its alloys, Ta and Nb, exhibit a better resistance than the stainless steel AISI 316L and a wrought CoNiCr alloy. The same ranking can be observed during the determination of the polarisation resistance of the various materials (Table 1.8) (Zitter and Plenk, 1987). Details of the corrosion behaviour of metallic materials are described in Chapter 4.

1.3.3 BIOLOGICAL PROPERTIES

The biological properties of the biomaterials are dominated by their chemical, physical and physicochemical properties. While the behaviour of the ceramics is bioinert or even bioactive (hydroxyapatite), the metallic materials have extremely

Table 1.8 Polarisation resistance R_p of metallic biomaterials in 0.9% NaCl (Zitter and Plenk, 1987)

	R_p (kΩ cm^{-2})
cp-Ta	1430
cp-T1	714
Ti6Al4V	455
cp-Nb	455
X2CrNiMo18135	4.38
Co20Cr35Ni10Mo	3.32

different biological properties. Bulk polyethylene is thought to induce only a little tissue reaction, while particular wear debris can produce a severe interaction and may even be a contributing factor in aseptic loosening of total joint replacements (Goodman *et al.*, 1990). The biological behaviour of the metallic biomaterials has been determined by various methods.

The level of toxicity of the various metallic elements was tested by investigating the reaction of salts of these elements with cells of the kidneys of green African monkeys. The CCR_{50} value, defined as the concentration of the studied substance that generates a reduction in survival of the renal cells of 50%, was measured. Of all the elements measured the lowest value of 3×10^{-2} µg ml^{-1} was observed for vanadium (Frazier and Andrews, 1979) (Table 1.9).

Various histological results were obtained after the insertion of wires of different metals into the epiphyseal region of rabbits and an exposure time of 15 months. With materials of inert or biocompatible behaviour the cells in the vicinity of the implant were still supplied with blood, while the cells in the neighbourhood of toxic materials underwent an inflammatory reaction and died. A few elements (Cr, Co, Ni and V) have toxic effects and a relatively low polarisation resistance. Ti and its alloys, Nb and Ta, which have a high polarisation resistance, exhibit an inert behaviour. Capsulated materials were found to have values in between. The results also show that not only the corrosion behaviour provided by the polarisation resistance is responsible for the biocompatibility of the material exposed to the tissue. The steel 316L and the CoCr alloy, which have a polarisation resistance similar to that of titanium, are capsulated by a tissue membrane and their behaviour is not inert (Figure 1.18) (Steinemann and Perren, 1985).

A sensitive and reproducible test of biocompatibility involves the cultivation of cells with an increasing content of fine metal powders (<20 µm). The survival rate

Table 1.9 Limit of toxicity CCR_{50} of different metal salts (Frazier and Andrews, 1979)

	Fe	Mn	Co	Ni	Cr	V
CCR_{50} (µg ml^{-1})	59	15	3.5	1.1	6×10^{-2}	3×10^{-2}

SELECTION OF MATERIALS

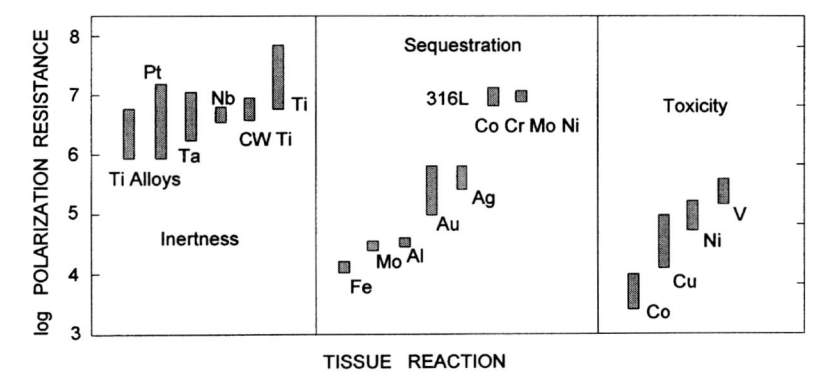

Figure 1.18 Corrosion resistance (0.5% NaCl, pH 7.4) and tissue reaction of various metallic biomaterials (Steinemann and Perren, 1985).

is measured after a constant exposure time. The limit of toxicity PE_{50} is defined as the value ($\mu g \ ml^{-1}$) of the powder concentration in the culture medium of cells that produces a dying off of 50% of the cells (Hildebrand, 1991) (see also Chapter 9). The following interactions can generate injuries in the implant–body system.

- An organic (direct) reaction of the implant or of primary corrosion products with proteins of the tissue takes place, causing, for example, inflammation.
- An inorganic (indirect) reaction of the implant or of primary corrosion products is caused by the solution of metal ions in the body fluid and transport to the various organs, where they are concentrated and can produce systematic or hypersensitive effects if the limit of toxicity for a certain metal is exceeded.
- The corrosion process produces a flow of electrons in the implant metal and a flow of ions in the surrounding tissue. The latter may disturb the physiological ion movement of the nerve cells.
- Generation of H_2O_2 by inflamed cells and decomposition of H_2O_2 by the formation of a hydroxyl radical causes injury in the biological system.

Whether one of these interactions occurs or not depends on the physical, chemical and physicochemical properties of the various materials. The heat of formation, solubility product, dielectric constant and, where possible, the acid–base properties of primary corrosion products are listed in Table 1.10.

Concerning organic or inorganic reactions, the primary corrosion products of the metallic implants are mainly responsible for the biocompatibility of the implanted metal because, owing to their large surfaces, they may interact with either the tissue or body fluid.

The primary corrosion products of the most important elements in metallic implant materials vary in their thermodynamic stability. While the oxides or hydroxides of Al, Cr, Nb, Ta, Ti and V are stable because of a more negative heat of formation than that of water, the oxides and hydroxides of Co and Ni are unstable because of a less negative heat formation than that of water (Kubashewski *et al.*,

Table 1.10 Dielectric constant ε, heat of formation ΔH and solubility p_k (negative log) of primary corrosion products compared with H_2O

Primary corrosion product	$-\Delta H^0_{298}$ (kJ mol)	p_k	ε
Ag_2O	32	7.7	
Al_2O_3	1675	+14.6	5–10
$Al(OH)_3$	916	32.3	
CoO	239	−12.6	
Cu_2O	168	>14	
CuO	162		
Cr_2O	1141	18.6	12
CrO_3	595		
$Cr(OH)_2$	988	−1.8	
FeO	267	−13.3	
Fe_2O_3	822	−14	100
$Fe(OH)_2$	568	+2.3	30–38
H_2O	273	+14	78
MoO_3	712	+3.7	
NiO	240	−12.2	
$Ni(OH)_2$	538	15.8	
NbO	486		
Nb_2O_5	1905	>20	280
Ta_2O_5	2090	>20	12
TiO	518		
TiO_2 anatas	935		
brookite		+18	78
rutile	943		110
VO	410		
V_2O_3	1560	+10.3	
WO_3	838	14	

1967). The interaction between the oxide or hydroxide and the body fluid is more probable if the heat of formation for oxide or hydroxide is increased. Therefore, the thermodynamically stable corrosion products have a low solution product and a low solubility in the body fluid. This is directly demonstrated by the p_k values (negative logarithm of the solution product of the primary corrosion products). While oxides of Ti, Ta, Nb and Cr have p_k values of >14, i.e. hydrolysis cannot play a role, oxides of Co, Fe and Ni may possess negative p_k values, which cause considerable solubility. In spite of a high negative heat of formation for Fe_2O_3, $Fe(OH)_2$ and $Cr(OH)_2$, negative p_k values and a high solubility are reported (Zitter, 1976). A remarkable solubility of Cr in serum has been observed, while titanium is practically insoluble owing to the formation of the thermodynamically very stable oxide TiO_2.

Thermodynamically stable primary corrosion products with a low solubility in body fluid are in stable equilibrium with only a low reactivity with the proteins of the surrounding tissue.

Ti, Ta and Nb are reported to be biocompatible because they form protective surface layers of semiconductive or non-conductive oxides. Because of their isolating effect, these oxides are able to prevent to a great extent an exchange of electrons and therefore a flow of ions through the tissue (Zettner *et al.* 1980). This isolating effect may be demonstrated by the dielectric constants of the different metal oxides. There are three groups of oxides. While TiO_2 (rutile), Fe_2O_3 and Nb_2O_5 have constants even higher than that of water, Al_2O_3, Cr_2O_3 and Ta_2O_5 have a lower isolating effect and a higher conductivity. For oxides of Ni and V dielectric constants are not available because of their high conductivity. The relatively low isolating effect of Ta_2O_5 is indirectly proved by the cytotronic effects of Ta on the membrane properties and on the growth of spinal ganglion cells during *in vitro* tests. In contrast, Ti showed no effect on either the membrane properties or the growth of ganglion cells (Bingmann and Tetsch, 1986).

The generation of H_2O_2, leading to the formation of an OH^o radical, plays only a subordinate role in the case of the highly reactive metals (Ti, Ta, Nb) because this radical will be trapped immediately after its formation.

The integration of metallic implants by ingrowth was studied for many different materials and implant systems. The osseointegration of miniplates of commercially pure titanium and of the stainless steel 316L was investigated after the implantation of these plates on the legs of Hanford minipigs. The miniplates were fixed to the legs of the pigs by screws. After removal following an exposure time of 8 weeks a histological examination was performed by fluorescence microscopy. In all animals where titanium plates had been used a new formation of bone could be observed in close contact to the surface of the screws and plates (Breme *et al.*, 1988). In contrast, when stainless steel was used, there was less new bone formation and, in addition, granulated tissue was found between the metallic surface and the surrounding bone (Breme *et al.*, 1988). This granulated tissue at the bone–implant interface has the disadvantage that it is not supplied with blood. Therefore, systematic treatment of the host tissue against inflammatory reactions in the neighbourhood of the implants by means of injections is not possible because the agent cannot be transported directly to the inflamed area. In addition, the granulated connective tissue is not able to sustain or transfer loads, so that a loosening of the implant will take place. Growth of the bone in close contact with the metal has been reported in several investigations (Schröder *et al.*, 1978, 1981; Kirsch, 1980; Simpson, 1981; Branemark *et al.*, 1983; Krekeler and Schilli, 1984) in which the area of contact of the tissue and implant was studied in detail. On the surface of the passive titanium oxide layer hydroxyl groups are generated as monolayers by the adsorption of water. This hydroxylated surface is able to cause bonding to the organic molecules and to metal ions by means of protonation and deprotonation, respectively. The deprotonation and protonation of the surface hydroxyl allows the chemisorption of cations such as Ca^{2+} and anions such as HPO_{4+}^{2-} and amino acids (Kennedy and Humphreys, 1976; Gold *et al.*, 1989; Listgarten *et al.*, 1992). This may explain the observation of blood and lymphatic vessels in the contact zone of the bone to titanium implants in a retrieval study. In the same study, with stainless steel and cobalt-base implants, no living tissue was observed in the neighbourhood of the implants (Simpson, 1981).

Table 1.11 Price of semiproducts (bar with a diameter of 20 mm) and volume price of various metallic biomaterials

	Price ($ kg^{-1})	Weight (kg dm^{-3})	Volume price ($ dm^{-3})
Stainless steel	10	8	80
CoCrNi	200	9.1	1820
cp-Ti	35	4.5	159
Ti6Al4V	53	4.43	235
cp-Nb	206	8.56	1762
cp-Ta	368	16.6	6103

1.4 CONCLUSIONS

From the discussion of the mechanical, chemical and biological properties it becomes clear that the titanium materials possess distinct advantages over other metallic biomaterials. Their processability is similar to that of the other materials. Because of their low specific weight, titanium and its alloys, along with stainless steels, are the least expensive materials especially if the volume price (dm^3) is calculated (Table 1.11).

NOMENCLATURE

BF   biofunctionality
E Young's modulus
I moment of inertia
K_{IC} fracture toughness
S stiffness
p porosity
σ_b rotating bending strength

REFERENCES

Bartel, D.L., Bicknell, V.L. and Wright, T.M. (1986) The effect of conformity, thickness and material on stresses in ultra-high molecular weight components for total joint replacement, *J. Bone Joint Surg.* **68A**, 1041–51.

Bingmann, D. and Tetsch, P. (1986) Untersuchungen zur Biokompatibilität von Implantatmaterialien, *Dt. Z. Zahnärztl. Implantol.* **2**, 190–4.

Branemark, P.I., Adell, R., Albrektsson, T., Lekhom, U., Lundkvist, S. and Rockler, B. (1983) Osseointegrated titanium fixtures in the treatment of edentulousness, *Biomaterials* **4**, 25–8.

Breme, J. and Schade, W. (1985) Phase transformation in TiAl5Fe2.5 alloy, in *Titanium, Science and Technology* (eds G. Lütjering, U. Zwicker and W. Bunk), DGM, Oberursel, pp. 1487–94.

Breme, J., Steinhäuser E. and Paulus, G. (1988) Commercially pure titanium Steinhäuser plate-screw system for maxillo facial surgery, *Biomaterials* **9**, 310–13.

Carter, D.R., Fyhrie, D.P. and Walden, R.T. (1987) Trabecular bone density and loading history: regulation of connective tissue biology by mechanical energy, *J. Biomech.* **20**, 785–94.

Cebon, D. and Ashby, M.F. (1994) *Cambridge Materials Selector Version 2.0*, Granta Design, Cambridge.

Christel, P., Meunier, A., Heller, M., Torre, J.P. and Peille, C.N. (1989) Mechanical properties and short-term *in-vivo* evaluation of yttrium-oxide partially-stabilized zirconia, *J. Biomed. Mater. Res.* **23**, 45–61.

Esslinger, J.O. and Rutkowski, E.J. (1973) Studies on the skeletal attachment of experimental hip prostheses in the pygmy goat and the dog, *J. Biomed. Mater. Res. Symp.* **4**, 187–93.

Fraker, A.C., Ruff, A.W., Sung, P., von Orden, A.C. and Speck, K.M. (1983) Surface preparation and corrosion behaviour of titanium alloys for surgical implants, in *Titanium Alloys in Surgical Implants* (eds H.A. Cuckey and F. Kubli), ASTM STP 796, American Society for Testing and Materials, West Conshohocken, PA, pp. 206–19.

Frazier, M.E. and Andrews, T.K. (1979) *In vitro* clonal growth assay for evaluating toxicity of metal salts, in *Trace Metals in Health and Disease* (ed. N. Karash), Raven Press, New York, p. 71.

Gold, J.M., Schmidt, M. and Steinemann, S.G. (1989) XPS study of amino acid adsorption to titanium surfaces, *Helv. Phys. Acta* **62**, 246–9.

Goodman, S.B., Fornasier, V.L., Kee, J. and Kei, G. (1990) The effects of bulk versus particulate titanium and cobalt chrome alloy implanted in the rabbit tibia, *J. Biomed. Mater. Res.* **24**, 5139–49.

Hart, R.T, Dava, D.T. and Heiple, K.G. (1984) Mathematical modeling and numerical solutions for functionally dependent bone, *Calif. Tissue Int.* **36** 11–18.

Helsen, J.A., Jaecques, S., Simon, J.-P. and Mattheuws, D. (1993) Biocompatibility testing of thermoplastic elastomers for use in hard tissue replacements, *Polym. Polym. Compos.* **2**, 399–405A.

Higham, P.A. (1985) *Proceedings of the Conference on Biomedical Materials*, Boston, December 1985, Society for Biomaterials, Minneapolis, p. 483.

Hildebrand, H.F. (1991) *DGM Hochschulseminar Biomaterialien*, Saarbrücken, Germany.

Jaecques, S.V., Helsen, J.A., Simon, J.-P. and Mattheuws, D. (1995) Development of an elastomer coated hip prosthesis, *J. Mater. Sci. Mater. Med.* **6**, 685–9.

Kennedy, J.F. and Humphreys, J.D. (1976) Active immobilized antibiotics based on metal hydroxides, *Antimicrob. Agents Chemother.* **9**, 767–70.

Kirsch, A. (1980) Titan-spritzbeschichtetes Zahnwurzelimplantat unter physiologischer Belastung beim Menschen, *Dt. Zahnärztl. Z.* **35**, 112–14.

Krekeler, G. and Schilli, W. (1984) Das ITI-Implantat Typ H: Technische Entwicklung, Tierexperiment und klinische Erfahrung, *Chir. Zahnheilk.* **12**, 2253–63.

Kubashewski, O., Evans, C.C.L. and Alcock C.B. (1967) *Metallurgical Thermochemistry*, Pergamon Press, London.

Kydd, W.L. and Daly, D.H. (1976) Bone titanium implant response to mechanical stress, *J. Prosthet. Dent.*, **35**, 567–71.

Lee, E.H., Rao, G.R., Lewis, M.B. and Mansur, L.K. (1993) Ion beam application for improved polymer surface properties, *Nucl. Instr. Meth. Phys. Res.* **74**, 326–30.

Liao, R.J.D. (1995) Modifications physico-chimiques et mécaniques du polythylène et du polypropylène par implantation ionique d'azote, plasma micro-ondes, bombardement d'électrons et irradiation', in *Projet de Thèse*, École nationale Supérieure des Mines de Saint-Etienne, Staint-Etienne, France.

Listgarten, M.A., Buser, D., Steinemann, S.G., Donath, K., Lang, N.P. and Weber H.P. (1992) Light and transmission electron microscopy of the intact interfaces between non-submerged titanium coated epoxy resin implants and bone or gingiva, *J. Dent. Res.* **71**, 364–71.

McKee, G.K. (1982) Total hip replacement – past, present and future, *Biomaterials* **3**, 130–5.

McKellop, H., Clark, I.C., Markolf, K.L. and Amstutz, H. (1981) Friction and wear properties of polymer metal and ceramic prosthetic joint materials evaluated on a multichannel screening device, *J. Biomed. Mater. Res.* **15**, 619–23.

Nagy, E. and Li, S. (1990) Environmental damaging of polyethylen implants, *Trans. Soc. Biomater.* **16**, 274.

Natali, A.N. and Meroi, E.A. (1989) A review of the biomedical properties of bone as a material, *J. Biomed. Engng.* **11**, 212–19.

Newcombe, W.R., Rep, R.U. and Eaton, N.B. (1987) A mechanical evaluation of an elastic femoral prosthetic stem, *J. Biomech.* **20**, 179–85.

Ondracek, G. (1988) The basis of microstructure-property-correlations, *Proceedings of the Colloquium Interfaces in Materials*, KAW, Brussels, 113–48.

Repo, R.U., Newcombe, W.R. and Occhionorelli, J. (1986) An elastic femoral replacement prosthesis. An experimental study, *Acta Orthop. Belg.* **52**, 217–27.

Roesler, H. (1987) The history of some fundamental concepts in bone biomechanics, *J. Biomech.* **20**, 1025–34.

Rubin, C.T., Kenneth, J. and Steven, D.B. (1990) Functional strains and cortical bone adaption: epegenetic assurance of skeletal integrity, *J. Biomech.* **23**, 43–54.

Schafmeister, P. and Ergang, P. (1938/39) Das Zustandsschaubild Eisen-Nickel-Chrom unter besonderer Berücksichtigung des nach Dauerglühungen auftretenden spröden Gefügebestandteiles, *Arch. Eisenhüttenw.* **12**, 459–64.

Schmidt, M., Weber, H. and Schön, R. (1996) Cobalt chromium molybdenum metal combination for modular hip prostheses, *Clin. Orthop. Relat. Res.* **329S**, S35–47.

Schröder, A., Stich, H. Strautmann, F. and Sutter, F. (1978) Über die Anlagerung von Osteozement an einem belasteten Implantatkörper, *Schweiz Mschr. Zahnheilk.* **4**, 1051–8.

Schröder, A., van der Zypen, E. and Sutter, F. (1981) The reaction of bone connnective tissue and epithelium to endosteal implants with titanium-sprayed surface, *J. Maxillofac. Surg.* **9**, 15.

Semlitsch, M., Staub, T. and Weber, H. (1985) Titanium–aluminium–niobium alloy, development for biocompatible, high strength surgical implants, *Biomed. Tech.* **30**, 334–9.

Simon, J.-P. (1994) Restoration of bone stock with impacted cancellous allografts and cement in revision of the femoral component in total hip arthroplasty, Thesis, *Geaggregeerde van het hoger onderwijs*, Department of Orthopaedic Surgery, K.U. Leuven.

Simpson, J.P. (1981) Retrieved fracture plates – implant and tissue analysis, *NBS Spec. Publ.* **601**, 395–422.

Smith, G.D. and Yates, D.H. (1968) High strength – ductility – corrosion resistance – multiphase alloys have all three, *Metal Progress* **93**, 100–2.

Steinemann, S.G. and Perren, S.M. (1985) Titanium alloys as metallic biomaterials, in *Titanium Science and Technology* (eds G. Lütjering, U. Zwicker and W. Bunk), DGM, Oberursel, pp.1327–34.

Streicher, R.M., Semlitsch, M., Schön, R., Weber, H. and Rieker, C. (1996) Metal-on-metal articulation for artificial hip joints: laboratory study and clinical results, *Proc. Inst. Mech. Engr.* **210**, 223–32.

Waterman, N.A. and Ashby, M.F., eds (1991) *Elsevier Materials Selector*, Elsevier Applied Science, London, pp. 1–3

Willert, H.G., Buchhorn, G.H. and Semlitsch, M. (1993) Particle disease due to wear of metal alloys, in *Biological, Material and Mechanical Considerations of Joint Replacement* (ed. B.F. Morres), Raven Press, New York, pp. 239–46

Williams, D.F. (1992) Biofunctionality and biocompatibility in materials science and technology, in *Medical and Dental Materials*, Vol. 14 (eds R.W. Cahn, O. Haasen and E.J. Kremer) VCH, Weinheim, pp. 1–27.

Williams, J.M. and Buchanan, R.A. (1985) Ion implantation of surgical Ti–6Al–4V, *Mater. Sci. Engng* **69**, 237–46.

Williams, P.L., Warwick, R., Dyson, M. and Bannister, L.H., eds (1989) *Gray's Anatomy*, 37th edn, Churchill Livingstone, Edinburgh.

Zettner, K., Plenk, H. and Stassl, H. (1980) Tissue and cell reactions *in vivo* and *in vitro* to different metals for dental implant, in *Dental Implants* (ed. G. Heimke), C. Hanser, München, p.15.

Zichner, L.P. and Willert, H.-G. (1992) Comparison of alumina–polyethylene and metal–polyethylene in clinical trials, *Clin. Orthop. Relat. Res.* **282**, 86–94.

Zitter, H. (1976) Schädigung des Gewebes durch metallische Implantate, *Unfallheilkunde* **79** (3), 91–100.

Zitter, H. and Plenk, H., Jr (1987) The electrochemical behaviour of metallic implant materials as an indicator of their biocompatibility, *J. Biomed. Materials Res.* **21**, 881–96.

Zwicker, U. and Breme, J. (1984) Investigations on the friction behaviour of oxidized TiAl5Fe2.5 surface layers of implant material, *J. Less Common Metals* **100**, 371–5.

Zwicker, U., Bühler, U., Müller, R., Beck, H., Schmid, H.J. and Ferstl, J. (1980) Mechanical properties and tissue reactions of a titanium alloy for implant material, in *Titanium '80 Science and Technology* (eds H. Kimura and O. Izumi), Kyoto, AIME, New York, pp. 505–18.

Zwicker, U., Etzold, U. and Moser, T. (1984) Abrasive properties of oxide layers on TiAl5Fe2.5 in contact with high density polyethylene, in *Proceedings of the 5th World Conference on Titanium*, Vol. 2, DGM, Oberursel, pp. 1343–50.

2
Metals and implants

H.J. BREME[1], V. BIEHL[1] AND J.A. HELSEN[2]
[1]University of the Saarland, Saarbrücken, Germany
[2]Catholic University of Leuven, Leuven, Belgium

2.1 INTRODUCTION

This chapter gives in tabular form the chemical composition, physical and mechanical properties, and recommendations for processing (deformation, machining, welding and brazing) the following groups of metals:

- stainless steels
- CoCr-based alloys
- titanium and titanium alloys
- dental restoration materials
- refractory materials.

The alloys with their most interesting properties located in and around a martensitic phase transition domain are discussed in Chapter 3, which is dedicated exclusively to shape memory metals.

To avoid confusion, each subclass of alloys is preceded, wherever possible, by a synoptic table containing the international standards paralleled by some national standards. In addition, some properties of bone are given. At the end of the chapter definitions, symbols, dimensions and units of the most important properties are listed.

2.2 STAINLESS STEELS

Tables 2.1–2.5 describe the chemical composition, Table 2.6 the physical properties, Tables 2.7–2.17 the mechanical properties and Tables 2.18–2.22 the processing recommendations.

2.3 CoCr-BASED ALLOYS

Tables 2.23–2.25 describe the chemical composition, Table 2.26 the physical properties, Tables 2.7–2.17 the mechanical properties and Tables 2.18–2.22 the processing recommendations.

Metals as Biomaterials ISBN 0 471 96935 4 Edited by J.A. Helsen and H.J. Breme. © 1998 John Wiley & Sons Ltd

Table 2.1 Comparison of international standard stainless steel alloy numbers for various medical applications (Wegst, 1989; Schäning, 1995; DIN, ASTM, AFNOR, BSI, JIS)

Alloy[a]	Germany[b] Alloy no.	USA[c] AISI/ SAE no.	France[d] AFNOR no.	Great Britain[e] BSI no.	Japan[f] JIS no.
X20Cr13 (cast)	1.4021	410CA-15	Z12Cr13	410C21	SUS410
X20Cr13	1.4021	420	Z20C13	420S27	SUS4020J1
X15Cr13	1.4024			420S29	
X46Cr13	1.4034		Z38C13M	(420S45)	
X20CrNi172	1.4057	431	Z15CN16.02	431S29	SUS431
X12CrMoS17	1.4104	430F/J405-89	Z10CF17	SUS430F	
X5CrNi1810	1.4301	304	Z6CN18-09	304S15	SUS304
		304H		304S16	
				304S31	
X10CrNiS189	1.4305	303	Z10CNF18.9	303S21	SUS303
X2CrNi1911	1.4306	304L/	Z2CNF18.9	304S12SUS19	
X2CrNi189 (cast)		J405-89	Z2CN19	304S11	SUS304L
X12CrNi177	1.4310	301	Z12CN17.07	301S21	SUS301
X5CrNiMo17122	1.4404	316	Z6CND17.11	316S16	SUS316
X5CrNiMo17133	1.4436		Z6CND17.12		
X2CrNiMo17132	1.4404	316L	Z2CND18.13	315S11	SUS316L
X2CrNiMo17130			Z2CND17.12	316S12	
X2CrNiMo1810 (cast)					
X2CrNiMoN17122	1.4406	316LN	Z2CND17.12Az	316S61	SUS316L
X2CrNiMoN17133	1.4429		Z2CND17.13Az	316S62	
			Z12CN18.07		
			Z2CN18.9	304C12	
X2CrNiMo18164	1.4438	317L	Z2CND19.15	317S12	SUS17L
X5CrNiMo1713	1.4449	317		317S16	SUS317
X6CrNiTi1810	1.4541	321	Z6CNT18.10	321S12	SUS321
				321S31	
X10CrNiNb189	1.4550	347	Z10CNNb18-10		
X10CrNiMoNb1810	1.4580	318	Z8CNDNb18-12		
X2CrNiN1810		XM-21			

[a]Chemical composition: figure following X = carbon content multiplied by 100, e.g. X2CrNiMo17132: C = 0.02%, Cr = 17%, Ni = 13%, Mo = 2%.
L, Low carbon content; Mo, S, N, Ti, Nb contain the mentioned element.
[b]Standardised in DIN 17440–17443; DIN 17440 will be replaced by DIN EN 10088.
[c]Also standardised in ASTM A276.
[d]Standardised in NFA 35-574, replaced by NF EN 10088-3.
[e]Standardised in BS 970/1.
[f]Standardised in JIS G4303.

Table 2.2 Chemical composition (wt%) of steels for medical instruments (DIN, 1977, 1996c, 1997a)

	C	Cr	Ni	Si	Mn	P	S	Mo	Application
Martensitic and austenitic free cutting steels									
X12CrMoS17	0.1–0.17	15.5–17.5	–	≤ 1.0	≤ 1.5	≤ 0.045	0.15–0.25	0.01	Handles, screws, nuts
X12CrNiS188	≤ 0.15	17–19	8–10	≤ 1.0	≤ 2.0	≤ 0.045	0.1–0.2		Handles, screws, bolts, probes
Austenitic steels									
X5CrNi1810	≤ 0.07	17–20	9–11.5	≤ 1.0	≤ 2.0	≤ 0.045	≤ 0.03	–	Pincettes, scissors, forceps
X12CrNi177	≤ 0.15 (AISI)	16–18	6–9	≤ 1.5	≤ 2.0	≤ 0.045	≤ 0.015	≤ 0.8	Handles, drills
X5CrNiMo17122	≤ 0.07	16.5–18.5	10.5–13.5	≤ 1.0	≤ 2.0	≤ 0.045	≤ 0.03	2–2.5	Pincettes, scissors, drills

Table 2.3 Chemical composition (wt%) of steels for medical instruments (Benjamin and Kirkpatrick, 1980; DIN, 1996c, 1997a)

	C	Cr	Ni	Si	Mn	P	S	V	Mo	Application
Martensitic steels										
X10Cr13	≤ 0.15	11.5 13.5	–	≤ 1.0	≤ 1.0	≤ 0.04	≤ 0.03	–	–	
X15Cr13	0.12–0.17	12–14	–	≤ 1.0	≤ 1.0	≤ 0.045	≤ 0.03	–	–	Pincettes, forceps, probes, suture hooks
X20Cr13	0.17–0.22	12–14	–	≤ 1.0	≤ 1.0	≤ 0.045	≤ 0.03	–	–	As above, curettes, drills
X40Cr13	0.4–0.5	12–14	–	< 1.0	≤ 1.0	≤ 0.045	≤ 0.03	–	–	Scissors, forceps, scalpels, drills
X20CrNi172	≤ 0.20	15.5–17.5	1.25–2.5	≤ 1.0	≤ 1.0	≤ 0.04	≤ 0.03	–	–	
X65CrMo17	0.60–0.75	16–18	–	≤ 1.0	≤ 1.0	≤ 0.04	≤ 0.03	–	0.75	
X38CrMoV15	0.35–0.4	14–15	–	0.3–0.5	0.2–0.4	≤ 0.045	≤ 0.03	0.1–0.15	0.4–0.6	Scissors, forceps, scalpels, curettes
X45CrMoV15	0.4–0.5	14–15	–	0.3–0.5	0.2–0.4	≤ 0.045	≤ 0.03	0.1–1.15	0.4–0.6	Scissors, forceps, scalpels, curettes
X20CrMo13 (cast)	0.15–0.18	12–14	≤ 1.0	≤ 1.0	≤ 1.0	≤ 0.045	≤ 0.03	–	0.9–1.3	Curettes, sharp spoons
X35CrMo17 (cast)	0.33–0.43	15.5–17.5	≤ 1.0	≤ 1.0	≤ 1.0	≤ 0.045	≤ 0.03	–	0.9–1.3	Curettes, sharp spoons

Table 2.4 Chemical composition (wt%) of austenitic stainless steels (Benjamin and Kirkpatrick, 1980)

	C	Cr	Ni	Si	Mn	P	S	Mo	Others
X12CrNi177	≤ 0.15	16.0–18.0	6.0–8.0	≤ 1.0	≤ 2.0	≤ 0.045	≤ 0.03	–	–
X5CrNi1810	≤ 0.08	18.0–20.0	8.0–10.5	≤ 1.0	≤ 2.0	≤ 0.045	≤ 0.03	–	–
X2CrNi1911	≤ 0.03	18.0–20.0	8.0–12.0	≤ 1.0	≤ 2.0	≤ 0.045	≤ 0.03	–	–
X25CrNi2522	≤ 0.25	24.0–26.0	19.0–22.0	≤ 1.5	≤ 2.0	≤ 0.045	≤ 0.03	–	–
X25CrNi2520	≤ 0.25	23.0–26.0	19.0–20.0	1.5–3.0	≤ 2.0	≤ 0.045	≤ 0.03	–	–
X5CrNiMo17133	≤ 0.08	16.0–18.0	10.0–14.0	≤ 1.0	≤ 2.0	≤ 0.045	≤ 0.03	2.0–3.0	–
X2CrNiMo17133	≤ 0.03	16.0–18.0	10.0–14.0	≤ 1.0	≤ 2.0	≤ 0.045	≤ 0.03	2.0–3.0	–
X5CrNiMo18164	≤ 0.08	18.0–20.0	11.0–15.0	≤ 1.0	≤ 2.0	≤ 0.045	≤ 0.03	3.0–4.0	–
X2CrNiMo18164	≤ 0.03	18.0–20.0	11.0–15.0	≤ 1.0	≤ 2.0	≤ 0.045	≤ 0.03	3.0–4.0	–
X6CrNiTi1810	≤ 0.08	17.0–19.0	9.0–12.0	≤ 1.0	≤ 2.0	≤ 0.045	≤ 0.03	–	Ti ≤ 5 × wt% C

Table 2.5 Chemical composition (wt%) of steels for implant surgery (DIN, 1997b)

	C	Cr	Ni	Si	Mn	P	S	Mo	N	Nb
X2CrNiMoN18133	≤ 0.03	17.0–18.5	13.0–14.5	≤ 1.0	≤ 2.0	≤ 0.025	0.01	2.7–3.2	0.14–0.22	–
X2CrNiMo18153	≤ 0.03	17.0–18.5	13.5–15.5	≤ 1.0	≤ 2.0	≤ 0.025	≤ 0.01	2.7–3.2	≤ 0.01	–
X2CrNiMoN18154	≤ 0.03	17.0–18.5	14.0–16.0	≤ 1.0	≤ 2.0	≤ 0.015	≤ 0.01	2.7–3.2	0.1–0.2	–
X2CrNiMnMo22136	≤ 0.03	21.0–23.0	10.0–16.0	≤ 0.75	5.5–7.5	≤ 0.025	≤ 0.01	2.7–3.2	0.35–0.5	0.1–0.25

The minimum content of Cr and Mo amounts to ≥ 26 according to the sum of efficacy which is given by 3.3 × %Mo + %Cr.

2.4 CP-TITANIUM AND TITANIUM ALLOYS

Tables 2.35–2.38 describe the chemical composition, Tables 2.39 and 2.40 the physical properties, Tables 2.41–2.46 the mechanical properties and Tables 2.47–2.51 the processing recommendations.

2.5 MATERIALS FOR DENTAL RESTORATION

Tables 2.52–2.58 describe the properties of precious metals, Tables 2.59 and 2.60 the properties of non-precious metals and Tables 2.61–2.63 the properties of amalgam.

2.6 REFRACTORY METALS

Tables 2.64–2.67 summarise the properties of niobium and tantalum and those of their alloys with potential biomedical importance. The use of refractory metals in biomedical applications is very limited. However, niobium and tantalum show high corrosion resistance and, moreover, a very good bone apposition when implanted in

Table 2.6 Physical properties of selected steels for medical instruments (DIN 1996c, 1997a)

	Density (g cm^{-3})	Thermal expansion coefficient between 70 and 300°C (10^{-6} K^{-1})	Thermal conductivity at 20°C (W m^{-1} K^{-1})	Specific heat capacity at 20°C (J kg^{-1} K^{-1})	Specific electrical resistance at 20°C (μΩ m)	Young's modulus (GPa)	Magnetic properties
X10Cr13	7.8	9.9	24.9		0.57	216	magnetisable
X15Cr13		11.5			0.60	216	magnetisable
X20Cr13	7.8	11.5	30	460	0.60	220	magnetisable
X40Cr13		11.5			0.60		magnetisable
X45CrMoV15		11.0			0.65	220	Ferromagnetic
X12CrMoS17	7.5	11.0	26.1	460	0.60	216	Ferromagnetic
X20CrNi172	7.5	12.1	20.2	460	0.72		Ferromagnetic

Table 2.7 Physical properties of selected steels for medical instruments (DIN, 1996c, 1997a)

	Density (g cm^{-3})	Thermal expansion coefficient between 70 and 300°C (10^{-6} K^{-1})	Thermal conductivity at 20°C (W m^{-1} K^{-1})	Specific heat capacity at 20°C (J kg^{-1} K^{-1})	Specific electrical resistance at 20°C (μΩ m)	Young's modulus (GPa)	Magnetic properties
X12CrNi177	8.0	17.0	16.2	500	0.72	193	Paramagnetic
X5CrNi1810	8.0	17.8	16.2	500	0.72	193	Paramagnetic
X2CrNi1810	8.0	17.8	16.2	500	0.72	193	Paramagnetic
X25CrNi2520	7.8	15.1	17.5	500	0.77	200	Paramagnetic
X5CrNiMo17133	8.0	15.9	16.2	500	0.74	193	Paramagnetic
X2CrNiMo17133	8.0	15.9	16.2	500	0.74	193	Paramagnetic
X2CrNiMoN17133	8.0	15.9	16.2	500	0.74	193	Paramagnetic
X2CrNiMo18164	8.0	15.9	16.2	500	0.74	193	Paramagnetic
X5CrNiMo18164	8.0	15.9	16.2	500	0.74	193	Paramagnetic
X6CrNiTi1810	8.0	16.6	16.1	500	0.72	193	Paramagnetic

Table 2.8 Mechanical properties of steels for medical instruments (DIN, 1997a)

Steel	Condition	Tensile yield strength (0.2%) (MPa)	Ultimate tensile strength (MPa)	Elongation at fracture (%)	Reduction of area (%)
Martensitic steels					
X15Cr13	As forged + annealed	–	≥720	–	–
X20Cr13	As forged + annealed	–	≥740	–	–
X45CrMoV15	As forged + annealed	–	≥900	–	–
X20CrMo13	As cast + annealed	–	≥800	–	–
X35CrMo17	As cast + annealed	–	≥950	–	–
Martensitic and austenitic free cutting steels					
X12CrMoS17	As forged + annealed	–	540–740	16	–
X12CrNiS188	As forged + quenched	195	500–700	35	–
Austenitic steels					
X5CrNi1810	As forged[a] + quenched	220–235	550–750	43–45	–
X5CrNiMo17122	As forged[a] + quenched	240–255	550–700	43–45	–
X12CrNi177	Wire, cold deformed	–	1250–2450[b]	–	>40

[a]Longitudinal/transversel.
[b]Depends on the degree of cold deformation.

bone (Gypen, 1979; Zitter and Plenk, 1987; Johansson 1990, 1991). The mechanical properties of both pure metals is hardly sufficient for orthopaedic or dental implants, but can be improved by cold working or alloying. As seen in Table 2.64, the melting points are extremely high and alloying will be an expensive operation. However, as powders are easily available, alloying by the powder metallurgical route seems to be promising. Mechanical alloying is a relatively inexpensive process and its feasibility has been demonstrated by Dessein (1996).

Table 2.9 Mechanical properties of austenitic stainless steels (minimum values at room temperature) (Benjamin and Kirkpatrick, 1980; Harris and Priebe, 1988; ASTM, 1992d)

	Condition	Ultimate tensile strength (MPa)	Tensile yield strength (MPa)	Elongation at fracture (%)	Reduction of area (%)
X12CrNi177	Annealed full hard	515	205	40	
	Full hard	1280	965	9	
X5CrNi1810	Hot finished + annealed	515	205	40	50
	Cold finished	620	310	30	40
X2CrNi1911	Hot finished + annealed	480	170	40	50
	Cold finished + annealed	620	310	30	40
X25CrNi2520	Hot finished + annealed	215	205	40	50
	Cold finished + annealed	620	310	39	40
X5CrNiMo17133	Hot finished + annealed	515	205	40	50
	Cold finished + annealed	620	310	40	50
X2CrNiMo17133	Hot finished + annealed	515	170	40	50
	Cold finished + annealed	620	310	30	40
X5CrNiMo1713	Hot finished + annealed	515	205	40	50
	Cold finished + annealed	620	310	30	40
X2CrNiMo18164	Annealed	585	240	55	65

METALS AND IMPLANTS

Table 2.10 Mechanical properties of martensitic stainless steels (minimum values at room temperature) (Benjamin and Kirkpatrick, 1980; DIN, 1997a)

	Condition	Ultimate tensile strength (MPa)	Tensile yield strength (MPa)	Elongation at fracture (%)	Reduction of area (%)
X10Cr13	Hot finished + annealed	485	275	20	45
	Cold finished + annealed	485	275	16	45
X20Cr13	Hardened + tempered, 204°C	1720	1480	8	25
X20CrNi172	Hardened + tempered, 260°C	1370	1070	16	55
	Hardened + tempered, 593°C	965	795	19	57
X65CrMo17	Hardened + annealed	725	415	20	–
	Hardened + tempered, 316°C	1790	1650	5	20

2.7 BONE PROPERTIES

Some of the properties of bone are compiled in Table 2.68 for comparison with metals. Only the properties of bone are listed and not those of soft tissue. The highest mechanical loads on implants are found in devices for the support or replacement of long bones.

2.8 DEFINITIONS, SYMBOLS, DIMENSIONS AND UNITS

Mechanical properties are not a unique function of a material but are a result of a given way of stressing a representative test piece of the material. For all properties listed the following assumptions have been made:

(1) all properties listed are determined below the creep range
(2) all materials listed are considered to be isotropic.

Table 2.11 Mechanical properties of steels for implant surgery (minimum values at room temperature) (DIN, 1997b)

	Condition	Ultimate tensile strength (MPa)	Tensile yield strength (MPa)	Elongation at fracture (%)
X2CrNiMoN18133	Solution treated	600–800	300	40
X2CrNiMo18153		490–690	190	40
X2CrNiMoN18154		590–800	285	40
X2CrNiMnMoN22136		850–1050	500	35

Special requirements:
1. Allowed melting procedures: vacuum arc furnace or electroslag remelting.
2. After the solution heat treatment the material must be free of delta-ferrite.
3. Grain size of at least ASTM4.
4. Resistance to intercrystalline corrosion determined according to Table 2.5.
5. Microscopic purity concerning inclusions of oxides and sulfides determined according to Table 2.5.

Table 2.12 Mechanical properties of wire for implant surgery (DIN, 1997b)

	Condition	Ultimate tensile strength (MPa)	Elongation at fracture[a] (%)
X2CrNiMoN18133	Solution treated	800–1000	30
X2CrNiMoNi18154	Solution treated	800–1000	40
X2CrNiMoNi18133	Cold worked	1350–1850	–
X2CrNiMoN18154	Cold worked	1350–1850	–

[a]Minimum values.
The values depend on the diameter of the wire (decrease in diameter and increase in degree of deformation = increase in value).

As an *aide-mémoire* the definitions of all properties listed in the tables are given, together with the dimensions and units. Some of the definitions are taken from or are according to those given by Waterman and Ashby (1978). They are based mainly on commonly accepted knowledge.

If possible, all units are given according to the International System of Units [Système International d'Unités (SI)]. For practical reasons the authors have deviated from this rule wherever other units are so common that it would be confusing to act otherwise; for example, density will be expressed in g cm^{-3}. The basic unit is given and, where useful, the most appropriate multiple. The dimension or dimensional product is the expression of a quantity as a product of powers of base quantities, omitting their vectorial or tensorial character, sign and numerical factors. These dimensions are useful when checking the result of combined calculations and the units attributed in the final result. The dimension is given between square brackets and the symbols used are: L, length; M, mass; T, time; θ, thermodynamic temperature; J, current; –, dimensionless.

Table 2.13 Mechanical properties of X2CrNiMo17133 stainless steel as a function of the degree of cold working (Cigada *et al.*, 1983)

Degree of cold working (%)	Ultimate tensile strength (MPa)	Tensile yield strength (MPa)
0	584	255
31	912	831
50	1138	1036
63	1255	1169
70	1344	1204
76	1421	1252

METALS AND IMPLANTS

Table 2.14 Influence of cold deformation on the mechanical properties of steels for implant surgery (DIN, 1997b)

	Condition	Ultimate tensile strength (MPa)	Tensile yield strength[a] (MPa)	Elongation at fracture[a] (%)
X2CrNiMoN22136	As cold, worked, dia. ≤ 19 mm	860–110	690	12
X2CrNiMo18154		860–110	650	12

[a]Minimum values.

2.8.1 DEFINITIONS: NAME (SYMBOL, [DIMENSION], UNITS)

Creep (ε or σ – or [$ML^{-1} T^{-2}$], % or MPa)

Creep is the plastic deformation of a material when it is constantly loaded for a relatively long period at a constant temperature. Around room temperature creep is important for polymers only, while for metals and ceramics it is measurable only at elevated temperatures. The creep resistance is determined by the stress σ producing a given ε in a given time at a constant temperature, e.g. $\sigma_{0.1/1000}$ is the stress that produced a creep of 0.1% in 1000 h or at a constant temperature.

Degree of deformation (ε, – , %)

The degree of deformation is determined as the reduction in thickness for sheet, and in section for rods and wire. Alternatively (symbol ρ), it is calculated as the natural logarithm of the ratio of thickness before and after deformation for sheet, or the ratio of section before and after deformation for rods and wire.

Table 2.15 Fatigue strength (rotating/bending; $N = 10^7$ cycles) of various stainless steels (Schmidt, 1981)

	Heat treatment	Testing condition			Fatigue strength (MPa)
		R	α_k	Medium	
X20Cr13	30 min/1020°C/oil + 2 h/550°C/air	−1	1	Air	481
			1	30% NaCl	69
			3.6	Air	206
			3.6	30%NaCl	49
X20Cr13	30 min/1020°C/oil + 2 h/625°C/air	−1	1	Air	412
			1	30% NaCl	78
			3.6	Air	177
			3.6	30% NaCl	29
X5CrNi1810	30 min/1050°C/water	−1	1	Air	220–550
X5CrNiMo17133	15 min/1050°C/water	−1	1	Air	265
				30% NaCl	216

α_k, Notch factor.

Table 2.16 Fatigue strength σ_f (Wöhler curves) and rotating bending fatigue strength σ_R of various stainless steels (Thull, 1979; Webster, 1988; Breme and Schmid, 1990)

	σ_f (MPa)	σ_R (MPa)	R
X2CrNiMo17133	250–320	250	−1
X2CrNiMo18153	–	250–320[a]	−1
		350–415[b]	
X2CrNiMnMoN22136	–	500–650[c]	−1

[a]Annealed.
[b]Cold worked.
[c]Hot forged.

Table 2.17 Fatigue strength (2×10^6 cycles) determined by the stair-case method[a] of X2CrNiMo17133 stainless steel (Cigada et al., 1993)

Degree of cold deformation (%)	Tensile strength (MPa)	Stress ratio R	Fatigue strength (MPa)
7	658	0	283
57	1211	0	362
57	1211	−1	505

[a]Explanation:
(1) Starting with a stress S_o.
(2) If specimen fails before 2×10^6 cycles → new specimen with a stress $S-\Delta S_o$. If specimen does not fail before 2×10^6 cycles → new specimen with a stress $S_o+\Delta S$.
(3) Perform (2) for 15–20 samples and evaluate with standard statistical methods.

Table 2.18 Processing of stainless steels (Heimann et al., 1985; Harris and Priebe, 1988)

Process	Conditions
Hot deformation	925–1100°C if δ-ferrite occurs
	925–1260°C if δ-ferrite does not occur
	Martensitic steels must be cooled slowly to 590°C
Descaling	Sand blasting using non-metallic blast material
	10% H_2SO_4 or
	10% HNO_3–2% HF or
	1.5–2% NaOH
Cold deformation	No problem for low C contents
	For ferritic steels 100–300°C is recommended and for high deformation rates an intermediate annealing at 750–800°C
	Lubricants: oil with graphite or MoS_2

METALS AND IMPLANTS

Table 2.19 Machining parameters for stainless steels (Kosa and Ney, 1989)

	Type of machining	Tool material	Depth of cut (mm)	Speed (m min^{-1})	Feed (mm rev^{-1})
Martensitic	Turning	HSS	0.75–3.8	20–38	0.18–0.38
		Carbide	0.75–3.8	80–180	0.18–0.38
Austenitic	Turning	HSS	0.75–3.8	23–20	0.18–0.38
		Carbide	0.75–3.8	100–160	0.025–0.46^a
Martensitic	Drilling	M1, M7, M10	–	3–12	–
Austenitic				4–8	
Martensitic	Tapping	M1, M7, M10	–	3–12	–
Austenitic				4–8	
Martensitic	Milling	M2, M7	–	27–34	0.025–0.15 mm tooth^{-1}
		C6	–	82–107	0.025–0.15 mm tooth^{-1}
		M2, M7	–	23–24	0.025–0.15 mm tooth^{-1}
		C6	–	79–82	0.025–0.15 mm tooth^{-1}
Martensitic	Powder			50–90 strokes min^{-1}	0.1 mm stroke^{-1}
Austenitic	Hardening				

HSS, High-speed steel.
^{a}Depending on hole diameter.

Density (ρ, [ML^{-3}], kg m^{-3}, g cm^{-3})

This property of matter, macroscopically measured by the mass per unit volume, is a function of the degree and/or the kind of order of its atoms or molecules.

Elongation at fracture (A, –,%)

The ductility of a material is measured in tensile tests by its elongation (relative to a standard gauge length) and is expressed as the percentage change in length. Elongation is a measure of the deformability or the ability of a material to accommodate stress concentrations, and it can be related to fracture toughness. In some instances, in addition to elongation tensile tests, the reduction in area in the necking zone is given. It is also a measure of the ductility of the material.

Table 2.20 Chemical composition (wt%) of filler metals and brazing temperature for brazing stainless steels (DIN, 1979; Mills *et al*., 1983)

	Ag	Cu	Zn	Cd	Ni	Sn	Mn	In	Brazing temperature range (°C)
AgCu	53–59	Balance	–	–	–	–	–	–	765–980
Ag55Sn	54–57	20–23	Balance	–	–	2.5	–	–	650
Ag56InNi	55–57	Balance	–	–	3.5–4.5	–	–	13–15	730
AgCuZn	20–70	20–40	14–40	–	≤ 3.5	≤ 5.5	–	–	650–870
AgCuZnCd	30–50	14–35	13–25	12–25	–	–	–	–	620–840
AgCuZnMn	20–50	15–40	21–37	–	≤ 2.5	–	1.5–8	–	700–870

Processes: furnace, torch, induction, resistance.
Fluxes: boric acid, borates, fluorides, fluoborates (not necessary with furnace brazing in argon or vacuum).

Table 2.21 Electrodes for arc welding of stainless steels (Mills et al., 1983; DIN, 1997b)

Steel	Condition of weld for service	Electrode or welding rod
X12CrNi177	As welded or annealed	X8CrNi2011
X5CrNi1810		
X2CrNi1911	As welded or stress relieved	X8CrNi1811
X2CrNi2520	As welded	X2CrNi2520
X5CrNiMo17133	As welded or annealed	X5CrNiMo17133
X2CrNiMo17133	As welded or stress relieved	X2CrNiMo17133
X5CrNiMo18164	As welded or annealed	X5CrNiMo18164
X2CrNiMo18164	As welded or stress relieved	X2CrNiMo18164
X6CrNiTi1810	As welded or stabilised and stress relieved	X8CrNi1811
X20Cr13[a]	Annealed or hardened and stress relieved	X20Cr13
X20CrNi1810[a]	As welded	X25CrNi2520 X8CrNi2011

[a]To avoid cracking: careful preheating to 260°C and slow cooling at $C > 0.2$ wt%; in addition, annealing at 1065–1120°C is required.

Fatigue strength (σ_f or σ_b, [ML^{-1} T^2], Pa, MPa)

Failures that occur as a result of dynamic periodic stressing are referred to as fatigue failures. Fatigue strength is defined as the highest periodic stress that does not initiate a failure of the material after a given number of cycles, e.g. $N = 10^7$. Fatigue failures occur only in the elastic region of the static loading. Therefore the fatigue strength is lower than the yield strength. σ_f is the fatigue strength under pulsating tension and compression; σ_b is the rotating-bending fatigue strength; R is the ratio of the lowest to the highest applied stress amplitude.

Fracture toughness (K, [ML$^{-1/2}$T^{-2}], N m$^{-3/2}$)

Resistance of a material to crack propagation is related to the stress intensity factor, K. The condition for failure is that K reaches a critical value K_c, the plane strain

Table 2.22 Recommended heat treatments for various stainless steels (DIN, 1996c, 1997a)

	Stress relief[a]	Soft annealing (°C)	Hardening (°C)	Hardening medium	Annealing[b] (°C)
X20Cr13	540–900	750–780	950–1000	Oil	650–700
X12CrMoS17	540–900	800–850	1020–1050	Oil	550–600
X5CrNiMo17133	540–900		1050–1100	Water, air	
X2CrNiMo17133	540–900		1000–1100	Water, air	
X5CrNi1810	540–900		1000–1050	Water, air	
X6CrNiTi1810	540–900		1020–1070	Water, air	

[a]540°C: 95 min/mm thickness; 900°C: 25 min/mm thickness.
[b]Tempering of martensite

METALS AND IMPLANTS

Table 2.23 Comparison of international standards for CoCr-based alloys (ISO, DIN, BSI, AFNOR, JIS, ASTM)

Alloy[a]	International Organisation for Standardisation (ISO)	Germany (DIN)[b]	Great Britain (BSI)[b]	France (AFNOR)[b]	Japan (JIS)	USA (ASTM)
Co29Cr5Mo (cast)	5832–IV	5832–4 13912–1	7252–4	Project S94–054	T6115	F75
Co29Cr5Mo (wrought/PM)	5832–XII	5832–12	7252–12	Project S94–053	T6104	F799
Co20Cr15W10Ni	5832–V	5832–5	7252–5	Project S90–406 NF ISO 5832–5		F90
Co20Cr35Ni10Mo	5832–VI	5832–6	7252–6	NFISO5832–6		F562
Co20Cr16Ni16Fe7Mo (wrought/cast)	5832–VII	5832–7	7252–7	Project S94–057		F1058
Co20Cr20Ni5Fe3Mo3W	5832–VIII	5832–8	7252–8	Project S94–058		F563

[a]Direct chemical composition, e.g. Co29Cr5Mo: 29 wt% Cr, 5 wt% Mo, balance Co.
[b]Exactly corresponding to ISO standard.

fracture toughness. It is measured by means of the different modes of loading. The most frequent mode is mode I and is loading the samples perpendicular to an initiated crack (K_{IC}).

Hardness (H, –, –)

For metals (and ceramics) hardness is best defined as the resistance of a material to permanent deformation by indentation. According to standards, the hardness should be dimensionless. For metals, four indentation bodies are mainly used:

ball (1–10 mm)	Brinell	HB
four-sided pyramid (top angle 136°)	Vickers	HV
ball (1/16″)	Rockwell B	HR_B
cone (120°)	Rockwell C	HR_C

Reduction in area: *see Elongation*

Specific electrical resistance (ρ [ML^3 T^{-3} A^{-2}], ·μΩ m)

This is the resistance of a block with a length of 1 m and a cross-section of 1 m^2, also called resistivity.

Table 2.24 Chemical composition (wt%) of cast CoCr alloys (DIN/ISO, 1980a, b; ASTM, 1992a)

Alloy	Co	Cr	Mo	Ni	Fe	C	Si	Mn	Ti
Co29Cr5Mo	Balance	26.5–30.0	4.5–7.0	≤ 2.5	≤ 1.0	≤ 0.35	≤ 1.0	≤ 1.0	–
CoCrMo[a]	33.0–75.0	15.0–32.5	4.0–7.5	≤ 2.0	≤ 1.5	≤ 0.05	≤ 1.0	≤ 1.0	≤ 5

[a]Alloys used for dental restoration (according to standards sum of Co + Cr ≥ 85%, Cr + Mo + Ti ≥ 25%, Be ≤ 0.01%).

Table 2.25 Chemical composition (wt%) of wrought CoCr alloys (DIN/ISO, 1980a, b, 1992c–e; ASTM, 1992c–e)

Alloy	Co	Cr	Mo	Ni	Fe	C	Si	Mn	P	S	W	Ti
Co20Cr15W10Ni	Balance	19.0–21.0	–	9.0–11.0	≤ 3.0	≤ 0.15	≤ 1.0	≤ 2.5	≤ 0.04	≤ 0.03	14.0–16.0	–
Co20Cr35Ni10Mo[a]	Balance	19.0–21.0	9.0–10.5	33.0–37.0	≤ 1.0	≤ 0.15	≤ 0.15	≤ 0.15	≤ 0.015	≤ 0.010	–	–
Co20Cr16Ni16Fe7Mo	39.0–42.0	18.5–21.5	6.5–8.0	14.0–18.0	Balance	≤ 0.15	–	1.0–2.5	≤ 0.015	≤ 0.015	–	≤ 1.0
Co20Cr20Ni5Fe3Mo3W	Balance	18.0–22.0	3.0–4.0	15.0–25.0	4.0–6.0	≤ 0.05	≤ 0.05	≤ 1.00	–	≤ 0.010	3.0–4.0	0.5–3.5

[a]Other elements: single ≤ 0.1, sum ≤ 0.4; Be ≤ 0.001.

Table 2.26 Physical properties of CoCr alloys (DIN/ISO, 1980a, b; Latrobe Steel, 1980)

	Density (g cm^{-3})	Thermal expansion coefficient 20–300°C (×10^{-6} K^{-1})	Thermal conductivity at 20°C (W m^{-1} K^{-1})	Specific heat capacity (J kg^{-1} K^{-1})	Specific electrical resistivity at 20°C (μΩ m)	Young's modulus	Melting point (interval) (°C)	Transformation temperature hcp→fcc (°C)
Co29Cr5Mo	8.2–8.4	14.2	14.8	420	0.91	210–230	1235 (eutectic) 1300–1400	890
Co20Cr15W10Ni	9.1	12.3	10.2	384	0.89	225		650
Co20Cr35Ni10Mo	8.43	13.1	11.1	390	1.03	235	1315–1427	650

METALS AND IMPLANTS

Table 2.27 Mechanical properties of cast CoCr alloys and alloys produced by powder metallurgy (DIN/ISO, 1980a,b; Pilliar, 1981; ASTM, 1992a)

	Condition	Ultimate tensile strength (MPa)	Tensile yield strength (0.2%) (MPa)	Elongation at fracture (%)	Reduction in area (%)
Co29Cr5Mo	As cast	≥ 665	≥ 450	≥ 8	≥ 8
CoCrMo(pm)[a]	HIP	1277	841	14	

[a]Powder metallurgical production.

Table 2.28 Mechanical properties of wrought CoCr alloys (Pilliar, 1981; DIN/ISO, 1992c–e; ASTM, 1995e)

	Condition	Ultimate tensile strength (MPa)	Tensile yield strength (0.2%) (MPa)	Elongation at fracture (%)	Reduction in area (%)
Co20Cr15W10Ni	As annealed	950–1200	450–650	30–60	
	17.5% cold worked	1350	1180	22	
Co20Cr35Ni10Mo	As annealed	800	300	40	
	50% cold worked	1000	650	10	
	Hard worked	1200	1000	10	
	Solution heat treated	793–1000	241–448	50	
Co20Cr16Ni16Fe7Mo	As annealed	550	450	65	
	30% cold worked	1450	1300	8	
	Heat treated	1650	1400	1	
	As annealed	600	276	50	65
Co20Cr20Ni5Fe3Mo3W	Cold worked or cold worked + aged	1000	827	18	50
	Moderately hard worked	1310	1172	12	45
	Hard worked	1580	1310	5	35
	Extra hard worked				

Table 2.29 Fatigue strength σ_f and rotating bending strength σ_R of various CoCr alloys (Thull, 1979; Pilliar, 1981)

	Condition	R	σ_f (MPa)	σ_R (MPa)
Co29Cr5Mo	As cast	−1	200–300	300
Co20Cr35Ni10Mo	As cast	−1	200–300	–
Co20Cr15W10Ni	Wrought	−1	540–600	500
pm-Co29Cr5Mo	Hot isostatic pressing	−1	370–430	725

Table 2.30 Influence of the heat treatment on the fatigue strength (10^7 cycles) of CoCr alloys (Lorenz et al., 1978; Pilliar, 1981)

	R	Heat treatment	Tensile fatigue strength (MPa)
Co29Cr5Mo	−1	As cast + polished	>200
	−1	As cast + shot peened	>260
	−1	Solution annealed (1230°C/1 h/water quenched)	220–280
	−1	Annealed 1170°C	280–350
Co20Cr15W10Ni	−1	Cold worked (17.5%)	490
	−1	Cold worked (44%)	587
Co20Cr35Ni10Mo	−1	Hot forged and annealed	440–450
	−1	Hot forged >650°C	520

Table 2.31 Processing of CoCr alloys (Mills et al., 1983; Bever, 1986)

Process	Conditions
Casting	Lost wax process, performed in vacuum temperature: 1350–1450°C Solution heat treatment 1200–1250°C must follow
Hot deformation	870–1125°C
Powder metallurgy	Hot isostatic pressing 1100°C/1000 bar
Descaling	Sand blasting using non-metallic blast material 10% HNO_3–2% HF
Cold deformation	No problem for fcc materials

Table 2.32 Machining parameters for CoCr alloys (Davis et al., 1989)

	Type of machining	Tool material	Depth of cut (mm)	Speed (m min^{-1})	Feed (mm rev^{-1})
Cast	Turning		2.5	3–15	0.13–0.18
Wrought	Finishing		5	5–17	0.25
Cast	Turning		0.8	3–18	0.13
Wrought	Finishing		0.8	6–27	0.13
Cast	Drilling	–	2–4.5	0.025–0.15	
Wrought		–	4.5–6	0.05–0.1	
Cast	Face milling	HSS	1–8	4.5–1.5	0.075–0.05
		carbide	1–4	14–9	0.15–0.13
Wrought	Face milling	HSS	1–8	6–4.5	0.1–0.005
		Carbide	1–4	20–18	0.15–0.13
Cast	Milling finish	HSS	0.5	3.0–3.6	0.025–0.05
		Carbide	0.5	12–18	
Wrought	Milling finish	HSS	0.5	3.6–4.5	0.025–0.05
		Carbide	0.5	18–21	

HSS, High-speed steel.

METALS AND IMPLANTS

Table 2.33 Chemical composition (wt%) of filler metals for brazing CoCr alloys (Mills et al., 1983)

Co	Cr	Ni	Si	W	Fe	B	C	P	S	Al	Ti	Zr
Balance	18–20	16–18	7.5–8.5	3.5–4.5	1.0	0.7–0.9	0.35–0.45	0.02	0.02	0.05	0.05	0.05

Furnace brazing in H_2 atmosphere or vacuum. For better wetting: Ni surface layers.
Other filler metals: Ni-based alloys or AuPd alloys.

Table 2.34 Recommended parameters for the welding of CoCr alloys by tungsten or metal inert gas (Mills et al., 1983)

Parameter	TIG	MIG
Power supply	DC transformer	DC transformer
Electrode diameter (mm)	1.1–1.6	0.9
Filler metal	–	According to base metal
Shielding gas	Ar, He	Ar, He
Welding position	Flat	Flat
Current (A)	12–70	130–160
Voltage (V)	10–20	22–25
Arc starting	High frequency	–
Welding speed (m min^{-1})	0.4–2.3	0.75

Careful cleaning by grinding or washing in a solvent; sand blasting should be avoided.
TIG, Tungsten inert gas welding; MIG, metal inert gas welding.

Table 2.35 Comparison of international standards for titanium and titanium alloys (ISO, DIN, BSI, AFNOR, JIS, ASTM)

Alloy[a]	International Organisation for Standardisation (ISO)	Germany (DIN)[b]	Great Britain (BSI)	France (AFNOR)	Japan (JIS)	USA (ASTM)
Ti-1	5832/II	5832-2 and 17850, respectively	2TA1	NF ISO 5832-2 and S90-404, respectively	H4600	F67/Grade 1
Ti-2			2TA2			F67/Grade 2
Ti-3			2TA6			F67/Grade 3
Ti-4						F67/Grade 4
Ti6Al4V	5832/III	5832-3 and 17851, respectively	2TA10, 2TA13	NF ISO 5832-3 and S94-080, respectively	H4607	F136
Ti5Al2.5Fe	5832/X	5832-10 and 17851, respectively	–	–	–	–
Ti6Al7Nb	5832/XI	5832-11 and 17851, respectively		XP S94-081	–	F1295

[a]Ti-1–Ti-4, Commercially pure titanium.
Others: direct chemical composition, e.g. Ti6Al4V: 6 wt% Al, 4 wt% V, balance Ti.
[b]Terms of delivery: DIN 17860, DIN 17862.

Table 2.36 Chemical composition (wt%) of cp-titanium (DIN, 1990c)

	Ti	Fe (max.)	O (approx.)	N (max.)	C (max.)	H (max.)
Grade 1	Balance	0.2	0.1	0.05	0.08	0.013
Grade 2	Balance	0.25	0.2	0.06	0.08	0.013
Grade 3	Balance	0.3	0.25	0.06	0.1	0.013
Grade 4	Balance	0.35	0.3	0.07	0.1	0.013

Table 2.37 Chemical composition (wt%) of ($\alpha+\beta$)-titanium alloys (Zwicker et al., 1980; Semlitsch et al., 1985; DIN, 1990d)

	Ti	Al	V	Fe	Nb	Ta	O[a]	N[a]	C[a]	H[a]
Ti6Al4V	Balance	5.5–6.75	3.5–4.5	0.3	–	–	0.2	0.05	0.08	0.015
Ti5Al2.5Fe	Balance	4.5–5.5	–	2.0–3.0	–	–	0.2	0.05	0.08	0.015
Ti6Al7Nb	Balance	5.5–6.5	–	0.25	6.5–7.5	0.5	0.2	0.05	0.08	0.009

Others: ≤ 0.1% each, ≤ 0.4% together.
[a]Maximum.

Table 2.38 Chemical composition (wt%) of examples of β- and near β-titanium alloys (Breme and Wadewitz, 1989; Mäusli et al., 1989; Steinemann et al., 1993; Wang et al., 1993; Mishra et al., 1996)

	Al	Mo	Zr	Ta	Nb	Sn	Fe	Ti
Ti15Mo5Zr3Al	3.8	15	5				0.2	Balance
Ti12Mo5Zr5Sn		11.5	5			4.5	0.2	Balance
Ti12Mo6Zr2Fe		12	6				2	Balance
Ti13Nb13Zr			13		13			Balance
Ti30Nb[a]					30		0.1	Balance
Ti30Ta[a]				30			0.1	Balance

[a]Experimental alloys.
C, O, N and H contents corresponding to Ti6Al4V.

Table 2.39 Physical properties of cp-titanium (DIN, 1990c; Boyer et al., 1994)

Young's modulus	105–110 GPa
Density	4.5 g cm^{-3}
Transformation temperature $\alpha \rightarrow \beta$	885°C
Crystal structure	>850°C β bcc <850°C α hex
Magnetic properties	Paramagnetic
Heat of transformation	67 kJ kg^{-1}
Thermal neutron-capture cross-section	5.8 × 10^{-22} cm^2
Specific heat at 15°C	520 J kg^{-1} K^{-1}
Heat fusion	419 kJ kg^{-1}
Thermal conductivity at room temperature	17 W m^{-1} K^{-1}
Thermal expansion coefficient between 20 and 200°C	9 × 10^{-6} K^{-1}
Specific electrical resistivity at 20°C	0.5 μΩ m

Table 2.40 Physical properties of titanium alloys (Semlitsch et al., 1985; DIN, 1990d; Wang et al., 1993; Boyer et al., 1994; Mishra et al., 1996)

	Ti6Al4V	Ti5Al2.5Fe	Ti6Al7Nb	Ti12Mo6Zr2Fe	Ti13Nb13Zr
Young's modulus (GPa)	100–110	110–116	110	74–85	64–83
Density (g cm^{-3})	4.43	4.45	4.52	5	5.3
Transformation temperature (°C)	990±15	950±15	1010±20	744±12	
Thermal conductivity at room temperature (W m^{-1} K^{-1})	6.5	–	–	–	
Coefficient of thermal expansion between 30 and 200°C (10^{-6} K^{-1})	8.6	9.3	-	8.8	
Specific heat at 20°C (kJ kg^{-1} K^{-1})	0.56	–	–	–	
Specific electrical resistivity at 20°C (μΩ m)	1.66	–	–	–	

Table 2.41 Mechanical properties of cp-titanium sheets as rolled (DIN, 1990c)

	Ultimate tensile strength (MPa)	Tensile yield strength (0.2%) (MPa)	Elongation at fracture[a] (%)	Reduction in area[a] (%)	Hardness (VHN)	Bend radius (105°) for sheet thickness	
						<2 mm	<5 mm
Grade 1	290–410	200	30	35	120	2t	3t
Grade 2	390–540	250	22	30	150	3t	4t
Grade 3	460–590	320	18	30	170	4t	5t
Grade 4	540–740	390	16	30	200	5t	6t

[a]Minimum values.

Table 2.42 Influence of cold deformation on the mechanical properties of cp-titanium (Ramsdell and Hull, 1960)

	Degree of cold deformation (%)	Ultimate tensile strength (MPa)	Tensile yield strength (0.2%) (MPa)	Elongation at fracture (%)
Grade 1	30	635	555	18
	40	645	560	16
	55	710	605	15
	60	725	620	14
	65	730	640	14.5
Grade 2	30	680	605	18
	40	740	645	17
	50	780	680	16
	60	795	685	16
	65	810	692	16.5

Table 2.43 Mechanical properties of (α+β)-titanium alloys (DIN, 1990d; Boyer et al., 1994)

	Condition: sheet as rolled thickness	Ultimate tensile strength (MPa)	Tensile yield strength (0.2%) (MPa)	Elongation at fracture (%)	Reduction in area[a] (%)	Hardness (VHN)	Bend radius (105°) for sheet thickness t	
							<2 mm	<5 mm
Ti6Al4V	–6	950	870	8	25	310	9t	10t
	6–100	920	830	8	25	310	9t	10t
	5 HTA[a]	1140	1070	8	20	–	–	–
Ti5Al2.5Fe	–6	860	780	8	25	310	9t	10t
Ti6Al7Nb	Extruded	896–1008	811–952	7–13	24–44	–	–	–
	Hot rolled + hot forged	869–1008	943–1008	11–16	40–55			
Ti6Mn	–6	1095	1058	11.5	26	360	–	–

[a]Solution heat treated and aged for 18–60 min, 800–200°C/H$_2$O + 2–4 h, 480 – 600°C/air.

Table 2.44 Mechanical properties of β- and near β-titanium alloys (experimental alloys) (Breme and Wadewitz, 1989; Steinemann, 1993; Wang et al., 1993; Mishra et al., 1996)

	Ultimate tensile strength (MPa)	Tensile yield strength (0.2%) (MPa)	Elongation at fracture[a] (%)	Reduction in area[a] (%)
Ti15Mo5Zr3Al	882–1117	870–1173	15–20	43–80
Ti12Mo5Zr5Sn	1010	1002	17.8	56
Ti12Mo6Zr2Fe	1060–1100	1000–1060	18–22	64–73
Ti13Nb13Zr	703–1034	433–906	11–29	28–74
Ti30Nb[b]	700	500	20	60
Ti30Ta[b]	740	590	28	58

[a]Minimum.
[b]Experimental alloys.

Table 2.45 Fracture toughness of titanium alloys (Borowy and Kramer, 1984; Steinemann et al., 1993; Wang et al., 1993, Mishra et al., 1996)

	Condition	Fracture toughness K_{IC} (N mm$^{-3/2}$)
Ti6Al4V	Annealed	1740
	Solution treated + annealed	2020
Ti15Al2.5Fe	Annealed (2 h/700°C/air)	1225
	Solution treated + annealed (1 h/900°C/water; 2 h/700°C/air)	1785
Ti5Mo5Zr3Al	Solution treated at 740°C	4580
	Solution treated at 740°C + annealed at 600°C	2430
	40% cold worked + annealed at 600°C	980
Ti12Mo6Zr2Fe	Solution treated + annealed	3880
Ti13Nb13Zr	Water quenched + aged	2150

METALS AND IMPLANTS

Table 2.46 Fatigue strength σ_f and rotating/bending fatigue strength σ_R of titanium and titanium alloys (Thull, 1979; Breme and Schmid, 1990; Wang et al., 1993; Mishra et al., 1996)

	R	σ_f (MPa)	σ_R (MPa)
cp-Ti	−1	230–280	200
Ti6Al4V	−1	400–450	500–660
notched $\alpha_K = 1.6$		320	280–350
Ti5Al2.5Fe	−1	–	450–550
Ti6Al7Nb	−1	–	450–600
Ti30Ta[a]	−1	–	400
Ti12Mo6Zr2Fe	−1	–	585
notched $\alpha_K = 1.6$		410	
Ti13Nb13Zr	0.1	425–500	
notched $\alpha_K = 1.6$		335	

[a]Experimental alloy.

Table 2.47 Processing of cp-titanium and titanium alloys (Zwicker, 1974; Hülse et al., 1989; Boyer et al., 1994)

Process	Conditions
Hot deformation	Ti-1 and 2: 650–870°C
	Ti-3 and 4: 700–930°C
	Ti alloys: 760–1050°C
Descaling	Sand blasting using non-metallic blast material
	20% HNO_3/2% HF
	Chromate
Cold deformation	No problem for Ti-1 and -2
	Moderately easy for Ti-3 and -4
	For deep drawing coatings in the form of polymer foils are effective
	Other lubricants: graphite or MoS_2

Table 2.48 Machining parameters for cp-titanium and titanium alloys (DIN, 1990f)

	Type of machining	Tool material	Depth of cut (mm)	Speed (m min^{-1})	Feed (mm rev^{-1})
cp-Ti	Turning	HSS	>2.5	4.0–7.5	0.1–1.25
	Roughening	Carbide		30–75	0.2–0.4
Ti alloys	Turning	HSS	>2.5	3–15	0.1–0.4
	Roughening	Carbide		15–25	0.2–0.4
cp-Ti	Turning	HSS	0.1–0.75	20–50	0.05–0.1
	Finishing	Carbide		60–100	0.075–0.3
Ti alloys	Turning	HSS	0.1–0.75	9–15	0.05–0.1
	Finishing	Carbide		20–70	0.075–0.3
cp-Ti	Milling	HSS	>2.5	15–30	0.1–0.2
		Carbide	Gear cutter	7.5–20	0.07–0.2

HSS, High-speed steel.

Table 2.49 Recommendations for the heat treatment of cp-titanium and titanium alloys (DIN, 1990f)

	Stress relief	Soft annealing	Solution annealing
Ti grades I–IV	15 min–2 h 450°C/air	15 min–8 h 650–750°C	–
Ti6Al4V	3 min/mm Min. 30 min Max. 4 h 500–600°C/air	Min. 15 min Max. 4 h 700–850°C Slow cooling rate to 550°C	15–60 min 820–950°C/H_2O + 2h 480–600°C/air
Ti5Al2.5Fe	3 min/mm Min. 30 min Max. 4 h 500–600°C/air	Min. 15 min Max. 4 h 700–850°C/air Slow cooling rate to 550°C	15–60 min 800–920°C/H_2O + 2–4 h 480–600°C

Table 2.50 Chemical composition (wt%) of filler metals for brazing cp-titanium and titanium alloys (Kosa and Ney, 1989)

Al	Ag	Be	Cu	Ga	Ni	Pd	Si	Sn	Ti	Zr
67			3				3.5	5		
77			16				3	4		
		4			0–2				48	48
			15–20		15–20				60–70	
	82			9		9				
5	95									
	90					10				

Furnace brazing in vacuum (10^{-4}–10^{-5} mbar) or in an inert atmosphere.

Table 2.51 Recommended parameters for the welding of cp-titanium and titanium alloys with tungsten, metal inert gas and plasma arc welding (Kosa and Ney, 1989)

TIG, MIG (MIG possible for sheets >3 mm, but TIG is usually preferred)	
Power supply	DC transformer
Tungsten electrode diameter (mm)[a]	1.6–0.9
Filler metal[a]	None[b] or according to the metal
Filler rod diameter (mm)[a]	0–4
Shielding gas (Ar, He) flow (m^3/h), backing gas is necessary	630–1400
Current (A)[a]	20–425
Welding speed (m min^{-1})	0.15
PAW	
Power supply	DC transformer
Shielding gas (Ar, He) flow (m^3 h^{-1})	2100
Current (A)[c]	185–250
Welding speed (m min^{-1})[c]	7–2.5

TIG, Tungsten inert gas;
MIG, metal inert gas;
PAW, plasma arc welding.

[a]According to sheet thickness, one pass for sheet 0.15–3.2 mm, two passes 4.8–9.5 mm.
[b]For sheet thickness 0.15–1.6mm, square groove for sheets 0.15–4.8 mm, V-groove for sheets >4.8 mm.
[c]According to sheet thickness, square groove for sheets 3–13 mm, V-groove 13 mm.
For all weldments a careful cleaning is necessary: alkaline or vapour degreasing, oxide removal by brushing, grinding or acid pickling (nitric–hydrofluoric acid or sodium dichromate).

Table 2.52 Chemical composition (wt%) of high and low gold-containing dental cast alloys according to standards: International Organisation for Standardisation, ISO 1562, 8891. Japan, JIS T6116, Germany, DIN 13906, DIN/EN 28891; France, AfNOR NF EN 21562 (S91-204)

	Au + Pt metals	Au	Pt	Pd	Ir	Rh	Ag	Cu	Zn	Others
HGC-1	88.6	87.5		1.0	0.1		11.5			
HGC-2	80.5–81.2	75.7–79.3	0.3–1.4	1.6–3.3			12.3–15.0	4.1–5.5	0.4–1.0	Ta 0–0.1
HGC-3	78.0–78.5	74.0–74.4	0–2.4	2.0–3.5			9.6–13.5	7.0–11.5	0.9–1.0	
HGC-4	75.5–80.0	65.5–71.0	4.4–12.9	0.0–2.0	0.1		10.0–14.0	8.2–10.0	0.5–4.0	
HGC-1-C	95.0–97.0	80.0–85.0	5.0–11.0	3.3–4.4	0.2	0–1.1	3.0–5.0			
HGC-2-C	95.0	70.0	7.5	15.0	0.5	1.6	5.0			
HGC-3-C	98.0–99.0	82.6–86.0	9.7–10.4	0–2.2	0.1–0.3	0–1.6				In 1–2
HGC-4-C	82.9–97.4	73.8–84.4	8.0–9.0	5.0–8.9	0.1		1.2–9.2	0.3–4.4	0–2.0	In 1.5–2.5 Re 0–0.2 Sn 0.5–0.8 Ta 0–0.2
LGC-4	48.0–66.7	40.0–62.2	0–4.4	0–9.9	0.1		23.3–35.0	7.0–12.0	0.4–3.5	In 0–0.5
LGC-4-C	74.8–89.8	43.0–55.1		29.0–38.5	0.1–0.2		0–19.5	0–0.3	In 0–9.0	Ga 0–1.5 Co 0–2.8 Re 0–0.2 Ta 0–0.1 Fe 0–0.2

HGC, high gold-containing (Au + Pt metals > 75 wt%, Pt, Ir, Rh, Re, Os).
LGC-4, low gold-containing, extra hard (60 wt% ≤ Au + Pt metals ≤ 75 wt%).
LGC-4, low gold-containing, extra hard fusible.
1, Soft; 2, medium hard; 3, hard; 4, extra hard.
C, Ceramic alloy (bonding with ceramic is possible).

Table 2.53 Chemical composition (wt%) of AgPd and Pd alloys (Degussa, 1993; Wieland, 1993)

	Au + Pt metals	Au	Pt	Pd	Ir	Ag	Cu	Sn	Zn	Others
AgPd-1	29.5	2.0		27.5		70.0		0.2	0.3	
AgPd-4	29.5–40.0	≤ 2.0		27.4–39.9	0.1	52.0–58.5	0–10.5	≤ 2.0	1.5–4.0	In≤ 2.0
Pd-4-C	52–88	0–17	≤ 1.0	25–70		7.2–38.0	0–11.6	1.9–7.5	≤ 2.0	In 0–4.0 Ga 0–7.2 Ge≤ 0.5 Ru≤ 0.8

Specific (thermal) heat capacity (c_p, [L2 T^{-1} θ^{-1}], J kg^{-1} K^{-1})

The specific heat at constant pressure is the quantity of heat necessary to produce unit change of temperature in unit mass (or in molar units when specified as specific molar heat capacity).

Tensile yield strength (YS, [ML^{-1} T^{-2}], Pa, MPa, N mm^{-2})

Tensile yield strength is a given value of stress where the stress–strain relationship departs from linearity. From this value one permanent set remains after removal of the stress. For practical reasons the stress inducing a plastic deformation of 0.2% is generally taken as the yield strength. YS can be determined by tensile or compression testing.

Table 2.54 Physical properties of precious dental alloys (Degussa, 1993; Wieland, 1993)

	Density (g cm^{-3})	Melting temperature (interval) (°C)	Thermal expansion coefficient 25–600°C ($\times 10^{-6}$/K^{-1})	Young's modulus (GPa)
HGC-1	17.2	1030–1080		
HGC-2	16.1–16.4	900–1040		92–95
HGC-3	15.6–15.8	900–975		
HGC-4	15.6–16.8	800–1000		98–109
HGC-1-C	18.3–18.6	1090–1370	14.1–14.8	
HGC-2-C	17.3	1285–1370	13.6	
HGC-3-C	18.4–19.5	1045–1220	14.2–14.7	100–105
HGC-4-C	16.7–18.1	900–1260	14.0–16.8	102–113
LGC-4	12.1–14.1	770–1065		94–106
LGC-4-C	14.0–14.8	1150–1315	13.8–14.8	
AgPd-1	11.1			
AgPd-4	10.6–11.1	950–1150		
Pd-4-C	11.2–12.2	1100–1290	14.0–15.4	122–126

METALS AND IMPLANTS

Table 2.55 Mechanical properties of high and low gold-containing dental cast alloys (Degussa, 1993; Wieland, 1993)

		Ultimate tensile strength (MPa)	Tensile yield strength (0.2%) (MPa)	Elongation at fracture (%)	Hardness (VHN)
HGC-1		170	80	45	55
HGC-2		370–390	180–240	35–45	95–110
HGC-3	s	460	330–350	35–40	145
	h	550–590	350–390	20–23	170–190
HGC-4	s	500–580	300–420	15–37	155–195
	h	710–879	540–780	5–18	225–295
HGC-1-C	s	220–280	90–130	29–38	60–75
	h	230–300	105–140	27–38	70–90
HGC-2-C	s	400	230	20	105
	h	410	240	18	125
HGC-3-C	s	460–515	370–420	8–15	150–160
	h	530–590	470–490	6–9	185–200
HGC-4-C	s	530–580	380–480	7–14	150–200
	h	550–650	470–600	3–6	220–230
LGC-4	s	480–510	310–400	18–43	155–170
	h	640–890	555–830	3–13	220–275
LGC-4-C	s	570–790	310–590	11–26	180–250
	h	710–900	55–700	6–18	235–285

s, Soft; h, hardened.

Table 2.56 Mechanical properties of AgPd and Pd alloys (Degussa, 1993; Wieland, 1993)

	Ultimate tensile strength (MPa)	Tensile yield strength (0.2%) (MPa)	Elongation at fracture (%)	Hardness (VHN)
AgPd-1	230	80	33	55
AgPd-4	510–950	285–595	3–31	140–310
Pd-4-C	630–900	340–630	8–30	180–285

Table 2.57 Recommendations for processing precious metals (Combe, 1984; Degussa, 1993; Wieland, 1993)

Casting	Lost wax process, centrifugal or vacuum pressure casting using graphite or ceramic crucibles
	Heating: resistance, torch (reducing flame), induction, electrical arc
	Temperature: 100–200°C above the melting interval (Table 2.54)
Heat treatment	Precipitation hardening 15 min at
	HGC: 400°C
	HGCC: 500–600°C
	LGC: 400–500°C
	LGCC: 600°C
	AgPd: 550°C
	Pd-C: 600°C
	Soft annealing 5 min at
	HGC: 700–800°C
	HGCC: 950°C
	LGC: 700–800°C
	LGCC: 850°C
	Pd-C: 950°C
Handling with ceramic	Surface roughening by sand blasting with alumina (100–150 µm, 2 bar)
	Cleaning with hot steam
	Annealing 10 min 980°C
	Bonding temperature 800–900°C

Table 2.58 Chemical composition (wt%) and brazing temperatures of various filler metals for high and low gold alloys (Degussa, 1993; Wieland, 1993)

	Brazing temperature (°C)	Au	Pt	Pd	Ir	Ag	Cu	Zn	In	Re
HGC, LGC	700–840	50–73	≤ 19	≤ 1.0	≤ 0.1	8.0–28	0–9.0	6.0–14	≤ 2.0	≤ 0.1
AgPd	760–820	73	0.9	1.0	0.1	13.0		12.0		
HGC-C, LGC-C	700–1120	50–73	≤ 1.9	≤ 1.0	≤ 0.1	10.0–28.0	0–5.0	12.0–14.0	≤ 2.0	≤ 0.1
Pd-4-C	1030–1120	50–73	≤ 1.9	≤ 1.0		10.0–28.0	3.0–5.0	12.0–14.0	≤ 2.0	

Table 2.59 Chemical composition (wt%) of the NiCr alloys used for dental restoration

Ni	Co	Fe	Cr	Mo	Nb	Ti	W	Be	Ga	Si	C
58–82	0–2	0–9	12–26	0.5–16	0–7	0–3	0–1.5	0–4	0–7.5	0–3	≤ 0.5

Others: Al, Ce, B, Mn, Sn, Ta, V, Cu, Y, La.
CoCr alloys: see Table 2.24.

METALS AND IMPLANTS

Table 2.60 Physical and mechanical properties of NiCr alloys used in dental restoration

Melting interval	940–1430°C
Young's modulus	170–220 GPa
Density	7.8–8.6 g cm^{-3}
Mean coefficient of linear thermal expansion between 25 and 600°C	13.9–15.5 × 10^{-6} K^{-1}
Tensile yield strength	255–800 MPa
Elongation at fracture	3–25%
hardness	160–325 VHN

CoCr alloys; see Table 2.27.

Table 2.61 Chemical composition (wt%) of dental amalgams[a] (Combe, 1984; Cahn et al., 1992)

Alloy powder	Ag	Sn	Cu	Zn	Hg
LCS	66–73	25–29	<6	<2	0–3
HCB	69	17	13	1	–
HCSS, HCSL	40–60	25–30	15–30	–	–

The mercury concentration after amalgamation is <50%.
LCS, Low-copper spherical; HCB, high-copper blended; HCSS, high-copper single-composition spherical; HCSL, high-copper single-composition lathe-cut.
[a]According to standards: International Organisation for Standardisation, ISO, 1559; Germany DIN 13904; France AFNOR NF EN 21559; Japan, JIS T6109.

Table 2.62 Physical and mechanical properties of amalgams (Combe, 1984)

Thermal expansion coefficient	25 × 10^{-6} K^{-1}
Thermal conductivity	23 W m^{-1} K^{-1}
Ultimate tensile strength	≥ 60 MPa
Ultimate compression strength	≥ 300 MPa
Fracture toughness K_{IC}	<1 N mm$^{-3/2}$

Table 2.63 Influence of hardening time on the mechanical properties of amalgams (Combe, 1984)

	Ultimate compression strength (MPa)		Creep (%) (7 days after amalgamation, pressure 38 MPa)
	After 1 h	After setting	
LCL	120–170	380–450	2.5–3.5
LCS	140–180	380–450	0.3–1.5
HCB	120–330	410–460	0.2–1.7
HCSS, HCSL ternary alloy	230–320	460–540	0.002–0.3
HCSS, HCSL quaternary alloy with indium	210–410	430–480	0.06–0.1

LCL, Low-copper lathe-cut; LCS, low-copper spherical; HCB, high-copper blended; HCSS, high-copper single-composition spherical; HCSL, high-copper single-composition lathe-cut.

Processing of amalgams: mixing with Hg (<50 wt%) immediately before application; pressing in the cavities in small portions with 40–50 N; removing the Hg-rich phase of the last portion; polishing after 24 h.

Table 2.64 Chemical composition of commercially refractory alloys (Waterman and Ashby, 1978)

Base	Designation	Composition (wt%)				
		C	Ti	Zr	Mo	W
Niobium	AS30	0.1	–	1	–	20
	F48	0.06	–	1	5	15
	D31	0.1	10	–	10	–
	Nb-Zr	–	–	1	–	–
	Nb-Ti	–	25	–	–	–
	Nb-Ti	–	40	–	–	–
	Nb1TiO$_2$	–	–	–	–	–
Tantalum	Ta-10W	–	–	–	–	10
	Ta-TaC$_2$[a]	–	–	–	–	–

[a]Under development (Axler, 1995).

Table 2.65 Physical properties of refractory metals (Sisco and Epremian, 1965; Waterman and Ashby, 1978; English, 1984; Davis et al., 1990; Tysma, 1993; Matucha, 1996)

	Melting point (°C)	Density (g cm^{-3})	Thermal expansion coefficient (273–373 K) ($\times 10^{-6}$ K^{-1})	Thermal conductivity at 20°C (W m^{-1} K^{-1})	Specific heat capacity at 20°C (J kg^{-1} K^{-1})	Specific electrical resistance (μΩ m)	Young's modulus (GPa)
Niobium	2468	8.57	7.3	53.7	272	0.13	110
Molybdenum	2610	10.2	4.9	138	242	0.047	324
Tantalum	2996	16.6	6.5	57.5	142	0.12	185
Tungsten	3380	19.3	4.4	130	138	0.055	411

METALS AND IMPLANTS

Table 2.66 Mechanical properties of cp refractory metals (Waterman and Ashby, 1978)

	Condition	Tensile yield strength (0.2%) (MPa)	Ultimate tensile strength (MPa)	Elongation at fracture (%)
Niobium	S	–	462	33
Molybdenum	T	1386	1540	15
Tantalum	S	–	770	40
	R	405	453	36
	C	755	755	–
	D	–	1694	1
Tungsten	T	–	3126[a]	0–3

S, Sheet from sintered stock, recrystallised.
T, Stress relieved.
R, High-purity sheet, recrystallised.
C, As R, but cold worked.
D, As S, but cold worked.
[a]Wire, cold deformed, recrystallised 600 MPa.

Table 2.67 Mechanical properties of commercially available refractory alloys (Woijcik, 1994)

Alloy	Composition (wt%)	Young's Modulus (GPa)	Ultimate tensile strength (MPa)	Tensile yield strength (0.2%) (MPa)	Elongation at fracture (%)
Niobium					
FS-85	Nb28Ta10W1Zr	140	570–585	462–475	23
Cb-752	Nb10W2.5Zr	110	540	400	–
PWC-11	Nb1Zr0.1C	–	320	175	26
Nb-1Zr	Nb1Zr	69–80	241–275	138–150	40
–	Nb1TiO$_2$ (CW)		1000–1050	940–980	10–15
–	Nb1TiO$_2$ (REC)		550–600	425–475	25–35
Tantalum					
Tantaloy 61	Ta7.5W	200	1035–1165	875–1005	–
Tantaloy 60	Ta10W	205	550	460	–
Tantaloy 63	Ta2.5W	195	345	230	–

CW, Cold worked; REC, recrystallised.

METALS AS BIOMATERIALS

Table 2.68 Properties of hard tissue

	Density (g cm^{-3})	Young's modulus (GPa)	Strength[d] (MPa)	Fatigue strength[e] (MPa)	Elongation at fracture (%)	Thermal expansion coefficient (×10^{-6} K^{-1})	Thermal Conductivity (W m^{-1} K^{-1})
Teeth[a]							
enamel	2.2	48[f]	241[f]	–	–	11.4	0.82
dentin	1.9	13.8[f]	138[f]	–	–	8.3	0.59
Long human bone[b,c]							
cortical parallel	–	14–22[g]	80–150[g]	30	0–2	–	–
			106–190[f]				
		4	157–181[h]				
cortical perpendicular	–		10–50[g]	–		–	–
			106–130[f]				

[a]Collection of data from Park and Lakes (1992), pp. 196–7.
[b]Collection of data from Martens (1985), pp. 9–14.
[c]Poisson ratio of cortical bone: 0.3–0.5
[d]Modulus, strength: [f]compressive, [g]tensile or [h]bending mode.
[e]Fatigue strength under compression swelling (Fleck, 1996).

Thermal conductivity (μ, [L^{2}T$^{-3}\theta^{-1}$], W m^{-1} K^{-1})

Thermal conductivity is the proportionality constant between heat flow density and the temperature gradient (change in temperature per unit length).

Thermal expansion coefficient (α [θ^{-1}], K^{-1})

The linear expansion coefficient is given in the tables. It is calculated from the slope of the increase in length as a function of temperature. The coefficient is constant only in a given temperature domain. The temperature range for which the listed value is valid is indicated in the tables.

Thermal neutron-capture cross-section (–, [L^2], cm^2)

To characterise the efficiency of an interaction between an atom and a thermal neutron (energy = 0.025 eV) an equivalent cross-section is used. This is the effective cross-section of an atom to capture a neutron.

Ultimate tensile strength (UTS, [ML^{-1}T^{-2}], Pa, MPa, N mm^{-2})

Ultimate tensile strength is the highest endurable stress at which the test specimen begins to neck in tensile tests. When the test is performed under compression (mainly for brittle materials), the stress at failure is called ultimate compression strength.

Young's modulus (E, [MLl^{-1}T^{-2}], Pa, GPa, N mm^{-2})

According to Hooke's law, the modulus of elasticity, E, is determined as the initial slope of the stress–strain curve. E is measured from the analysis of the stress–strain curve (deflection per unit of stress in the tensile, compression or bend test over the range where strain is effectively proportional to stress) or calculated from measurements of specific gravity and sound velocity in the material. It is an important parameter because it controls many modes of failure (e.g. deflection under load, resistance to buckling, frequency of vibration).

The rigidity modulus (G) is calculated from E and ν (Poisson ratio) by the formula: $G = E/2(1 + \nu)$. The Poisson ratio ν is the ratio radial strain divided by longitudinal strain at a given stress. Its value is 0.3 for most metals in the elastic range.

NOMENCLATURE

A	elongation at fracture
c_p	specific heat capacity
E	Young's modulus
G	rigidity modulus
H	hardness
K	fracture toughness
UTS, R_m	ultimate tensile strength
YS, $R_{p0,2}$	tensile yield strength
α	thermal expansion coefficient
ε	degree of deformation
μ	thermal conductivity
ν	Poisson ratio
ρ	density
ρ	specific electric resistance
$\sigma_{0.1/1000}$	creep resistance
σ_f, σ_b	fatigue strength

REFERENCES

American Society for Testing and Materials (ASTM), West Conshohocken, PA
A276	(1996)
F55	(1991a, discontinued)
F67 Grade 4	(1995a)
F67 Grade 3	(1995b)
F67 Grade 2	(1995c)
F67 Grade 1	(1995d)
F75	(1992a)
F90	(1992b)
F136	(1992c)
F138	(1992d)
F562	(1995e)
F563	(1995f)
F799	(1995g)
F1058	(1991b)
F1295	(1992e).

Association Française de Normalisation (AFNOR), La Défense, Paris
A35–574 (1990)
NF EN 10088–3 (1995)
NF EN 21562 (1989)
NF IS0 5832–2 (1997a)
NF ISO 5832–3 (1987a)
NF ISO 5832–5 (1997)
NF ISO 5832–6 (1987b)
S90–404 (1987c)
S90–406 (Project)
S91–204
S94–053 (Project) (1997b)
S94–054 (Project) (1993a)
S94–057 (Project) (1997c)
S94–058 (Project) (1993b)
S94–080 (1997d)
XPS 94–081 (1996).

Axler, K.M. (1995) *Engineered Materials for Application in Severe Metallurgical Environments: Tantalum–Carbon Alloy Development*, LA-12876-T, UC-704, Los Alamos, NM.

Benjamin, D. and Kirkpatrick, C.W., eds (1980) *ASM Metals Handbook*, Vol. 3, *Properties and Selection: Stainless Steels, Tool Materials and Special-purpose Metals*, ASM, Metals Park, OH.

Bever, M.B., ed. 1986 *Encyclopedia of Materials Science and Engineering*, Pergamon Press, Oxford.

Borowy, K.H. and Kramer, K.H. (1984) On the properties of a new titanium alloy TiAl5Fe2.5 as implant material, in *Proceedings of the 5th World Conference on Titanium*, Vol. 2 (eds G. Lütjering, U. Zwicker and W. Bunk), pp. 1381–6.

Boyer, R., Welsch, G. and Collings, E.W. eds (1994) *Materials Properties Handbook: Titanium Alloys*, ASM, Metals Park, OH.

Breme, J. and Schmid, H.-J. (1990) Criteria for the bioinertness of metals for osseo-integrated implants, in *Osseo-Integrated Implants*, Vol. 1 (ed. G. Heimke), CRC Press, Boca Raton, FL.

Breme, J. and Wadewitz, V. (1989) Comparison of Ti–Ta, Ti–Nb alloys, *J. Oral Max. Implants* **4**, 113–18.

British Standards Institution (BSI), London
2TA1 (1974a)
2TA2 (1973a)
2TA6 (1973b)
2TA10 (1974b)
2TA13 (1974c)
BS 7252–4 (1997a)
BS 7252–5 (1994a)
BS 7252–6 (1990a)
BS 7252–7 (1994b)
BS 7252–8 (1990b)
BS 7252–12 (1997b)
BS 970/1 (1996).

Cahn, R.W., Haasen, P., Kramer, E.J. and Williams, D.F., eds (1992) Medical and dental materials, in *Materials Science and Technology*, Vol. 14, VCH Munich.

Cigada, A., De Soutis, G., Gratti, A.M., Roos, A. and Zaffe, D. (1993) *In vivo* behaviour of a high performance duplex stainless steel, *J. Appl. Biomater.* **4**, 39–46.

Combe, E. (1984) *Zahnärztliche Werkstoffe*, Hanser, Munich.

Davis, J.R. et al., eds (1989) *ASM Metals Handbook*, Vol. 16, *Machining*, ASM, Metals Park, OH.
Davis, J.R. et al., eds (1990) *ASM Metals Handbook*, Vol. 2, *Properties and Selection: Nonferrous Alloys and Pure Metals*, ASM, Metals Park, OH.
Davis, J.R. (1990) Properties and selection: nonferrous alloys and special-purpose materials, in *Metals Handbook*, 10th edn, Vol. 2, (eds J.R. Davis et al.), ASM, Metals Park, OH, pp. 557–73.
Degussa Product Information (1993) Degussa, Hanau.
Dessein, K. (1996) Tantalus geholpen? Fabricage en evaluatie van poedermetallurgische niobium- en tantaallegeringen voor biomedische toepassingen, Graduate Thesis, Catholic University of Leuven, Faculty of Engineering, Leuven, Belgium.
Deutsches Institut für Normung (DIN), Beuth, Berlin

DIN/ISO 5832-2	(1992a)
DIN/ISO 5832-3	(1992b)
DIN/ISO 5832-4	(1980a)
DIN/ISO 5832-5	(1992c)
DIN/ISO 5832-6	(1980b)
DIN/ISO 5832-7	(1992d)
DIN/ISO 5832-8	(1992e)
DIN/ISO 5832-10	(1992f)
DIN/ISO 5832-11	(1994)
DIN/ISO 5832-12	(1996a)
DIN 8513	(1979)
DIN 13906	(1990a)
DIN 13912	(1996b)
DIN 17440	(1996c)
DIN 17441	(1997)
DIN 17442	(1977b)
DIN 17443	(1997)
DIN 17840	(1990b)
DIN 17850	(1990c)
DIN 17851	(1990d)
DIN 17864 (draft)	(1990e)
DIN 17869 (draft)	(1990f)

DIN/EN 28891.
English, C.A. (1984) The physical, mechanical and irradiation behaviour of niobium and niobium-base alloys, in *Niobium, Proceedings of the International Symposium* (ed. H. Stuart), The Metallurgical Society of AIME, New York, pp. 239–324.
Fleck, C. (1996) Struktur und mechanische Eigenschaften des kortikalen Knochens unter quasistatischen und zyklischen Beanspruchung, *Werkstoffkundliche Berichte* (ed. D. Eifler), Universität Kaiserslautern.
Gypen, L. (1979) Mechanische eigenschappen en korrosiegedrag van substitutionele tantaallegeringen, Ph.D. thesis, Catholic University of Leuven, Faculty of Engineering, Leuven, Belgium.
Harris, T. and Priebe, E. (1988) Forging of stainless steels, in *ASM Metals Handbook*, Vol. 14: *Forming and Forging* (eds J.R. Davis et al.), ASM, Metals Park, OH.
Heimann, W., Oppenheim, R. and Weizling, W. (1985) Nichtrostende Stähle, in *Werkstoffkunde Stahl*, Vol. 2, *Anwendungen*, Springer, Berlin.
Hülse, K., Kramer, K.-H. and Breme, J. (1989) Influence of small additions of Fe, Cr and Ni on the recrystallisation behaviour of cp-Ti, *Proceedings of the 6th Internernational Conference on Titanium* (eds P. Lacombe, R. Tricot and G. Béranger), Les Editions de Physique, Les Ulis, pp.1675–83.

International Organisation for Standardisation (ISO), Geneva

ISO 1562	(1993a)
ISO 5832–II	(1993b)
ISO 5832–III	(1996a)
ISO 5832–IV	(1996b)
ISO 5832–V	(1993c)
ISO 5832–VI	(1980)
ISO 5832–VII	(1994a)
ISO 5832–VIII	(1987)
ISO 5832–X	(1996c)
ISO 5832–XI	(1994b)
ISO 5832–XII	(1996d)
ISO 8891	(1993d)

Japanese Industrial Standards (JIS), Tokyo

G4303	(1991a)
H4600	(1993)
H4607	(1991b)
T6104	(1994)
T6115	(1985)
T6116	(1995)

Johansson, C.B. (1990) Qualitative interfacial study between bone and tantalum, niobium and commercially pure titanium, *Biomaterials* 11, 227–8.

Johansson, C.B. (1991) A removal torque and histomorphometric study of commercially pure niobium and titanium implants in rabbit bone, *Clin. Oral Implant Rev.* 2, 24–9.

Kosa, T. and Ney, R.P. (1989) *Machining of Stainless Steels*, in *ASM Metals Handbook*, Vol. 6, *Welding, Brazing and Soldering* (eds K. Mills, J.R. Davis, and B.R. Sanders), ASM, Metals Park, OH.

Latrobe Steel (1980) Multiphase MP35N Alloy, Technical Data, Latrobe Steel Co., Latrobe, PA.

Lorenz, M., Semlitsch, W., Panic, B., Weber, H. and Willert, H.G. (1978) Fatigue strength of cobalt–base alloys with high corrosion resistance for artificial hip joints, *Engng Med.* 7, 241.

Martens, M.A. (1985) Mechanical properties of human bone, Ph.D. thesis, Catholic University of Leuven, Faculty of Medecine, Leuven, Belgium.

Matucha, K.H. (1996) Structure and properties of nonferrous alloys, in *Materials Science and Technology, A Comprehensive Treatment*, Vol. 8 (eds. R.W. Cahn, P. Haasen and E.J. Kramer), VCH, New York.

Mäusli, P.-A., Steinemann, S.G. and Simpson, J.P. (1989) Properties of surface oxides on titanium and some titanium alloys, in *Proceedings of the 6th World Conference on Titanium* (eds P. Lacombe, R. Tricot and G. Béranger), Les Editions de Physique, Les Ulis. Cedex.

Mills, K., Davis, J.R. and Sanders, B.R., eds ASM Committee of Brazing of Heat-resistant Alloys (1983) Brazing of heat-resistant alloys, in *ASM Metals Handbook*, Vol. 6, *Welding, Brazing and Soldering*, ASM, Metals Park, OH.

Mishra, A.K., Davidson, J.A., Poggie, R.A., Kovacs, P. and FitzGerarld, T.J. (1996) Mechanical and tribological properties and biocompatibility of diffusion hardened Ti-13Nb-13Zr – a new titanium alloy for surgical implants, in *Medical Applications of Titanium and its Alloys: The Material and Biological Issues*, ASTM STP 1272 (eds S.A. Brown and J.E. Lemons), ASTM, West Conshohocken, PA.

Park, J.B and Lakes, R.S. (1992) *Biomaterials: An Introduction*, Plenum Press, New York.

Pilliar, R.M. (1981) Manufacturing processes of metals: the processing and properties of metal implants, in *Metal and Ceramic Biomaterials*, Vol. 1, *Structure*, CRC Press, Boca Raton, FL.

Ramsdell, J.D. and Hull, E.D. (1960) Characteristics of cold-rolled and annealed Ti, Bureau of Mines, Report of Investigation 5656, Pittsburgh, PA.

Schäning, K. (1995) Internationaler Vergleich von Standard-Werkstoffen, Beuth, Berlin.
Schmidt, W. (1981) Werkstoffverhalten bei schwingender Beanspruchung, *Thyssen Edelst. Techn. Berl.* **7**, 55–71.
Semlitsch, M., Staub, F. and Weber, H. (1985) Development of a vital, high-strength titanium–aluminium–niobium alloy for surgical implants, *Proceedings of the 5th European Conference on Biomaterials*, Paris, 4–6 September.
Sisco, F.T. and Epremian, E. (1965) *Colombium and Tantalum*, Wiley, New York.
Steinemann, S.G., Mäusli, P.-A., Szmukler-Moncler, S., Semlitsch, M., Pohler, O., Hintermann, H.-E. and Perren, S.M. (1993) Beta-titanium alloy for surgical implants, *Proceedings of the 7th World Conference on Titanium* (eds F.H. Fraes and L. Caplan), TMS, Warendale, pp. 2689–96.
Thull, R. (1979) Eigenschaften von Metallen für orthopädische Implantate und deren Prüfung, *Orthopädie* **7**, 29–42.
Tysma, S. (1993) *Polytechnisch Zakboekje*, 45e druk, Koninklijke PBNA, Arnhem.
Wang, K., Gustavson, L. and Dumbleton, J. (1993) Low modulus, high strength, biocompatible titanium alloy, in *Proceedings of the 7th World Conference on Titanium* (eds F.H. Froes and L. Caplan), TMS, Warendale, pp. 2689–96.
Waterman, N.A. and Ashby, M.F., eds (1978) *Elsevier Materials Selector*, Vols 1–3, Elsevier Applied Science, London.
Webster, J.G., ed. (1988) *Encyclopedia of Medical Devices and Instrumentation*, Vol. 1, Wiley-Interscience, New York.
Wegst, C.W. (1989) *Stahlschlüssel*, Stahleisen, Düsseldorf.
Wieland Product Information (1993) Wieland Edelmetalle, Pforzheim.
Wojcik, C.C. (1994) Processing, properties and applications of high temperature niobium alloys, in *High Temperature Silicides and Refractory Alloys, Materials Research Society Symposium Proceedings*, Vol. 322, (eds C.L. Briant, J.J. Petrovic, B.P. Bewlay, A.K. Vasudevanand and H.A. Lipsitt), MRS, Pittsburgh, PA, pp. 519–30.
Zitter, H. and Plenk, H., Jr (1987) The electrochemical behavior of metallic implant materials as an indicator of their biocompatibility, *J. Biomed. Mater. Res.* **21**, 881–96.
Zwicker, U. (1974) *Titan und Titanlegierungen*, Springer, Berlin.
Zwicker, U., Bühler, U., Müller, R., Beck, H., Schmid, H.J. and Festl, J. (1980) Mechanical properties and tissue reactions of a titanium alloy for implant material, in *Titanium '80 Science and Technology* (eds H. Kimura and O. Izumi), pp. 505–18.

3
Shape memory alloys

J. VAN HUMBEECK[1], R. STALMANS[1] AND P.A. BESSELINK[2]
[1]Catholic University of Leuven, Leuven, Belgium
[2]Memory Metal Holland, Enschede, The Netherlands

3.1 MARTENSITIC TRANSFORMATION

The distinctive functional properties of shape memory alloys (SMA) are closely linked to a solid–solid phase transformation occurring in a metastable solid state of some specific alloys. It occurs without diffusion and is therefore called martensitic and the solid phase obtained during cooling is called martensite. The parent phase in which the transformation occurs is very often called the beta (β)-phase (Funakubo, 1984; Ahlers, 1986; Delaey, 1991). The temperature at which the transformation occurs can be chosen within a temperature range between −150°C and 200°C, depending on the composition and microstructural constitution, the latter being determined mainly by thermomechanical processing.

The temperature-induced transformation is characterised by four temperatures: M_s and M_f during cooling, and A_s and A_f during heating. M_s and M_f indicate the temperatures at which the transformation from the parent phase (β-phase) into martensite starts and ends, respectively (Figure 3.1). A_s and A_f indicate the temperatures where the reverse transformation (martensite to beta) starts and ends, respectively. The overall transformation describes a hysteresis in the order of 10–50°C.

At a temperature above the A_f temperature (limited to a few tens of °C), the martensitic phase can also be induced by straining the sample (Figure 3.2). After reaching a critical stress, $\sigma^{p\text{-}m}$, the sample will start to transform into martensite. The value of $\sigma^{p\text{-}m}$ increases linearly with the temperature (on an average 5 MPa K^{-1}), starting from zero at the M_s temperature. During further straining, the stress at which the transformation occurs is almost constant until the material is fully transformed. Further straining will now lead to elastic loading of the martensite, followed by plastic deformation. When the strain is limited to the start of elastic loading of the martensite and the applied stress is again released, the reverse transformation will occur at a lower stress level than during loading, leading to the reverse movement of the first induced strain. The material is said to be superelastic. Reversible strains up

---

Metals as Biomaterials ISBN 0 471 96935 4 Edited by J.A. Helsen and H.J. Breme. © 1998 John Wiley & Sons Ltd

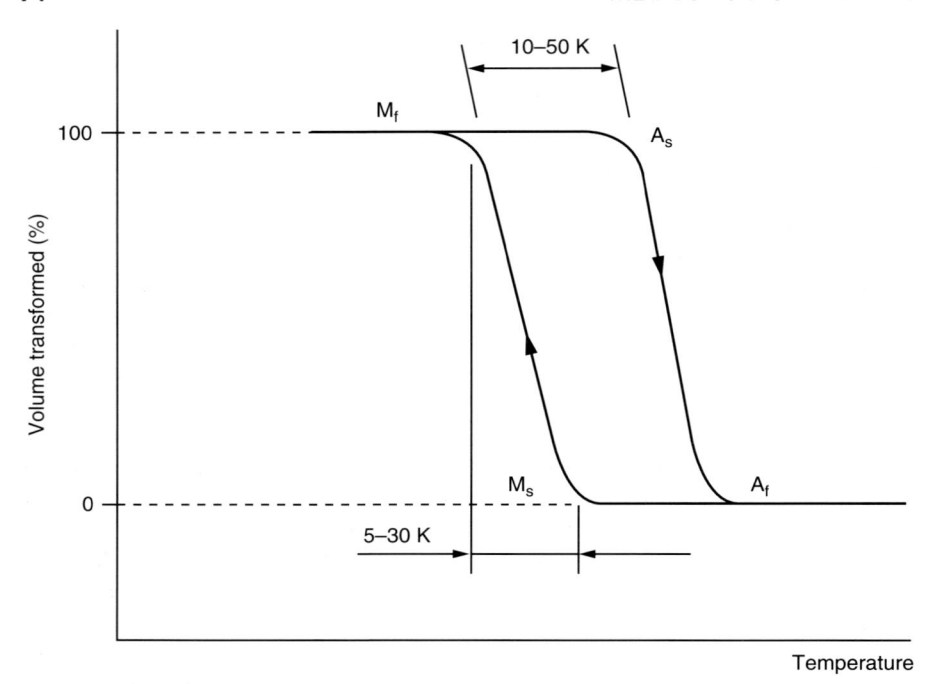

Figure 3.1 Schematic representation of the volume transformed as a function of the temperature.

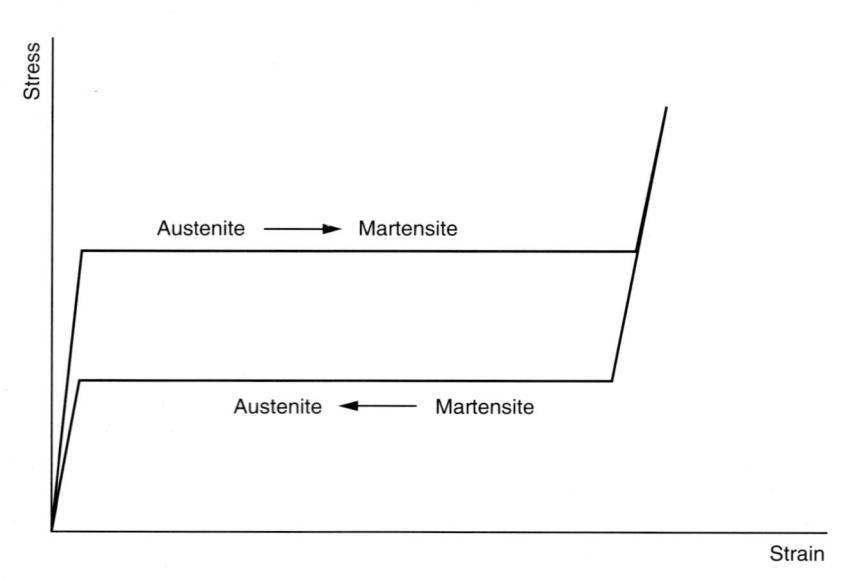

Figure 3.2 Superelastic behaviour at constant temperature due to stress-induced transformation.

SHAPE MEMORY ALLOYS

to 8% of the initial length can be obtained, compared with the normal 0.2% elastic strain of normal metallic material. Since this superelastic effect is due to phase transformation, it is also often called pseudoelasticity, pseudoelastic effect or superelasticity. The reverse deformation occurs at a lower stress plateau than during loading and thus shows a hysteresis, analogous to the temperature-induced transformation, but with a size of 50–300 MPa.

It follows that the temperature- or stress-induced transformation cannot be characterised by a single value of temperature or stress and the volume fraction transformed. It is important to note that many characteristics such as Young's modulus and the electrical resistivity change drastically during transformation. These changes can be used in specific applications and also for feedback control of SMA actuators.

Many alloy systems (Delaey, 1991) show shape memory behaviour but only a few of them have been developed on a commercial scale (NiTi, NiTi–X, Cu–Zn–Al). At present more than 90% of new SMA applications are based on NiTi or ternary NiTi–Cu and NiTi–Nb alloys. Other SMA are close to market introduction (Cu–Al–Ni, Fe–Mn–Si) while still others have interesting potential but are difficult to produce or suffer from brittleness (Ni–Al, NiTi–Zr).

Although NiTi SMA are more expensive and more difficult to machine than Cu-based, there are several reasons why virtually only NiTi SMA are used in new developments. NiTi SMA allow much higher working stresses and strains, NiTi SMA generally show a higher stability in cyclic applications, NiTi SMA are available in the shape of thin wires and thin films, and NiTi SMA have a higher electrical resistivity, making electrical activation much simpler. The requirements for medical applications also eliminate the Cu-based alloys in most cases. Therefore only NiTi-based SMA will be discussed in the remainder of this chapter. For some reasons, mainly Ni but also Ti can be partially (a few per cent) replaced by Cu, Co, Fe, Nb or Mo. These elements can improve the hysteresis (stress and/or temperature hysteresis), corrosion behaviour, control of transformation temperatures, fatigue behaviour, etc.

3.2 FUNCTIONAL PROPERTIES

Temperature-induced transformation is the basis of the one- and two-way memory effect, the generation of recovery stresses and work production. Stress-induced transformation is the basis of the superelastic effect (Stöckel, 1992).

When the material is martensite it is said to be in its cold shape, whereas in the β-phase it is said to be in its hot shape. The initial shape that the material obtains after processing is always the hot shape, and therefore after cooling into martensite the defined cold shape is equal to the initial hot shape. This shape can now be further deformed to the final cold shape (limited to less than 10% strain deformation of the initial shape) to induce the specific properties now described. The specific functional properties of SMA are six-fold and are illustrated in Figure 3.3–3.7 using the example of a shape memory spring.

(1) In the martensitic state, the shape memory element can easily be deformed from a fixed 'hot shape', retained after cooling to almost any 'cold shape' (Figure 3.3). The only restriction is that the deformations must not exceed a certain strain limit (up to 8%). These apparent plastic deformations can be completely recovered during heating, resulting in the original hot shape. This effect is called the **one-way memory effect**, since only the hot shape is memorised. The transition temperatures between the cold shape condition and hot shape condition are determined by the alloying and processing parameters and can be varied by the SMA suppliers.

(2) The **two-way memory effect** refers to the memorisation of two shapes (Figure 3.4). A cold shape is obtained spontaneously during cooling. In contrast to the one-way memory effect, no external forces are required to obtain the memorised cold shape. During subsequent heating the original hot shape is restored. The two-way memory effect is obtained only after a specific thermomechanical treatment, called training, which can be applied by the SMA supplier.

(3) When the shape recovery from the cold shape to the hot shape is impeded, high **recovery stresses** are gradually generated during heating (Figure 3.5). Stresses up to 800 MPa can be obtained.

(4) The shape recovery during heating can be biased by an external force (Figure 3.6). The resulting motion against a bias force corresponds to **work production**, up to 5 J g^{-1}.

(5) The shape memory effects described above require temperature changes. In contrast, the **superelastic effect** (Figure 3.7) is isothermal in nature and involves the storage of potential energy. Isothermal loading of the shape memory element in the hot shape condition results in large reversible deformations (up to 8%) at

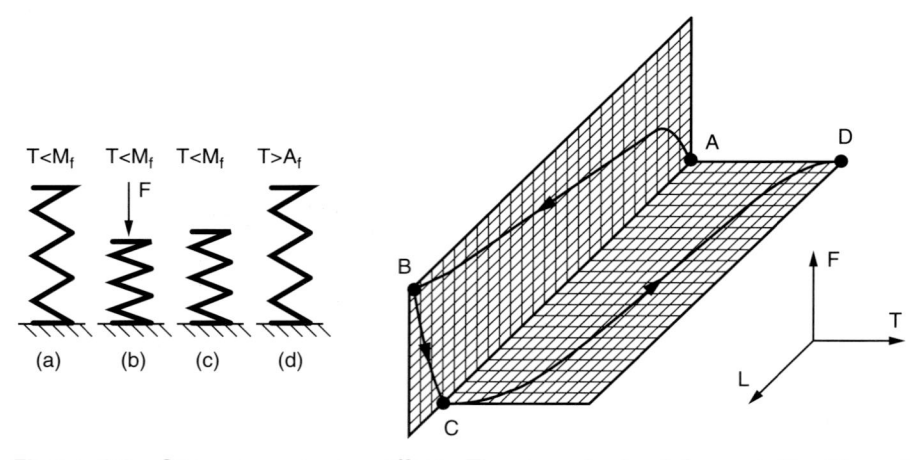

Figure 3.3 One-way memory effect. The sample is deformed (A→B) and unloaded (B→C) at a temperature below M_f. The apparent plastic deformation is restored during heating to a temperature above A_f (C→D). Length change, load and temperature are indicated by L, F and T, respectively.

SHAPE MEMORY ALLOYS

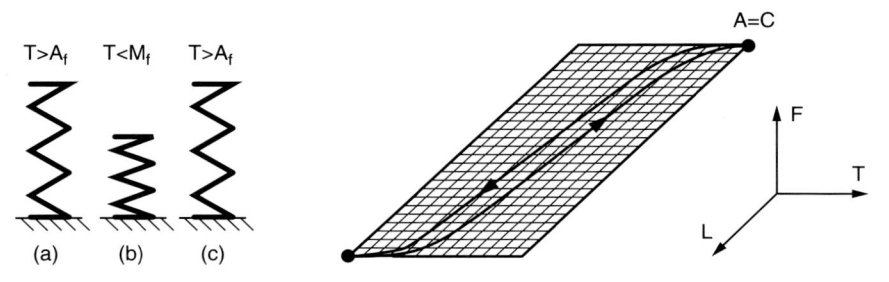

Figure 3.4 Two-way memory effect. A spontaneous shape change occurs during cooling to a temperature below M_f (A→B). This shape change is recovered during subsequent heating to a temperature above A_f (B→C).

nearly constant stress levels (see also Figures 3.2 and 3.9). The deformations are completely recovered at a lower stress level during unloading. These stress levels are alloy and temperature dependent. In general, the stress levels increase linearly (2–15 MPa K^{-1}) with increasing temperature.

(6) SMA also have a **high damping capacity** in the martensitic state and two-phase conditions. These alloys show in the cold shape condition a strong amplitude-dependent internal friction (Van Humbeeck, 1986). For impact loads, the

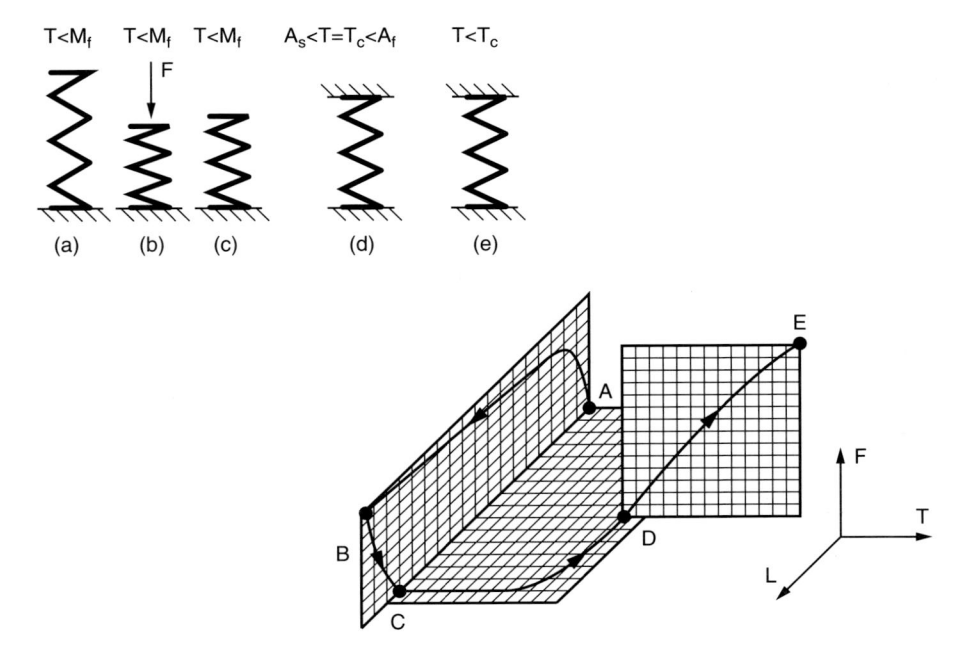

Figure 3.5 Generation of shape recovery stresses. The sample is deformed (A→B) and unloaded (B→C) at a temperature below M_f. Recovery stresses are generated during heating (D→E) starting from the contact temperature T_c (D), situated between A_s and A_f.

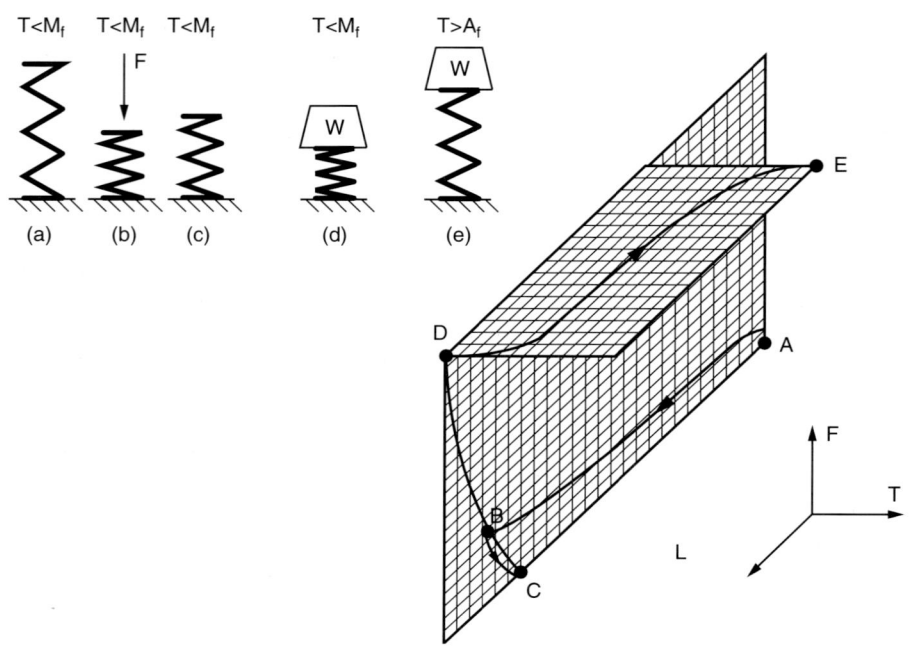

Figure 3.6 Work output. The sample is deformed at a temperature below M_f (A→B), followed by unloading (B→C) and repeated loading with a bias weight W (C→D). Shape recovery occurs at an opposing force W during heating to a temperature above A_f (D→E), so work is done.

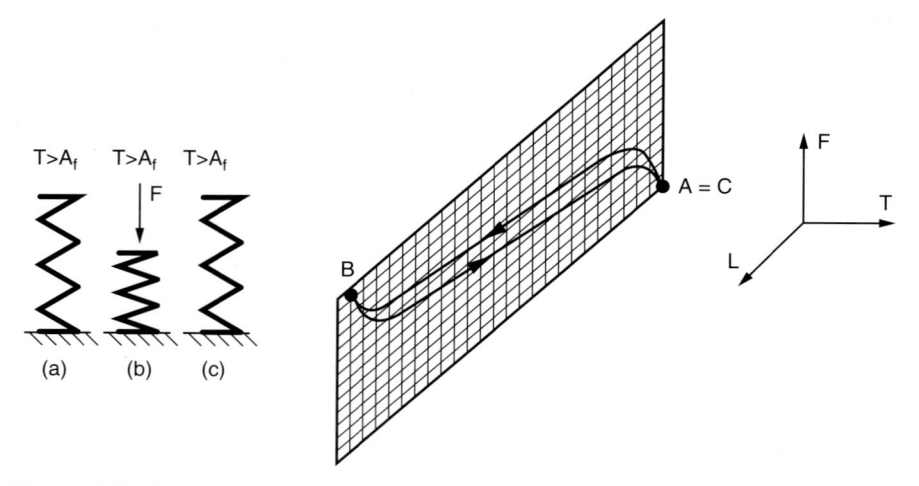

Figure 3.7 Superelastic effect. The sample is strongly deformed (A→B) at a temperature above A_f. During subsequent unloading a complete shape recovery occurs (B→C). The area enclosed between the loading and unloading curves is a measure of the energy dissipated in one superelastic cycle.

SHAPE MEMORY ALLOYS

specific damping capacity can be as high as 90%. In the hot shape condition, energy is dissipated during superelastic cycling as a result of the stress hysteresis between superelastic loading and unloading (Figure 3.2).

The functions and applications linked with these properties can be divided into five categories.

(1) The one- and two-way memory effect can be used for **free recovery applications**. This refers to applications in which the single function of the SMA element is to cause motions without any biasing stress. Examples can be found in gadgets and toys (e.g. flower with opening/closing petals during heating/cooling; Van Humbeeck et al., 1991), temperature indicators (e.g. the thermomarker; Raymont and Weynant, 1991), space antennae (Krupp, 1973) and the vena cava filter (Simon et al., 1977).
(2) The generation of recovery stresses can be used for diverse **clamping and fixation devices**, such as SMA couplings and SMA connectors, ranging from very small (<1 mm) to very large diameters (>1 m) (Schetky, 1995).
(3) Diverse **actuation applications** have been developed based on the work production capacity of SMA.
(4) Pseudoelasticity is used in many **biomedical and other superelastic applications** where high reversible strains have to be combined with high stress plateaux.
(5) **Damping applications** can be developed based on the high damping capacity of SMA. The high damping capacity of the cold shape has been used in spacecraft (AMT, 1993). The superelastic hysteresis might be interesting for earthquake damping and isolation purposes (Whitthaker et al., 1995).

In the past few years, SMA have found their specific niches in many domains of industrial activities. A steadily growing number of different SMA applications now exists in large-scale production. Detailed descriptions of many successful or potentially successful applications can be found in recent conference proceedings (Duerig et al., 1990; Wayman and Perkins, 1993; Pelton et al., 1995; Gotthardt and Van Humbeeck, 1995).

3.3 SHAPE MEMORY ALLOY DATA AND DESIGN WITH SHAPE MEMORY ALLOY ELEMENTS

Designing with SMA is very different from designing with conventional structural materials. First, the mechanical and physical properties change to a large extent during transformation, so that single property values cannot be used. Secondly, SMA are used because of their six functional properties and, as indicated above, these functional properties can be substantially modified by alloy composition, thermomechanical treatment, etc. Thirdly, the thermomechanical behaviour is non-linear and temperature dependent with hysteresis. Therefore, the design of shape memory applications requires either (1) a thorough knowledge of shape memory behaviour,

(2) close co-operation with a SMA supplier, or (3) the use of specific computer programs (Stalmans et al., 1989) which might evolve to expert systems.

Table 3.1 summarises the most important property values of binary NiTi alloys. The data given in the table are based on an evaluation of results in literature and the authors' experimental results. They give only a first estimate and should be handled carefully. A more detailed and regularly updated table can be found on the World Wide Web at http://www.mtm.kuleuven.ac.be/Research/Physical/smatab.htm.

Table 3.1 Property values of NiTi shape memory alloys

Property	Unit	Value
Physical		
melting point	°C	1250
density	10^3 kg m^{-3}	6.5
Thermal conductivity	W m^{-1} K^{-1}	
of austenite		18
of martensite		8.6
Coeficient of thermal expansion	10^{-6} K^{-1}	
of austenite		11
of martensite		6.6
Specific heat	J kg^{-1} K^{-1}	500
Transformation enthalpy	J kg^{-1}	15 000
Corrosion performance		Similar to 300 series stainless steel
Wear resistance		Good
Electromagnetic		
Resistivity	10^{-6} Ω m	
of austenite		1.0
of martensite		0.8
Magnetic permeability		<1.002
Magnetic susceptibility	emu g^{-1}	3×10^6
Mechanical		
Young's modulus (austenite)	GPa	80
G (austenite)	GPa	27
Ultimate tensile strength	MPa	700–1100 (annealed) 1300–2000 (not annealed)
Elongation at failure	%	30–50
Fatigue strength $N=10^6$	MPa	350
Shape Memory		
Transformation temperatures	°C	–100 to 100
Hysteresis	°C	5–50
One way memory strain	%	3–8
Maximum temperature (short time)	°C	300
Damping capacity	%SDC	15
Superelastic strain	%	6–8
Superelastic energy storage	J g^{-1}	6.5
Maximum recovery stress	MPa	600–900
Stress rate	MPa K^{-1}	5–15
Work output	J g^{-1}	4

SHAPE MEMORY ALLOYS

3.4 TEMPERATURE-ACTIVATED APPLICATIONS

Temperature-activated applications can be divided into clamping devices and actuation devices. As stated above, the stresses generated by constrained SMA elements during heating can be used for clamping, fixation or stiffening purposes. There are numerous examples in the biomedical field, including dental root implants, stents and staples for the connection of fractures.

Most SMA actuators are used for on/off applications. Commercial on/off applications are available in very small sizes such as a miniature actuator (Van Moorleghem *et al.*, 1992), also used in Braille systems, for loads up to 1 N and with an activation time of 0.1 s. At the other extreme one also finds large actuators for loads up to 400 N (Maclean *et al.*, 1991). Recently, many research efforts have been directed towards continuous position and force control of SMA actuators (Reynaerts and Van Brussel, 1995).

3.4.1 ADVANTAGES

SMA offer the following important advantages in these types of devices.

3.4.1.1 Simplicity, Compactness and Reliability

In many cases the device can be reduced to a single SMA element, e.g. an electrically activated SMA wire can be used as a direct linear actuator. The stroke and force exerted by the device can be easily modified by the selection of the SMA element, e.g. a SMA wire can be selected for a combination of high force and low stroke, and a helical SMA spring for a high stroke and lower force. Additional parts such as reduction gears are not required. The result is a much more simplified, more compact and more reliable device. Ease of installation is an important advantage in fixation devices, e.g. the SMA dental root implant fastens itself firmly during heating to body temperature, without the necessity of auxiliary instruments.

3.4.1.2 Creation of Clean, Silent and Spark-free Working Conditions

Friction is almost absent in activated SMA elements and no lubrication is required. Hence, the production of waste products can be avoided. NiTi SMA are highly corrosion resistant and can therefore operate in nearly any environment without protection, including in corrosive liquids and tissues.

SMA actuators can be controlled in such a way that very smooth movements are generated. Since there are no additional vibrating parts, the activation is almost completely silent. While no high-voltage or electrical switches are required, SMA actuators can operate completely spark free, allowing them to be used in highly inflammable environments.

3.4.1.3 High Power/Weight (or Power/Volume) Ratios

Ikuta (1990) compared all types of actuating technologies (from small dc motors to gas turbines) and concluded that SMA actuators offer the highest power to weight ratio at low levels of weight (below 100 g) (Figure 3.8). Therefore, it is expected that SMA actuators will become a very important design tool in the important and rapidly growing field of microactuation. Examples of prototypes have already been described (Walkers *et al.*, 1990; Ikuta *et al.*, 1991; Johnson *et al.*, 1992). Examples in the biomedical field can be found in drug-delivery systems and various laparoscopic instruments. One of the challenges in this field is the production of high-quality and reliable thin foils of NiTi–X by magnetron sputtering (Johnson, 1991; Miyazaki *et al.*, 1992, 1995) or melt spinning (Wang *et al.*, 1994).

3.4.2 DISADVANTAGES

Some important drawbacks, which limit the use of SMA actuators to specific niches, should also be considered.

3.4.2.1 Low Energy Efficiency

It can be easily calculated that the maximum theoretical efficiency (work output/heat input) of an SMA actuator is of the order of 10%. In reality, the conversion of heat into mechanical work occurs much less efficiently, with the result that the real

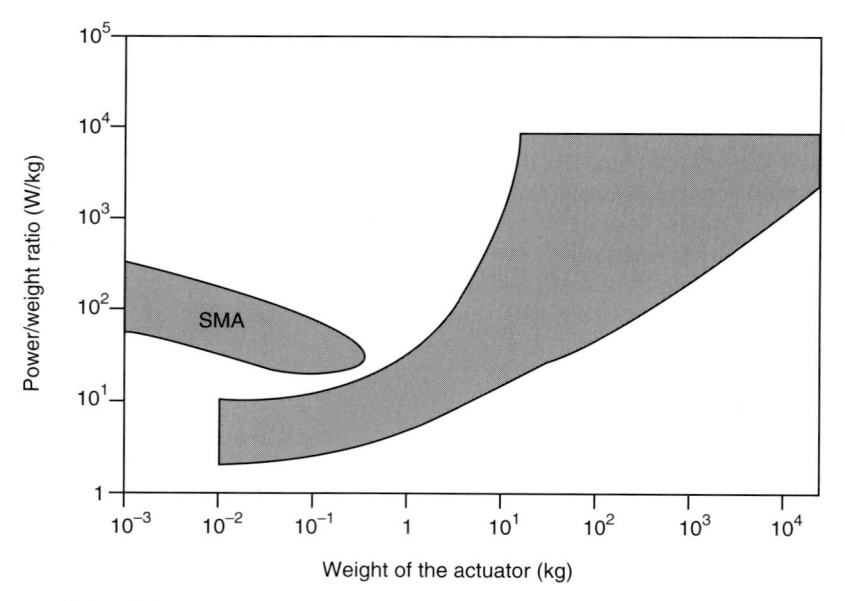

Figure 3.8 Schematic representation of the locus of SMA actuators in a power/weight ratio vs weight of actuator. The area enclosed between the two border lines indicates where other types of actuators are situated (ac and dc motors, rotary and piston engines, turbines, etc.). (After Ikuta, 1990.)

SHAPE MEMORY ALLOYS

efficiency is at least one order smaller than the theoretical value. This efficiency is also to a large extent determined by the design and shape of the SMA actuator. For example, the stress and strain distribution over the cross-section of a helical spring decreases from the maximum value in the outer layer to zero at the neutral axis. This inhomogeneous distribution has a negative effect on the efficiency and the bandwidth of the spring-based actuator because, for the same output, a larger material volume has to be heated and cooled. Therefore, SMA actuators contain mostly SMA wires or ribbons since this offers the advantage of optimum use of the material.

3.4.2.2 Limited Bandwidth, Mainly Due to Cooling Restrictions

SMA can be heated in different ways: by radiation or conduction (thermal actuators) and by inductive or resistive heating (electrical actuators). For a fast and homogeneous response, resistive heating offers the most attractive solution and is therefore widely used. The response speed of a SMA actuator is limited mainly by the cooling capacities. In addition, the martensitic transformation is exothermic (± 15 J g^{-1}), which means that extra heat has to be removed during cooling. The limited cooling speed can be increased by (1) the use of rectangular flat strips rather than round wires, (2) forced cooling by a moving liquid, and (3) miniaturisation of the SMA elements.

3.4.2.3 Degradation and Fatigue

The reliability of shape memory devices depends on their global lifetime performance (Van Humbeeck, 1991). The failure of SMA elements is completely different from the failure of conventional materials. SMA can fail owing to a decrease of the stroke during repeated actuation, a shift in the transformation temperatures, etc. Moreover, degradation and fatigue are influenced in a complex way by many parameters. Time, maximum temperature, maximum stress, maximum strain, strain mode and the amount of cycles are important external parameters in this respect. Important internal parameters that may have a strong influence on the lifetime are alloy system, alloy composition, heat treatment and processing. For general purposes, the maximum memory effect, strain and/or stress, will be selected depending on the required number of cycles. There have been significant improvements with respect to fatigue properties in the past few years and, properly designed and treated, SMA can even run for millions of cycles.

3.4.2.4 Complex Control

SMA show a complex three-dimensional thermomechanical behaviour with hysteresis. Moreover, this behaviour is influenced by a large number of parameters. It follows that there are, in general, no direct and simple relations between the temperature and the position or force. Therefore, accurate position or force control of SMA devices requires the use of powerful controllers and the experimental determination of complex data. Many mathematical models are being developed by different research groups to overcome this important limitation.

Because of these drawbacks, it is unlikely that SMA will be used as conventional actuators other than in specific niches, such as in microactuation (Melton, 1994).

3.5 SUPERELASTIC APPLICATIONS

Superelastic behaviour creates new design opportunities, as will become clear in the following paragraphs. Two important concomitant effects should receive due attention.

(1) The stress at which the superelastic straining occurs increases with increasing temperature. The superelasticity is also limited in temperature range, and applying the effect at too high temperatures can result in permanent plastic deformation.
(2) As also already mentioned, the superelastic effect shows a hysteresis: the stress during loading is higher than during unloading. This stress difference can be partially controlled by the composition or processing of the alloy.

3.6 BIOMEDICAL APPLICATIONS

Most of the earlier developments of SMA applications were linked with the thermally activated functions of actuation and coupling. In recent years, however, it has become clear that the largest commercial successes of SMA are linked to biomedical applications (Melton, 1994; Pelton *et al.*, 1994; Besselink and Sachdeva, 1995). The combination of good biocompatibility, good strength and ductility with the specific functional properties such as the shape memory effect and superelasticity creates a unique material for medical applications.

In particular, the superelastic effect of SMA results in a unique combination of high strength, high stiffness and high pliability, and no other material or technology can offer this unique combination. The temperature-dependent character of the superelastic effect, which is disadvantageous in other application areas, is of less importance in the biomedical field because of the stable temperature of the human body. NiTi with proper surface treatment shows an excellent biocompatibility (Shabalovskaya, 1995). The concept of a metallic material with an extreme elasticity and nearly constant stress levels over a large strain area can be tackled more easily by designers than the concepts related to temperature-activated shape memory effects (Melton, 1994). As a consequence, regarding the specific functional properties, the largest commercial successes of SMA are linked with the use of superelasticity (Pelton *et al.*, 1994).

SHAPE MEMORY ALLOYS

The following paragraphs illustrate present developments of applications in the biomedical field that obtain added value from the functional properties of SMA.

3.6.1 APPLICATIONS IN ORTHODONTICS

Orthodontic archwires were the first mass biomedical application (Sachdeva and Miyazaki, 1990; Duerig et al., 1990; Fukuyo and Sachdeva, 1992). While in the case of stainless steel wires the forces quickly relax during movement of the teeth, concomitantly retarding this movement, NiTi wires allow the teeth to move under almost constant force over a long treatment time and a much larger displacement of the teeth before the orthodontist has to retighten the wires. The stored elastic energy for the same maximum stress is much larger for superelastic material than for steel (Figure 3.9). Depending on the desired constant force a wire with a specific plateau stress can be chosen.

The plateau stress depends on the relative difference between the ambient temperature and the transformation temperature. The value is high for wires with a low transformation temperature. This makes the wire more sensitive to small temperature changes in the mouth, which causes intermittent forces on the teeth. A new type of orthodontic wire has a transformation temperature just below the body temperature and thus has a very low plateau stress. The advantages are obvious: the treatment requires less chair time and is thus less expensive, and the force remains constant and does not reach the point of causing pain. Different grades of wire stiffness are now available, with round and rectangular sections, and variation in diameters and thus in strength (Sachdeva et al., 1990b; Tuissi et al., 1995). Since NiTi archwires were introduced in the late 1970s, over 30% of the archwires used today are NiTi (Duerig et al., 1998).

Besides archwires, specific endosseous implants based on the shape memory effect have also been developed. These implants can be in blade or rod form, depending on whether several teeth or one single tooth has to be inserted. After insertion, the predeformed shapes are heated by warm saline or by an induction coil apparatus to a temperature not above 50°C, but above the A_f temperature of the material (Fukuyo and Sachdeva, 1982; Sachdeva et al., 1990a).

Other common devices for applications in orthodontics are listed below:

- dental root implants for a stable attachment in the bone. The memory metal root deforms and locks itself firmly in the bone after reaching body temperature
- adjustable dental abutments with self-locking temperature-sensitive ball joints (Figure 3.10)
- adjustable telescopic head gears for reposition of the molars. This device uses a memory metal locking ring that prevents relative motion between the inner head gear wire and the head gear tube. Adjustment of the length or angle is easily accomplished by cooling the locking ring
- small superelastic tension and compression springs to create space or close gaps between the elements in the mouth (Figure 3.11)

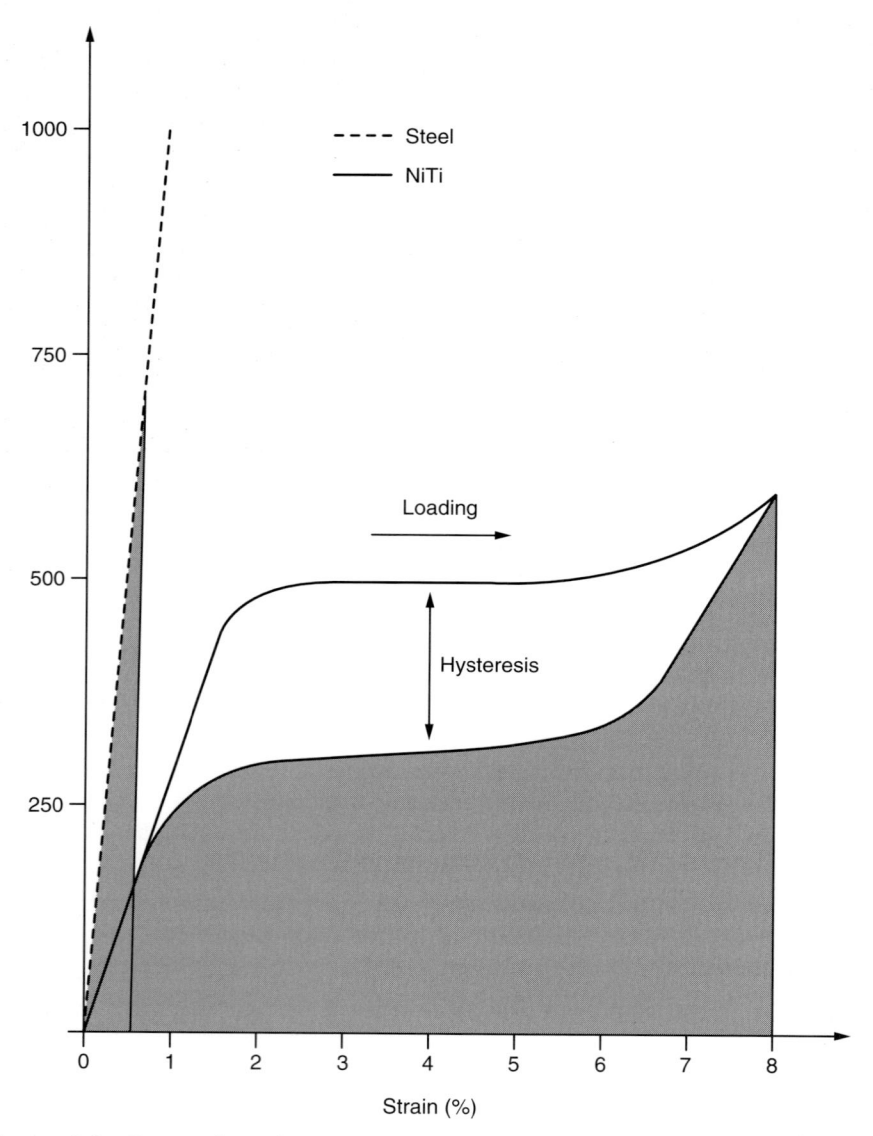

Figure 3.9 Comparison between the stored elastic energy for steel (linear stress–strain relationship) and for superelastic NiTi (non-linear hysteretic relationship) for the same maximum stress. The dashed area under the stress–strain curve represents this amount of energy.

SHAPE MEMORY ALLOYS

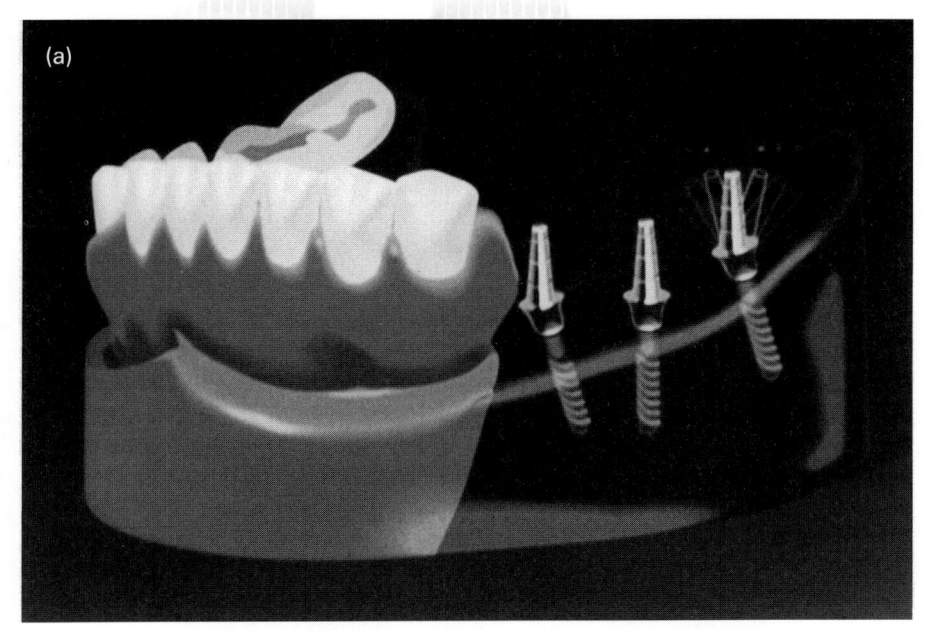

Figure 3.10 Dyna adjustable abutment for use in combination with dental root implants. The ball joint is cooled with cooling spray, then it can be adjusted to any angle within ± 15°. (a) Position of the abutment in a model; (b) shown overleaf. (Photograph from Dyna Dental Engineering, MMH.)

- heavy suture expanders with superelastic springs to change the width of the mandible
- martensitic, very shapeable wires and strips for retention of the teeth after correction
- special connectors with a wedge shape to hold two teeth tightly together
- adjustable orthodontic brackets with torque and angulation control
- connectors for threadless anchoring of abutments to dental root implants.

3.6.2 STENTS

Intravascular scaffolding using various designs is a technique that is significantly expanding (Figure 3.12). The devices used are generally called stents, based on the name of the nineteenth-century London dentist, Charles Stent. Besides many types of endovascular stents, stents for non-circulating conduits have been developed such as bronchial stenting, biliary stenting, oesophageal stenting and stenting of the ureter (Sigwart, 1996).

The specific functional properties of NiTi alloys add unique values to stent technology. Two types of NiTi stents are distinguished: permanent stents and remov-

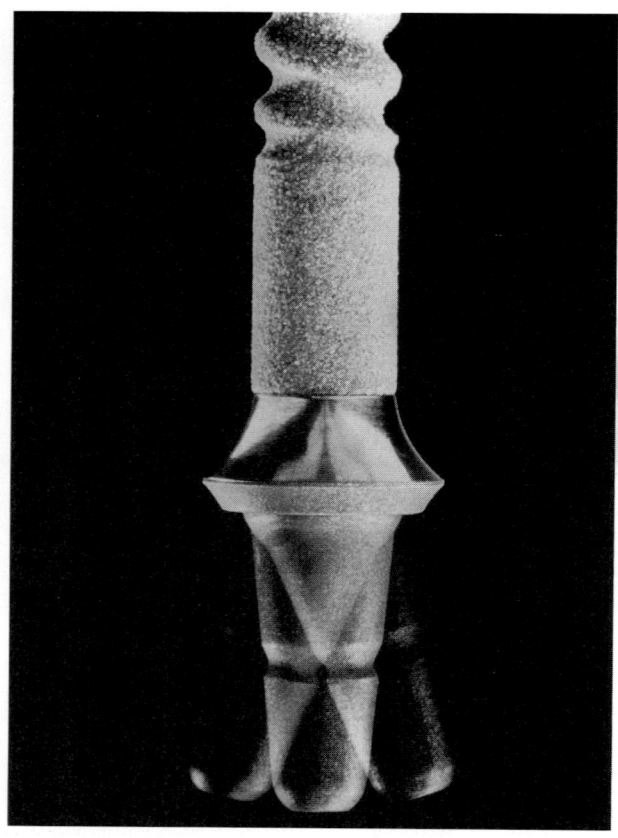

Figure 3.10 (*Continued*) (b) Possible adjustability. (Photograph from Dyna Dental Engineering, MMH.)

able stents (Makkar *et al.*, 1996). Permanent stents can be placed by different methods: (1) self-expansion based on the superelastic properties; (2) balloon expansion in the martensitic state; or (3) use of the shape memory effect by slightly heating the stent after positioning (Makkar *et al.*, 1996; Beyar, 1996). The advantage of self-expansion and the shape memory effect is that (almost) no recoil of the stent occurs, thus avoiding the overstraining required by balloon expansion.

Removable (heat-shrinkable) stents are devices which, deployed in the vessel after balloon expansion in the martensitic state, can be removed by a specially designed recovery catheter, coaxially placed in the stent in combination with an infusion of normal saline at 55°C to heat the stent so that shape recovery can occur. Apart from the advantage that a foreign object can be removed after healing, other potential applications include the prospect of using local drug or radiation therapy (Makkar *et al.*, 1996).

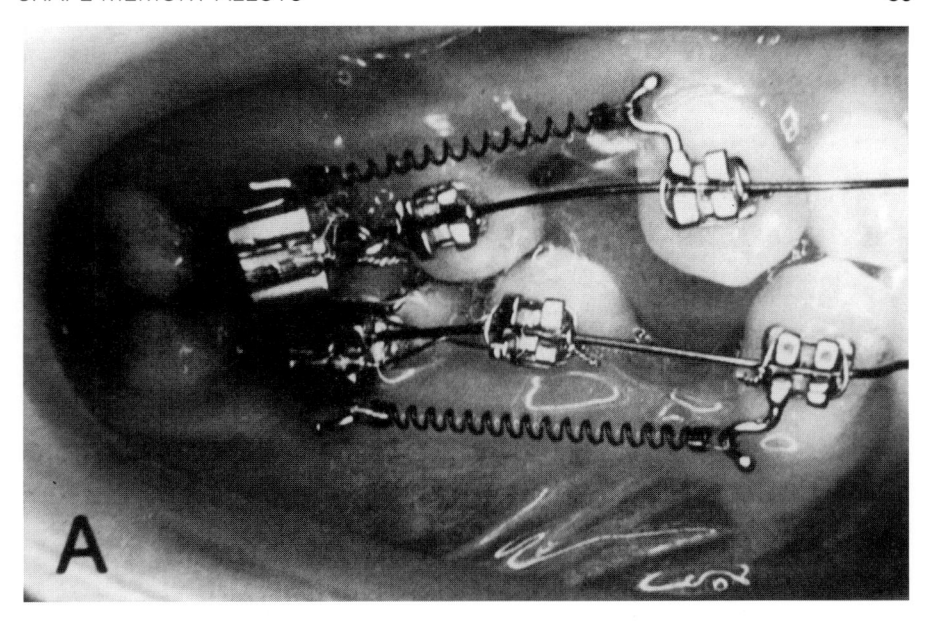

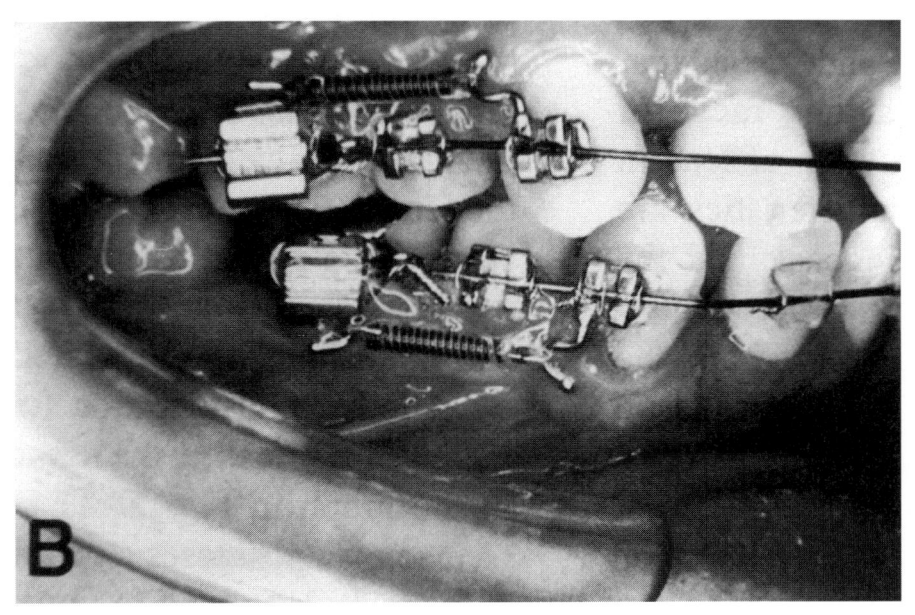

Figure 3.11 Superelastic expansion springs for tooth movement. (A) Critical position and (B) new situation after 6 weeks without further adjustment by the dentist. (Photographs from Miura, MMH.)

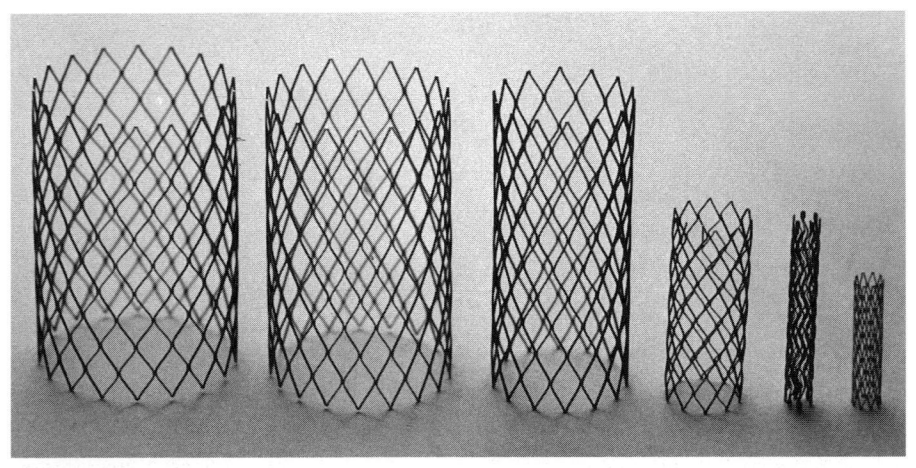

Figure 3.12 Self-expanding Nitinol stents laser cut from Nitinol tubing. (Photograph from NDC.)

3.6.3 APPLICATIONS IN ORTHOPAEDICS

In this field, many applications have been designed, explored and tested. The list below is certainly not exhaustive but summarises the present ideas, most of which are developing into large-scale standardised applications:

- miniature bone anchors with superelastic prongs for the reattachment of soft tissues to bone by means of sutures
- superelastic or shape memory cerclage wires for a tight connection of bone parts
- shape memory locking mechanisms for the adjustment of tension in cerclage wires
- shape memory locking rings for the fixation of liners in the cups of hip prostheses (Figure 3.13).
- intramedullary fixation nails with self-expanding memory metal elements that adapt to the local diameter for the fixation of fractures in long bones. This nail has a very low insertion force, as opposed to conventional systems which have an invariable and more or less cylindrical shape
- implantable bone distraction devices used for an Illizarov method to change the length of a bone. This device can also be used for a growing bone prosthesis for children
- osteosynthesis bone staples for a stable reposition and fixation of two bone parts after fracture or corrective osteotomy
- osteosynthesis compression plates
- superelastic rods for gradual correction of scoliosis by means of relaxation of the body tissue. In conventional systems much greater forces and thus heavier rods are required to obtain the same results during this operation

SHAPE MEMORY ALLOYS

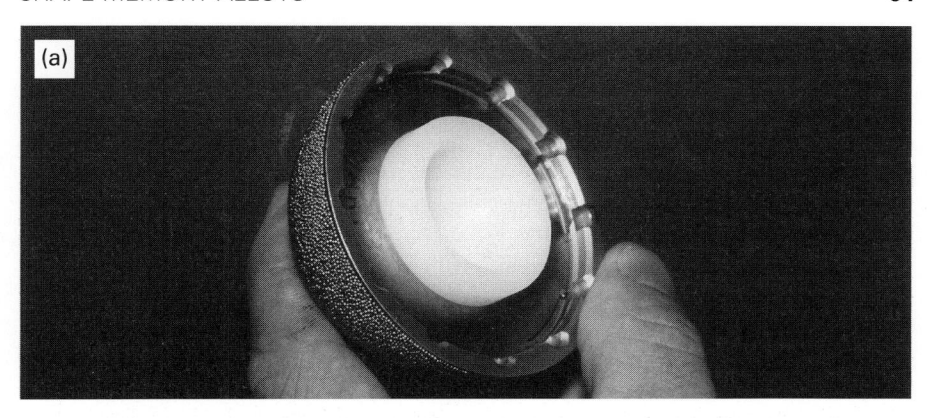

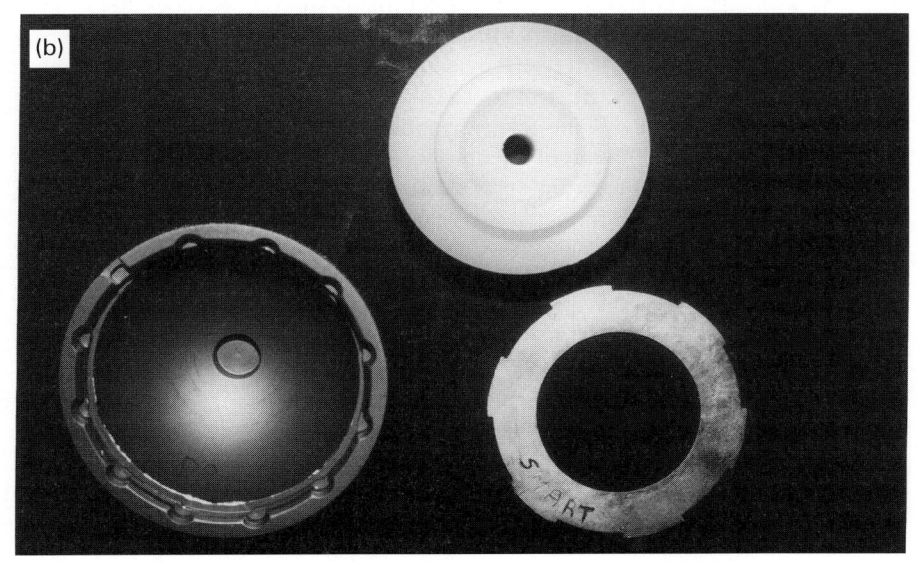

Figure 3.13 Shape memory locking ring for the fixation of a liner in the cup of a hip prosthesis. The cup, liner and disc-shaped NiTi ring are shown separately and assembled. (Photographs from MMH.)

- tools for the removal of broken bone screws
- straight superelastic tension wires for the fixation of hip implants to the bone. In the case of bone resorption the force in the wire and thus the stability of the connection are not influenced because of the constant plateau stress
- external fixators with a high grade of adjustability, locked by temperature-sensitive rings and ball joints
- external distraction devices with shape memory actuators
- connectors for modular orthopaedic implants.

3.6.4 MEDICAL INSTRUMENTS AND TOOLS

The development of minimal invasive surgery created a market push as well as a market pull on the development of new instruments, mainly on the basis of the superelastic properties (Melzer and Stoeckel, 1995). Complex but very flexible and tactile instruments, which are even capable of going around corners, are now used and can perform complex and delicate tasks through a trochar (a tube with a diameter of 5–10 mm) (Figure 3.14).

One of the main advantages is the use of hingeless instruments (Figure 3.15). In instruments used for minimal invasive surgery functions such as endoscopy, tomography and radiology, the demand for flexibility and steerability led to the use of superelastic wires, strips and tubes. These superelastic elements can be deformed by at least a factor of 10 more than conventional materials and the kinking resistance is excellent. Miniature cutters and grippers are normally made of several parts, which makes production and sterilisation complicated. A new type of hingeless gripper is made entirely of one single part and the beaks have to be heat treated to remember the open position (Figure 3.16). The beaks can be closed by advancing a tube over the flexible part of the jaws. The relative motion between the central superelastic memory metal part and the delivery tube is controlled very accurately by the proximal handpiece. This tool can be kept clean very easily because of its simple construction and it allows a further scaling down to extremely fine instruments.

NiTi alloys are also used in needles (Figure 3.17), stylets, guidewires, catheters, stents, filters, tissue anchoring and connection, flow control devices, rhinosurgical

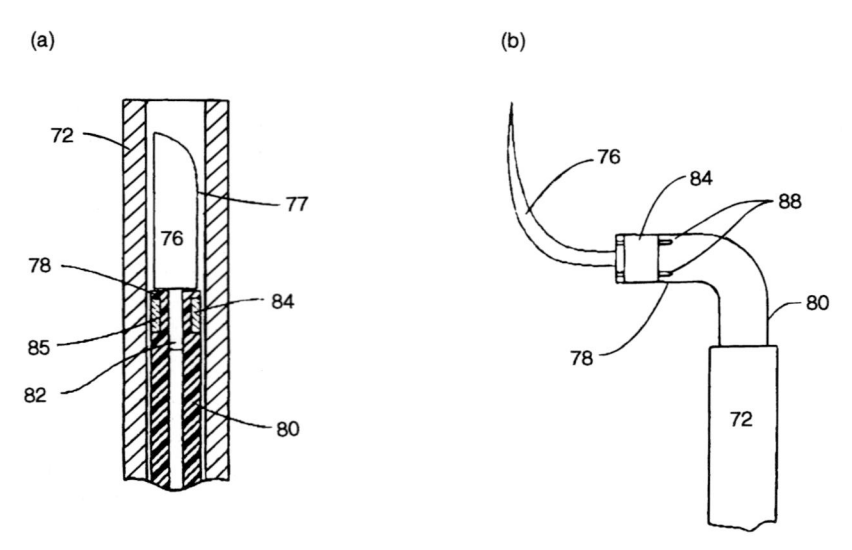

Figure 3.14 Steerable knife for minimal invasive surgery, using superelasticity. Either knife 76 or rod 80 returns into the programmed curved shape upon leaving the straight delivery tube 72. (Diagram from MMH.)

SHAPE MEMORY ALLOYS

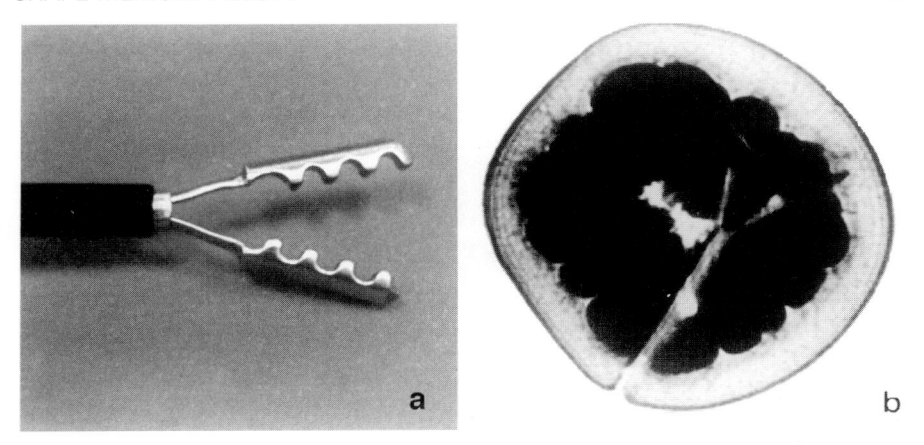

Figure 3.15 Superelastic hingeless forceps for endoscopic gall bladder surgery made from Nitinol and magnetic resonance image of the forceps. (Photographs from NDC.)

instruments, etc. (Pelton *et al.*, 1995). Very thin tubes (OD ≤ 100 µm) can be used in arteries or the application of small stents for angioplasty. The possibility of removal after healing avoids the problems associated with permanent implants, i.e. long-term anticoagulation medication and excessive cell growth around a foreign body.

The following list of present applications is certainly not exhaustive but illustrates clearly the growing importance of these alloys:

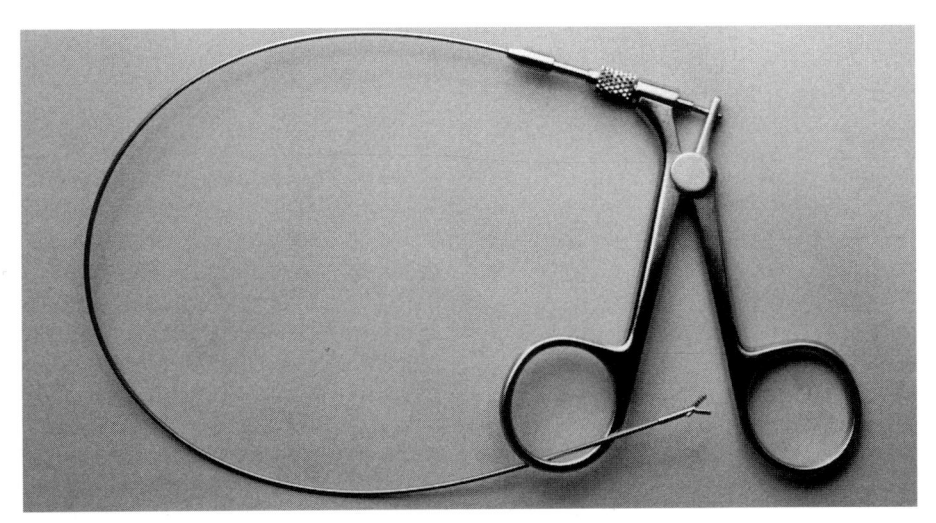

Figure 3.16 Superelastic micrograsper using Nitinol tubing. (Photograph from NDC.)

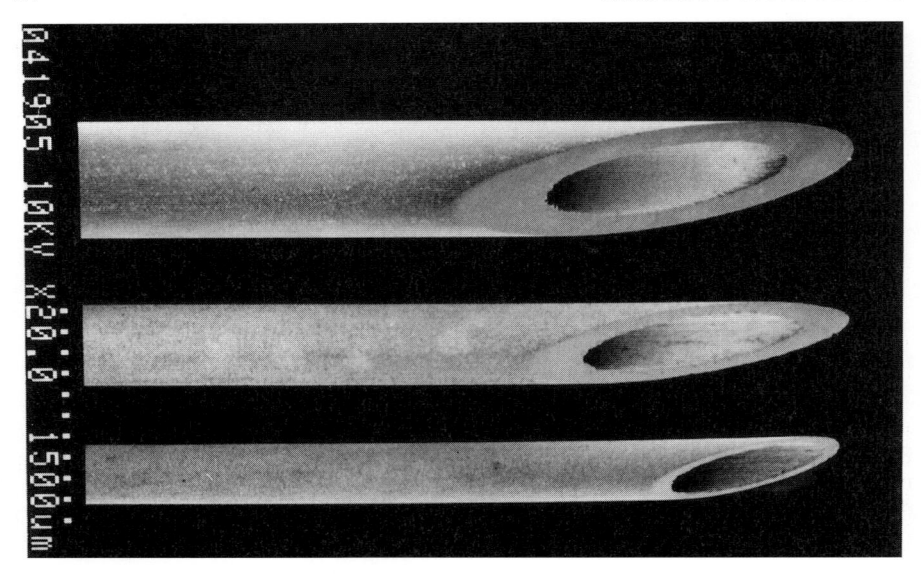

Figure 3.17 NiTi superelastic needles. (Photograph from Furukawa.)

- superelastic massive or tubular guide wires. Some of these guidewires have an optical system and a steerable tip
- steerable lasers with superelastic, bending housing in an endoscope
- catheters with a basket for catching stone fragments from the gallbladder (Figure 3.18)
- curved locator wires for non-palpable breast lesions. The wire is inserted through a straight needle and curls around the lesion when it leaves the needle
- self-fixating needles, electrodes and sensors with a tip that changes shape during insertion into the body
- vena cava filters for the prevention of recurrent pulmonary embolism. These filters are inserted into the veins in a straight shape by means of a catheter (Figure 3.19)
- intraocular lenses (for cataract patients) with fixation loops that are temporarily collapsed during insertion into the eye
- clips for aneurisms and sterilisation
- artificial sphincters for stress incontinence
- temperature indicators for the control of the maximum temperature level of blood, organs, etc., during transportation and storage
- instrument boxes with a heat-sensitive lock that can be opened only if the sterilisation temperature is reached
- self-locking instruments that cannot be reused without sterilisation
- miniature endoscopic suturing instruments
- endoscopic superelastic knives with an angle that can be continuously varied by changing the relative position between the knife and delivery tube

SHAPE MEMORY ALLOYS

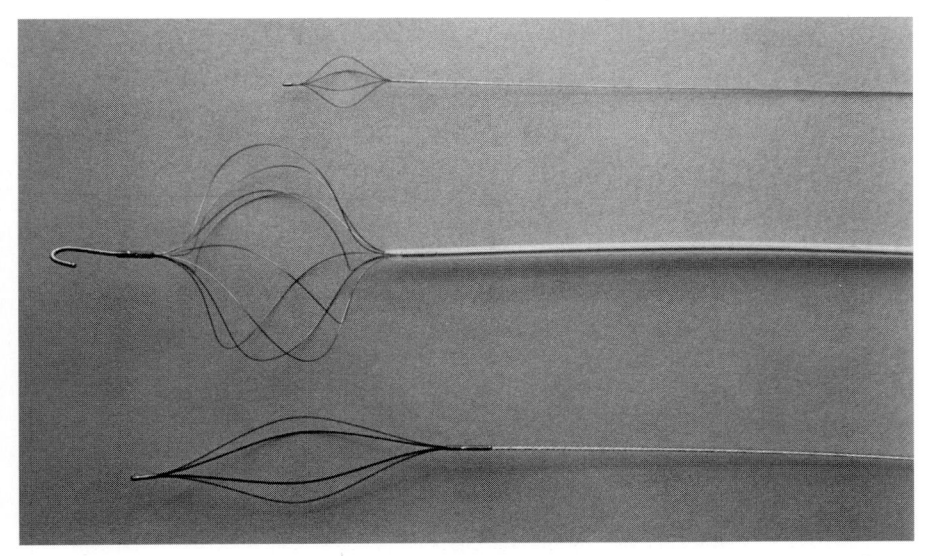

Figure 3.18 Baskets made from superelastic Nitinol wires. (Photograph from NDC).

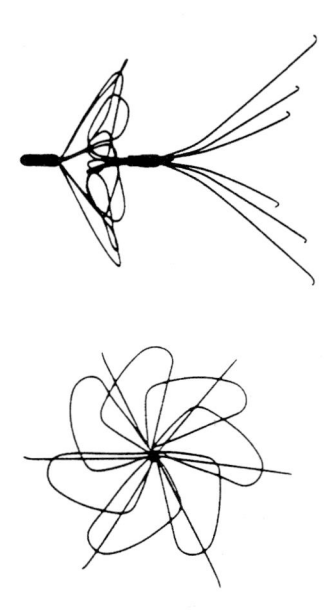

Figure 3.19 The Simon Nitinol filter (SNF) is implanted in the vena cava via the shape memory effect to entrap blood clots and prevent pulmonary embolisms. (Diagram from SMA).

- steerable endoscopic instrument holders with a shape memory locking ring in the tip for rapid changing of tools
- microactuators for Braille systems or implantable microvalves
- active ortheses for the treatment of rheumatic joints. By an alternating change in the temperature of the memory elements the device makes continuous movements
- superelastic deployable umbrellas for atrial septal defect occlusion (Figure 3.20).

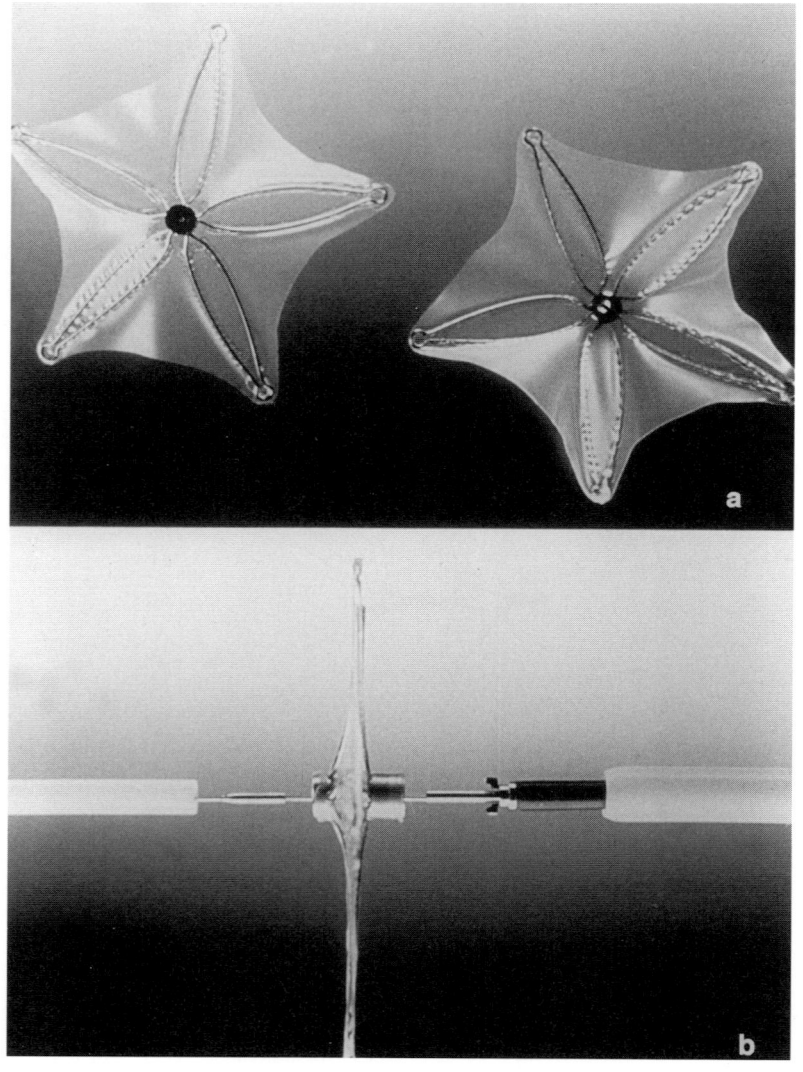

Figure 3.20 Superelastically deployable umbrellas for atrial septal defect occlusion. (Photographs from Osypka/NDC.)

3.7 BIOCOMPATIBILITY OF NiTi ALLOYS

NiTi alloys are considered to be highly corrosion resistant, biocompatible materials. The elements Ni and Ti form an intermetallic stoichiometric compound $Ni_{0.5}Ti_{0.5}$. Off-stoichiometric alloys will contain no more than a few tenths of an atomic per cent of Ni in solid solution.

Extensive *in vivo* experience in the human body with implants, mainly related to dentistry, especially orthodontic wires, but also in orthopaedics, stenting or other medical branches has thus far not revealed any special problems.

Regarding its biocompatibility, NiTi can be compared with stainless steel (grade 316 L), CoCr alloys and even pure Ti. The origin of these properties is mainly related to the passivation layer of TiO_2. To obtain a good passivation care must be taken in the final treatment to avoid small islands of pure Ni at the surface or mixtures of NiO and Ti_2O, which may create favoured sites for selective dissolution in crystals (Chan *et al.*, 1990; Oshida *et al.*, 1992).

In this respect surface conditions are extremely important. These surface conditions are controlled by the specific thermomechanical treatments that NiTi alloys must undergo in order to achieve optimal performance. Further processing and mounting should be performed with care in order not to damage the TiO_2 layer.

More detailed information and discussion on the biocompatibility of NiTi alloys can be found in several publications (Catright *et al.*, 1973; Castleman *et al.*, 1976; Oshida *et al.*, 1990; Oshida and Miyazaki, 1991; Dutta *et al.*, 1993; Shabalovskaya, 1995) and dedicated conference proceedings (Pelton, 1994).

3.8 CONCLUSIONS

The functional properties of SMA offer unique opportunities in many fields of industrial activity. Most of the recent commercial successes are related to the use of superelasticity in biomedical applications.

Moreover, NiTi alloys are considered to be good corrosion-resistant and even biocompatible materials. With the increasing number of applications, more attention is now devoted to this particular property, although no definite classification as a full biocompatible material is yet available.

It is also important to note that the design for shape memory applications always requires a specific approach, completely different from that of conventional structural materials. This requires experienced designers who are familiar with the physical and mechanically non-linear behaviour of these materials.

ACKNOWLEDGEMENTS

R. Stalmans and J. Van Humbeeck acknowledge the Fund for Scientific Research, Flanders, for a grant as Postdoctoral Fellow and Research Director, respectively.

NDC (Fremont, CA, USA), SMA (Santa Clara, CA, USA), Furukawa (Yokohama, Japan) and MMH (Enschede, The Netherlands) are kindly acknowledged for providing pictures of some of their products.

NOMENCLATURE

A_f temperature at which the reverse transformation (martensite → beta) is completed during heating

A_s temperature at which the reverse transformation (martensite → beta) starts during heating

M_f temperature at which the forward transformation (beta → martensite) is completed during cooling

M_s temperature at which the forward transformation (beta → martensite) starts during cooling

$\sigma^{p\text{-}m}$ critical stress to start the forward transformation

REFERENCES

Ahlers, M. (1986). Martensite and equilibrium phases in Cu–Zn and Cu–Zn–Al alloys, *Prog. in Mater. Sci.* **30** (3), 135–86.

AMT (1993) Commercial brochures of AMT on *High Damping* and *High Damping Metals with Emphasis to Cu–Zn–Al (PROTEUS) Shape Memory Alloys*, AMT, Herk-de Stad, Belgium.

Besselink, P.A. and Sachdeva, R.C.L. (1995) Applications of shape memory effects, *J. Phys. IV*, (Suppl. III 5), C8-111–116.

Beyar, R. (1996) Self-expanding Nitinol stents, in *Endoluminal Stenting* (ed. U. Sigwart), W.B. Saunders, London, pp. 154–9.

Castleman, L.S., Molzkin, S.M., Alicandri, F.P., Bonavit, V.L. and Johnson, A.A. (1976) Biocompatibility of nitinol alloy as an implant material, *J. Biomed. Mater. Res.* **10**, 695–731.

Catright, D.E., Bhaskar, S.N., Johnson, R.M. and Corvan, G.S.M. (1973) Tissue reaction to Nitinol wire alloy, *Oral Surg.* **35**, 578–84.

Chan, C.M, Trigwell, S. and Duerig, T. (1990) Oxidation of an NiTi alloy, *Surf. Intern. Anal.* **15**, 349–54.

Delaey, L. (1991) Diffusionless transformations, in *Materials Science and Technology*, Vol. 5, *Phase Transformations in Materials* (ed. P. Haasen), VCH Verlagsgesellschaft, Weinheim, pp. 339–404.

Duerig, T.W., Melton, K.N., Stöckel, D. and Wayman, C.M., eds (1990) *Engineering Aspects of Shape Memory Alloys*, Butterworth-Heinemann, London.

Duerig, T.W., Pelton, A.R. and Stöckel, D. (1998) The use of superelasticity in medicine, in *Proceedings of the Wayman Symposium* Warrendale, TMS, to be published.

Dutta, R.S., Madangopal, K., Gadiyar, H.S. and Banergy, S. (1993) Biocompatibility of NiTi shape memory alloy, *Br. Corros. J.* **28**, 217–21.

Fukuyo, S. and Sachdeva, R., eds (1982) Periot root implant and medical application of shape memory alloy, in *Proceedings of the First Conference of the International Academy of Shape Memory Material for Medical Use*, Nihon University, Tokyo.

Funakubo, H. (1984) *Shape Memory Alloys*, Gordon & Breach, New York.

Gotthardt, R. and Van Humbeeck, J., eds (1995) Session VI: Applications of martensite, in *Proceedings of the ICOMAT 95, J. Phys. IV, Colloque C8*.

Ikuta, K. (1990) Micro/miniature shape memory alloy actuator, in *Proceedings of the IEEE Workshop*, pp. 2156–61.

Ikuta, K., Tsukamoto, M. and Hirose, S. (1991) Shape memory alloy servo actuator system with electric resistance feedback and application for active endoscope, in *Proceedings of the IEEE MEMS Workshop*, pp. 103–8.

Johnson, A.D. (1991) Vacuum-deposited TiNi shape memory thin film: characterization and applications in microdevices, *J. Micromech. Microengng.* **1**, 34–41.

Johnson, A.D., Bush, J.D., Curtis, A.R. and Sloan, C. (1992), Fabrication of silicon-based shape memory alloy micro-actuator, in *Materials Research Society Symposium Proceedings*, Vol. 276, MRS, Pittsburgh, PA, pp. 151–9.

Krupp-Untersuchsbericht UB1022/73 (1973), *Experimentalstudie über die Memory Legierung NiTi als Antrieb für die Entfaltung von Antennen oder Solarzellenauslegen*, Krupp, Essen.

Maclean, J.B., Draper, J.L. and Misra, M.S. (1991) Development of a shape memory material actuator for adaptive truss applications, *J. Intell. Mater. Syst. Struct.* **2**, 261–80.

Makkar, R., Eigler, N., Forrester, J.S. and Litwach, F. (1996) Technical and engineering aspects of stents which may be either permanent or removable, in *Endoluminal Stenting* (ed. U. Sigwart), W.B. Saunders, London, pp. 230–7.

Melton, K.N. (1994) Engineering design and application of shape memory materials, in *Shape Memory Materials '94* (eds C. Yougi and T. Hailing), International Academic Publishers, Beijing, pp. 523–9.

Melzer, A. and Stöckel, D. (1995) Performance improvement of surgical instrumentation through the use of NiTi materials, in *Proceedings of SMST-94 (Shape Memory and Superelastic Technologies)* (eds A. Pelton, D. Hodgson and T. Duerig), MIAS, Monterey, pp. 401–9.

Miyazaki, S., Ishida, A. and Takei, A. (1992) Development and characterization of Ti–Ni shape memory thin films, in *Proceedings of the International Symposium on Measurement and Control of Robotics (ISMCR '92)*, AIST Research Centre, Tsukuba, pp. 495–500.

Miyazaki, S., Nomura, K. and Zhirong, H. (1995) Shape memory effect and superelasticity developed in sputter-deposited NiTi thin films, in *Proceedings of SMST-94 (Shape Memory and Superelastic Technologies)* (eds A. Pelton, D. Hodgson and T. Duerig), MIAS, Monterey, pp. 19–24.

Oshida, Y. and Miyazaki, S. (1991) Corrosion and biocompatibility of shape memory alloys, *Corros. Engng* **40**, 1009–25.

Oshida, Y., Sachdeva, R.C.L. and Miyazaki, S. (1992) Microanalytical characterization and surface modification of TiNi orthodontic archwires, *Bio-Med. Mater. Engng* **2**, 51–9.

Oshida, Y., Sachdeva, R., Miyazaki, S. and Fukuyo, S. (1990) Biological and chemical evaluation of NiTi alloys, *Mater. Sci. Forum* **56–8**, 705–10.

Pelton, A. R., Hodgson, D. and Duerig, T. eds (1995) *Proceedings of SMST-94 (Shape Memory and Superelastic Technologies)*, MIAS, Monterey, 527 pp.

Raymont, M. and Weynant, E. (1991) Testing of the thermomarker: importance of hysteresis, *J. Phys. IV, Colloque* C4, 169–74.

Reynaerts, D. and Van Brussel, H. (1995) Shape memory alloy based electrical actuation for robotic applications, in *Proceedings of SMST-94 (Shape Memory and Superelastic Technologies)* (eds A. Pelton, D. Hodgson and T. Duerig), MIAS, Monterey, pp. 271–5.

Sachdeva, R., Fukuyo, S., Suzuki, K., Oshida, Y. and Miyazaki, S. (1990a), Shape memory NiTi alloys – applications in dentistry, *Mater. Sci. Forum* **56–8**, 693–8.

Sachdeva, R.C.L. and Miyazaki, S. (1990) Superelastic NiTi alloys in orthodontics, in *Engineering Aspects of Shape Memory Alloys* (eds T.W. Duerig, K.N. Melton, D. Stoeckel and C.M. Wayman), Butterworth-Heinemann, London, pp. 452–69.

Sachdeva, R., Oshida, Y., Fukuyo, S. and Miyazaki, S. (1990b) NiTi alloys in orthodontics: a clinical and thermomechanical evaluation, in *Proceedings of the International Conference on Medical Applications of Shape Memory Alloys* (ed. Jin Jia Ling), Shanghai Iron and Steel Research Institute, Shanghai, pp. 187–98.

Schetky, McD.L. (1995) The application of constrained recovery shape memory devices for connectors, sealing and clamping, in *Proceedings of the First International Conference on Shape Memory and Superelastic Technologies* (eds A.R. Pelton, D. Hodgson and T. Duerig), MIAS, Monterey, pp. 239–43.

Shabalovskaya, S.A. (1995) Biological aspects of TiNi alloy surfaces, in *Proceedings of ICOMAT '95* (eds R. Gotthardt and J. Van Humbeeck), *J. Phys.* IV, *Colloque* C8, pp. 1199–204.

Sigwart, U., ed. (1996) *Endoluminal stenting*, W.B. Saunders, London, 601 pp.

Simon, M., Kaplow, R., Salzman, E. and Freiman, D. (1977) A vena cava filter using thermal shape memory alloy. *Radiology*, **125**, 88.

Stalmans, R., Van Humbeeck, J. and Delaey, L. (1989) CADSMA: computer aided design of shape memory alloys, in *The Martensitic Transformation in Science and Technology* (eds E. Hornbogen and N. Jost), DGM, Oberursel, pp. 207–13.

Stöckel, D. (1992) Status and trends in shape memory technology, in *Proceedings of Actuator 92* (Eds. H. Borgmann and K. Lenz), VDI/VDE-Technologiezentrum Informationstechnik, Berlin, pp. 79–84.

Tuissi, A., Ranucci, T., Ceresara, S., Coluzzi, B., Biscarini, A., Mazzolai, F.M., Staffaloni, N., Guerra, M. and Santoro, M. (1995) Pseudoelasticity and transformation features of some NiTi orthodontic commercial wires, in *Proceedings of ICOMAT '95* (eds R. Gotthardt and J. Van Humbeeck), *J. Phys.* IV, *Colloque* C8, pp. 1229–34.

Van Humbeeck, J. (1986) High Damping Capacity due to Microstructural Interfaces, in *Roles of Interfaces on Material Damping* (eds B.B. Rath and M.S. Misra), ASM, Metals Park, Ohio, pp. 5–24.

Van Humbeeck, J. (1991) Cycling effects, fatigue and degradation of shape memory alloys, *J. Phys.* IV, *Colloque* C4, 189–97.

Van Humbeeck, J., Chandrasekaran, M. and Delaey, L. (1991) Shape memory alloys: materials in action, *Endeavour, New Series* **15**, 148–54.

Van Moorleghem, W., Reynaerts, D., Van Brussel, H. and Van Humbeeck, J. (1992) General discussion: The use of shape memory actuators, in *Proceedings of the International Conference on New Actuators, Actuator '92* (ed. Axon GmbH), Axon GmbH, Bremen, 24–26 June 1992, pp. 225–7.

Walkers, J.A., Gabriel, K.J. and Mehregang, M. (1990) Thin-film processing of TiNi shape memory alloy, *Sens. Act.* **A21**, 243–6.

Wang, S.D., Wu, X.Z., Zhang, J.P., Su, H.Q., Jin, J.L. and Song, B.T. (1994) Phase transformations of rapidly solidified TiNi shape memory alloy, in *Advanced Materials '93 V-B: Shape Memory Materials and Hydrides* (eds. K. Otsuka, C.T. Liu, K. Shimizu, Y. Suzuki, J. Van Humbeeck, Y. Fukai, S. Ono and S. Sudo), *Trans. Mater. Res. Soc. Jpn*, Elsevier Science, Amsterdam, pp. 1061–4.

Wayman, C.M. and Perkins, J. eds (1993) Session V6: Engineering and application of shape memory alloys, in *Proceedings of ICOMAT '92*, Montrey Institute of Advanced Studies, Carmel, NY, pp. 1217–335.

Whitthaker, A.S., Krumme, R., Hayes, J.R. (1995) Structural control of building response using shape-memory alloys, Report Nr. TR95, 22, (ed. National Technical Information Service), Springfield, VA, p. 224.

4
Degradation
(*in vitro–in vivo* corrosion)

D. SCHARNWEBER
Technical University of Dresden, Dresden, Germany

4.1 INTRODUCTION

This chapter deals with the degradation of metallic biomaterials. It proceeds from the advantages of metallic biomaterials described in the previous chapters, such as good processability, weldability and mechanical properties adjustable within a wide area (stiffness and elastic modulus). These mechanical properties, however, are mostly disadvantageous and very different from those of bones. According to the connotation of the late Latin word *degrado* (disparage, demote, degrade), degradation in the context of biomaterials means the deterioration of characteristic properties.

Compared with the definitions formulated at the Chester Consensus Conference (Williams, 1988), in this chapter the subject will be restricted to those metallic biomaterials used for the production of implants. The terms 'metallic biomaterial' and 'implant (material)' will be used synonymously in this chapter.

As the subject of this book is restricted to metallic biomaterials, this chapter will summarise the degradation phenomena occurring from interactions of metallic biomaterials with the bioenvironment with regard to both the implant and the recipient's body (Figure 4.1), and test methods for assessing the degree of influence of these phenomena. Recent summaries on degradation are published in Winter *et al.* (1980), Hench and Ethridge (1982), Lycett and Hughes (1984), Barbosa (1992) and Wintermantel and Suk-Woo Ha (1996).

In this context, the term 'degradation behaviour of metallic biomaterials in a bioenvironment' combines corrosion and wear behaviour (see page 111). The degradation of the bioenvironment results from the interaction with the surface of the biomaterial or with particles emitted by the biomaterials owing to corrosion and wear. Essential interacting mechanisms between the metallic biomaterial and the bioenvironment are caused by

- biomaterial to bioenvironment interactions
    - the emission of metal ions in the corrosion process as well as by the emission of particles (oxide or metal) caused by mechanical effects

---

Metals as Biomaterials ISBN 0 471 96935 4 Edited by J.A. Helsen and H.J. Breme. © 1998 John Wiley & Sons Ltd

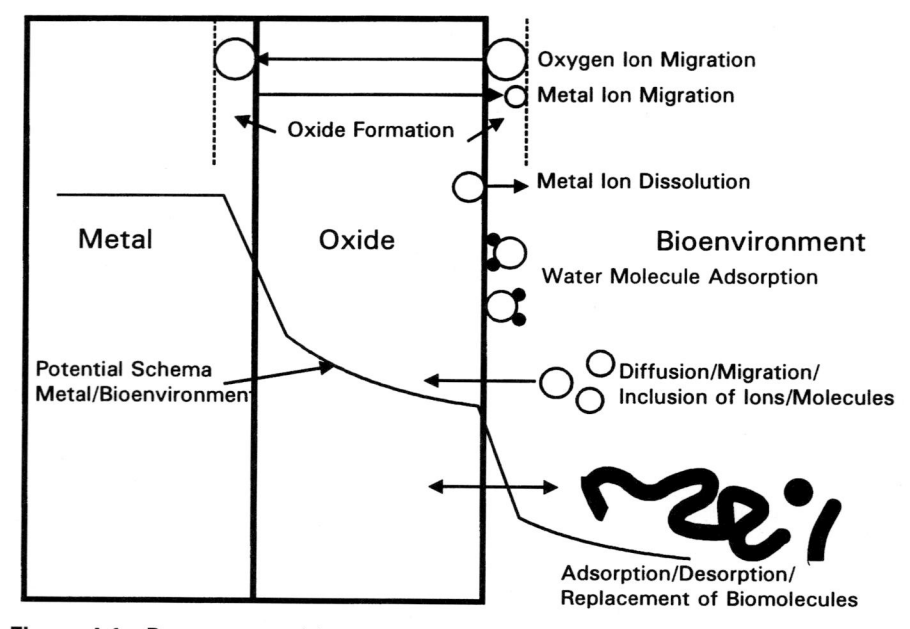

Figure 4.1 Processes and interactions occurring at the metal oxide/bioenvironment interface. (Based on *Biomaterials*, Vol. 15, Browne and Gregson, Surface Modification of titanium alloy implants, pp. 894–8, 1994, with permission from Elsevier Science.)

- alterations to the bioenvironment as a result of locally predominating partial reactions of the electrochemical corrosion process on the biomaterial surface (increase or decrease in pH caused by local corrosion, lowering the partial pressure of oxygen by a dominating cathodic partial reaction)
- the influence of adsorbed biomolecules by interaction forces, electric fields on the biomaterial surface (Helmholtz layer) as well as of surrounding cells by electric currents caused by galvanic corrosion
- bioenvironment to implant interactions
  - decrease in pH caused by local inflammation of the damaged tissue.

The biomaterial properties can be classified into four categories, according to the degree of degradation of the surrounding tissue caused by the interactions with the biomaterial (Table 4.1). It should be pointed out that even a purely adsorptive interaction of components of the bioenvironment with the surface of a biomaterial causing a disadvantageous change to the properties of this component is a degradation phenomenon (Jenissen, 1988). This subject is dealt with in Chapter 10, Tissue–implant interaction, and will be referred to in this chapter only as far as corrosion processes are concerned.

Looking at the development of metallic biomaterials from a historical point of view, the initial selection of materials for implantation was determined by the search for the least reactive materials, so gold had became the preferred material. In the field

Table 4.1 Tissue reactions caused by biomaterials and implants (Hench and Wilson, 1993)

Biomaterial properties	Tissue reaction
Toxic	Tissue necrosis
Inert	Tissue forms non-adherent connective tissue capsule around the material/implant
Bioactive	Tissue bonds directly to the material/implant
Degradable	Tissue replaces material/implant

of dental surgery, this situation has held to this day and alloys with a high gold content are mainly applied. Owing to the often insufficient mechanical properties of these materials, in later developments an attempt was made to optimise them. This resulted in the use of stainless steels and cobalt-based alloys in the implantation, although improved mechanical properties were achieved at the expense of the biocompatibility, when compared with gold. With the treatise of Leventhal, beginning in the 1940s (Ungethüm and Winkler-Gniewek, 1984; Semlitsch and Weber, 1992), the use of titanium as an implant material forged ahead so that at present titanium and its alloys are often the implant materials of choice from a medical point of view. In spite of this development, the majority of biomaterials in use in the field of implantation have not been developed exclusively for this application.

In this context, an intermediate stage in the development involves coatings, e.g. of Al_2O_3 (Brown, 1984; Brossa et al., 1987) or TiO_2 (Brossa et al., 1987) on implants made of stainless steels or rather cobalt-based alloys to improve their biocompatibility and to reduce the release of metallic ions.

Recently, in several research projects further optimisation of interactions arising between the implant surface and the biosystem has been dealt with, referring to the level attained in the mechanical, corrosive and chemical properties of the implant materials. Where possible, priorities are established by the active arrangement of these interactions. One trend of work aims at definitely adjusted physical–chemical surface properties of the implant (Andrade, 1985; Jenissen, 1988; Thull, 1990, 1994, 1995), while another includes significant organic substances (proteins, growth factors, etc.) for the cell colonisation and differentiation by the bioenvironment (Mikulec and Puleo, 1996; Richter et al., 1996; Scharnweber et al., 1997; Worch and Scharnweber, 1998).

In this chapter the position of an element or an alloy in the electrochemical series offers itself as a classification of the metallic biomaterials. Thus, statements on corrosion resistance from the thermodynamic point of view can be derived. This point of view, however, disregards that in many cases corrosion stability can be determined kinetically as a result of the ability of a metallic material to form tight oxide layers, affording protection from further corrosion (i.e. passive layers). For example, gold and platinum, as well as the alloys derived in each case, are part of the first mentioned group of metallic materials (thermodynamically caused corrosion stability). The second group comprises typical metallic biomaterials such as CoCrMo alloys, austenitic and ferritic highly alloyed steels and titanium and its alloys.

Further criteria that can be used for the classification of metallic biomaterials are wear resistance, the extent of reactions of the biosystem on particles and ionic species released by the materials, and the intended length of time the implant remains in the biosystem (temporary or permanent implants).

The next section will proceed from several generalised statements on the kinetics of corrosion processes and deal with passivity as well as local corrosion. The third section covers the methods used to measure and test corrosion and wear processes, and the fourth section discusses important groups of metallic biomaterials from the point of view of corrosion, chemistry, physicochemical properties of surfaces and wear behaviour.

4.2 CORROSION PROCESSES: KINETICS AND PHENOMENA

4.2.1 CORROSION PROCESSES

In general, corrosion processes on metals in metal–fluid systems can be described as destruction of the material based on electrochemical processes and starting on the surface. On closer examination, one must distinguish between (1) uniform corrosion, uniformly attacking the whole surface, and (2) localised corrosion, which is caused for several reasons (see Section 4.2.3) and creates a locally restricted attack preferably acting into the depth.

4.2.1.1 Fundamentals: Definitions

The terms 'electrochemical reaction' and 'electrode' are the basis for better understanding and should be defined as an introduction to this chapter.

An electrochemical reaction is a heterogeneous reaction between components contacting electrically conducting phases (I and II) during which a transfer of charge carriers at different places in the phase boundary takes place, creating a current flow through the phase boundary.

The reaction system consisting of both phases (I and II) is designated as the 'electrode'. In at least one of the phases, ion conduction should be achieved. One of the important features of an electrode is the potential difference across the phase boundary. However, this quantity cannot be measured directly, but only with respect to a reference electrode. Here it will be termed the electrochemical potential. Specifying the reference electrode used as an index, 'E_{SCE}' means, for example, that the potentials are referred to the saturated calomel electrode $Hg/Hg_2Cl_2,KCl$ (saturated solution).

The 'equilibrium potential' and the 'open circuit potential' should be distinguished as follows.

In the 'equilibrium potential', anodic and cathodic partial reactions are equal to each other but of opposite direction and are (on average) of equal rate. There is no gross turnover. In this case, the potential of a metal in a solution of its salt is determined by the metal ion activity and is described by the Nernst equation:

$$E = E^{\ominus} + \frac{RT}{zF}\ln\frac{a_{ox}}{a_{red}}. \quad (4.1)$$

This equation can be derived from the equilibrium case of the Butler–Volmer development (Bockris and Reddy, 1970). At the same time this equation describes the redox potential in solutions of redox systems such as O_2/OH^- and Fe^{2+}/Fe^{3+}. The standard potentials of elements relevant to metallic biomaterials are given in Table 4.2.

In the 'open circuit potential' (OCP) (mixed potential, rest potential), anodic and cathodic partial reactions are (on average) of equal rate but are different processes (gross turnover). In corrosion processes potentials are practically always mixed potentials. The corrosion current density (corrosion rate) of an electrode corroding at the open circuit potential is therefore equal to the rate of the anodic partial reaction, which is in turn equal to the rate of the cathodic partial reaction (Figure 4.2). It follows that the partial reactions may be far from equilibrium. The corrosion rate may be anodically or cathodically controlled depending on the slope of the current–potential curves of the partial reactions.

It should be pointed out that anodic and cathodic partial reactions are equal in amount to each other considering the total electrode area. However, this does not apply from a microscopic point of view, a situation of special importance and an essential prerequisite for localised corrosion.

In general, the anodic partial reaction can be written as

$$Me \rightarrow Me^{z+} + ze^-. \quad (4.2)$$

The cathodic partial reactions that can take place are hydrogen evolution:

$$2H^+ + 2e^- \rightarrow H_2 \quad (4.3a)$$

Table 4.2 Standard electrode potentials at 25°C (Kaesche, 1990)

Element	Standard potential $E^{\ominus}_{SCE}/V$
Ti/Ti^{2+}	−1.63
Cr/Cr^{3+}	−0.74
Co/Co^{2+}	−0.277
Ni/Ni^{2+}	−0.250
Hg/Hg^{2+}	0.789
Ag/Ag^+	0.7991
Pd/Pd^{2+}	0.987
Pt/Pt^+	1.2
Au/Au^{3+}	1.5
Au/Au^+	1.7

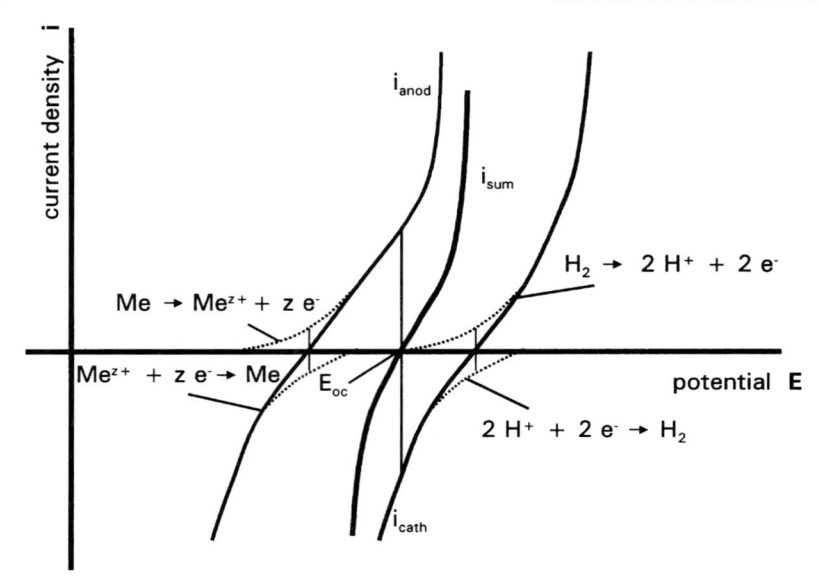

Figure 4.2 Schematic representation of current–potential curves in the case of mixed potential and corrosion of a metal with hydrogen evolution.

or oxygen reduction

$$O_2 + 4e^- + 2H_2O \rightarrow 4OH^- \quad (4.3b)$$

depending on the pH value, the oxygen partial pressure and the overvoltage of the reaction concerned at the respective surfaces.

The gross transfer of charge carriers at an electrode leads to a transfer of substance (mass, m; amount of substance, n). These quantities are related by Faraday's law

$$Q = nzF, \quad (4.4)$$

which allows a calculation of the corrosion rate from the corrosion current density. Additionally, the relation between the transferred charge quantity and the transferred substance is used in the electrochemical method of coulometry.

4.2.2 KINETICS OF CORROSION

To realise our intention, i.e. to determine the electrochemical reaction rate for determination of the corrosion rate of materials, it is necessary to examine more closely the relation between current density and overpotential at corroding electrodes. The term 'overpotential' in this context describes the potential difference between the potential of an electrode with current flowing into the (corrosion) cell

DEGRADATION (IN VITRO–IN VIVO CORROSION)

and the potential without that current. This relation is of central importance for the case that the transfer of electric charge carriers over the electric double layer determines the rate of the overall reaction. A typical case is the process of anodic metal dissolution in which no protective layers are formed.

The relation between the current density and the overpotential η is described by

$$i = i_0 \left[e^{\left(\frac{\alpha|z|F\eta_t}{RT}\right)} - e^{\left(\frac{(1-\alpha)|z|F\eta_t}{RT}\right)} \right]. \tag{4.5}$$

The derivation of this equation can be found in the specialised literature (Vetter, 1967; Bockris and Reddy, 1970).

The two exponential expressions in parentheses describe the anodic or cathodic partial reaction at the electrode and are equivalent to the anodic and cathodic partial current density in Figure 4.2. The current flowing in an external circuit is the sum of both current densities according to

$$i_{tot} = i_{anod} + i_{cath}. \tag{4.6}$$

At the open circuit potential are valid

$$i_{tot} = 0 \tag{4.7}$$

and

$$i_{anod} = |i_{cath}|. \tag{4.8}$$

For several metals and alloys of technical importance (see Sections 4.4.2 and 4.4.3), for higher overpotentials the anodic partial current curve is influenced by the formation of oxidic layers on the surface causing an increasingly reduced slope of the curve. Further anodic polarisation results in a complete oxide coverage of the surface, causing a strong negative slope of the current density. This behaviour is termed 'passivity'. The course of a current–potential curve of a passive metal is shown schematically in Figure 4.3.

The size of the potential region of passivity is mainly determined by the type of conduction of the passive layer. For electron-conducting passive layers (see Section 4.4.2), oxygen develops anodically to the potential of the oxygen electrode in the electrolyte solution ($E^\ominus = 820$ mV$_{NHE}$ for pH 7), whereas pure ion-conducting and n-semiconducting passive layers (i.e. Ti, Ta, Al) can be polarised nearly without limit (up to 200 V), forming thick anodic oxide layers (the layer thickness is proportional to the voltage).

Metals and alloys that passivate by themselves under the respective corrosion conditions are of technical importance. Such behaviour can be described by an inequality according to Equation (4.9), valid in the region of active dissolution

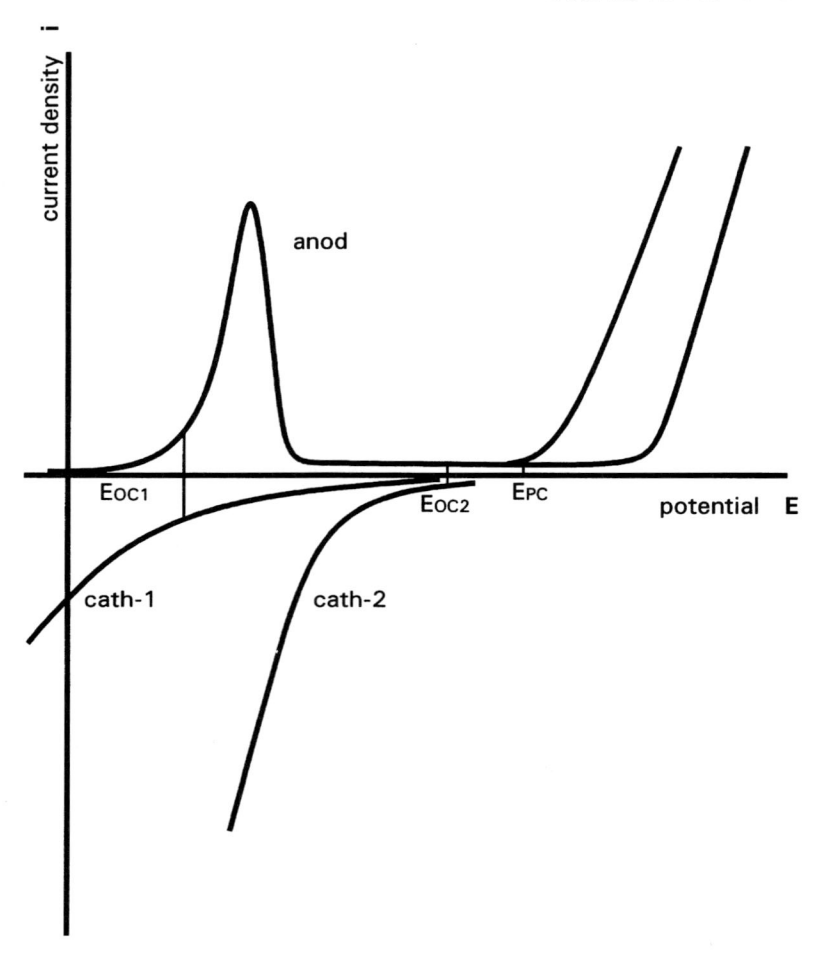

Figure 4.3 Schematic current–potential curve of a passive metal.

$$i_{anod} < |i_{cath}|. \qquad (4.9)$$

In Figure 4.3 the cathodic partial current density of curve 2 causes passivity. An open circuit potential (E_{oc2}) in the passive region is established, whereas curve 1 causes strong anodic dissolution at the open circuit potential E_{oc1}. It follows clearly from the figure that the formation of a passive layer brings about a drastic change in the corrosion properties of the metals and alloys concerned.

4.2.3 LOCALISED CORROSION

In many cases, uniform corrosion is under control in its effects on the mechanical

DEGRADATION (IN VITRO–IN VIVO CORROSION)

stability of the implant, and can be taken into consideration in the phase of construction, whereas localised corrosion is often decisively involved in the failure of components or implants. Silva et al. (1985) and Cook et al. (1987) published studies on the retrieval of implants and found the incidence of corrosion to be 70% (Silva et al.) and 89% (Cook et al.). According to Silva et al. the vast majority of cases of corrosion was due to crevice corrosion or fretting corrosion. Both forms of corrosion were responsible for 86% of cases, while stress corrosion cracking, corrosion fatigue and pitting corrosion accounted for only 14%.

The reasons for the occurrence of localised corrosion can be classified into the following three groups.

(1) Local changes in the corrosion conditions caused by geometric effects result in local alterations to the corrosion environment and thus in locally different corrosion rates (corrosion under layers or in crevices, concentration polarisation, etc.)
(2) A macroscopic or microscopic coupling of materials with different standard potentials results in a preferred corrosion attack of the less noble material (galvanic corrosion, intercrystalline corrosion or alloy corrosion).
(3) Proceeding from the passive region, the locally irreversible or cyclic abolition of the passivity caused by chemical or mechanical influences produces considerable local corrosion (pitting corrosion, stress corrosion cracking, fatigue corrosion, fretting corrosion)

The most important types of local corrosion occurring on biomaterials will be discussed, regarding causes and effects. For mechanistic details the reader should refer to the specialist literature (Kaesche, 1990). In practice, overlapping of several kinds of local corrosion processes is usually observed (e.g. pitting corrosion and crevice corrosion, grain boundary attack and galvanic corrosion).

4.2.3.1 Pitting Corrosion

Pitting corrosion occurs on passive metals as a steep slope of the current–potential curve in the passive region (at potentials anodically to the pitting potential E_{pc}) caused by local destruction preferably at weak points of the passive layer by aggressive anions. The following corrosive attack of the basic metal starts with the formation of pits followed by holes varying greatly in size (micrometre to millimetre) and shape (hemispherical to highly irregular).

The partial current density (curve 2 in Figure 4.3) demonstrates the current–potential function in the case of pitting corrosion.

The value of the pitting potential of a material (a measure of the resistance against pitting corrosion) depends on metallurgical factors (impurities, unfavourable heat treatment) and especially on the pH of the solution and the type and concentration of the pitting-creating anion. Because of the existence of about 0.15 mol l^{-1} chloride in each biological system, as far as the electrolyte conditions are concerned, pitting corrosion can, in principle, occur.

In a series of investigations the pitting potentials of metallic biomaterials have been investigated comparatively in a physiological NaCl solution as well as in Ringer's solution (Hench and Ethridge, 1975; Fraker *et al.*, 1980; Zitter and Plenk, 1987). The value of the minimum pitting potential as a measure of resistance against pitting corrosion in a bioenvironment cannot be given in a simple manner. E_{pc} values between 400 and 600 mV$_{NHE}$ for austenitic stainless steels and cobalt-based alloys (Fraker *et al.*, 1980) are, in contrast to titanium, of the same order as the resting potential (Speck and Fraker, 1980; Williams, 1981) and can be reached in biological systems under unfavourable conditions. The pitting potentials of more than 2 V$_{NHE}$ (Hench and Ethridge, 1975) usually measured for titanium and its alloys are far removed from realistic potentials in biosystems. Thus, these values, on the one hand, indicate the high resistance against pitting corrosion of these materials and, on the other hand, question the efforts towards further improvement of this parameter.

4.2.3.2 Crevice Corrosion

Crevice corrosion as a local corrosion phenomenon is linked with the occurrence of special geometries, which can emerge from structures and are generated by coatings or layers. The reasons for this type of corrosion are crevices or cavities where an exchange of material with the bulk electrolyte is limited. This causes a depletion of the depolariser responsible for the cathodic partial reaction in the crevice followed by an anodic polarisation of the crevice surface with respect to the surface outside, finally forming a corrosion element (see Section 4.2.3.3). The short-circuit currents inevitably connected to the corrosion element cause a decrease in pH in the crevice by hydrolysis of the corrosion products and anion migration into the crevice.

The appearance of aggressive anions (see Section 4.2.3.1) enhances the conditions for pitting corrosion in the crevice. In the final stage of crevice corrosion caused by a decrease in the pH (up to several units) and increased anion concentrations (up to several orders of magnitude) the corrosion conditions in the crevice are extremely aggravated compared with the bulk electrolyte, and the metal surface is subject to an equivalent corrosion attack.

4.2.3.3 Galvanic Corrosion

By electron-conducting contact between metals with different corrosion potentials a corrosion element is formed where the metal with the more negative corrosion potential acts as the local anode and undergoes preferred anodic corrosion. However, the preferred course of the cathodic partial reaction may also act as the real corrosion failure owing to hydrogen embrittlement. Possible reasons for different corrosion potentials of metals and materials are:

- different metals (materials) (different standard potentials)
- different concentrations of redox systems (pH, oxygen partial pressure) at different places on a metal (material) (concentration polarisation).

DEGRADATION (IN VITRO–IN VIVO CORROSION)

Selective corrosion of two-phase alloys as well as grain boundary attack (see Section 4.2.3.4) may be considered as special cases of the first reason.

Whether galvanic corrosion is initiated upon electronic coupling of two metals or materials depends significantly on the anodic partial current density curve of the metal or surface region with the more negative corrosion potential, but also on the properties of the metal or surface region acting as the local cathode. It is required that galvanic corrosion processes can take place without completely abolishing the potential difference. Therefore, critical situations in the sense of generating galvanic corrosion are:

- local anode in the region of active dissolution
- local anode in the passive region close to the pitting potential
- small local cathode in the region of hydrogen evolution.

From this point of view metals with pure ion-conducting or n-semiconducting oxide layers are completely uncritical as local anodes, whereas critical situations caused by hydrogen embrittlement may arise in the case of metals with n-semiconducting oxide layers (titanium) as local cathodes.

The extent of galvanic corrosion is determined by the surface ratio of the anode to the cathode as well as by the conductivity of the electrolyte. A small ratio of the anode to the cathode surface leads to considerable corrosion caused by high local current densities at the anode. Similarly, a high conductivity of the electrolyte (at least the circuit of the galvanic corrosion is short-circuited by the ohmic resistance of the electrolyte) accelerates the corrosion rate. At the same time this explains the preferred corrosion attack of the local anode immediately on the local cathode (geometrically caused lowest ohmic resistance of the electrolyte).

4.2.3.4 Grain Boundary Attack

Finally, a local attack of grain boundaries is caused essentially by an unfavourable metallographic structure of the material, mainly due to unsuitable heat treatment or thermal joint methods. The reason for the grain boundary attack is the precipitation of phases in the grain boundaries where these phases can be either more or less noble than the matrix. In the first case, the regions close to the grain boundaries are preferably attacked, while in the second case the precipitations are attacked. Both varieties are summarised by the term 'grain boundary attack' because of their extensively similar macroscopic appearance (see page 101).

Besides a series of aluminium alloys, CrNi-stainless steels are especially susceptible to grain boundary corrosion where, at least, the chromium content is responsible for spontaneous passivation (see Figure 4.3). When these steels are heat treated in the temperature range of 500–800°C, chromium carbides ($Cr_{23}C_6$) are formed in the grain boundaries and, therefore, chromium is depleted in the regions close to the grain boundaries. Consequently, these regions behave as local anodes (local cathodes are the grain areas) and are the sites of preferred corrosion attack. This type of corrosion, caused by the extreme surface ratio of the local anode and the local cathode and the small geometric distances (micrometre range), is anodically determined and brings about very severe attacks.

Besides a drastic diminution in the carbon level, low concentrations of strong carbide formers (Ti, Nb) are well established as metallurgical protective processes in the case of CrNi-steels. Because of their high affinity to carbon, the formation of chromium carbides and the depletion of chromium as reasons for the corrosive attack are prevented in the regions near the grain boundaries.

4.2.3.5 Local Corrosion Processes Under the Influence of Mechanical Loading

In this subsection, corrosion processes caused by stress corrosion cracking, fatigue corrosion and fretting corrosion will be discussed.

Stress corrosion cracking is related to the formation and spreading of cracks in a material as a result of the eclipsing of a static internal or external tensile load and a corrosive attack. The formation of cracks can be initiated at preformed notches caused by improper surface finishing and by unfavourable structural features, and also by dislocation movements in the material and the breakthrough of these dislocations to the surface of the material. Essential factors for this phenomenon are metallurgical parameters such as precipitations and impurities, as well as corrosion processes influencing the mechanical properties (hydrogen embrittlement). From the point of view of fracture mechanics, additional corrosive influences are considered using variable stress intensity factors K_{IC}. In the case of compressive stresses, corrosion cracking is inhibited.

Fatigue corrosion is widely based on the same mechanisms as stress corrosion cracking and is initially caused by a cyclic mechanical load. Owing to a resulting fatigue compared with stress corrosion cracking, in principle, all materials can be attacked by fatigue corrosion. In addition, the chemical conditions in the region of the crack tip, as well as the frequency and amplitude of the acting mechanical load, can influence the corrosion progress significantly.

Fretting corrosion is mainly caused by relative movements of metallic compounds in mechanical contact. This causes permanent local destruction of passive layers and, therefore, results in accelerated corrosion in these areas. Supplementary galvanic effects between areas of intact layers or a considerably destroyed passive layer may cause a further aggravation of the corrosion situation. Moreover, fretting corrosion may cause an emission of particles (oxide or metal). Typical situations for the appearance of fretting corrosion are metal/metal-fretting pairings in artificial hip prostheses (Jacobs et al., 1996) and the contact areas between marrow nail/fixation bolts and osteosynthesis plates/screw heads in accident surgery (Hughes and Jordan, 1972).

4.3 EXPERIMENTAL PROCEDURES

The recommended experimental methods aim at assessing the biocompatibility of a material with regard to its tendency to degradation, i.e. its interactions with the

DEGRADATION (*IN VITRO–IN VIVO* CORROSION)

surrounding medium under the real conditions of exposure as well as the resulting deterioration of both components.

Unfortunately, the experimental measurements are restricted in that while there are powerful on-line methods for *in vitro* examinations, the transformation of the real *in vivo* conditions for designing appropriate model conditions is very difficult or even impossible owing to the extremely complex composition of the respective media occurring *in vivo*. Here, substances present in very low concentrations may play an important role in the degradation behaviour of the metallic biomaterial. This statement is especially true for species that

- will form strong complexes with metal ions
- influence the redox properties of the system and, hence, change the OCP
- modify the frictional and wear behaviour.

For this reason, a comprehensive presentation of the behaviour of metallic biomaterials in biomedia is impossible, unlike the practice for the assessment of the corrosion behaviour of metals in inorganic fluids, for instance, by means of the well-known Pourbaix diagrams (Pourbaix, 1963). Otherwise, it is hardly possible to follow *in vivo* experiments in detail or on-line. The obtainable results often represent a collection of snapshots based on varying conditions. Therefore, the assessment of the degradation tendency of metallic biomaterials should consist of the following examination stages, which are characterised by a decreasing amount of the materials involved:

- *in vitro* corrosion and wear examination in an inorganic medium
- *in vitro* corrosion and wear examination in a mixed inorganic–organic medium
- examinations using cell and organ cultures
- *in vivo* examinations based on implantation in animal organisms.

During the last few years, as a result of the unsatisfactory situation mentioned above, many activities have been aimed at combining the advantages of on-line electrochemical measuring methods with cellular biological investigations (Schade and Liefeith, 1995). Accordingly, Liefeith *et al.* (1994) and Hildebrand *et al.* (1995) developed a measuring system with which *in vitro* corrosion tests can be performed in biological electrolytes. An extension of this system as a bioreactor (see Figure 4.4) also yields information on cell adhesion using fluorescence microscopy. With the use of laser-induced fluorescence spectroscopy it is also possible to assess the physiological condition of test organisms as a function of the material in contact.

4.3.1 IN VITRO *METHODS*

Following the general discussion of the advantages and disadvantages of *in vitro* methods in the field of degradation examination, this subsection critically presents the procedures concerned, focusing first on corrosion and subsequently on wear behaviour. In many cases, electrochemical measurements are carried out in *in vitro* corrosion examinations. In some respects they are superior to gravimetric methods and to those analysing the examination medium after having finished the test.

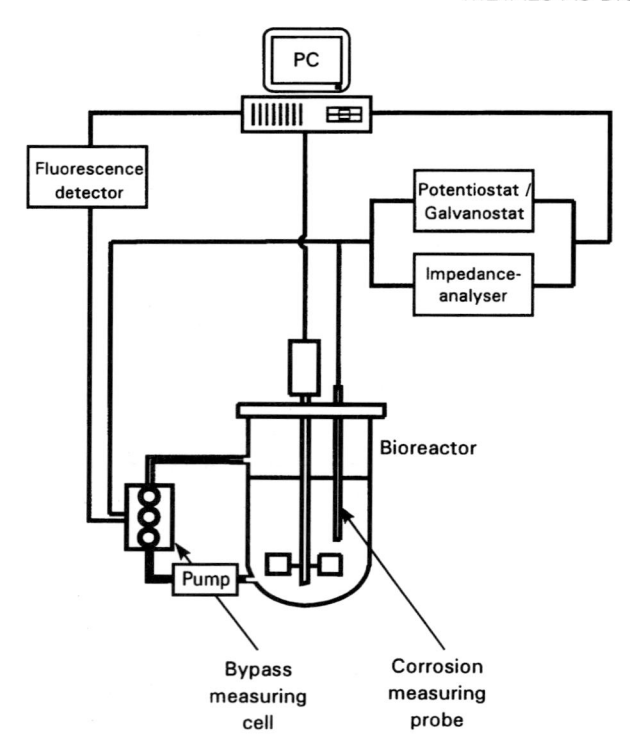

Figure 4.4 Schematic diagram of an *in vitro* measuring system for biocompatibility testing of biomaterials. (Reproduced by permission of K. Liefeith, IBA Heiligenstadt.)

4.3.1.1 Electrochemical Methods for the Assessment of Corrosion Behaviour

Within electrochemical investigations for the determination of the corrosion rate it is often necessary to impose definite conditions (potential or current) on the specimen to be examined. In doing so, the appropriate arrangement involves three electrodes. Besides the specimen as a working electrode (WE) and a reference electrode (RE) for adjusting or measuring the potential of the WE, an auxiliary electrode (AE) is necessary for the currents flowing through the cell. The RE is unable to do this, because a current flow via the RE would change its potential or even lead to its irreversible deterioration and, hence, prevent a correct measurement of the WE's potential. The RE may be positioned far from the WE, if a capillary probe (Haber–Luggin capillary) is used, which ends about 1 mm in front of the WE. Figure 4.5 outlines schematically the difference between a simple two-electrode arrangement, e.g. for galvanic baths, and a three-electrode arrangement.

As mentioned above, there are two different experimental approaches, which differ in the quantity (potential or current) to be controlled. When the potential is kept

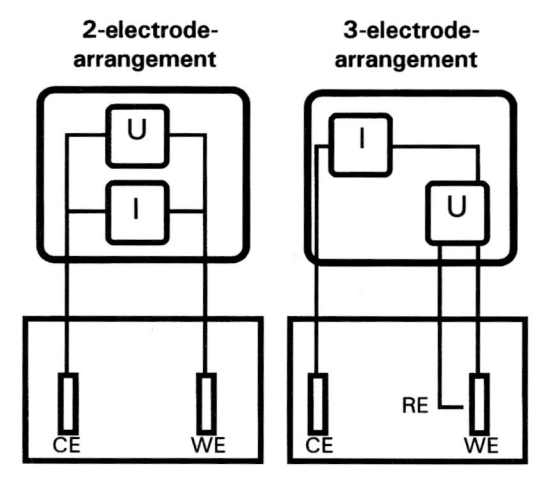

Figure 4.5 Schemes of two-electrode and three-electrode arrangements.

constant, the method is termed a 'potentiostatic polarisation', whereas a measurement with a constantly changing potential dE/dt is termed a 'potentiodynamic polarisation'.

Potentiostatic measurements are used to study stationary processes or to obtain stationary data on the processes occurring on the WE, and are often a prerequisite for accurate analysis. For example, the investigation of charge transfer polarisation is based on stationary current–potential relationships. Potentiostatic measurements are often very time consuming, which may be a strong disadvantage.

Potentiodynamic measurements may be carried out in order to obtain quasi-potentiostatic characteristics. In that case, the potential range of interest must be scanned with a decreasing polarisation rate. If the characteristic parameters of the current–potential relationship become constant, quasi-potentiostatic conditions will have been achieved. Such an approach is absolutely necessary when determining critical potential data, such as pitting potentials or potentials resulting from the onset of crevice corrosion. Generally, quasi-potentiostatic conditions can be expected only for dE/dt < 1–3 mV s^{-1}.

Galvanostatic methods with a controlled current are especially advantageous in comparison to potentiodynamic polarisation where critical potentials such as the pitting potential are to be determined. Whereas by potentiodynamic polarisation (depending on the scan rate) the risk is taken of determining too-positive potentials, this is generally avoided by the galvanostatic method.

Evaluation of the current–potential curves for the determination of the corrosion rate

For higher polarisations of more than 200 mV cathodically or anodically to the OCP, the current of the opposite process (anodic and cathodic, respectively) vanishes. For this case, Equation (4.5) can be written in the following manner (Tafel equation)

$$|\eta_t| = b \log\frac{|i|}{i_0} = b \log i_0 + b \log|i| = a + b \log|i|, \quad (4.10)$$

where

$$b_a = \frac{2.303\, RT}{\alpha_a |z_a| F} \quad (4.11\text{a})$$

and

$$b_c = \frac{2.303\, RT}{(1-\alpha_c)|z_c| F} \quad (4.11\text{b})$$

are the anodic and cathodic Tafel constants.

Under the provision of pure charge transfer control of the overall process, the Tafel plot of $\log |i|$ vs $E - E_{oc}$ (stationary data) reveals linear sections in these regions, the slopes of which may be utilised for the determination of the b values. The intersection of the straight lines results in the corrosion current (density), as shown in Figure 4.6. The Tafel constants express the kinetics of the respective partial reactions. Typical values are 20–40 mV for the charge transfer of metal ions, whereas 120 mV was often measured for the cathodic hydrogen evolution. A detailed analysis of these data is beyond the scope of this chapter. However, a principal disadvantage of such an approach is that information on the kinetics of the electrode reactions and the corrosion rate is obtained from higher polarisation and current densities, which may be greater than i_{corr} by orders of magnitude. Thus, the applicability of this method is restricted to conditions where the mechanisms of the reactions will be unchanged during polarisation.

A second approach is based on the evaluation of the (stationary) current–potential curve of the specimen in a potential range of approximately 10 mV around E_{oc}. For this case, the exponential functions can be approximated by power series neglecting the third and later terms ($e^x \approx 1 + x$)

$$i = i_0\left[1 + \frac{\alpha|z_a|F\eta_t}{RT} - 1 + \frac{(1-\alpha c_c)|z_c|F\eta_t}{RT}\right]. \quad (4.12)$$

Insertion of the Tafel constants and rearrangement lead to the following equation first derived by Stern and Geary (cited in Heitz and Schwenk, 1976), where the slope di/dE can be easily determined from the experimental curve around E_{oc}

$$R_t = \left(\frac{d\eta_t}{di}\right)_{i=0} = \frac{1}{i_0}\frac{b_a b_c}{2.303(b_a + b_c)}. \quad (4.13)$$

With $b_a = 30\text{–}40$ mV and $b_c = 120$ mV, the quantity B is in the range of 10–13 mV.

$$B = \frac{b_a b_c}{2.303(b_a + b_c)}. \quad (4.14)$$

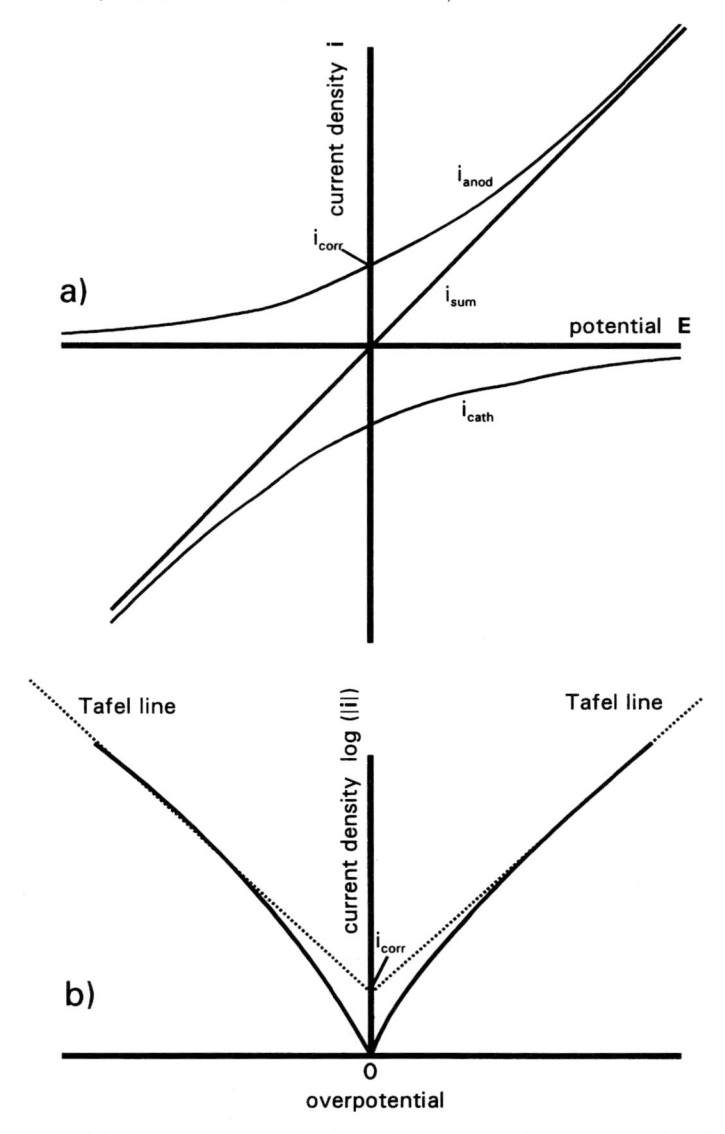

Figure 4.6 Tafel plot and determination of the corrosion current density: (a) i–E plot; (b) $\log(|i|)$–E plot.

Thus, differences in the anodic reaction mechanism, which are expressed in the given range of b_a, have only a slight influence on B.

This is also true in the case of a diffusion-controlled cathodic reaction ($b_c \to \infty$) giving $B = b_a/2.303 = 13$–17.5 mV

$$i_{corr} = \frac{b_a}{2.303} \frac{di}{dE}. \quad (4.15)$$

This means that B is relatively tolerant towards changes in the mechanisms of the partial reactions occurring on the corroding electrode.
Features of this method are:

- its small polarisation range
- its applicability for many systems
- that the Tafel constants or B must be known, where the latter may also be derived from gravimetric corrosion measurements.

A further method (Metikos-Hukovic and Zevnik, 1982; Rochini, 1984a–c) for the determination of parameters of charge transfer reactions [see Equation (4.5)] is based on a non-linear regression of the stationary experimental data in the polarisation range of 50–60 mV, referring to Equations (4.11a) and (4.11b). Using

$$\eta = E - E_{oc} \quad (4.16)$$

Equation (4.5) can be written as

$$i = i_0 \left[e^{\left(\frac{2.303(E-E_{oc})}{b_a}\right)} - e^{\left(\frac{-2.303(E-E_{oc})}{b_c}\right)} \right] \quad (4.17)$$

and non-linear regression results in the determination of all necessary parameters

$$E_{oc},\ b_a,\ b_c,\ i_0 = i_{corr}$$

simultaneously. The advantages of this method are the good theoretical foundation and the relatively narrow polarisation range.

Impedance spectrometry

Electrochemical impedance spectrometry (EIS) represents a recent method for determining the corrosion rate (Göhr, 1981; Jüttner et al., 1985). EIS aims to determine the transfer function of the WE, from which the charge transfer resistance and, hence, the corrosion rate can be derived. Moreover, the transfer function provides additional information on the processes of occurrence. The method is characterised by the measurement of the complex resistance of an electrochemical system. This is accomplished by applying an alternating (mostly sinusoidal) signal in a wide frequency range (typically <1 mHz–1 MHz). Similar to dc methods, either the WE potential or the current between WE and AE may be superimposed by this signal. To obtain significant spectra, the impedance should be determined at a minimum of five frequencies per decade. The potential change connected with the alternating polarisation must not exceed the linear range of the current–potential relationship around the rest potential (approximately ±10 mV) concerned, because all of the theoretical considerations are based on this prerequisite.

DEGRADATION (IN VITRO–IN VIVO CORROSION)

The measurements are performed using the three-electrode arrangement (see Figure 4.5). The determined impedance therefore contains an ohmic resistance corresponding to the solution between the capillary tip and the WE, as well as the phase boundary impedance of the WE. Two different forms of graphic representation have been introduced. The Nyquist plot (Figure 4.7) represents a complex plane (imaginary part Im vs real part Re) based on the equation

$$Z(\omega) = \text{Re} + j\,\text{Im}. \tag{4.18}$$

The more explicit form of this equation can be found in Chapter 14 (Equation 14.1). With equal scales of the axes, single features may be easily identified, e.g. R_iC combinations or diffusion elements. A drawback of this type of diagram is revealed when the system impedance spans a very wide range, so that low-impedance features may be overlooked.

In the second type of diagram, the Bode plot (Figure 4.8), log |Z| and φ or log (Re) and log (Im) are plotted in pairs against log f. These quantities are related to the components of the complex impedance by

$$|Z| = \sqrt{(\text{Re})^2 + (\text{Im})^2} \tag{4.19}$$

$$\varphi = \arctan(\text{Im}/\text{Re}). \tag{4.20}$$

In this manner, a uniform precision of the impedance spectrum is achieved throughout the total frequency range. The value of the graphic representations may be increased by plotting pseudo-three-dimensional graphs, for example, with log f on the abscissa, Re on the y-axis and Im on the z-axis.

Starting from a physically founded combination of impedance elements, an

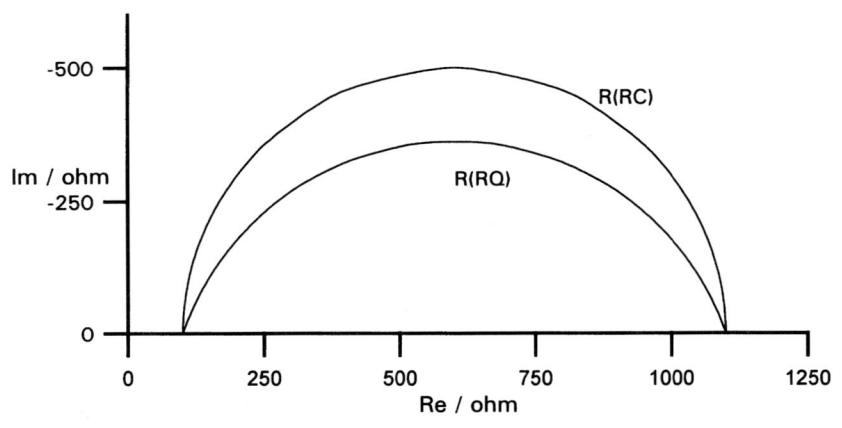

Figure 4.7 Nyquist plot: $R(RC)$: $R_{outer} = 100\ \Omega$, $R_{inner} = 1000\ \Omega$, $C = 10\ \mu F$; $R(RQ_{CPE})$: $R_{outer} = 100\ \Omega$, $R_{inner} = 1000\ \Omega$, $Q_{CPE} = 10^{-5}\ \Omega^{-1}$, $n_{CPE} = 0.8$.

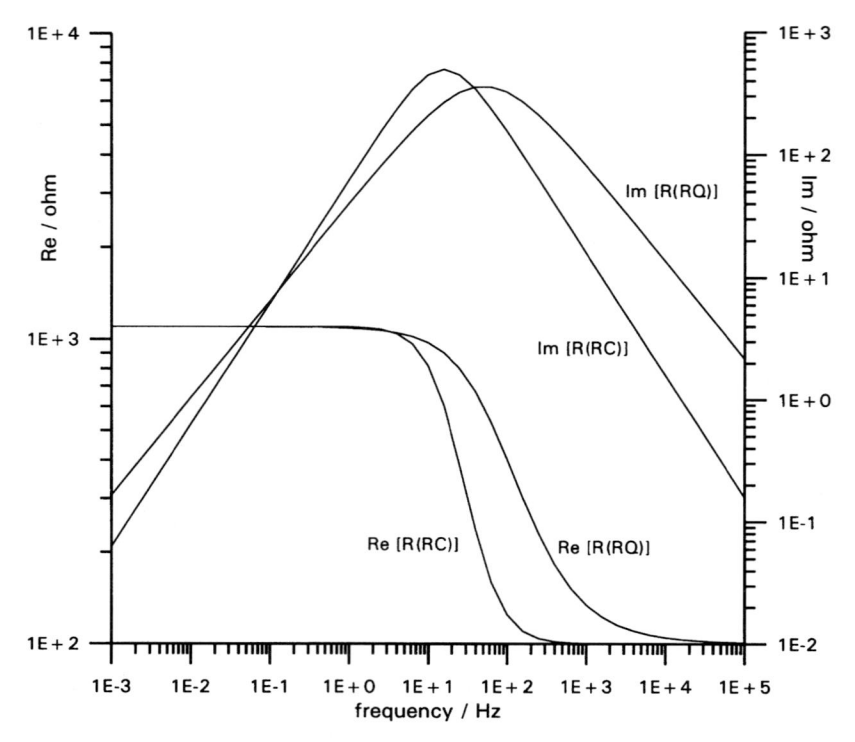

Figure 4.8 Bode plots: (a) log (Re) – log (Im) vs log (f) plot; (b) see opposite.

appropriate WE transfer model is developed and the parameter fit performed via non-linear regression using modern computation (Boukamp, 1993). It should be noted that the development and improvement of the transfer model is the decisive step in obtaining accurate results in the analysis of the measured impedance spectrum. This is due to the fact that a spectrum may be equally well described by different models of greater or lesser significance. Therefore, a maximum of information on the system under consideration should be integrated.

The most important electrochemical impedance elements will be presented and their transfer functions are compiled in Table 4.3. In usual transfer models the ohmic resistance R_i exists as either the electrolyte resistance or the charge transfer resistance, which is usually sought. A single ohmic resistance is reflected as a point on the real axis of a Nyquist plot, whereas in the log (Re) – log f and the log $|Z|$ – log f diagrams, a straight line parallel to the abscissa is formed. Im and φ are equal to zero over the whole frequency range.

At every metal–electrolyte interface a double layer is formed which can be modelled by a capacity. This element gives a line on the Im axis of the Nyquist plot ($Z = -j/\omega C$). In the log $|Z|$ – log f plot a capacity forms a straight line with a slope of -1. The phase angle is always $-90°$.

The simplest model of the transfer function of an electrode consists of a parallel

DEGRADATION (IN VITRO–IN VIVO CORROSION)

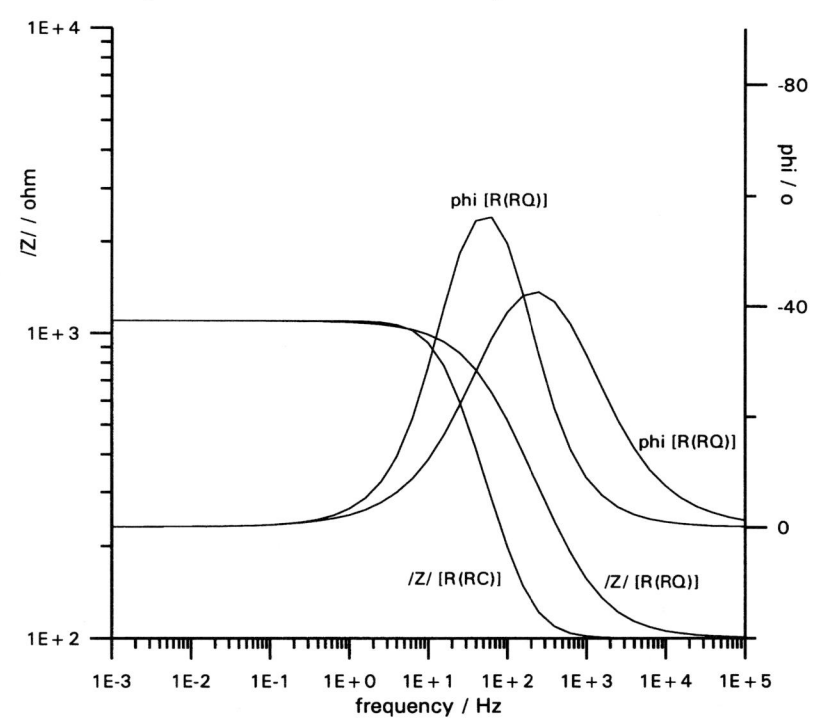

Figure 4.8 (*Continued*) (b) Log ($|Z|$) – phi vs log (f) plot. $R(RC)$: R_{outer} = 100 Ω, R_{inner} = 1000 Ω, C = 10 μF; $R(RQ_{CPE})$: R_{outer} = 100 Ω, R_{inner} = 1000 Ω, Q_{CPE} = 10^{-5} Ω^{-1}, n_{CPE} = 0.8.

arrangement of the transfer resistance R_t and the double layer capacity C_d, complemented by the electrolyte resistance R_e in series to the former (Figure 4.9). In the Nyquist plot, the spectrum of $\{R_e(R_iC_d)\}$ has the form of a semicircle (Figure 4.7, upper curve) with its ends at R_e (infinite frequency) and $R_s + R_t$ ($f \to 0$).

On the Bode plot (Figure 4.8), log (Re) shows two sections parallel to the abscissa with $|Z|$ = Re = $R_t + R_e$ and $|Z|$ = Re = R_e. In the region in between, the slope amounts to −1. The data for the model of Figures 4.7 and 4.9 are R_e = 100 Ω, R_t = 1000 Ω, and C_d = 10 μF.

In addition, a generally small inductive contribution L may occur at high frequencies owing to the leads contacting the cell. The graphic representations are similar to a capacity result (φ = +90°, slope +1).

The constant phase element (CPE) Q_{CPE} was introduced because in many cases of impedance measurements the centres of the Nyquist curves were found to be *below* the real axis (Figure 4.7, depressed semicircle $\{R_e(R_tQ)\}$ curve). It is obvious that modelling using only traditional elements is not successful.

The nature of the CPE is less clear. Experimentally, it could be indicated that the depression angle is related to the roughness of the WE (varying the final grain size

Table 4.3 Impedance elements and their transfer functions

Element	Symbol	Transfer function	Parameter
Resistance	R_i	R_i	R_i
Capacity	C	$-\dfrac{j}{\omega C}$	C
Inductivity	L	$j\omega L$	L
CPE	Q_{CPE}	$\dfrac{(j\omega)^{n_{CPE}}}{Y_o}$	Y_o, n_{CPE}
Warburg impedance	W	$\dfrac{1}{Y_o\sqrt{j\omega}}$	Y_o
Finite diffusion impedance	O	$\dfrac{\tanh\left[B_o\sqrt{j\omega}\right]}{Y_o\sqrt{j\omega}}$	Y_o, B_o

ω, Angular frequency, with $\omega = 2\pi f$. j, Imaginary unit, with $j = (-1)^{0.5}$.

during mechanical pretreatment) (Rammelt and Reinhard, 1990). Further, the concept of the fractal dimension of the surface was tentatively considered to interpret these findings (Pajkossy, 1991). At any rate, for $n_{CPE} = -1$ (Table 4.3) the transfer function is identical to that of a capacity, for $n_{CPE} = 0$ a simple resistance and for $n_{CPE} = 1$ an inductivity result.

The $\{R_e(R_tQ)\}$ model was also displayed in the Bode plot (Figure 4.8). Characteristic features are the reduced slopes occurring in the intermediate region of the log (Re) – log f curve and in both branches of the log (Im) – log f curve (for $f < f_{max}$ +0.8, for $f > f_{max}$ −0.8 corresponding to the figure of the exponent). Thus, this plot makes it possible to analyse the impedance behaviour if a CPE is involved.

The Warburg impedance W describes a classical diffusion process assuming that the concentration profile of the species concerned extends infinitely into the solution for $f \rightarrow 0$. In the Nyquist plot a straight line with a slope of 45° is formed (see Figure 4.7). Formally, this element is identical to a CPE of $n_{CPE} = -0.5$.

There is an important special case abbreviated with the letter O according to Boukamp, 1993, which applies to finite-length diffusion. This means that the concentration of the species at a definite distance from the phase boundary is considered to be equal to that in the bulk of the solution. Correspondingly, the limit of impedance for $f = 0$ is finite, achieved by an additional *tanh* factor in the transfer function. For high frequencies, O is identical to the Warburg impedance (decreasing diffusion length). The two diffusion impedance types are compared in Figure 4.9.

DEGRADATION (IN VITRO–IN VIVO CORROSION)

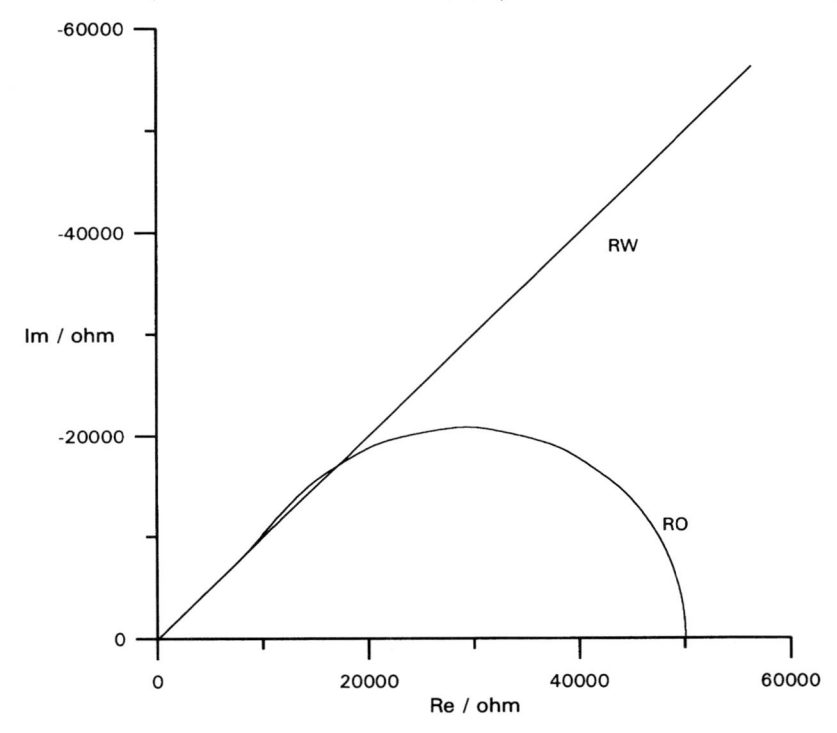

Figure 4.9 Comparison of the Warburg impedance and the finite-length diffusion impedance: RW: $R_i = 100\ \Omega$, $W = 10^{-5}\ \Omega^{-1}$; RO: $R_i = 100\ \Omega$, $Y_o = 10^{-5}\ \Omega^{-1}$, $B_o = 0.5\ s^{0.5}$.

Finite-length diffusion impedance was found to be operative in oxygen type of corrosion or in cases where diffusion was hindered by films on a metal surface. Impedance elements and their transfer functions are summarised in Table 4.3.

Impedance spectra of different oxide layers on titanium are compared in Figure 4.10 using Bode plots. Whereas the spectrum for the air-formed oxide layer shows only one time constant (one maximum in phase angle) the spectrum for the anodically formed oxide layer is more complex. This indicates that this oxide layer has a two-layer structure and that diffusion processes are taking place in the outer part of the oxide layer (Nocke et al., 1996).

Electrochemical noise measurements

This type of method is characterised by the measurement of low inherent potential or current fluctuations of an electrode. The electrode is not excited by an outer signal, unlike the methods discussed above, and will be examined practically by a non-destructive method. However, the very high resolution concerning both time and the electrical signal requires special electronic instrumentation and a

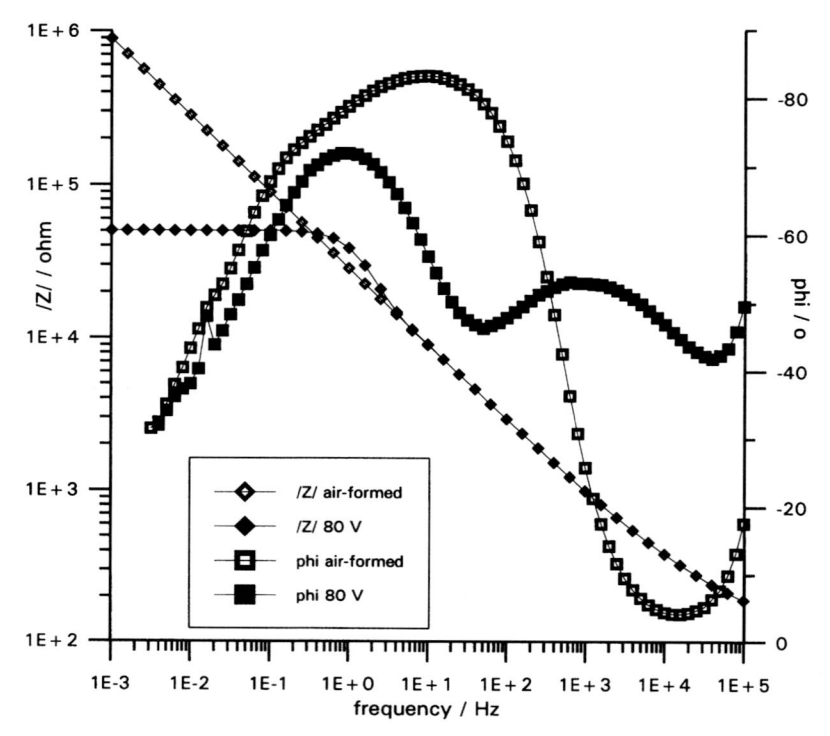

Figure 4.10 Bode plots of oxide layers on titanium (cf. Figure 4.17): (a) air formed oxide layer; (b) oxide layer formed anodically (formation voltage 80 V).

considerable expenditure on data analysis. These circumstances have prevented a broader application up to now. However, in principle this method is also suitable for *in vivo* applications, although no practical applications in this field could be found in the literature. Nevertheless, this promising method will be presented within this chapter.

The reason for the electrochemical noise will be explained for the case of an electrode corroding at the OCP. Over time, the average rates of the anodic and cathodic partial reactions are equal in amount. By recording the course of the potential with a high resolution, it is found that both partial reactions have undergone small fluctuations in intensity. For example, if the current produced by the cathodic reaction increases for a short time, the open circuit potential will become somewhat more positive and vice versa. In the case of a potentiostatic control of the open circuit potential, fluctuations may be seen in the net current around zero.

Electrochemical noise measurements are preferentially used for the detection of initial phases of local corrosion (see Section 4.2.3). It is possible to indicate the first changes in the electrode state well before a rise in the total current (as for until the onset of pitting (Hashimoto *et al.*, 1992a–c) or crevice corrosion (Pohl, 1996)) occurs.

DEGRADATION (*IN VITRO–IN VIVO* CORROSION)

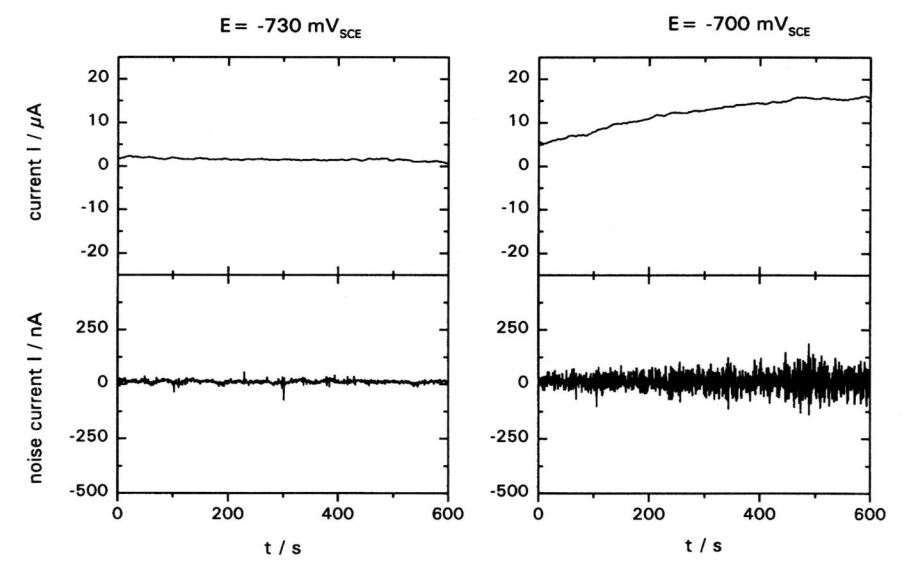

Figure 4.11 dc Current–time (upper) and noise current–time (lower) plots for the system Al/artificial sea water at different potentials (Pohl, 1996): (left) $E = -730$ mV$_{SCE}$, no crevice corrosion conditions; (right) $E = -700$ mV$_{SCE}$, crevice corrosion conditions.

Two types of graphic representation are in general use. Plots of signal amplitude vs time (Figure 4.11) often make it possible to derive initial conclusions on the nature of the processes and detailed information may be gained. Alternatively, after Fourier transformation into the frequency domain noise spectra are displayed by plotting the power density I^2/f or V^2/f vs f. Besides a more visual evaluation, classification after the generation of the probability of electrochemical noise events is used.

For a similar system, Figure 4.12 reflects the influence of the crevice width on the form of the power density spectra. It should be noted that the power density of noise increases with decreasing distance to the crevice corrosion potential. In contrast to the clear indication of anodic corrosion processes on the electrode, the dc signal was found to be nearly unchanged for all conditions so that information on the corrosion progress could not be derived from this quantity.

Application of the Scanning Kelvin Probe

The development of the scanning Kelvin microprobe as a tool for local corrosion studies is connected with the work of Stratmann (Stratmann and Streckel, 1990a, b; Stratmann *et al.*, 1990), which is in turn based on the studies of Gomer and Tryson (1977). The latter authors succeeded in relating the Volta potentials of metals, which depend on their work functions, to the electrochemical potentials. They indicated,

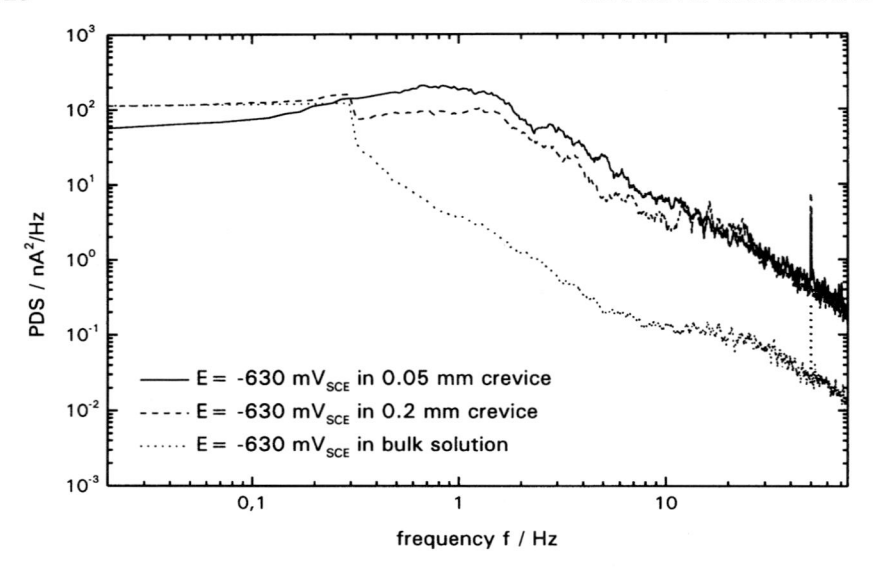

Figure 4.12 Power density spectra for the Al/artificial sea water system at constant potential and varying crevice widths (Pohl, 1996).

for example, that the potential of the standard hydrogen electrode at 298 K corresponds to a Volta potential of -4.73 ± 0.05 V.

Stratmann's work aimed at developing a method to permit the investigation of corrosion processes on metals covered with extremely thin adsorbed electrolyte layers, where conventional electrochemistry is not possible. The method utilises the contactless measurement of the Volta potential between two metals, one of them being the specimen to be investigated. Moreover, if the probe is made of a fine wire, a potential distribution can be recorded by scanning the surface of the specimen.

The electrical set-up may be roughly outlined as follows (see Figure 4.13). The probe and the specimen are connected in an outer circuit. Between them is a voltage which is identical to the Volta potential difference $\Delta\psi$, because their Fermi levels are equal. The probe is forced to perform a sinusoidal vibration perpendicular to the sur-

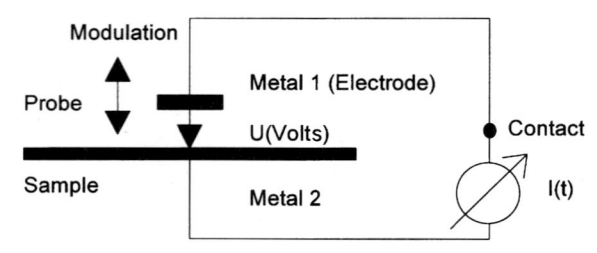

Figure 4.13 Scheme of the measuring principle of the Kelvin probe. (Reproduced by permission of UBM Messtechnik GmbH, Ettlingen.)

DEGRADATION (IN VITRO–IN VIVO CORROSION)

face of the specimen, with the vibration amplitude being smaller than the intermediary distance. This vibration causes a corresponding change in the capacitance C across the gap and an alternating current i

$$i = (\Delta\Psi\ E)\frac{dc}{dt}. \qquad (4.21)$$

By varying the outer voltage U until $i = 0$, U becomes equal to $\Delta\psi$. Based on the potential correlation mentioned above, a contactless determination of the electrochemical potential and its lateral distribution is achieved.

This technique may be applied in the following fields involving metallic biomaterials:

- investigation of the adsorption of biomolecules (see Chapter 6, Special thin organic coatings)
- modelling of galvanic corrosion phenomena in the oral cavity, i.e. under the conditions of thin electrolyte films
- investigations directed at the assessment of the quality and stability of oxide and other layers.

Figure 4.14 shows an example illustrating the latter topic. The diagrams indicate that mechanical damage to an anodically produced oxide layer on titanium (thickness approximately 200 nm) leads to a complete repassivation in air (Nocke et al., 1997). However, a considerably thinner film was formed because no interference colours appeared in the repassivated area. From investigations on the structure of the anodically formed oxide layers (Richter et al., 1996) it can be concluded that only a thin inner part of the oxide layer will be mainly responsible for passive behaviour. This is in good agreement with measurements on the structure and stability of oxide layers on aluminium (Hitzig et al., 1986). Also, in view of the assessment of biomaterials and their modification (Worch, 1996), much attention is paid to issues concerning the structure and properties of oxide layers (Nocke et al., 1996).

4.3.1.2 Other Methods for the Assessment of Corrosion Behaviour

At present, the European standards (i.e. EN ISO 1562, 1993; EN ISO 8891, 1995) in the field of metallic dental materials include a simple corrosion test of these materials, consisting of an immersion of specimens into a solution of 0.1 mol l^{-1} lactic acid and 0.1 mol l^{-1} NaCl (pH 2.2) at a temperature of 37°C for 7 days. The total amount of released metal ions in this period is measured either gravimetrically (EN ISO 8891) or by solution analytics, with AAS or OES, respectively (EN ISO 1562). According to *Dental Vademekum* (1995, p. 714), alloys with concentrations of <100 µg cm^{-2} are defined as being corrosion resistant. A conversion into corrosion currents assuming divalent metal ions of a molecular weight of 60 results in corrosion current densities of about 0.25 µA cm^{-2}.

The two standards differ in the shape of the test specimens and in the oxygen content of the test solutions. Whereas EN ISO 1562 prescribes testing in a closed

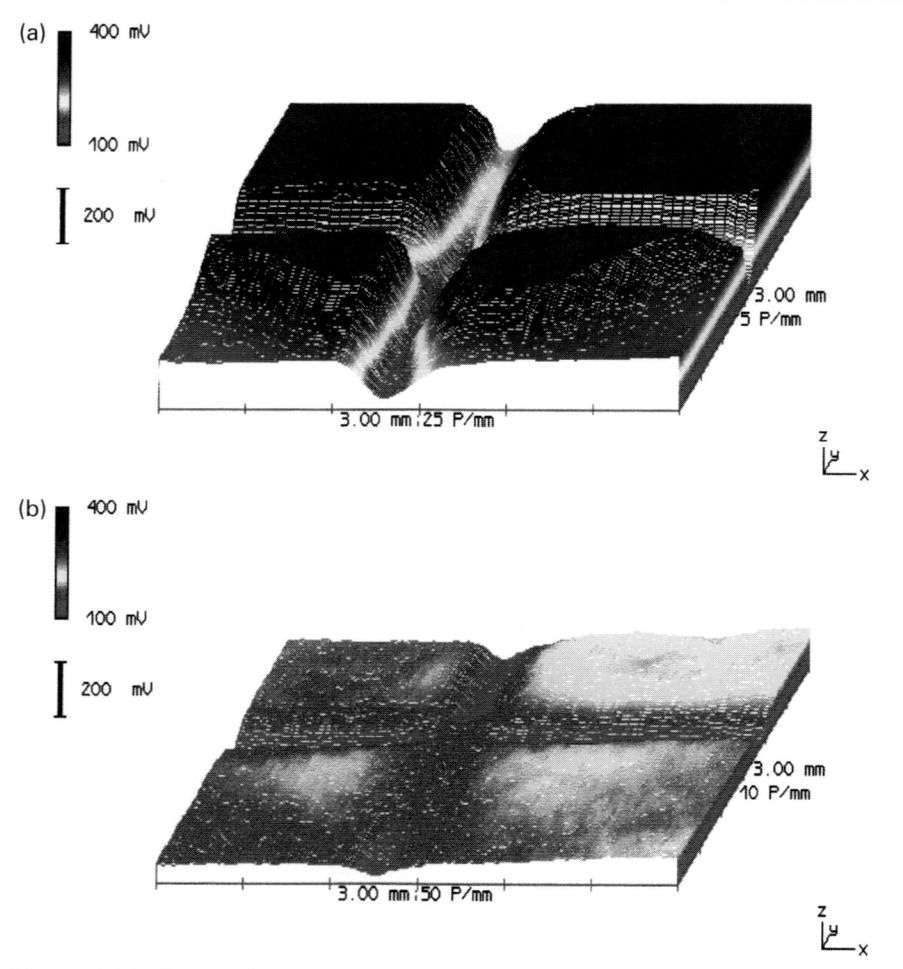

Figure 4.14 Potential distribution on scratched oxide-covered titanium based on the application of the scanning Kelvin microprobe: (a) 1 h after scratching; (b) 24 h after scratching; (c) see opposite.

container, standard EN ISO 8891 (1993) prescribes a continuously aerated solution. For materials with a high hydrogen overpotential (mercury alloys), where in comparatively acid solutions oxygen reduction is the dominating cathodic partial reaction, this should influence the results significantly. Because very thin electrolyte films are present on materials in the mouth cavity, for dental surgery testing according to EN ISO 8891 should be preferred. In addition to the real corrosion testing, the standard EN ISO 8891 includes a visual test of tarnish resistance as an immersion cyclic test in a 0.1 mol l^{-1} Na_2S solution.

DEGRADATION (IN VITRO–IN VIVO CORROSION)

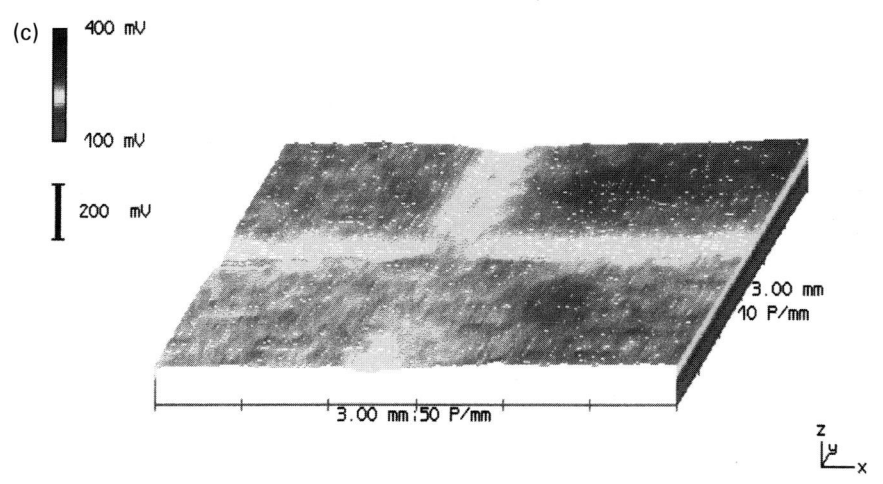

Figure 4.14 (*Continued.*) (c) 240 h after scratching.

4.3.1.3 Methods for the Investigation of Wear Behaviour

A detailed discussion of wear mechanisms will not be carried out in this chapter and can be found in the specialised literature (Zum Gahr, 1987; Lim and Ashby, 1987). The most important wear situations of metallic biomaterials, resulting from the fixation of implants using bone cement, screws and bolts, and in the hinge region of artificial implants are dealt with here.

The wear behaviour of artificial hip prostheses has been reviewed by Willmann (1996). Semlitsch and Weber (1992) have also discussed the wear behaviour of artificial hip prosthesis components and pointed out coating technologies for improved wear resistance.

Useful tribological test procedures (Unsworth, 1995) in this field, in the sense of screening methods, are the pin-on-disc and the ring-on-disc method. The ring-on-disc method is standardised according to DIN ISO 6474 (1992), and the pin-on-disc method according to ASTM G 99-90 (1990) and DIN 50324 (1992).

For usual testing media for wear resistance experiments see Section 4.3.1.4. Good *et al.* (1996) compared wear tests in water and bovine serum. They emphasise that for water-based tests these data raise serious doubts as to the validity of testing implant and material combinations as a predictor of clinical performance. Franke *et al.* (1996) used oscillating equipment operating without a medium for tribological investigations.

In summary, for these tests, it has to be pointed out that because the lubricating behaviour of synovial liquid can hardly be reproduced, comparative measurements will give only an initial indication of the *in vivo* behaviour.

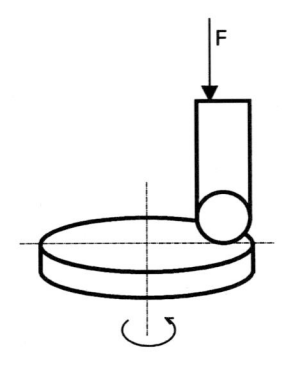

Figure 4.15 Schematic diagram of the pin-on-disc method.

4.3.1.4 Testing Media

Inorganic media

Investigations using purely inorganic testing media represent the simplest tests and at least provide a meaningful degree of testing the degradation behaviour of metallic biomaterials. Nevertheless, preliminary statements can be made especially on the stability against pitting corrosion followed by a selection of unfavourable materials.

Typical media are:

- isotonic NaCl solution
  9 g l^{-1} NaCl
- Ringer's physiological solution, pH 6.7 (Roche, 1993)
  8.00 g l^{-1} NaCl
  0.20 g l^{-1} CaCl$_2$
  0.20 g l^{-1} KCl
  1.00 g l^{-1} NaHCO$_3$.
  Ringer's physiological solution is often used in an acidic version (pH lowered to 2.5 by HCl) to simulate decreases in pH caused by inflammation processes.
- Hanks' balanced salt solution, pH 7.4 (Hanks and Wallace, 1949)
  0.185 g l^{-1} CaCl$_2$
  0.40 g l^{-1} KCl
  0.06 g l^{-1} KH$_2$PO$_4$
  0.10 g l^{-1} MgCl$_2 \cdot$6H$_2$O
  0.10 g l^{-1} MgSO$_4 \cdot$7H$_2$O
  8.00 g l^{-1} NaCl
  0.35 g l^{-1} NaHCO$_3$
  0.48 g l^{-1} Na$_2$HPO$_4$
  1.00 g l^{-1} D-glucose
  A similar solution with reduced concentrations of Ca^{2+} and HPO$_4^{2-}$ ions has also been used by Hanawa and Ota (1991).

Inorganic–organic media

- artificial saliva (Elagli *et al.*, 1993)
- bovine serum (Browne and Gregson, 1994; Good *et al.*, 1996)
- modified Eagle's medium (MEM) (Lacy *et al.*, 1996)
- Dulbecco's modified Eagle's medium (DMEM) (Lacy *et al.*, 1996)

4.3.1.5 Cell Line and Organ Culture Investigations

Cell-line and organ-culture investigations are situated in the boundary region between degradation and biocompatibility testing. Therefore, in this section only a short summary will be given. A detailed survey of the area of biocompatibility is given in Chapter 9 and also by Wintermantel and Suk-Woo Ha (1996). Experiments for testing the degradation of metallic biomaterials in cell lines and organ cultures are an important link between classic *in vitro* and *in vivo* investigations, in which organ-culture investigations are more convincing than cell-line experiments (Davies *et al.*, 1990).

Standard tests are fixed in both European and US standards (ASTM 813-83, 1992; DIN EN 30993, 1993; DIN V 13930, 1990).

The significance of the findings of related investigations is strongly influenced by the type of cell line used. Permanent lines have the advantage of comparability of the results between several laboratories without any difficulties (Table 4.4).

Primary cell cultures have the decisive advantage of their properties being far closer to those of a complete biosystem. Thus, the results are also more significant. Recently, there has been a significant trend towards the use of primary cell cultures. Table 4.5 gives a short survey of recent investigations. However, these investigations still show some disadvantages, in particular that the redox potential of a complete biosystem is not realised in cell-culture experiments.

The evaluation of cell-line experiments can be made with different specifications. Whereas, to some extent, only the shape and adhesion of cells (testing in flow equipment) are measured, more detailed investigations assess the proliferation and differentiation behaviour as well as the extent of protein synthesis and, in the case of osteoblasts, the appearance of a calcified matrix.

Table 4.4 Survey of frequently used permanent cell lines

Permanent cell cultures	Characteristics
MG 63	Human osteoblast-like (Martin *et al.*, 1995)
Balb/c 3T3	Fibroblasts (Wataha *et al.*, 1993; Richards *et al.*, 1995; Grant *et al.*, 1996)
MOLT 4	Human fibroblast-like (Berstein *et al.*, 1992)
X3T3 F10	Keratinocytes (Lacy *et al.*, 1996)
L-929	Mouse fibroblasts (Gebauer-Hartung *et al.*, 1995; Lacy *et al.*, 1996)

Table 4.5 Survey of frequently used primary cell lines

Primary cell cultures	Application
Human bone marrow cells	Response to Co–Cr corrosion products (Tomas et al., 1996)
	Attachment and adhesion (Verrier et al., 1996)
Human bone-derived cells	Initial cell attachment on different materials (Howlett et al., 1994)
Human tissue mast cells	Response to various metal cations (Schedle et al., 1995)
Human gingival fibroblasts	Structure and chemistry of Ti surfaces (Kononen et al., 1992)
	Topography of Ti surfaces (Chou et al., 1995)
	Comparative effects of Ninitol, Ni and Ti (Putters et al., 1992)
	Response to various metal cations (Schedle et al., 1995)
Rat calvarial osteoblasts	Expression of genes for cellular phenotype determining proteins on Ti6Al4V, hydroxyapatite and polystyrene (Puleo et al., 1993)
	Characterisation of titanium implant surfaces (Keller et al., 1994)
Rat gingival epithelial cells	Effect of scaling procedures on Ti (Kuempel et al., 1995)
Rat fibroblasts	Cell damage caused by direct contact with alloys (Evans, 1994)
Rat bone marrow cells	Interface to Ti (Davies et al., 1990)
	Osteogenic potential of Ca/P coatings (Hulshoff et al., 1995)

4.3.2 IN VIVO *INVESTIGATIONS*

The investigation of degradation processes in metallic implants is of special interest in the case of permanent implants. To some degree, pronounced degradation phenomena arising in temporary implants, as a result of friction and wear on bone marrow nails in the tibia region between the marrow nail and the fixative bolt, have so far been investigated only from the immunological point of view because of the comparatively short period of storage. These aspects are described in detail in Chapters 9, 10 and 12.

The main method of investigation for *in vivo* degradation is the determination of the concentrations of essential constituents of the implant material in the direct implant environment as well as in body fluids (e.g. serum and urine). In this way Michel *et al.* (1984, 1987, 1991) performed long-term studies on the release of heavy metals from cobalt–chromium alloys from hip joint prostheses.

Such investigations are being carried out because of the comparatively frequent appearance of particulate polyethylene generation when this material is used in sliding pairings of hip joint endoprostheses. In connection with considerations regarding the repeated use of metal/metal sliding pairings, which was typical in the 1970s, the patient groups involved are being investigated more intensively. According to the investigations of Jacobs *et al.* (1996) patients who had had artificial hip joints (McKee–Farrar implants) with CoCr–metal/metal sliding pairings for more than 20 years showed increased serum concentrations (nine times higher) and even more increased urine chromium concentrations (35 times higher) compared with control groups without artificial hip joints. The serum cobalt concentrations were only about three times higher. The values of a patient group with implant storage periods of <2 years were about three to four times higher than those of a group with implant periods of >20 years.

Recent studies of animal models in which different materials were investigated comparatively are given in Table 4.6. These studies reflect the tendency in the development of new implant materials towards titanium and titanium alloys as well as coated materials, as supported by testing in comparison with classical materials.

4.4 METALLIC BIOMATERIALS

At present, around 930 alloys (including solders) are used in Germany in the field of dental prosthetics (*Dental Vademekum*, 1995, p. 1040). Therefore, this chapter will concentrate on the most important groups of metallic biomaterials.

At first glance, some confusion may be caused by the following classification of metallic biomaterials into

Table 4.6 Degradation of metallic biomaterials in animal tests

Animal model	Materials under investigation
Rabbit tibia	NiTi, vitallium, cp–titanium, SAF, 316L (Berger-Gorbet *et al.*, 1996)
	Ti alloys, coatings of TiO_2 and Ti_5Si_3 (Kitsugi *et al.*, 1996)
Rabbit femoral cortical bone	cp-Ti, TiO_2/hydroxyapatite-ceramics (Fartash *et al.*, 1995)
	cp-Ti with different values of surface roughness (Wennerberg *et al.*, 1995)
Skin and deep tissue of hamsters	Distribution of Ni and Co ions (Lacy *et al.*, 1996)
Goat maxilla	Different CaP-coated implants, cp-titanium (Hulshoff *et al.*, 1996)
Sheep tibia diaphyses	Stainless steel with and without hydroxyapatite coating (Stea *et al.*, 1995)

- noble metals, derived alloys and amalgams
- materials of elements of the VIth–VIIIth group of d-elements of the periodic system
- titanium and its alloys

but this classification proves meaningful for electrochemical and thermodynamic reasons and considering the properties of passive layers.

The degradation stability of noble metals and derived alloys is caused mainly thermodynamically (strongly positive standard potentials). The stability of the following two groups can be derived from dense thin oxide layers (passive layers) on the surface of these materials which effectively protect against corrosion.

However, the properties of the passive layers of the materials consisting of elements of the VIth–VIIIth group of d-elements differ significantly from those of titanium and its alloys. This is of special importance because only the surfaces of biomaterials interact with the bioenvironment.

Figure 4.16 shows a comparison of the current density–potential curves of gold, iron-based and cobalt-based alloys, Ti6Al4V and some valve metals (Ta, Nb) in a NaCl solution containing the redox system $Fe(CN)_6^{3-}/Fe(CN)_6^{4-}$. Whereas in the cathodic region all materials show significant current densities (reduced for Ta), in the anodic region the redox system does not react with the valve metals (or, scarcely worth mentioning, Ti6Al4V). This behaviour is caused by the different conduction mechanisms in the passive layers of the materials. The passive layers formed on materials of elements of the VIth–VIIIth group of d-elements are electron conducting, i.e. there is an equilibrium between the energy levels of the electrons in the metal and at the phase boundary of the oxide/electrolyte, and the redox system can be oxidised or reduced.

Based on the electronic properties of its oxide layers, titanium belongs to the valve metals (like aluminium, tantalum, niobium and zirconium). The oxide layers of these metals are n-type semiconductors or isolators, respectively. In anodic polarisation at least, as is the normal case in a bioenvironment because of the typical redox potential of about 200 mV_{SCE} in biosystems, such oxide layers are only ion conducting and no electronic charge transfer is possible, i.e. the redox system can be reduced but cannot be oxidised. This is of great importance for the behaviour of these types of biomaterial in a bioenvironment and is discussed in the corresponding chapters of this book.

Apart from the above-named materials, the search for the replacement of amalgams in the field of dental surgery has led to various new developments (e.g. gallium alloys). These materials and other special developments will be discussed in a separate section.

The coating of metallic biomaterials has various aims. Besides aesthetic effects, particular emphasis is placed on the improvement in biocompatibility, increased degradation stability, the optimisation of physicochemical surface properties and the improvement of wear resistance.

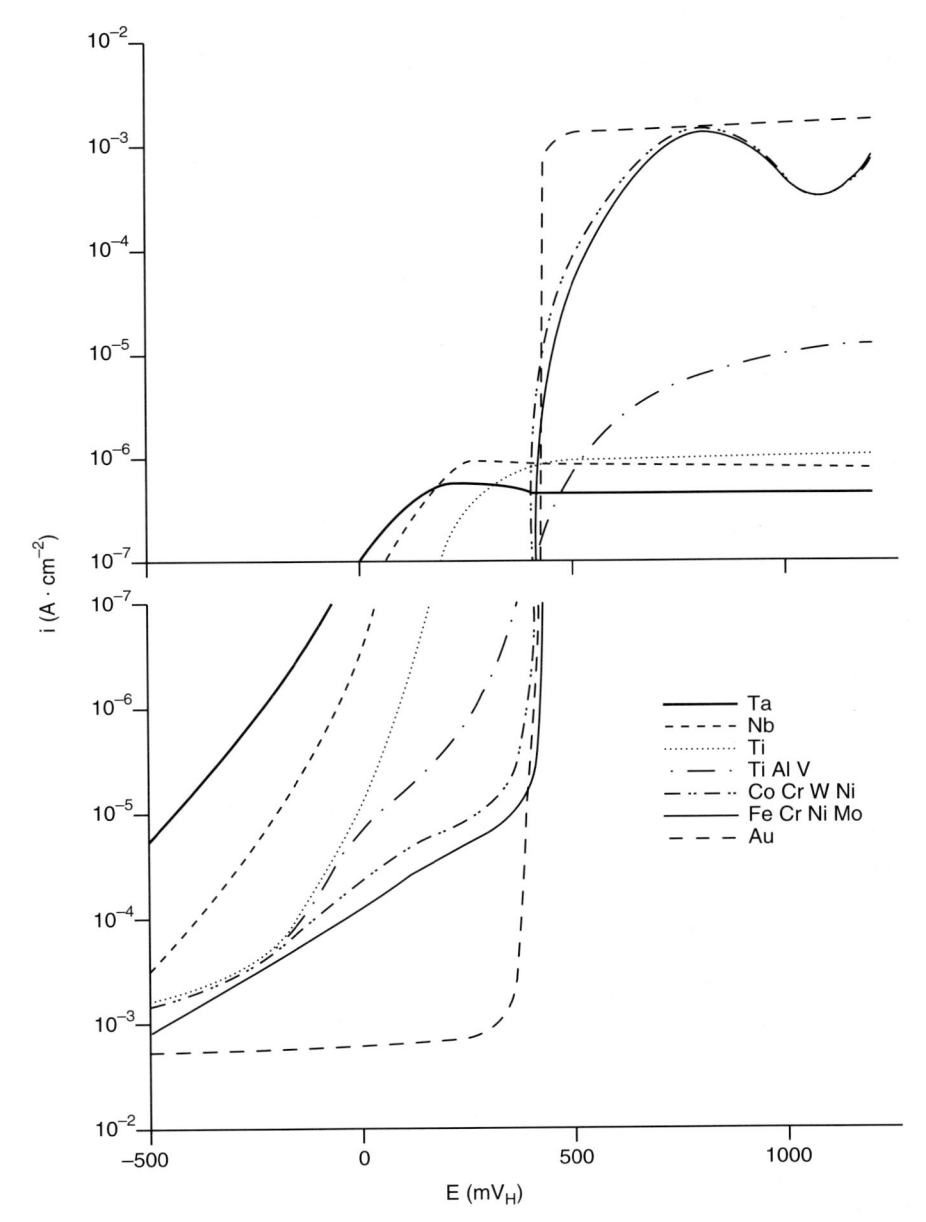

Figure 4.16 Current density–potential curves of the tested metals in saline with a stable redox system. Polarisation rate: 600 mV h^{-1}. (Reproduced with permission from Zitter and Plenk, 1987.)

4.4.1 NOBLE METALS, DERIVED ALLOYS AND AMALGAMS

Several authors (Mann and Lenz, 1992; Canay and Oktemer, 1992) have investigated comparatively the electrochemical corrosion behaviour of prostodentic alloys. Following a classification into high-gold, low-gold and palladium–silver groups, and using nickel–chromium-based alloys as a reference, the authors found very different corrosion behaviour. Whereas high-gold alloys were extremely resistant to corrosion, the resistance of the other alloys decreased from palladium–silver, low-gold to nickel–chromium alloys. The determination of the type of corrosion attack revealed pitting corrosion for nickel–chromium alloys and the selective dissolution of the phases rich in silver for the palladium–silver alloys. The corrosion resistance of the noble alloys was far superior to that of the nickel–chromium-based alloys.

In the dental laboratory the influence of casting on the corrosion behaviour of 45 palladium-based alloys was investigated by Brauner and Haussner (1989). Based on the results of potentiodynamic polarisation under quasi-potentiostatic conditions, the alloys were classified as:

- type 1: showing a flat curve without pronounced corrosion peaks, corresponding to high-gold alloys
- type 2: showing one marked peak
- type 3: having several pronounced corrosion peaks, resembling the well-known silver-based alloys.

Casting changed the corrosion behaviour in types 2 and 3 more significantly than in type 1. Alloys of types 1 and 2 alloys contained gallium.

Sliding-induced wear tests have been performed by Satoh et al. (1992) using a modified pin-on-disc method. In a comparison of three types of high-strength denture teeth, three types of conventional plastic denture teeth, porcelain teeth and metal teeth (Pd alloy), the metal showed the worst behaviour in both wear depth and weight loss.

The response of different cell types to various metal ions potentially released from dental alloys has been investigated by Schedle et al. (1995). The rank order of potency (lowest observed level) for human gingival fibroblasts was:

$$Pt^{4+} > Ag^+ > Au^{3+} > Sn^{3+} > Ga^{3+} > Ni^{2+} > Co^{2+} > Zn^{2+}$$
$$> Cu^{2+} > Cr^{3+} > Pd^{2+} > Mo^{5+} > Sn^{2+}.$$

A similar rank order was found for L-929 fibroblasts. In primary human mast cells in the dose range tested (3.3 µM–1 mM) only Ag^+ and Au^{3+} caused dose-dependent histamine release. In these tests, Pd showed good behaviour compared with other alloy components (such as Ag, Au and Pt) used in dental applications. However, because for several reasons palladium has started to displace both amalgam and gold in dental fillings, the sensitisation rate for palladium is increasing (2.8% according to a European study; 8.3% in Austria) (Aberer et al., 1993).

4.4.2 MATERIALS OF ELEMENTS OF THE VITH–VIIITH GROUP OF D-ELEMENTS OF THE PERIODIC SYSTEM

The corrosion behaviour of these materials, which also belong to the classic metallic biomaterials and are less often applied, is based on the formation of electron-conducting passive layers. The stability of these passive layers decisively dominates the corrosion processes, which is due to the interaction with the bioenvironment.

The main groups of materials groups are (see Chapters 1 and 2):

- stainless steels 304L, 316L and comparable compositions
- cobalt-based alloys of the CoCrMo and CoCrWNi type, with some restrictions
- nickel-based alloys of the NiCrMo type.

A detailed survey of investigations into the corrosion of these materials is given by Steinemann (1980).

The upper limiting concentrations of carbon (≤ 0.03 and 0.02 wt%), phosphorus and sulfur in the preferably used 316L steel as well as the duplex type 25Cr7Ni4MoN steel are considerably diminished (Kohn, 1992). This leads to a distinct decrease in the susceptibility of these materials to local corrosion. Additionally, the molybdenum content of the duplex steel induces a positivation of the pitting potential. Nevertheless, for these materials both pitting corrosion and crevice corrosion were observed (Williams, 1981).

The corrosion rates of CoCrMo alloys and stainless steels were compared to those of titanium and its alloys *in vivo* by Steinemann (1980). Whereas the values for steels and Co-based alloys were 20–26 $\mu g\ cm^{-2}\ day^{-1}$, for titanium and its alloys values of about 11 $\mu g\ cm^{-2}\ day^{-1}$ were determined. Taking the values of corrosion resistance of metallic biomaterials in the field of dental surgery required by the European standards of $<14.3\ \mu g\ cm^{-2}\ day^{-1}$ (see Section 4.3.1.2.) as a basis, only titanium and its alloys meet these standards.

In 1993, the Bundesgesundheitsamt (Federal Health Department) made recommendations (*Dental Vadenekum*, 1995, p. 1042) for minimum alloy compositions of the materials in the field of dental surgery. Consequently, nickel-based alloys should contain at least 20 wt% of chromium and 4 wt% of molybdenum, whereas nickel, cobalt and chromium should comprise in total at least 85 wt% of the composition. For cobalt-based alloys at least 25 wt% of chromium and 4 wt% of molybdenum as well as a total amount of cobalt, nickel and chromium of at least 85 wt% are recommended.

4.4.3 TITANIUM AND ITS ALLOYS

Proceeding from first clinical applications in 1951 (Laing, 1979), titanium and its alloys have in recent years become increasingly established as metallic biomaterials. Besides the high-strength alloy Ti6Al4V, which has not been developed specifically for medical use, at present there is a trend for substituting vanadium as a stabiliser of the β-phase with iron or niobium, because of vanadium's toxic properties (Semlitsch and Weber, 1992).

The primary reasons for the widespread and increasing use of these materials are their excellent corrosion behaviour and biocompatibility. The corrosion stability of titanium is due to an n-semiconducting passive layer of the formula $Ti_{1+\delta}O_2$ on the surface. The thickness of an air-formed passive layer is less than 20 nm. At normal potential conditions of the bioenvironment, this passive layer is completely ion conducting, in contrast to the passive layers discussed in Section 4.4.2. The dissolution rate of $Ti_{1+\delta}O_2$ of about 0.043 nm day^{-1} (Allard et al., 1975) at the physiological pH value of 7.4 is of minor importance for medical use because the body fluids are saturated with titanium ions (Maeusli et al., 1986).

Starting from the fact that the surface properties of a biomaterial mainly determine its interactions with the bioenvironment, these relations will be pointed out exemplarily for titanium. This is supported by the fact that the excellent biocompatibility is frequently considered with respect to the surface chemistry of the passive layer (Schmidt, 1992; Thull, 1995).

It is well known that under atmospheric conditions the surface of titanium is always covered with an oxide layer of TiO_2. This oxide layer, with a thickness of several nanometers, is amorphous, and thickening, e.g. by anodic electrochemical polarisation depending on the potential, leads to the appearance of crystalline phases (rutile and anatase). By reduction starting from TiO_2, a series of understoichiometric titanium oxides of the general formula Ti_nO_{2n-1}, the magneli phases, can be produced.

According to Boehm (Boehm and Hermann, 1967; Hermann and Boehm, 1969; Flaig-Baumann et al., 1970; Hermann et al., 1970; Boehm, 1971) the surface of titanium oxide in aqueous solutions is hydroxylated. Here, two types of OH groups existing nearly to the same extent with different pK values (pK_1 = 2.9, pK_2 = 12.7) have to be distinguished. The groups of alkaline character singly co-ordinated to titanium cations can be exchanged by other anions in acid solutions. The H$^+$ of the double co-ordinated acid OH groups can be exchanged by other cations in alkaline solutions.

The isoelectric point measured for pure crystalline TiO_2 to pH 6.4 (positive surface charge for pH < 6.4 and negative surface charge for pH > 6.4) (Janssen and Stein, 1986) coincides well with the pK values of the surface OH groups. Nevertheless, the present crystalline titanium oxide phase scarcely influences the isoelectric point in spite of the different band gaps for anatase (3.3 eV) and rutile (3.1 eV). However, pollution of the titanium oxide can cause shifts in the isoelectric point up to 2 pH units into the alkaline region (Janssen and Stein, 1986). This was also confirmed by Schröder (1988), who showed that the isoelectric point of TiO_2 can be shifted considerably by coating.

Until now, no cases have been reported for titanium and its alloys in which biodegradation without mechanical damage or fretting corrosion would have caused implant failure. However, because of the improper use of Ti6Al4V for cemented artificial hip implants, a series of drastic failures caused by fretting corrosion and crevice corrosion have been documented (Willert et al., 1996). The primary reason for failure is the higher hardness and stiffness of polymethylmetacrylate (PMMA) in

DEGRADATION (IN VITRO–IN VIVO CORROSION)

comparison with the titanium alloy. Starting with a crevice formation followed by fretting corrosion of the titanium alloy caused by the PMMA in the proximal region, heavy crevice corrosion is finally initiated in the distal region. The necessary revision of the implant frequently within a year is the serious consequence.

The very good *in vivo* corrosion stability of titanium and its alloys can be further improved by increasing the thickness of the passive layer (Browne *et al.*, 1996). The use of electrochemical methods (Figure 4.17) offers the advantage that the procedure works at nearly physiological conditions (Born *et al.*, 1998). In this way, the optimised interaction of amphoteric surface OH groups of the titanium oxide with the bioenvironment shown by Browne *et al.* (1996) can be further improved.

Pan *et al.* (1994) reported of the occurrence of dark pigmented layers when titanium implants with air-formed passive layers were used *in vivo*. They succeeded in reproducing analogous layers *in vitro* by storage of implants in H_2O_2 containing solutions for a period of several weeks. It seems to be obvious that the layers *in vivo* were generated under similar conditions, i.e. in the presence of oxygen or OH radicals.

Souto and Burstein (1996) carried out preliminary comparative *in vitro* corrosion investigations on wires of cp-titanium (dia. 50 µm) and Ti6Al4V (dia. 250 µm) in Ringer's physiological solution. They found that, in contrast to cp-titanium in the alloy, transient microscopic breakdowns of the passive state occurred. The duration

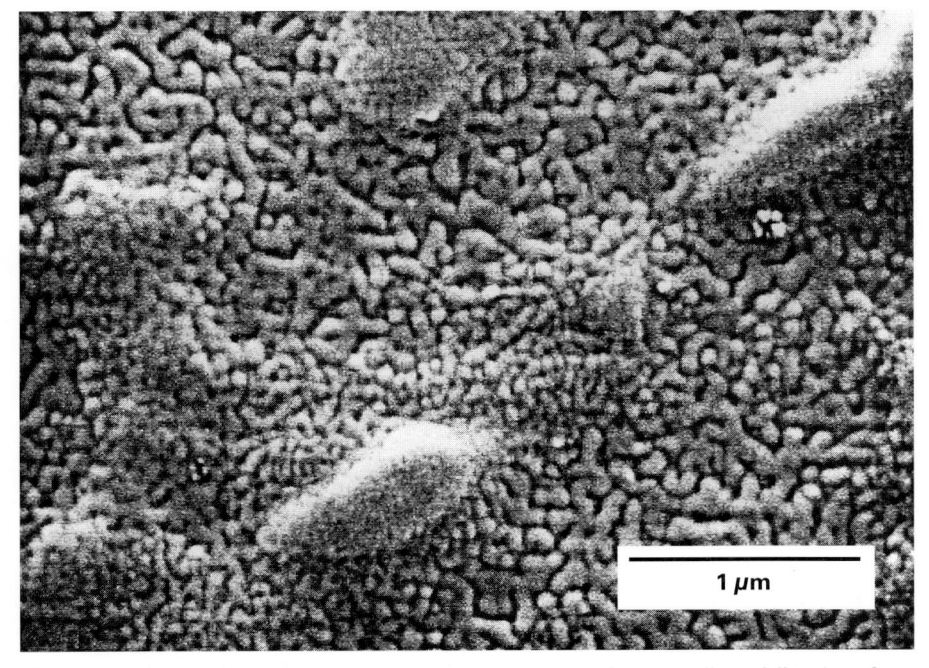

Figure 4.17 Scanning electron-microscopic image of an anodic oxidised surface of Ti6Al4V (formation voltage 80 V; oxide thickness ≈ 200 nm): nm structure of the oxide layer surface (cf. Figure 4.10).

of the single events was significantly shorter than 1 s and typical repassivation currents were of about 0.7 nA (maximally 3 nA). The calculation of typical charge quantities (~50 pC) and the assumption of complete transfer to TiO_2 gives about 2×10^6 nm^3 (density rutile 4.26 g cm^{-3}; Lide, 1993). The additional assumption that local corrosion forms hemispherical pits corresponds to diameters of about 200 nm.

Because of the very different diameters of the wires used in the investigations and because no metallographic investigations were conducted, besides the influence of the composition, an effect of the microscopic structure of the materials (grain boundary density) on the results of the investigations has to be taken into consideration.

For the alloy Ti6Al4V a negative influence of high surface vanadium content caused by unfavourable heat treatments is repeatedly discussed as being potentially toxic (Breme, 1989). Other investigations have shown that the vanadium content in the oxide layers is strongly diminished compared with that in the alloy (Hanawa and Ota, 1991; Leitao et al., 1995; Browne et al., 1996; Stölzel, 1996).

Ducheyne and Healy (1988) investigated the corrosion of Ti6Al4V in *in vitro* immersion experiments in Hanks' balanced solution with 1.5 mM EDTA, pH 6.4. These investigations also showed that the emission of vanadium ions from the alloy is considerably lowered compared with the portion of vanadium in the metallic phase (Table 4.7).

Keller *et al.* (1994) investigated cp-Ti and the alloy Ti6Al4V by means of a series of surface characterisation techniques [X-ray photoelectron spectroscopy (XPS), wetting angle], together with short-term *in vitro* biological assays to assess the effects of the material selection on osteoblast-like cell responses. The XPS measurements showed an enrichment of aluminium by a factor of about 5, whereas there was a depletion of vanadium in the oxide layers by a factor of more than 2. Determinations of equilibrium wetting angles for the two materials revealed insignificant differences for smooth, polished surfaces (cp-Ti 52 ± 2°, Ti6Al4V 56 ± 4°). The levels of cell attachment and adaptation of the attached cells to the surfaces of both materials were similar.

McGovern *et al.* (1996) studied the *in vivo* wear behaviour of femoral heads of 'monobloc' Ti6Al4V artificial hip implants in a retrieval study (implants retrieved after periods of 78–131 months). No consistent correlations were found between

Table 4.7 Corrosion of Ti6Al4V in HBSS with 1.5 mM EDTA, pH 6.4 (Ducheyne and Healy, 1988)

Immersion duration (weeks)	Ions in solution (ng ml^{-1} normalised)		
	Ti	Al	V
1	28.2 (90)	0.8 (2.55)	Not detectable
2	59.2 (90)	1.5 (2.28)	1.1 (1.67)
4	78.3 (90)	3.6 (4.13)	1.5 (1.72)

DEGRADATION (IN VITRO–IN VIVO CORROSION)

classical surface roughness parameters and the clinical parameters studied (patient's gender, weight and height, primary diagnosis, implantation time, etc.). They concluded that wear mechanisms *in vivo* are complex and that wear of the femoral heads under investigation can be attributed to a combination of an imperfect nature of the surface before implantation, removal of the oxide layer causing abrasion of the alloy, subsequent deformation of the bearing surface and, to a very small degree, patient parameters.

4.4.4 SPECIAL MATERIALS

In dental surgery a number of projects has been aimed at developments replacing amalgams with gallium-based alloys because of concerns about mercury toxicity (see Chapters 1 and 2). Oshida and Moore (1993) investigated the anodic polarisation behaviour of a gallium-based alloy in deoxygenated Ringer's solution at 37°C, either uncoupled or coupled with high-copper dental amalgam. For the uncoupled gallium-based alloy at low overpotentials a selective dissolution of divalent tin ions, followed by a dissolution of Ga, was detected. Furthermore, the uncoupled gallium-based alloys and the gallium alloy coupled with amalgam showed anodic current densities 10^3–10^4 times higher than that of an uncoupled amalgam, suggesting very poor corrosion stability.

Concerning possible toxic consequences, Chandler *et al.* (1994) compared the cytotoxicity of gallium and indium ions with that of mercuric ions in a concentration range of 1 μM–1 mM using L-929 mouse fibroblasts. Whereas for mercuric ions a 50% inhibition concentration of 0.35 mM was found, gallium and indium ions did not significantly inhibit dehydrogenase activity in either the growing or the confluent phase. These results are more critical than those of Oshida and Moore (1993), especially concerning the concentration range tested.

Furthermore, Okamoto and Hidaka (1994) studied the effects of metal ions used in dental materials on the conversion of amorphous calcium phosphate to hydroxyapatite *in vitro*. According to effects on both the rate of hydroxyapatite transformation and the induction time, metal ions were classified into three types:

- inhibitory (in the order Ni, Sn, Co, Mn, Cu, Ga, Th, Mo, Cd, Sb, Mg, Hg)
- ineffective (Cs, Ti, Cr, Fe^{2+})
- stimulatory (Fe^{3+}, In).

Although the possible conclusions of these findings are not yet completely clear, this investigation indicates possible negative effects, when using gallium-containing dental materials of unfavourable corrosion behaviour.

4.4.5 COATED METALLIC BIOMATERIALS, SURFACE FINISHING

Processes for coating biomaterials are discussed in detail in Chapter 5. This section covers the corrosion and wear processes related to biomaterials modified by coating processes.

The application of coatings for biomaterials has a variety of objectives, such as:

(1) improvements to the aesthetic properties
(2) improvements in the corrosion behaviour
(3) optimised wear resistance
(4) improvements in physicochemical and biochemical properties
(5) use of ceramic coatings (e.g. dental surgery and hydroxyapatite coating for implants).

For this reason, a great number of coating processes are used, and ion implantation will also be included in this chapter.

Because of the very complex strains acting on the biomaterials in a bioenvironment, optimised properties for a specific strain profile will often not have an overall improving effect but will frequently be connected with disadvantages in other profiles. In this way, improved mechanical properties resulting from coatings often lead to a lowered corrosion stability of the treated surfaces.

Examples of a combination of objectives (1), (2) and (3) are nitride layers on CoCr-based alloys, which are often used in dental surgery. Objective (4) also includes processes aimed at coating with porous layers for improved ingrowth of bones into implant surfaces and therefore improved mechanical conditions in the bone–implant interface (Ducheyne, 1983; AESCULAP, 1989). Related coating processes as well as the advantages and disadvantages of modified implants, including mechanical and chemical results due to corrosion, are reviewed by Pilliar (1987).

A similar method to the use of porous coatings is surface treatment of implants using blasting abrasives such as corundum and related materials. This treatment aims at an enlargement of the contact area between the implant and bone in order to optimise the interaction with the bioenvironment. Occasionally in blasting treatments, the blasting material is incorporated into the implant surface (Figure 4.18), so that thorough cleaning after the blasting treatment is absolutely necessary.

Leitao et al. (1995) investigated the influence of N^+ implantation on the corrosion behaviour of Ti6Al4V in Hanks' solution. For implantation energies of 40 keV they observed a minimum of the corrosion current density in the passive region for doses of 10^{16} ions cm^{-2} N^+. For lower doses no effect was seen, whereas for higher doses the corrosion current density increased significantly.

Ducheyne and Healy (1988) investigated *in vitro* the effect of plasma-sprayed calcium phosphate ceramic coatings on the metal ion release from porous Ti6Al4V and cobalt–chromium alloys. After immersion in Hanks' balanced solution with 1.5 mM EDTA, pH 6.4, a decrease in the titanium ion emission of about one to two orders of magnitude was measured, while the emission of aluminium ions was only lowered by a factor of about 2. A decrease was also observed for vanadium ions, but could hardly be quantified because of the low overall concentrations, which were always close to the detection limit.

Plasma spraying of cobalt–chromium alloys did not bring about any decrease in ion emission.

DEGRADATION (*IN VITRO–IN VIVO* CORROSION) **143**

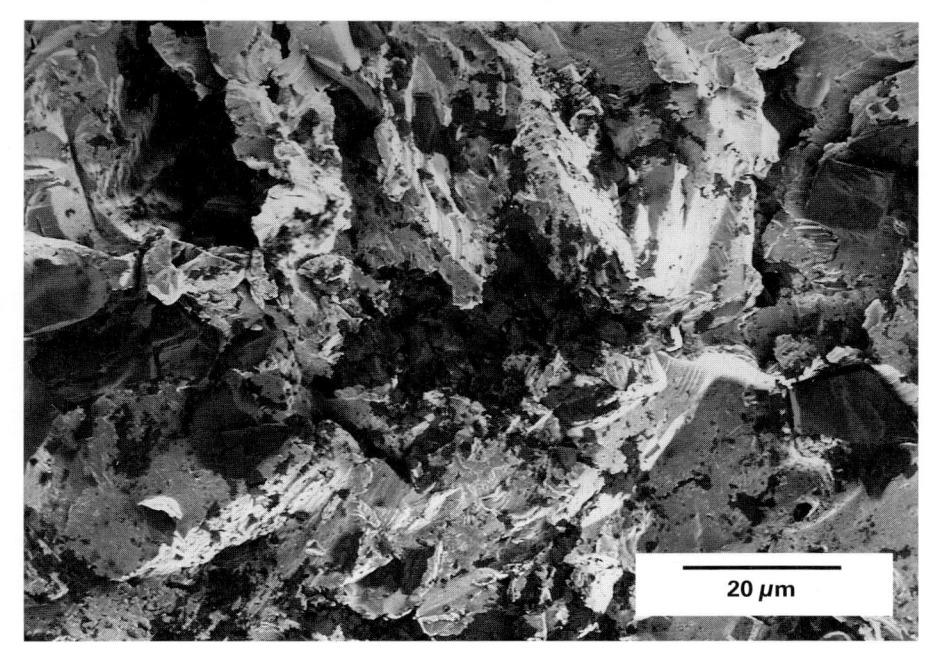

Figure 4.18 SEM image of corundum inclusions in a blasted Ti6Al4V surface (dark phases).

4.4.6 COMBINATIONS OF METALLIC BIOMATERIALS

As already mentioned in the first part of this chapter, local corrosion effects are one of the main reasons for the failure of metallic biomaterials. Besides pitting corrosion, intergranular corrosion and crevice corrosion, galvanic corrosion causes drastic local corrosion, mainly generated by an electron-conducting connection of different materials.

In Section 4.2.3.3, the electrochemical boundary conditions for the occurrence of galvanic corrosion in combinations of materials were given. In the field of dental surgery, the more craftsman-like techniques used in the dental laboratory may cause additional supplementary disadvantageous changes in the structure of the materials as a result of heat treatment during welding or soldering.

In a recent contribution, Romann (1995) investigated short-circuit potentials and local currents combining titanium with several other alloys in a 1% NaCl solution (pH 6.3), in part with 10% lactic acid (pH 1.81).

The main results may be summarised as follows:

- in combination with noble metal alloys, titanium acts as the local anode, and because of the stability of the ion-conducting passive layer no increased corrosion takes place

- in combination with nickel-based alloys, titanium acts as the local cathode, and because of the *n*-semiconducting properties of the titanium passive layer increased corrosion appears. This causes corrosion attack of the nickel-based alloys and, in the case of unfavourable surface ratios, damage to titanium due to hydrogen embrittlement.

Reclaru and Meyer (1994) and Iimmuro *et al.* (1993) coupled metallic materials conventionally used for dental treatment in electrochemical investigations and studied galvanic corrosion attack as well as the occurrence of other types of localised corrosion. Using 15 different galvanic couples (Ti/gold-based alloys, Ti/palladium-based alloys and Ti/non-precious alloys), titanium was under either cathodic or anodic control. According to Reclaru, an alloy is potentially useable for superstructures in galvanic coupling with titanium when it fulfils the following conditions:

- in a coupling titanium must have a weak anodic polarisation
- the galvanic cell current density must also be weak
- the crevice corrosion potential must be markedly higher than the coupling potential.

NOMENCLATURE

a	activity (mol l^{-1})
b_a, b_c	anodic and cathodic Tafel factors (V)
B	coefficient in Stern and Geary equation (V)
B_o	impedance parameter ($s^{0.5}$)
C	capacity (As V^{-1})
C_d	double layer capacity (As V^{-1})
E	electrode potential (V)
$E^\ominus$	standard electrode potential (V)
E_{oc}	open circuit potential (V)
E_{pc}	pitting potential (V)
f	frequency (s^{-1})
F	Faraday's constant (96 486 As/Equivalent)
i	current density (A cm^{-2})
i_0	exchange current density at an electrode for $\eta = 0$ (A cm^{-2})
i_{corr}	corrosion current density (A cm^{-2})
Im	imaginary part of the impedance (Ω)
j	imaginary unit
K_{IC}	stress intensity factor (MPa $mm^{0.5}$)
L	inductivity (Wb A^{-1})
n	substance transfer (mol)
n_{CPE}	impedance parameter (dimensionless)
O	limited diffusion impedance (Ω)
OCP	open circuit potential
Q	charge (As)

Q_{CPE} impedance element (Ω^{-1})
R universal gas constant (8.315 J mol^{-1} K^{-1})
Re real part of the impedance (Ω)
R_e electrolyte resistance (Ω)
R_i resistance (impedance element) (Ω)
R_t charge transfer resistance (Ω)
T absolute temperature (K)
W Warburg impedance (Ω)
Y_o impedance element (Ω^{-1})
z number of transferred charge units (dimensionless)
$|Z|$ impedance modulus (Ω)
$Z(\omega)$ impedance (Ω)
α transfer factor: part of the overpotential over the phase boundary at the point of maximum energy (dimensionless)
$\Delta\Psi$ Volta potential difference (V)
η_t overpotential (for the charge transfer determining process) (V)
ω angular frequency $\omega = 2\pi f$ (s^{-1})
φ phase angle phi (°)

REFERENCES

Aberer, W., Holub, H., Strohal, R. and Slavicek, R. (1993) Palladium in dental alloys – the dermatologists responsibility to warn?, *Cont. Dermat.* **28**, 163–5.

AESCULAP (1989) *Wissenschaftliche Informationen*. Die Plasmapore-Beschichtung für zementlose Gelenkendoprothesen, Tutlingen 11/89.

Allard, K.D., Ahrens, M. and Heusler, K.E. (1975) Wachstum und Auflösung anodisch erzeugter Oxidschichten auf Titan, *Werkstoffe Korrosion* **16**, 694–9.

Andrade, J.D. (1985) Principles of protein adsorption, in *Surface and Interfacial Aspects of Biomedical Polymers*, Vol. 2, *Protein Adsorption* (ed. J.D. Adrade), Plenum Press, New York, pp. 1–80.

ASTM G 99-90 (1990) Test method for wear testing with a pin-on-disk apparatus.

ASTM F 813-83 (Reapproved 1992) Standard practice for direct contact cell culture evaluation of materials for medical devices.

Barbosa, M.A. (1992) Surface layers and the reactivity of metallic implants, in *Biomaterials – Hard Tissue Repair and Replacement* (ed. D. Muster), Elsevier, Amsterdam, pp. 257–83.

Berger-Gorbet, M., Broxup, B. and Yahia, L.H. (1996) Biocompatibility testing of NiTi screws using immunohistochemistry on sections containing metallic implants, *J. Biomed. Mater. Res.* **32**, 243–8.

Berstein, A., Bernauer, I., Marx, R. and Geurtsen, W. (1992) Human cell culture studies with dental metallic materials, *Biomaterials* **13**, 98–100.

Bockris, J.O.M. and Reddy, A.K.N. (1970) *Modern Electrochemistry*, Plenum Press, New York.

Boehm, H.P. (1971) Acidic and basic properties of hydroxylated metal metal oxide surfaces, *Disc. Faraday Soc.* **52**, 264–75.

Boehm, H.P. and Hermann, M. (1967) Über die Chemie des Titandioxids I. Bestimmung des aktiven Wasserstoffs, thermische Entwässerung und Rehydroxylierung, *Z. anorg. allg. Chem.* **352**, 156–67.

Born, R., Scharnweber, D., Rößler, S., Stölzel, M., Thieme, M., Wolf, C. and Worch, H. (1998) Surface analysis of metallic biomaterials, *Fresenius J. Anal. Chem.* **361**, in press.

Boukamp, B.A. (1993) *Equivalent Circuit*, Version 4.51, University of Twente.

Brauner, H. and Haussner, T. (1989) Zum Korrosionsverhalten von Palladiumbasislegierungen, *Dtsch. Zahnrtzl. Z.* **44**, 119–21.

Breme, J. (1989) Le titane et les alliages de titane, biomateriaux de choix, *Mem. et Études Sci. Rev. de Metall.* **10**, 627–37.

Brossa, F., Looman, B., Pietra, R., Sabbioni, E., Gallorini, M. and Orvini, E. (1987) The use of titania and alumina as protective coatings on metallic prosthesis to prevent metal release, in *High Tech Ceramics* (ed. P. Vincenzini), Elsevier, Amsterdam, pp. 99–109.

Brown, S.D. (1984) The medical-physiological potential of plasma-sprayed ceramic coatings, *Thin Solid Films* **119**, 127–39.

Browne, M. and Gregson, P.J. (1994) Surface modification of titanium alloy implants, *Biomaterials* **15**, 894–8.

Browne, M., Gregson, P.J. and West, R.H. (1996) Characterization of titanium alloy implant surfaces with improved dissolution resistance, *J. Mater. Sci. Mater. Med.* **7**, 323–9.

Canay, S. and Oktemer, M. (1992) *In vitro* corrosion behaviour of 13 prosthodontic alloys, *Quint. Int.* **23**, 279–87.

Chandler, J.E., Messer, H.H. and Ellender, G. (1994) Cytotoxicity of gallium and indium ions compared with mercuric ion, *J. Dent. Res.* **73**, 1554–9.

Chou, L., Firth, J.D., Uitto, V.J. and Brunette, D.M. (1995) Substratum surface topography alters cell shape and regulates fibronectin mRNA level, mRNA stability, secretion and assembly in human fibroblasts, *J. Cell Sci.* **108**, 1563–73.

Cook, S.D., Thomas, K.A., Harding, A.F., Collins, C.L., Haddad, R.J., Jr, Milicic, M., Fischer, W.L. (1987) The *in vivo* performance of 250 internal fixation devices: a follow up study, *Biomaterials* **8**, 177–184.

Davies, L.E., Lowenberg, B. and Shiga, A. (1990) The bone–titanium interface *in vitro*, *J. Biomed. Mater. Res.* **24**, 1289–306.

Dental Vademekum (1995) Hrsg.: Bundeszahnärztekammer und Kassenzahnärztliche Vereinigung, Deutscher Ärzte-Verlag Köln, 1980, 1995.

DIN 50324 (1992) Prüfung von Reibung und Verschleiß.

DIN EN 30993 (1993) Biological evaluation of medical devices.

DIN V 13930 Vornorm (1990) Biologische Prüfungen von Dentalwerkstoffen.

DIN ISO 6474 Entwurf (1992) Implants for surgery; ceramic materials based high purity alumina.

Ducheyne, P. (1983) *In vitro* corrosion study of porous metal fibre coatings for bone ingrowth, *Biomaterials* **4**, 185–91.

Ducheyne, P. and Healy, K.E. (1988) The effect of plasma-sprayed calcium phosphate ceramic coatings on the metal ion release from porous titanium and cobalt–chromium alloys, *J. Biomed. Mater. Res.* **22**, 1137–63.

Elagli, K., Traisnel, M. and Hildebrand, H.F. (1993) Electrochemical behaviour of titanium and dental alloys in artificial saliva, *Electrochim. Acta* **38**, 1769–74.

EN ISO 1562 (1993) Dental casting gold alloys.

EN ISO 8891 (1995) Dental casting alloys with noble metal content of 25% up to but not including 75%.

Evans, E.J. (1994) Cell damage *in vitro* following direct contact with fine particles of titanium, titanium alloy and cobalt–chrome–molybdenum alloy, *Biomaterials* **15**, 713–17.

Fartash, B., Liao, H., Li, J., Fouda, N. and Hermansson, L. (1995) Long-term evaluation of titania based ceramics compared with commercially pure titanium *in vivo*, *J. Mater. Sci. Mater. Med.* **6**, 451–4.

Flaig-Baumann, R., Hermann, M. and Boehm, H.P. (1970) Über die Chemie des Titandioxids. III. Reaktionen der basischen Hydroxylgruppen auf der Oberfläche, *Z. anorg. allg. Chem.* **372**, 296–307.

Fraker, A.C., Ruff, A.W., Sung, P., van Orden, A.C. and Speck, K.M. (1980) *Ti 80, Science and Technology*, Plenum Press, New York, p. 2447.
Franke, R., Haase, I., Bäther, K.H. and Thomas, G. (1996) Erhöhung der Verschleißfestigkeit der TiAl6V4-Legierung durch Implantieren mit Stickstoff-Ionen, *Mat.-wiss. Werkstofftech.* **27**, 9–13.
Gebauer-Hartung, P., Kaden, P., Richter, H.A. and Mittermayer, Ch. (1995) Die Zellzahl – ein essentieller Faktor in der Biokompatibilitätsprüfung, *BIOforum* **18**, 488–92.
Göhr, H. (1981) Über Beiträge einzelner Elekrodenprozesse zur Impedanz, *Ber. Bunsenges. Phys. Chem.* **85**, 274–80.
Gomer, R. and Tryson, G. (1977) An experimental determination of absolute half-cell emfs and single ion free energies of solvation, *J. Chem. Phys.* **66**, 4413.
Good, V.D., Clarke, I.C. and Anissian, L. (1996) Water and bovine serum lubrication compared in simulator PTFE/CoCr wear model, *J. Biomed. Mater. Res.* **33**, 275–83.
Grant, D.M., Lo, W.J., Parker, K.G. and Parker, T.L. (1996) Biocompatible and mechanical properties of low temperature deposited quaternary (Ti, Al, V) N coatings on Ti6Al4V titanium alloy substrates, *J. Mater. Sci. Mater. Med.* **7**, 579–84.
Hanawa, T. and Ota, M. (1991) Calcium phosphate naturally formed on titanium in electrolyte solutions, *Biomaterials*, **12**, 767–74.
Hanks, J.H. and Wallace, R.E. (1949) Relation of oxygen and temperature in the preservation of tissues by refrigeration, *Proc. Soc. Exp. Biol. Med.* **71**, 195–200.
Hashimoto, M., Miyajima, S. and Murata, T. (1992a) A stochastic analysis of potential fluctuation during passive film breakdown and repair on iron, *Corrosion Science* **33**, 885–904.
Hashimoto, M., Miyajima, S. and Murata, T. (1992b) An experimental study of potential fluctuation during passive film breakdown and repair on iron, *Corros. Sci.* **33**, 905–16.
Hashimoto, M., Miyajima, S. and Murata, T. (1992c) A spectrum analysis of potential fluctuation during passive film breakdown and repair on iron, *Corros. Sci.* **33**, 917–25.
Heitz, E. and Schwenk, W. (1976) Theoretical basis for the determination of corrosion rates from polarisation resistance, *Br. Corros. J.* **11**, 74–7.
Hench, L.L. and Ethridge, E.C. (1975) Biomaterials – the interfacial problem, *Adv. Biomed. Eng.* **5**, 35–150.
Hench, L.L. and Ethridge, E.C. (1982) *Biomaterials – An Interfacial Approach*, Academic Press, New York.
Hench, L.L. and Wilson, J. (1993) *An Introduction to Bioceramics*, World Scientific Publishing, Singapore.
Hermann, M. and Boehm, H.P. (1969) Über die Chemie des Titandioxids II. Saure Hydroxylgruppen auf der Oberfläche, *Z. anorg. allg. Chem.* **368**, 73–86.
Hermann, M., Kaluza, U. and Boehm, H.P. (1970) Über die Chemie des Titandioxids IV. Austausch von Hydroxidionen gegen Fluoridionen, *Z. anorg. allg. Chem.* **372**, 308–13.
Hildebrand, G., Kraft, D., Liefeith, D., Mann, E. and Lenz, E. (1995) Vergleichende Korrosionsprüfung von dentalen Legierungen im Laborbioreaktor, *Mater. and Corros.* **46**, 157–64.
Hitzig, J., Jüttner, K., Lorenz, W.J. and Paatsch, W. (1986) AC-impedance measurements on corroded porous aluminium oxide films, *J. Electrochem. Soc.* **133**, 887–92.
Howlett, C.R., Evans, M.D., Walsh, W.R., Johnson, G. and Steele, J.G. (1994) Mechanism of initial cell attachment of cells derived from human bone to commonly used prosthetic materials during cell culture, *Biomaterials* **15**, 213–22.
Hughes, A.N. and Jordan, B.A. (1972) Metallurgical observations on some metallic implants which failed *in vivo*, *J. Biomed. Mater. Res.* **6**, 33–48.
Hulshoff, J.E., van Dijk, K., van der Waerden, J.P., Ginsel, L.A. and Jansen, J.A. (1995) Biological evaluation of the effect of magnetron sputtered Ca/P coatings on osteoblast-like cells *in vitro*, *J. Biomed. Mater. Res.* **29**, 967–75.
Hulshoff, J.E., van Dijk, K., van der Waerden, J.P., Kalk, W. and Jansen, J.A. (1996) A histological and histomorphometrical evaluation of screw-type calciumphosphate (Ca-P) coated

implants; an *in vivo* experiment in maxillary cancellous bone of goats, *J. Mater. Sci. Mater. Med.* **7**, 603–9.

Iimuro, F.T., Yoneyama, T. and Okuno, O. (1993) Corrosion of coupled metals in a dental magnetic attachment system, *Dent. Mater. J.* **12**, 136–44.

Jacobs, J.J., Skipor, A.K., Doorn, P.F., Campbell, P., Schmalzried, T.P., Black, J. and Amstutz, H.C. (1996) Cobalt and chromium concentrations in patients with metal on metal total hip replacements, *Clin. Orthop.* **329**, 256–63.

Janssen, M.J.G. and Stein, H.N. (1986) The TiO_2/electrolyte solution interface. I. Influence of pretreatment conditions and of impurities, *J. Coll. Interface Sci.* **109**, 509–16.

Jenissen, H.P. (1988) General aspects of protein adsorption, *Macromol. Chem. Macromol. Symp.* **17**, 111–34.

Jüttner, K., Lorenz, W.J., Paatsch, W., Kendig, M. and Mansfeld, F. (1985) Bedeutung der dynamischen Systemanalyse für Korrosionsuntersuchungen in Forschung und Praxis, *Werkstoffe Korros.* **36**, 120–30.

Kaesche, H. (1990) *Die Korrosion der Metalle*, Springer, Berlin, p. 30.

Keller, J.C., Stanford, C.M., Wightman, J.P., Draughn, R.A. and Zaharias, R. (1994) Characterizations of titanium implant surfaces. III., *J. Biomed. Mater. Res.* **28**, 939–46.

Kitsugi, T., Nakamura, T., Oka, M., Yan, W.-Q., Goto, T., Shibuya, T., Kokubo, T. and Miyaji, S. (1996) Bone bonding behaviour of titanium and its alloys when coated with titanium oxide (TiO_2) and titanium silicate (Ti_5Si_3), *J. Biomed. Mater. Res.* **32**, 149–56.

Kohn, D.H. (1992) Materials for bone and joint replacement, in *Materials Science and Technology, a Comprehensive Treatment*, Vol. 14, *Medical and Dental Materials* (ed. D.F. Williams), VCH, Weinheim, pp. 31–109.

Kononen, M., Hormia, M., Kivilahti, J., Hautaniemi, J. and Thesleff, I. (1992) Effect of surface processing on the attachment, orientation, and proliferation of human gingival fibroblasts on titanium, *J. Biomed. Mater. Res.* **26**, 1325–42.

Kuempel, D.R., Johnson, G.K., Zaharias, R.S. and Keller, J.C. (1995) The effects of scaling procedures on epithelial cell growth on titanium surfaces, *J. Periodontol.* **66**, 228–34.

Lacy, S.A., Merritt, K., Brown, S.A. and Puryear, A. (1996) Distribution of nickel and cobalt following dermal and systemic administration with *in vitro* and *in vivo* studies, *J. Biomed. Mater. Res.* **32**, 279–83.

Laing, P.G. (1979) Clinical experience with prosthetic materials; historical perspectives, current problems and future directions, *ASTM-STP* **684**, 199–201.

Leitao, E., Sa, C., Silva, R.A., Barbosa, M.A. and Ali, H. (1995) Electrochemical and surface modifications on N^+ ion implanted Ti–6Al–4V immersed in HBSS, *Corr. Sci.* **37**, 1861–6.

Lide, D.R., ed. (1993) *CRC Handbook of Chemistry and Physics*, 73rd edn, CRC Press, Boca Raton, FL, pp. 4–108.

Liefeith, K., Hildebrand, G., Kraft, D., Lenz, E. and Mann, E. (1994) *In-vitro* Korrosionsprüfung von Dentallegierungen in biologischen Elektrolyten – Methodenentwicklung und Eignungsnachweise, *Swiss Dent.* **15** (3), 7–11.

Lim, S.C. and Ashby, M.F. (1987) Wear-mechanism maps, *Acta Metall.* **35**, 1–24.

Lycett, R.W. and Hughes, A.N. (1984) Corrosion, in *Metal and Ceramic Biomaterials*, Vol. II, *Strength and Surface*, Chap. 4 (eds P. Ducheyne and G.W. Hastings), CRC Press, Boca Raton, FL.

Maeusli, P.A., Bloch, P.R., Geret, V. and Steinemann, S. (1986) Surface characterisation of titanium and Ti-alloys, in *Biological and Biomechanical Performance of Biomaterials, Proceedings of the Fifth European Conference on Biomaterials*, Paris, 4–6 September 1985 (eds P. Christel, A. Meun and A.J.C. Lee), Elsevier, Amsterdam, pp. 57–62.

Mann, E. and Lenz, E. (1992) Vergleichende elektrochemische Korrosionsuntersuchungen an Gold und Palladiumbasislegierungen, *Swiss Dent.* **13**, 17–18.

Martin, J.Y., Schwartz, Z., Hummert, T.W., Schraub, D.M., Simpson, J., Lankford, J., Dean, D.D., Cochran, D.L. and Boyan, B.D. (1995) Effect of titanium surface roughness on

proliferation, differentiation, and protein synthesis of human osteoblast-like cells, *J. Biomed. Mater. Res.* **29**, 389–401.
McGovern, T.E., Black, J., Jacobs, J.J., Graham, R.M. and LaBerge, M. (1996) In vivo wear of Ti6Al4V femoral heads: a retrieval study, *J. Biomed. Mater. Res.* **32**, 447–57.
Metikos-Hukovic, M. and Zevnik, C. (1982) Determination of polarization resistance and corrosion rate by using pulse method, polarization curves and AAS, *Werkstoffe Korros.* **33**, 661–8.
Michel, R., Hofmann, J., Löer, F. and Zilkens, J. (1984) Trace element burdening of human tissues due to corrosion of hip joint prostheses made of cobalt–chromium alloys, *Arch. Orthop. Trauma Surg.* **103**, 85–95.
Michel, R., Löer, F., Nolte, M., Reich. M. and Zilkens, J. (1987) Neutron activation analysis of human tissues, organs and body fluids to describe the interaction of orthopaedic implants made of cobalt–chromium alloys with the patients organism, *J. Radioanal. Nucl. Chem.* **113**, 83–95.
Michel, R., Nolte, M., Reich, M. and Löer, F. (1991) Systemic effects of implanted prostheses made of cobalt–chromium alloys, *Arch. Orthop. Trauma Surg.* **110**, 61–74.
Mikulec, L.J. and Puleo, D.A. (1996) Use of p-nitrophenyl chloroformate chemistry to immobilize protein on orthopedic biomaterials, *J. Biomed. Mater. Res.* **32**, 203–8.
Nocke, K., Scharnweber, D., Rößler, S. and Worch, H. (1997) Investigations of modified Titanium surfaces by impedance spectroscopy and scanning Kelvin probe, in *Proceedings of the 5th European Conference on Advanced Materials and Processes and Applications*, Vol. 3 (eds L.A.J.L. Sarton and H.B. Zeedijk), Maastricht, 21–23 April 1997, pp. 559–64.
Nocke, K., Scharnweber, D. and Worch, H. (1996) Untersuchungen von modifizierten Titanoxidschichten mit Hilfe der Impedanzspektroskopie, in *Proceedings Werkstoffwoche '96*, Vol. 4, *Werkstoffe für die Medizintechnik* (ed. J. Breme), DGM-Informationsgesellschaft, Oberursel, pp. 117–22.
Okamoto, Y. and Hidaka, S. (1994) Studies on calcium phosphate precipitation: effects of metal ions used in dental materials, *J. Biomed. Mater. Res.* **28**, 1403–10.
Oshida, Y. and Moore, B.K. (1993) Anodic polarization behaviour and microstructure of a gallium-based alloy, *Dent. Mater.* **9**, 234–41.
Pajkossy, T. (1991) Electrochemistry at fractal surfaces, *J. Elechochem. Soc.* **300**, 1–11.
Pan, J., Thierry, D. and Leygraf, C. (1994) Electrochemical and XPS studies of titanium for biomaterial applications with respect to the effect of hydrogen peroxide, *J. Biomed. Mater. Res.* **28**, 113–22.
Pilliar, R.M. (1987) Porous-surfaced metallic implants for orthopedic applications, *J. Biomed. Mater. Res. Appl. Biomater.* **21A**, 1–33.
Pohl, H. (1996) Anwendung des Elektrochemischen Rauschens zur Früherkennung und Charakterisierung von Spaltkorrosionsprozessen an Aluminiumwerkstoffen, Diplomarbeit, TU Dresden.
Pourbaix, M. (1963) *Atlas d'Equilibres Electrochimiques*, Gautier-Villars, Paris.
Puelo, D.A., Preston, K.E., Shaffer, J.B. and Bizios, R. (1993) Examination of osteoblast–orthopaedic biomaterial interactions using molecular techniques, *Biomaterials* **14**, 111–14.
Putters, J.L., Kaulesar Sukul, D.M., de Zeeuw, G.R., Bijma, A. and Besselink, P.A. (1992) Comparative cell culture effects of shape memory metal (Nitinol), nickel and titanium: a biocompatibility estimation, *Eur. Surg. Res.* **24**, 378–82.
Rammelt, U. and Reinhard, G. (1990) On the applicability of a constant phase element to the estimation of roughness of solid metal electrodes, *Electrochim. Acta* **35**, 1045–9.
Reclaru, L. and Meyer, J.M. (1994) Study of corrosion between a titanium implant and dental alloys, *J. Dent.* **22**, 159–68.
Richards, R.G., Rahn, B.A. and Gwynn, I.A.P. (1995) Scanning electron microscopy of the undersurface of cell monolayers grown on metallic implants, *J. Mater. Sci. Mater. Med.* **6**, 120–4.

Richter, S., Stölzel, M., Scharnweber, D. and Worch, H. (1996) Biologisierung von Implantatoberflächen durch Immobilisierung von Biopolymeren, in *Proceedings Werkstoffwoche '96*, Vol. 4, *Werkstoffe für die Medizintechnik* (ed. J. Breme), DGM-Informationsgesellschaft, Oberursel, pp. 123–7.

Hoffman-La Roche A.G., ed. (1993) *Roche Lexikon Medizin*, Schwarzenberg & Urban, München, p. 1437.

Rochini, G. (1984a) Determination of corrosion current density by the INTOL code, in *Proceedings of the 9th International Congress on Metallic Corrosion*, Toronto, 3–7 June 1984, pp. 436–42.

Rochini, G. (1984b) A new way of introducing linear polarization response, in *Proceedings of the 9th International Congress on Metallic Corrosion*, Toronto, 3–7 June 1984, pp. 563–70.

Rochini, G. (1984c) SOFTCOR-DC-1 a code for evaluating polarization resistance, in *Proceedings of the 9th International Congress on Metallic Corrosion*, Toronto 3–7 June 1984, pp. 571–7.

Romann, V. (1995) Entwicklung und Anwendung voltammetrischer Analysenmethoden für Titan und Nichtedelmetallegierungen zum Studium der Korrosion metallischer Biomaterialien, Dissertation, Humboldt-Universität Berlin.

Satoh, Y., Nagai, E., Maejima, K., Ohyama, T., Ito, S., Toyoma, H., Ohwa, M., Kobayashi, E., Ohki, K., Kaketani, M. (1992) Wear of denture teeth by use of metal plates. Part 3: Abrasive wear of posterior teeth and wear of opposing metal plates, *J. Nihon Univ. Sch. Dent.* **34**, 249–64.

Schade, R. and Liefeith, K. (1995) Technische Konzepte zur *in-vitro*-Prüfung von Biomaterialien, in *Proceedings Werkstoffprüfung*, Bad Nauheim, 5–6 December 1995, pp. 181–8.

Scharnweber, D., Stölzel, M., Thieme, M., Rößler, S., Eichler, H. and Worch, H. (1997) Biologisierte Knochenimplantate – ein neuer Weg zur Langzeitstabilität, *Wiss. Z. Techn. Univ. Dresden* **46** (3), 16–23.

Schedle, A., Samorapoompichit, P., Rausch-Fan, X.H., Franz, A., Fureder, W., Sperr, W.R., Sperr, W., Ellinger, A., Slavicek, R., Boltz-Nitulescu, G. and Valent, P. (1995) Response of L-929 fibroblasts, human gingival fibroblasts, and human tissue mast cells to various metal cations, *J. Dent. Res.* **74**, 1513–20.

Schmidt, M. (1992) Spezifische Adsorption organischer Moleküle auf oxidiertem Titan: 'Bioaktivität' auf molekularem Niveau, *Osteologie* **1**, 222–35.

Schröder, J. (1988) Surface treatment of pigments, *Prog. Org. Coat.* **16**, 3–17.

Semlitsch, M. and Weber, H. (1992) Titanlegierungen für zementlose Hüftprothesen, in *Die zementlose Hüftprothese*, Demter, Gräfelfingen, pp. 18–26.

Silva, R.A., Barbosa, M.A., Costa, A.S. and Ribeiro, J.A.C. (1985) Estudo analitico de implantes e proteses ortopédicas, *Proceedings of the 2nd Meeting of the Portuguese Materials Society*, Vol. V, Sociedade Protuguesa de Materials.

Souto, R.M. and Burstein, G.T. (1996) A preliminary investigation into the microscopic depassivation of passive titanium implant materials *in vitro*, *J. Mater. Sci. Mater. Med.* **7**, 337–43.

Speck, K.M. and Fraker, A.C. (1980) Anodic polarization behavior of Ti–Ni and Ti–6Al–4V in simulated physiological solutions, *J. Dent. Res.* **59**, 1590–5.

Stea, S., Visentin, M., Savarino, L., Donati, M.E., Pizzoferrato, A., Moroni, A. and Caja, V. (1995) Quantitative analysis of the bone–hydroxyapatite coating interface, *J. Mater. Sci. Mater. Med.* **6**, 455–9.

Steinemann, S.G. (1980) Corrosion of surgical implants – *in vivo* and *in vitro* tests, in *Evaluation of Biomaterials* (eds G.D. Winter, J.L. Leray and K. de Groot), Wiley, London, pp.1–34.

Stölzel, M. (1996) Untersuchungen zur Entwicklung eines Materialverbundes von Titan mit Komponenten des Knochens, Diplomarbeit, TU Dresden.

Stratmann, M. and Streckel, H. (1990a) On the atmospheric corrosion of metals which are covered with thin electrolyte layers – I. Verification of the experimental technique, *Corr. Sci.* **30**, 681–96.

Stratmann, M. and Streckel, H. (1990b) On the atmospheric corrosion of metals which are covered with thin electrolyte layers – II. Experimental results, *Corr. Sci.* **30**, 697–714.

Stratmann, M., Streckel, H., Kim, K.T. and Chrockett, S. (1990) On the atmospheric corrosion of metals which are covered with thin electrolyte layers – III. The measurement of polarisation curves on metal surfaces which are covered by thin electrolyte layers, *Corr. Sci.* **30**, 715–34.

Thull, R. (1990) Semiconductive properties of passivated titanium and titanium based hard coatings on metals for implants – an experimental approach, *Med. Prog. Tech.* **16**, 225–34.

Thull, R. (1994) Naturwissenschaftliche Aspekte von Werkstoffen in der Medizin, *Naturwissenschaften* **81**, 481–8.

Thull, R. (1995) Oberflächen biokompatibler Funktionswerkstoffe, *DGM-Fortbildungsseminar Biomaterialien*, Saarbrücken, 8–10 October 1995.

Tomas, H., Carvalho, G.S., Fernandes, M.H., Freire, A.P. and Abrantes, L.M. (1996) Effects of Co–Cr corrosion products and corresponding separate metal ions on human osteoblast-like cell cultures, *J. Mater. Sci. Mater. Med.* **7**, 291–6.

Ungethüm, M. and Winkler-Gniewek, W. (1984) *Metallische Werkstoffe in der Orthopädie und Unfallchirurgie*, Georg Thieme, Stuttgart.

Unsworth, T. (1995) Wear, retrieval and simulators for artificial joints, *Orthop. New Prod. News* March/April, 30–4.

Verrier, S., Bareille, R., Rovira, A., Dard, M. and Amedee, J. (1996) Human osteoprogenitor responses to orthopaedic implant: mechanism of cell attachment and cell adhesion, *J. Mater. Sci. Mater. Med.* **7**, 46–51.

Vetter, K.J. (1967) *Electrochemical Kinetics*, Academic Press, London.

Wataha, J.C., Hanks, C.T. and Craig, R.G. (1993) The effect of cell monolayer density on the cytotoxicity of metal ions which are released from dental alloys, *Dent. Mater.* **9**, 172–6.

Wennerberg, A., Albrektsson, T. and Andersson, B. (1995) An animal study of c.p. titanium screws with different surface topographies, *J. Mater. Sci. Mater. Med.* **6**, 302–9.

Willert, H.G., Brobäck, L.-G., Buchhorn, G.H., Jensen, P.H., Köster, G., Lang, I., Ochsner, P. and Schenk, R. (1996) Crevice corrosion of cemented titanium alloy stems in total hip replacements, *Clin. Orthop. Relat. Res.* **333**, 51–75.

Williams, D.F. (1981) Electrochemical aspects of corrosion in the physiological environment, in *Fundamental Aspects in Biocompatibility I* (ed. D.F. Williams), CRC Press, Boca Raton, FL, pp. 11–42.

Williams, D.F. (1988) Consensus and definitions in biomaterials, in *Advances in Biomaterials* (eds C.K. de Putter, K. de Lange, K. de Groot and A.J.C. Lee), Elsevier, Amsterdam, pp. 121–36

Willmann, G. (1996) Hüftgelenkersatz – eine tribologische Herausforderung, *Mat.-wiss. Werkstofftech.* **27**, 199–205.

Winter, G.D., Leray, J.L. and de Groot, K., eds (1980) *Evaluation of Biomaterials*, Wiley, London.

Wintermantel, E. and Suk-Woo Ha (1996) *Biokompatible Werkstoffe und Bauweisen*, Springer, Berlin.

Worch, H. (1996) Patent DE 196 43 555, Metallischer Gegenstand mit einer dünnen mehrphasigen Oxidschicht sowie Verfahren zu dessen Herstellung.

Worch, H. and Scharnweber, D. (1998) Biologisierte Titanwerkstoffe – Werkstoffwissenschaft im Grenzbereich zwischen belbter und unbelebter Materie, *Z. Metallkd.* **89**, 153–63.

Zitter, H. and Plenk, H., Jr (1987) The electrochemical behavior of metallic implant materials as an indicator of their biocompatibility, *J. Biomed. Mater. Res.* **21**, 881–96.

Zum Gahr, ed. (1987) *Microstructure and Wear of Materials*, Elsevier, Amsterdam.

5
Surfaces, surface modification and tailoring

H.J. BREME
University of the Saarland, Saarbrücken, Germany

5.1 INTRODUCTION

The success of a replacement by implantation depends strongly on the interaction between the living and synthetic material, whereby totally different effects can be achieved. While, for instance, for implants remaining in contact with the blood, e.g. stents, haemocompatible behaviour with a minimum of interaction is normally required (see Chapter 8), osseointegated implants must show a maximum interaction producing a high adhesion strength. The osseointegration can be influenced by both the structure and the composition of the surface.

In the following sections, examples of both influences are given.

5.2 INFLUENCE OF THE SURFACE STRUCTURE

The surface structure of an implant has a significant influence on both its anchorage and the strength of adhesion to the tissue. Since this strength is defined as the ratio of the loading force to the area on which the force is exerted, the load under service conditions can be greater the larger the area. From this simple consideration it is clear that a smooth implant surface with a small area of contact with the tissue will show a lower adhesion strength than a structured surface. This behaviour was demonstrated in rabbits by implanting flattened cylinders made of titanium alloys and of varying surface roughness into the legs. After exposure times of 84 and 168 days, the tensile strength was measured in tear-off tests, the results of which are shown in Figure 5.1. A measurable adhesion strength to the bone was present only when a certain degree of surface roughness (>22 µm) existed. With increasing roughness the tensile strength was enhanced. Consequently, it was shown that the tear-off force was increased owing to the increase in the contact area by holes being drilled in the flattened cylinder surface. However, with respect to the enlargement of

---

Metals as Biomaterials ISBN 0 471 96935 4 Edited by J.A. Helsen and H.J. Breme. © 1998 John Wiley & Sons Ltd

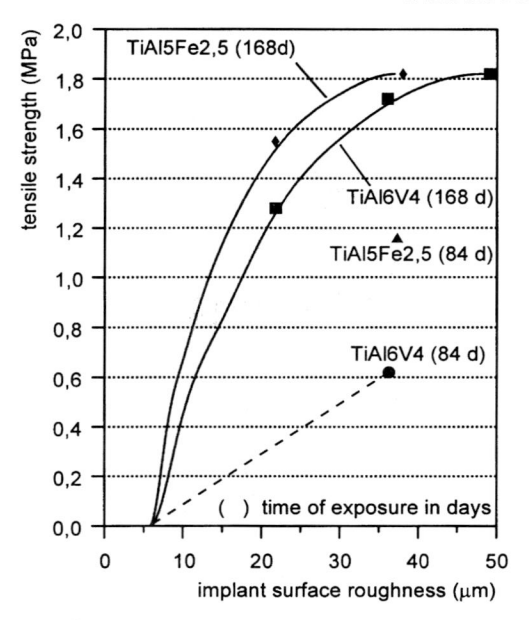

Figure 5.1 Influence of the surface roughness of implants on the tensile strength of bone–implant (Schmitz et al., 1988).

the area, a similar tensile strength was calculated (Schmitz et al., 1988). In addition, the adhesion strength depends on the time of exposure. The bone requires a certain amount of time to bridge the gap to the implant and grow into the surface crevices, causing a mechanical bonding to the implant. This requirement was confirmed in many different investigations (Brunski et al., 1979; Kirsch, 1980; Hansson et al., 1983; Krekeler et al., 1984).

From the point of view of applied mechanics, the ingrowth of the bone into surface cavities has a favourable influence, as shown schematically in Figure 5.2. The shear stress, which is generated by the functional loading of the implant at the implant–bone interface, is decreased because, similarly to the thread of a screw, the load at this interface causes, in addition to the normal stress perpendicular to the inclined area, only a small shear stress effective in the inclined area. This perception finally led to the cementless implantation, which in turn resulted in a wide range of proposals and originations for structuring implant surfaces, including structuring by casting, surface roughening, lacunae holes and porous coating produced by sintering or plasma spraying. Structuring by casting is a widespread practice for CoCr alloys. By the use of corresponding wax models a roughened surface or special open-celled, porous, spongy structure can be produced by investment and precision casting, respectively. On the shafts of hip prostheses, for example, the spongy structure has a preferred depth of 3–5 mm (Henssge et al., 1985; Henssge and Peschel, 1987). For titanium and its alloys, casting plays a subordinate role because of the high reactivity

SURFACES, SURFACE MODIFICATION AND TAILORING

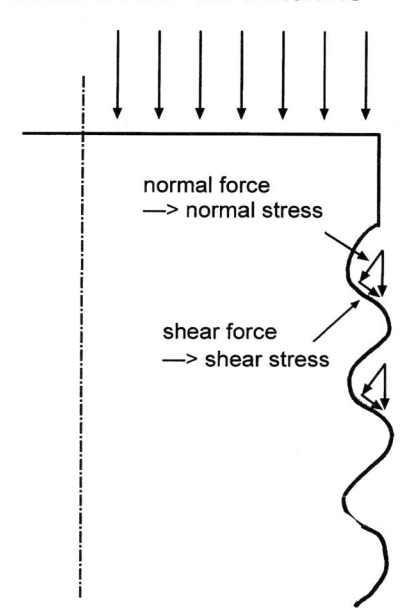

Figure 5.2 Influence of implant surface cavities on stress distribution (schematic).

of the melt which may produce, with the embedding material, the α-case, which is an oxygen-rich surface layer with low ductility (Schädlich-Staubenrauch *et al.*, 1988; Feagin, 1986). Therefore, for titanium implants the remaining methods of surface structuring, which nevertheless are also applied for CoCr implants, are preferred.

Besides the favourable influence on the implant anchorage, there is a further important advantage in the use of surface structuring. The ingrown bone, which will be subjected to strain by compression or tension, produces calcium, resulting in the stimulation of new bone formation. It is clear that the appearance of this phenomenon will be enhanced in proportion to the improvement of the load transfer. As shown schematically in Figure 5.3, the surface structure itself plays an important role. In areas that are unaffected by the stresses, no strain field will exist and, as a result, decalcification of the bone will occur together with the formation of soft tissue. These load-shadowed areas cause a disuse atrophy (Heimke *et al.*, 1980, 1982; Heimke, 1990). From the mechanical point of view, the load transfer will improve as the stiffness of the implant decreases in the area of the ingrown bone. The stiffness S can be described by the product of the moment of inertia and Young's modulus E (Chapter 1). Since the moment of inertia is given in most cases by the geometry of the landscape, the Young's modulus value of the material must be lowered in order to decrease the stiffness of the implant in the direction of the bone. As can be seen from the schematic diagram in Figure 5.4, a drastic change in

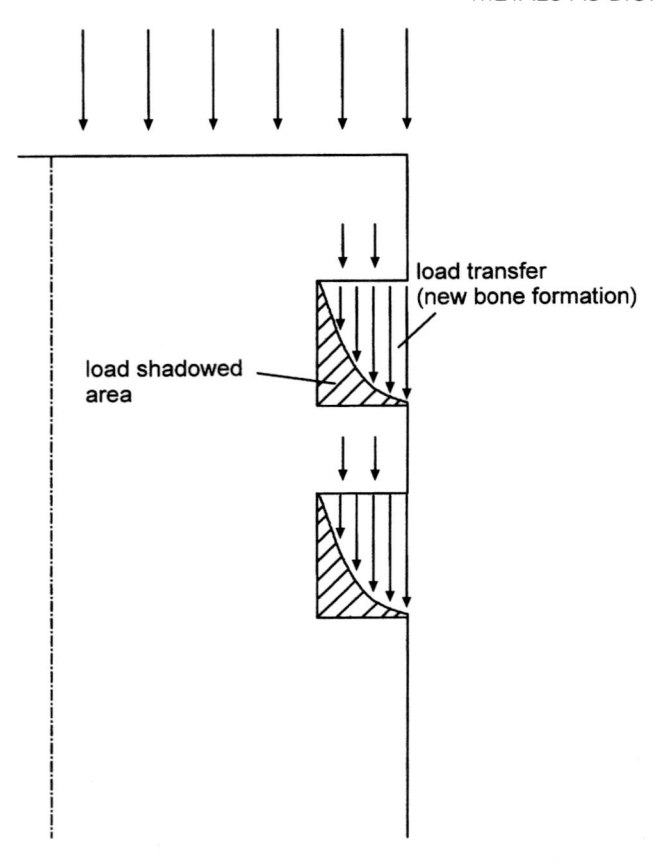

Figure 5.3 Unfavourable surface structure (schematic) producing load shadowed areas (according to Heimke, 1990).

Young's modulus from the implant to the bone should be avoided because the difference in the elastic deformation can cause delamination stresses in the interface. By comparison, a gradual transition in Young's modulus (Figure 5.4b) from the bone to the implant or even isoelastic behaviour in the area of the ingrown bone, which can be achieved by porous surface layers, helps to avoid these delamination stresses. Moreover, in addition to an improved anchorage of the implant, the reduced stiffness in this area provides the necessary good load transfer and the stimulation of new bone formation.

Because of the value of Young's modulus for titanium and its alloys, which amounts to only about 50% of that of the CoCr alloys and stainless steel, it is possible to produce with titanium a stiffness in the porous surface layer with a lower porosity than with the other materials. This is of great importance for the mechanical properties. This concept of an isoelastic implant or implant surface can be successful

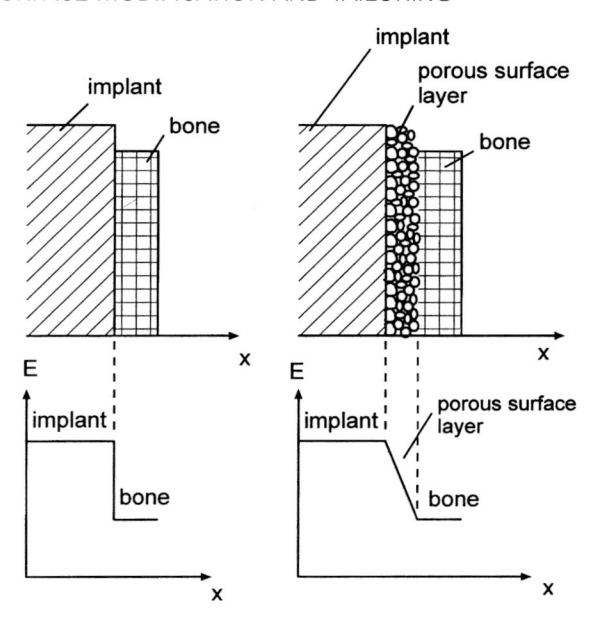

Figure 5.4 Change in Young's modulus at the bone–implant interface with a smooth and a porous implant surface, respectively (schematic).

only if an open porosity is obtained which provides a total ingrowh of the bone, producing a composite material (metal–bone). The isoelastic concept with a good load transfer will function only if the metallic scaffold is totally filled by ingrown bone (Griss and Heimke, 1976). The concept of isoelasticity was implemented in a prosthesis by R. Mathys in Switzerland (Morscher et al., 1976). This company commercialised a hip prosthesis made of polyacetal resin with a metal core. The Young's modulus of polyacetal is 5–10 MPa, quite comparable to that of bone. Durability, wear and pressure resistance, and biocompatibility were considered sufficient for this type of prosthesis (Kinzi et al., 1976) and the initial results were encouraging (Bombelli and Mathys, 1982). As discussed in Chapter 1, a potentially good concept does not necessarily lead to excellent biological performance because the response of the body is neither fully understood nor predictable. The same is true here: the prosthesis had only limited success and the long-term results proved to be less favourable (Niinimäki et al., 1994). The micromovements between the Mathys prosthesis and the bone were not as perfect as originally assumed by the designers.

The reduction in both implant stiffness and Young's modulus by porous sintering results in a change in the remaining mechanical properties, especially in a decrease in the strength properties. Titanium and its alloys are known to show a certain amount of notch sensitivity which causes a deterioration of the fatigue behaviour. Under alternating bending stresses the fatigue strength is reported to be reduced for titanium alloys after heat treatment, producing a porous surface layer by sintering to more than 75% if the sintering operation is performed above the (α+β/β) transition temperature (Henssge et al., 1990). Besides the factor of the notch sensitivity, this effect can be explained by the change in the microstructure. Annealing or deformation in the β-phase field produces a coarse β-grain which has a diminished fatigue strength. By comparison, sintering below the transition temperature results in a loss of fatigue strength of about 40%, while CoCr alloys with sintered porous surface layers show a drop of only 3–30% (Henssge et al., 1990). Better results have been obtained with titanium alloys using plasma spraying as a surface-coating procedure. The fatigue strength was reduced by about 10% (Plitz and Böhme, 1988). When this method is used, another problem, that of a poor adhesion strength of the porous layer to the bulk material, can arise because of the low substrate temperature during spraying. This problem can be overcome by careful preparation of the implant surface and the use of special spray powders.

Porous surface layers on the stems of hip prostheses made from titanium alloys, for example Ti6Al4V, are industrially produced by means of vacuum plasma spraying (VPS) of a commercially pure titanium hydrogenisation–dehydrogenisation (HDH) powder. Owing to the high plasma temperature of more than 20 000°C the powder may be partially melted at the surface, by means of which a sufficient bonding to the substrate can be achieved. In addition, by the use of vacuum spraying, impurification of the powder by the atmosphere is avoided, and the bonding strength of the porous layer to the implant will be improved compared with techniques operating under atmospheric conditions. Samples with plasma-sprayed porous titanium surface layers have been tested in animal experiments. Using the press fit method, cylindrical implants were inserted into the distal femur of canines and histological slices prepared after 12 weeks. Comparison with implanted cylinders with a polished ($R_t > 1$ μm) and a roughened ($R_t = 20$ μm) surface, respectively, showed significantly more favourable behaviour of the implants with a porous surface layer. In the case of the latter samples, bone trabeculae were orientated perpendicular to the implant surface, while in the case of the implants with the smooth and roughened surfaces the trabeculae formed a concentric frame around the implants. In addition, between these implants and the bone a gap consisting of soft tissues was observed, whereas the sample with the porous surface layer showed a close contact to the bone due to the stimulation by the load transfer. Consequently, the adhesion strength measured by means of the pull-out test amounted to 2.5–5.5 MPa in the case of the implants, with failure occurring in the bone, while the implants with a smooth and a roughened surface had an adhesion strength of less than 0.5 MPa. The animal experiments have been confirmed by clinical results (Winkler-Gniewek et al. 1991; Fink, 1996).

Since dental implants are subjected to relatively low loads under service conditions, the isoelastic concept is easily realised with this type of implant. A titanium alloy, Ti30Ta, has been developed which can be directly diffusion welded with alumina (see Chapter 8). Owing to a high proportion of the β-phase this alloy has a decreased Young's modulus ($E = 80\ 000$ GPa) compared with cp-titanium. In the martensitic structure, which can be produced by annealing in the β-phase field at 900°C and subsequent water quenching, Young's modulus amounts to only about

Table 5.1 Influence of microstructure and porosity on the mechanical properties of Ti30Ta (Breme et al., 1993)

	Porosity (%)	Compression yield strength (MPa)	Young's modulus (GPa)
cp-Ti		250–300	105.0
Ti30Ta (α+β)		610	81.2
Ti30Ta (martensitic)		598	63.7
Ti30Ta (α+β)	12.3	520	59.4
Ti30Ta (martensitic)	12.3	515	50.0
Ti30Ta (α+β)	24.4	385	41.8
Ti30Ta (martensitic)	24.4	378	35.3
Ti30Ta (α+β)	30.4	203	25.5
Ti30Ta (martensitic)	30.4	189	23.6

60 GPa and is already very similar to that of the cortical bone (10–20 GPa). In order to achieve an isoelastic behaviour to the bone a further decrease in Young's modulus has been obtained by porous sintering (Table 5.1) (Breme et al., 1993). A powder was produced from Ti30Ta by means of the HDH procedure. For this purpose the alloy produced by electron arc melting was annealed in a reactor in a hydrogen atmosphere. The pick-up of hydrogen causing the formation of TiH_2 and the pinning of dislocation by hydrogen on the slip planes causes an embrittlement of the alloy, so that the material can be milled to produce the desired grain size. The dehydrogenisation of the powder was performed in the same reactor in a vacuum at 500–600°C (Renpo et al., 1985). The irregularly shaped powder can easily be pressurised to produce a green body for sintering in a vacuum or high vacuum. By varying the sintering parameters (pressure, temperature, time and powder grain size) porous samples with different mechanical parameters were produced. Young's modulus and the yield strength, measured with strain gauges, depend on the porosity

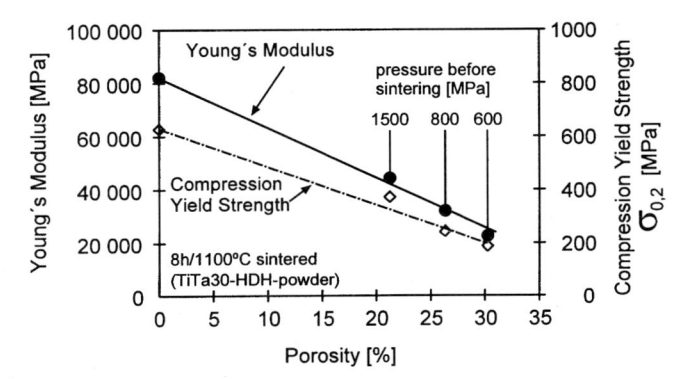

Figure 5.5 Influence of the porosity of Ti30Ta samples on the compression yield strength and on Young's modulus (Breme et al., 1993).

of the sintered samples (Table 5.1 and Figure 5.5). The yield strength decreases with increasing porosity. At a porosity of 30% the yield strength amounts to 190 MPa, a value which is sufficient for application as a dental implant because, even in the case of the maximum measured biting force of 800 N (Schwickerath, 1976), the compression stress is not greater than 50 MPa. For Young's modulus good agreement was found between the measured values and those calculated according to Equation (1.3) (see Chapter 1). Therefore, samples and implants can be produced with a specific porosity whereby the strength properties can be optimised by the sintering parameters. In addition to the porosity itself, the pore size plays an important role. It must be sufficiently large (approximately 50–100 μm) to allow the ingrowth of the bone (Hulbot et al., 1970). In order to determine the fatigue strength, a pneumatic testing apparatus, which is able to simulate the chewing forces under a pressure swelling load, was developed. Since the dental implants are dynamically stressed, the fatigue strength of the material is another important characteristic value. Figure 5.6 shows the results of tests performed with an increasing swelling load (10 MPa after 200 000 cycles) as a function of the porosity of the samples. As one may expect, the stress producing a 0.2% plastic deformation as well as the stress necessary to cause fracture of the sample will decrease with increasing porosity. Nevertheless, even for an entirely porous sample with a porosity of >30%, the stresses measured are high enough for dental implant applications because this stress is not reached at the maximum biting force of 800 N (Wack et al., 1997). Another important result of the investigation was the fact that the static mechanical properties did not depend on the grain size of the powder used for the production of the samples. By comparison, for the dynamic behaviour of the samples, the grain size and especially the notch factor play an important role (Figure 5.7). With samples of a decreasing powder grain size the fatigue strength is increased.

Besides the porous sintered implants, another type of implant with a special surface structure decreasing the implant stiffness and imitating the natural anchorage of teeth has been developed. A spiral of cp-titanium wire was diffusion welded (24 h at 1100°C) on a core consisting of the alloy Ti30Ta. The ingrowth of the bone into

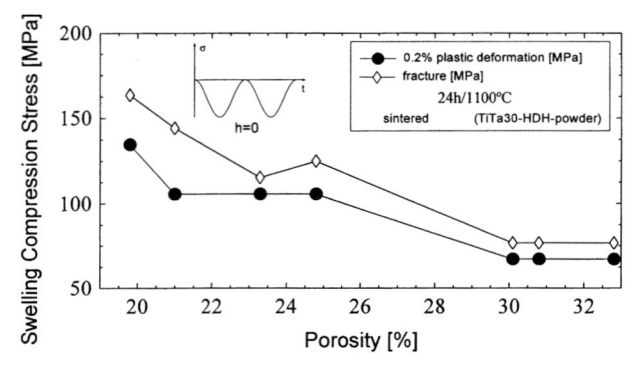

Figure 5.6 Influence of the porosity of Ti30Ta samples on the fatigue behaviour (Wack et al., 1997).

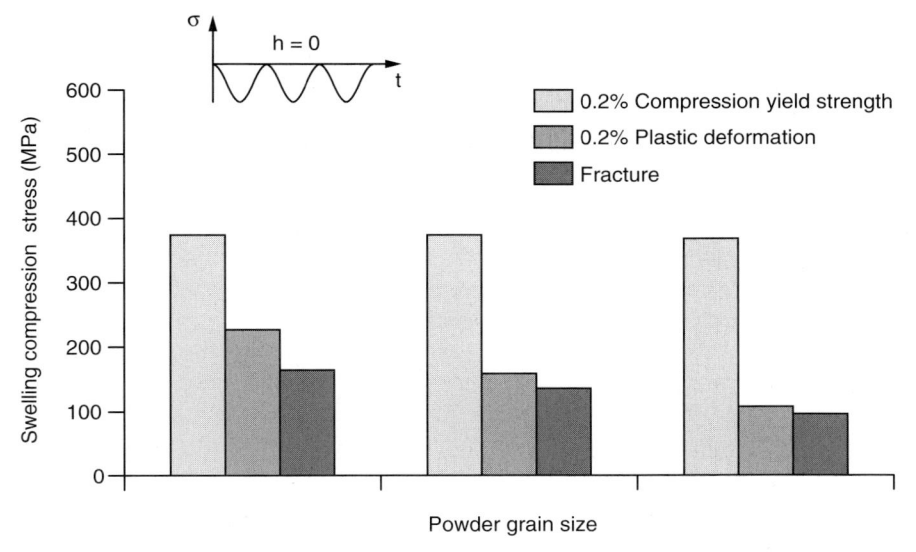

Figure 5.7 Influence of the powder grain size of sintered Ti30Ta samples on the mechanical properties (Wack *et al.*, 1997).

the produced loops imitates the natural suspension by transmitting a damping capacity to the implant similar to the Sharpey fibres of the tooth (Breme *et al.*, 1991). The adhesion strength of the titanium loops to the core of the Ti30Ta alloys was measured in push-out tests. The force amounted to 4500 N. This value is sufficient for functional loading compared with the highest measured chewing forces (Schwickerath, 1976). The functionality of both implant types was determined *in vitro* as well as *in vivo*. For the *in vitro* experiments an artificial jaw was constructed from a plastic material with the same elastic properties and geometry as a human jaw with the inner part ($E = 3$ GPa) corresponding to the spongy bone and the outer part (12 GPa) corresponding to the cortical bone (Breme *et al.*, 1992a). The implants were inserted in the model. The model and the implants were loaded in a testing apparatus in which the strain, and therefore the stresses, of both were measured by means of strain gauges. In order to achieve a clear result concerning the influence of the stiffness of the implant, a systematic change in Young's modulus was studied by a comparison of implants consisting of various materials (alumina, steel, cp-titanium and the isoelastic implants). Figure 5.8 shows the artificial jaw with different implants. The measurement of the *in vitro* functionality of implants embedded in an artificial jaw showed that the implant with the loops on the surface has an elasticity very similar to that of the bone (Figure 5.9). The stresses measured with strain gauges at the jaw during the loading of different implants demonstrate that the load transfer is more effective with decreasing values of Young's modulus. In particular, those samples with values below 50 GPa which are obtained by porous sintering show high compression stress, which is required for the stimulation of new bone formation (Figure 5.10).

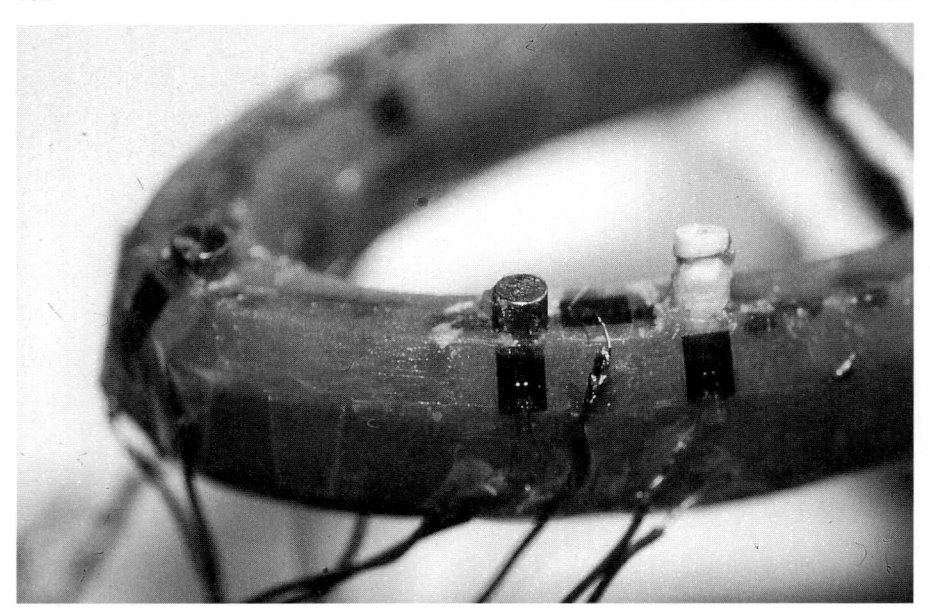

Figure 5.8 Artificial jaw consisting of a core with a modulus (3 GPa) corresponding to that of spongy bone and a surface area with a modulus (128 GPa) corresponding to that of cortical bone (Breme et al., 1991).

In another experiment the biting forces were introduced in the area of the incisor teeth, while strain and stress were measured in the neighbourhood of implants inserted in the area of the molar teeth. The results were similar to those obtained with direct loading. With decreasing values of Young's modulus the compression stress

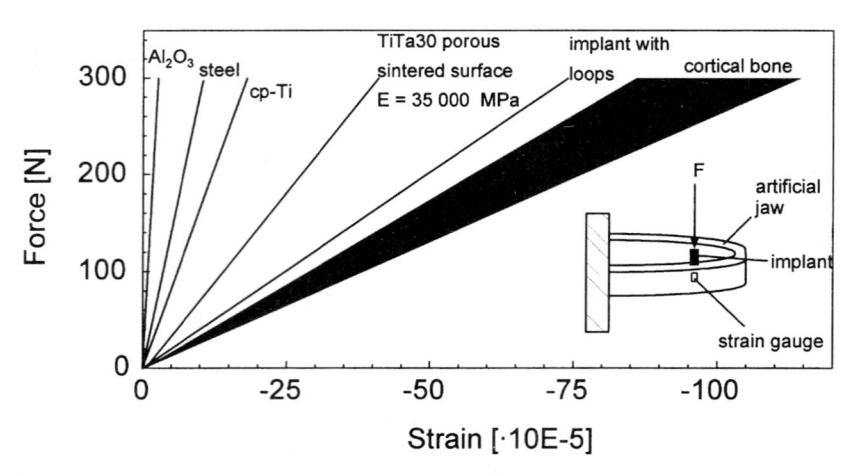

Figure 5.9 Influence of the material on the strain and stress, respectively, measured under functional load at the artificial jaw (Breme et al., 1991).

SURFACES, SURFACE MODIFICATION AND TAILORING

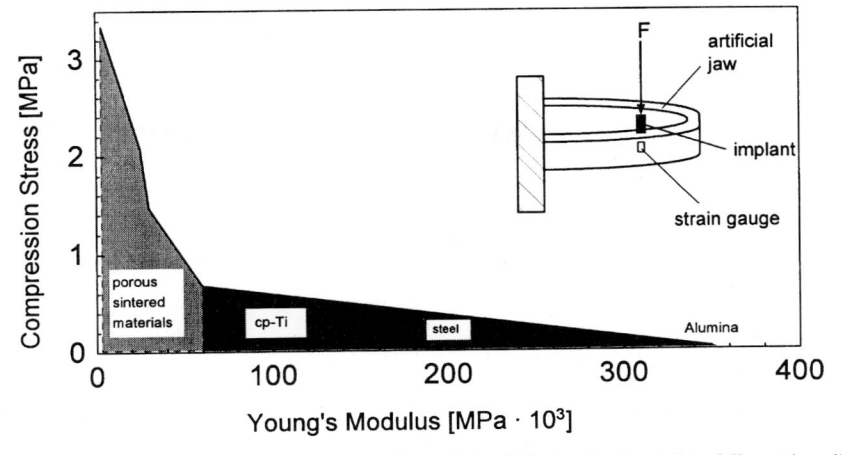

Figure 5.10 Compression stress as a function of Young's modulus (direct loading of the implant) (Breme et al., 1991).

increases (Figure 5.11). Because of this effect Young's modulus also has an influence during the unloaded healing period after implantation, producing stress conditions by which the new bone formation is governed (Biehl et al., 1996). For the functional loading during the *in vivo* tests in adult dogs a special design, shown schematically in Figure 5.12, was necessary. The surface layers of the implants for the animal experiments had a porosity of 20%, a pore size of 103 µm, a Young's modulus value of 45 GPa and a yield strength of 340 MPa. The layers were produced from Ti30Ta powder with a grain size of 200–315 µm by sintering at 1100°C for 24 h in an argon atmosphere. The implants (Figure 5.13) were inserted into the lower jaws of the dogs. After a healing period of 3 months the implants were provided with a dental

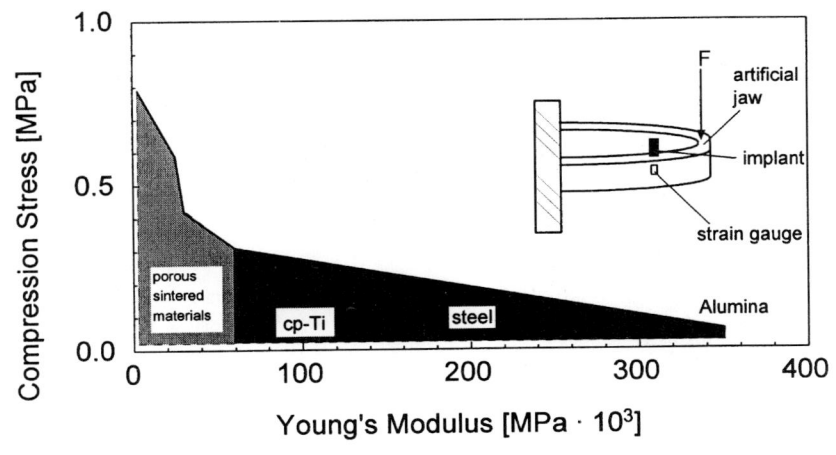

Figure 5.11 Compression stress as a function of Young's modulus (indirect loading of the implant) (Breme et al., 1991).

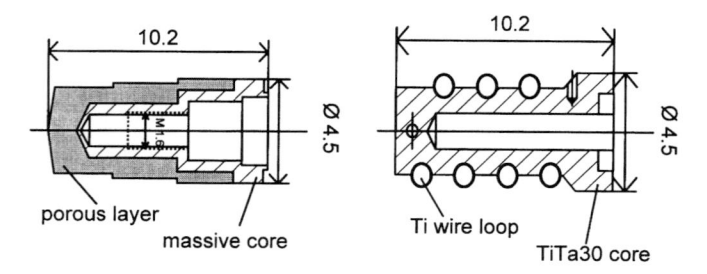

Figure 5.12 Drawings of implants with a porous surface layer (left) and with surface loops (right) (Biehl et al., 1996).

prosthesis. After functional loading for a period of 6 months the implants underwent histological investigation which was preceded by the preparation of microsections according to the method proposed by Donath (1985). Figures 5.14 and 5.15 show the results of the animal experiments. In all implants good interlocking of the bone and close bone contact to the implant surface were observed. Implants with a porous surface layer showed bone ingrowth into the open porosity. Ingrowth of bone was observed, especially in the implants with surface loops. In another study it was shown that the bone had already entered the loops after an implantation duration of

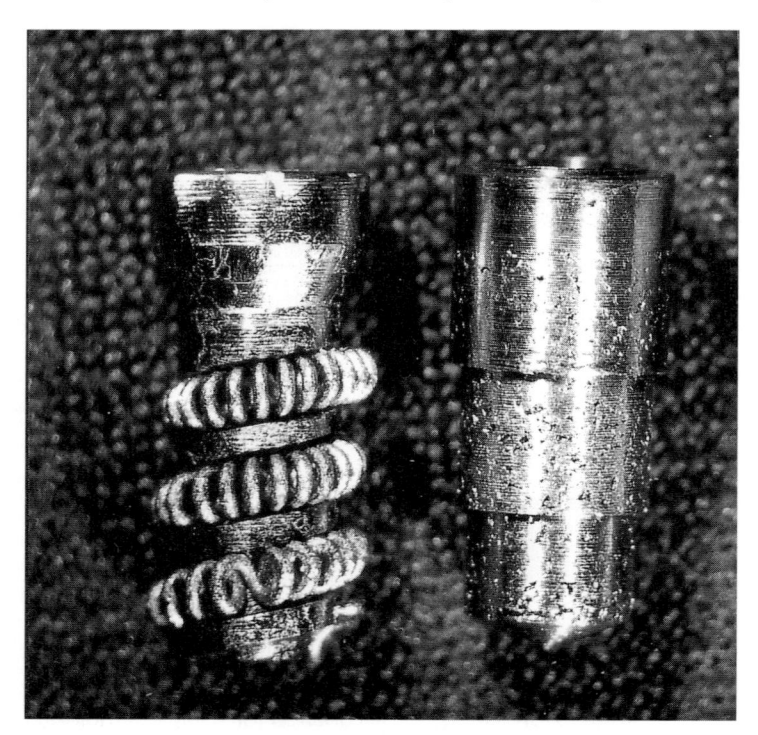

Figure 5.13 Photographs of the implants (Biehl et al., 1996).

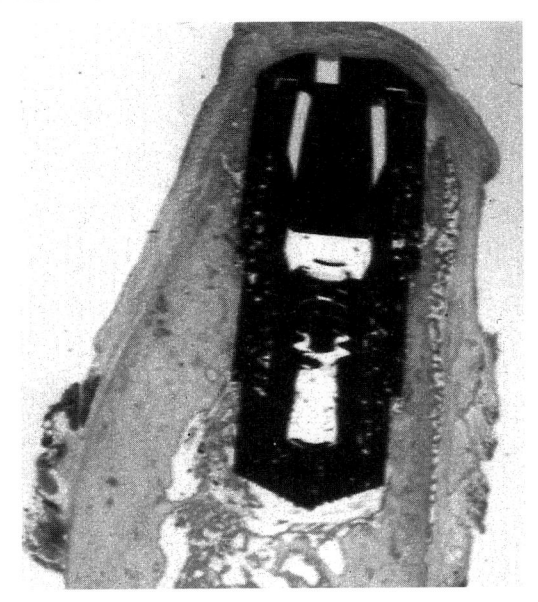

Figure 5.14 Histological slice of an implant with a porous surface (Biehl *et al.*, 1996).

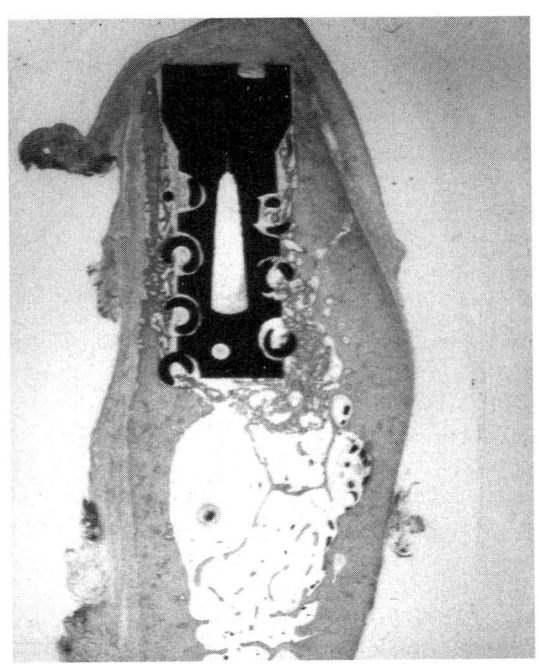

Figure 5.15 Histological slice of an implant with surface loops (Breme *et al.*, 1992a).

only 2 months and no significant difference between the Ca:P ratio of the ingrown bone and the initial bone could be analysed (Breme et al., 1992a, b). For more details on the interaction between dental implants, occlusal forces and tissue reactions, refer to the thesis of Barbier (1995) in which the adaptive bone remodelling around Ti plasma-sprayed oral implants under centric and eccentric loading is discussed in great detail. The author performed very extensive quantitative histology around these implants and, moreover, simulated the system by finite element analysis. This study is one of the (infrequent) publications in which the relation is given between *in vivo* observations and the finite element analysis.

Not only the macrostructure, but the microstructure of the implant surface is of great importance. For example, a dental implant that passes through the gingiva must have a good sealing to the gingiva in order to avoid the migration of bacteria from the oral cavity to the implant bed in the jaw, which would cause inflammation (Guy et al., 1993). This sealing, as well as the adhesion strength, can be improved by a suitable surface structure. From the first contact to a strong adhesion between the biomaterial and, for example, a fibroblast a number of different stages is involved (Alberts and Bray, 1990). At the beginning, the cell has only a weak contact with the substrate. A conducting seam has many focal contacts. In order to locate favourable adhesion conditions the cells move over the surface of the substrate. The direction of the movement is determined by chemical messengers, e.g. fibronectin, or by a direction where the cells register favourable conditions from a guiding structure of the biomaterial (Hynes and Yamada, 1982). After this period of movement the fibroblasts acquire a favourable orientation on the substrate. In order to minimise the forces acting on the cytoskeleton they show an alignment along surface structures like grinding marks (Clark et al., 1991). After this orientation the cells secrete an extra-cellular matrix which depends on the cell type and acts as a bonding agent. Therefore, if implants are coated with molecules (e.g. fibronectin) which are components of the extracellular matrix, an improved adhesion strength is observed (Friedländer et al., 1988; Lotz et al., 1989). In order to study the influence of the surface structure in samples of different metallic materials a defined surface roughness was produced by grinding with SiC paper of various grain sizes. The surface structure was measured with a profilometer. Figure 5.16 shows an example of such a measurement. After cleaning in an ultrasonic bath, the samples were cultured with cells for 2 days, then incubated in a culture medium consisting of gingival biopsies obtained after oral surgical procedures. The test cells of the fourth passage grown in culture flasks were used, and showed a tendency towards alignment along the grinding marks. A cell is considered to be orientated when its longitudinal axes deviate by less than $\pm 10°$ from the deviation of the guidance structure (Eisenbarth et al., 1996). It was shown that the orientated cells on a structured surface (Figure 5.17) possess more focal contacts than round cells on a polished substrate (Figure 5.18). Therefore, a better adhesion strength can be expected for the elongated cells. In addition, the contact area of the cells to the surface is increased by a factor of 1.3–1.6 because the cells are able to grow into the grooves and fill them. The portion of orientated cells depends, within certain limits, on the surface roughness (Figure 5.19).

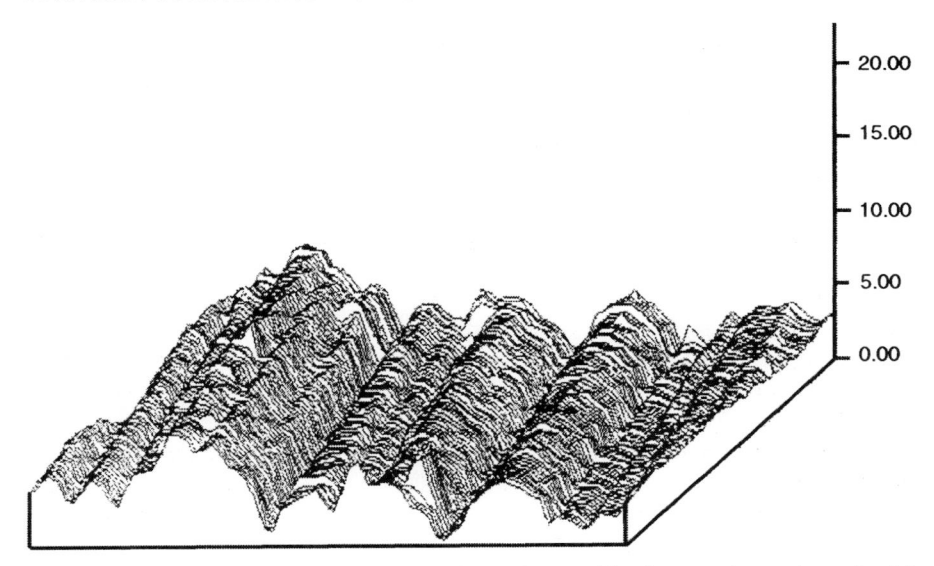

SURFACES, SURFACE MODIFICATION AND TAILORING 167

Figure 5.16 Example of the roughening of a cp-Ti plate to be cultured with fibroblasts (Eisenbarth et al., 1996).

Other investigations demonstrated similar cell behaviour (Meyle et al., 1993). It has been shown that even very small changes in the roughness cause cell reactions. A structure in the range of 130 nm was already sufficient to induce a contact guidance (Curtis and Clark, 1990; Clark et al., 1991). In another study with microstructured material which was implanted subcutaneously, it was shown that changes

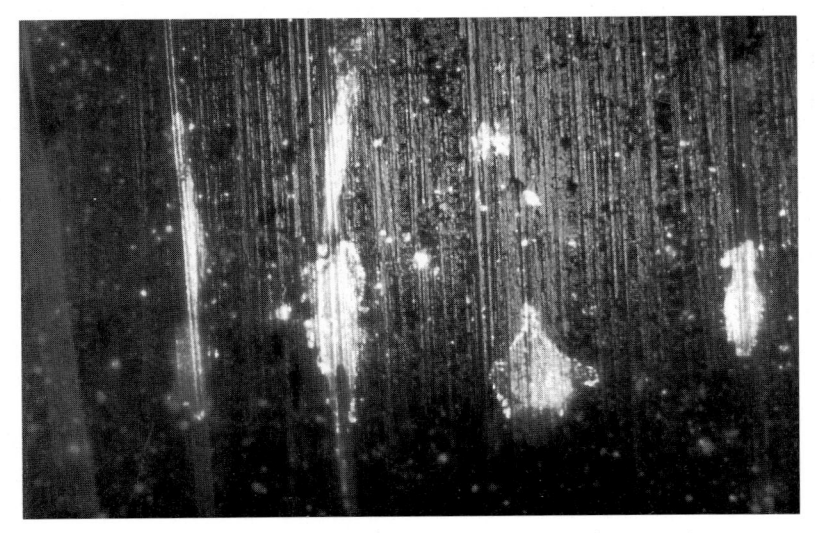

Figure 5.17 Aligned fibroblasts on a ground cp-Ti sample.

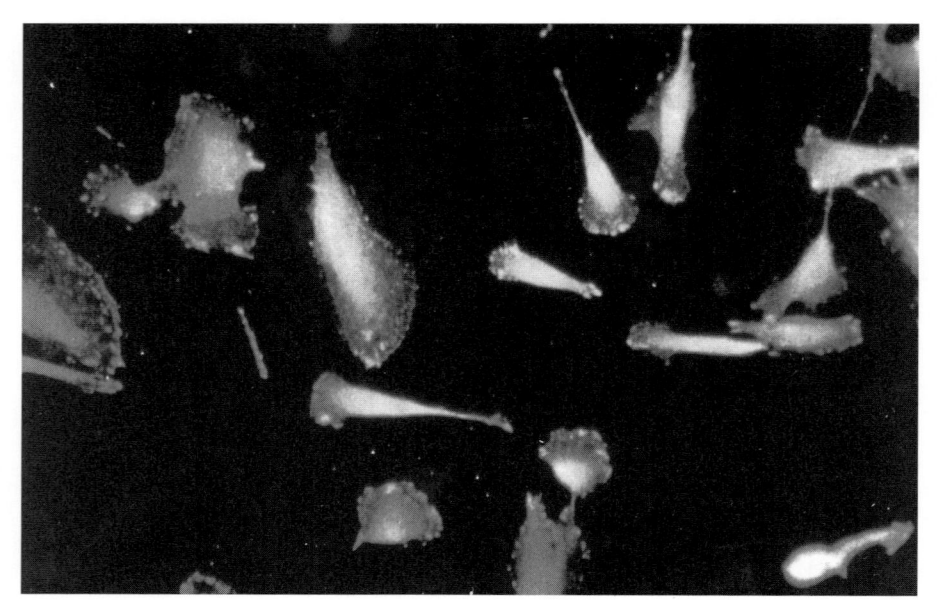

Figure 5.18 Fibroblast on a polished cp-Ti sample.

in the surface pattern in the micrometre range can cause a different tissue reaction (Campbell and van Recum, 1989). It is clear that an average roughness that is excessively high does not allow the cells to enter the grooves.

The ability to orientate along guidance structures depends on the cell type. In comparison with fibroblasts the epithelial cells show a tendency to pass over the grooves of the substrate surface, as shown schematically in Figure 5.20 (Clark *et al.*, 1991).

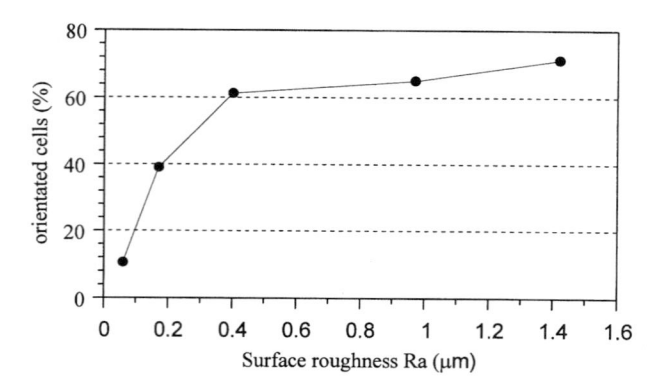

Figure 5.19 Influence of the surface roughness of cp-Ti samples on the orientation of fibroblasts (Eisenbarth *et al.*, 1996).

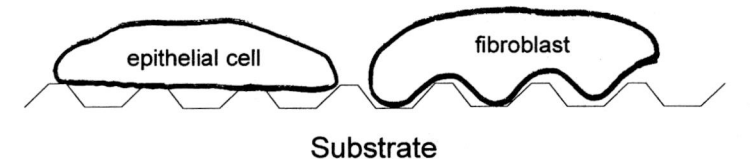

SURFACES, SURFACE MODIFICATION AND TAILORING 169

Figure 5.20 Behaviour of epithelial cells (left) and fibroblasts (right) on a roughened surface (schematic) (Clark *et al.*, 1991; Eisenbarth *et al.*, 1997).

5.3 INFLUENCE OF THE SURFACE COMPOSITION

In order to study the influence of the composition of the substrate on the orientation of the cell, samples of cp-Ti, Ti30Ta and Ti6Al4V were prepared by grinding to the same surface roughness and cultivated with fibroblasts. After a cultivation time of 2 days no substantial difference was observed. The number of orientated cells was similar for all materials within the limit of error (Figure 5.21). Therefore, with

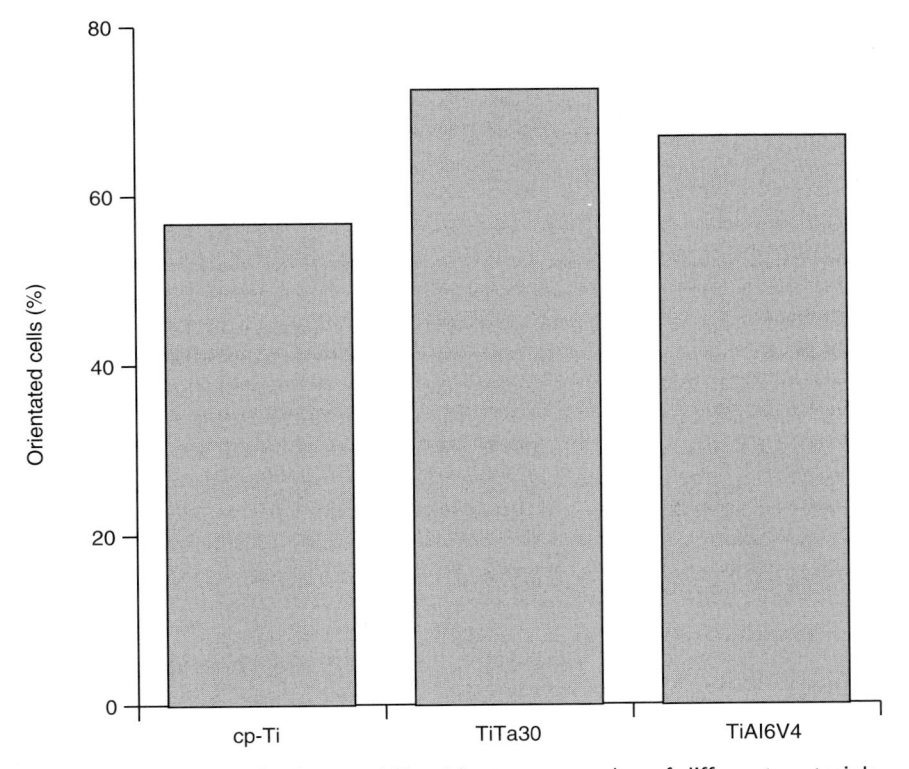

Figure 5.21 Portion of orientated fibroblasts on samples of different materials.

polished samples of the same materials, the period of cultivation was extended to 14 days. In addition, as a further criterion of orientation, the morphology of the cells was determined by measuring their area A and circumference C. By means of these data a shape factor S_f was calculated as follows:

$$S_f = \frac{C}{2\sqrt{\pi A}} - 1. \qquad (5.1)$$

For an exactly round cell the factor amounts to zero. The more aligned the cells, the higher the S_f value. The retention of the aligned cell shape, which stands for a high adhesion strength to the substrate, takes place with a consumption of metabolic energy. As a consequence, impairment of the metabolism of the cells by toxic alloying elements has an influence on the cell morphology and therefore on the adhesion strength. Fibroblasts which become round in shape have decreased vitality and adhesion strength. After an incubation period of 2 days the calculated shape factor was similar but after 14 days a significant difference was observed (Figure 5.22). The cells grown on samples of cp-Ti and Ti30Ta were still aligned with a shape factor of 1.76 and 1.58, respectively (Figure 5.23), whereas the cells on samples of Ti6Al4V had a shape factor of only 0.93 (Figure 5.24). This unfavourable

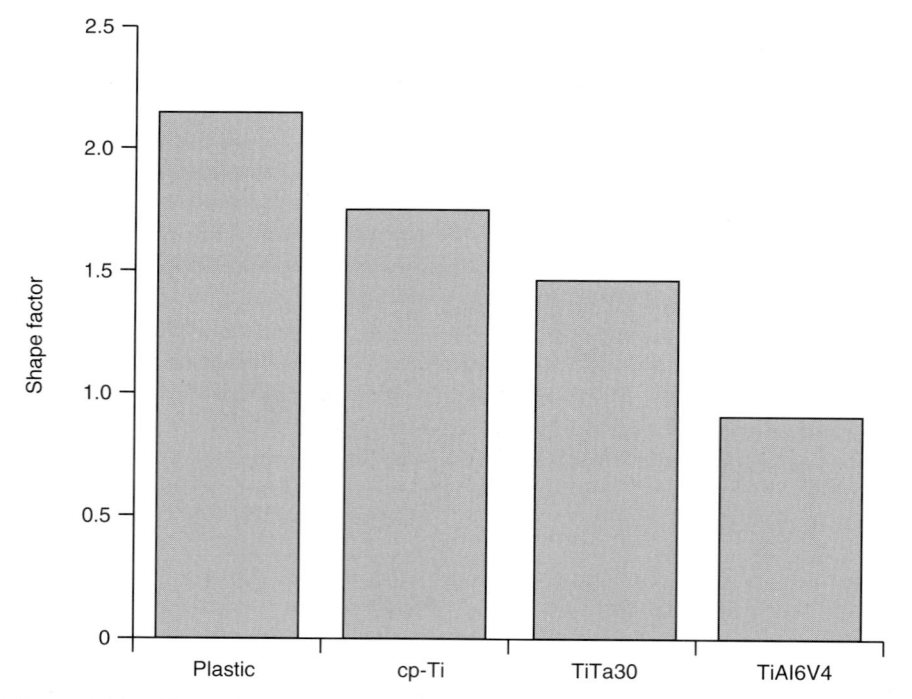

Figure 5.22 Shape factor of fibroblasts on samples of different materials.

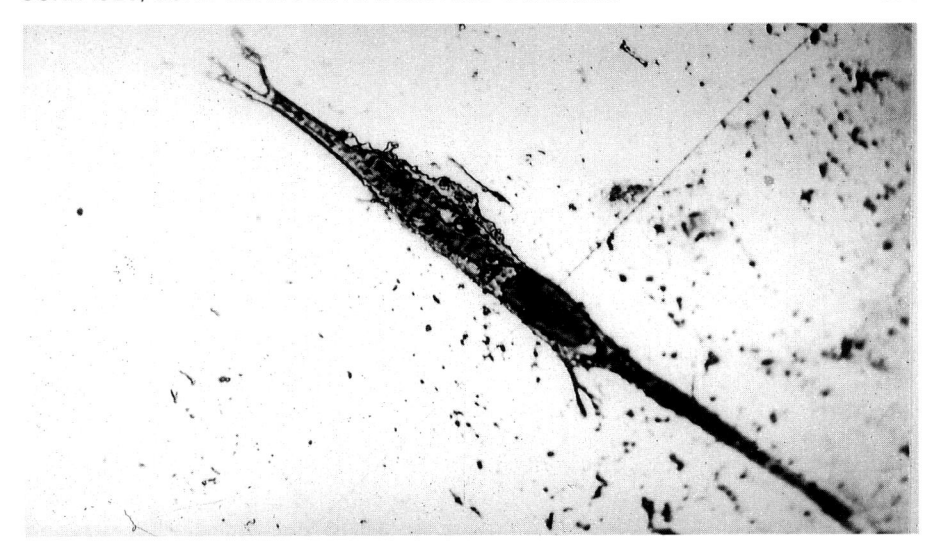

Figure 5.23 Fibroblast on a Ti30Ta sample after 14 days' culture (Eisenbarth et al., 1997).

behaviour in the case of the Ti6Al4V samples signifies an interaction with the cells which is observed only after the longer incubation time. The reason for this behaviour may be a local enrichment of vanadium from which ions can be set free

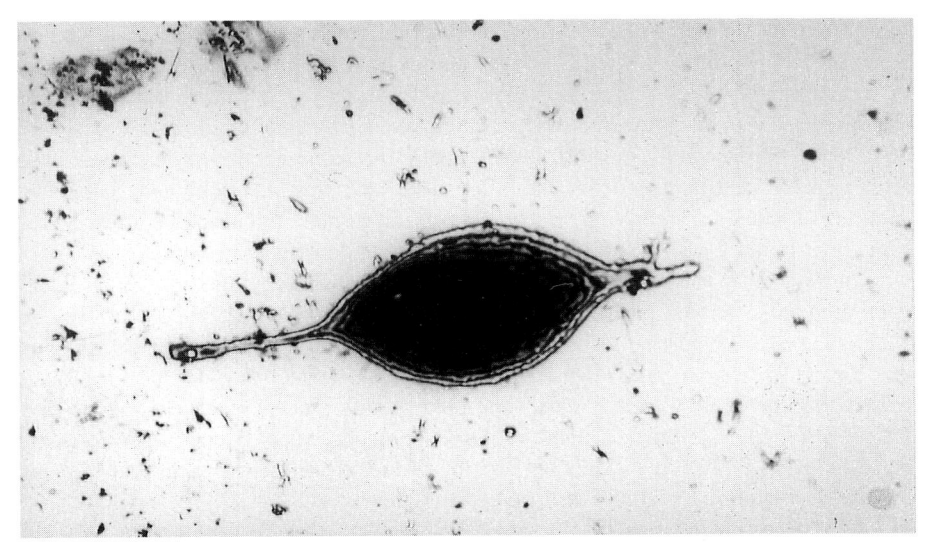

Figure 5.24 Fibroblast on a Ti6Al4V sample after 14 days' culture (Eisenbarth et al., 1997).

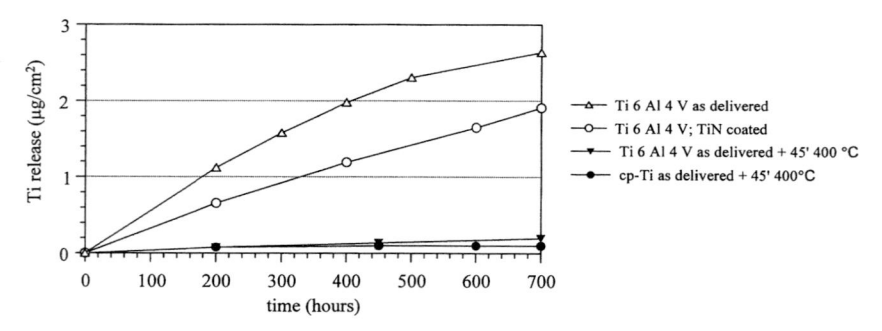

Figure 5.25 Influence of the TiO_2 surface layer on titanium samples on the Ti ion release in bovine serum (Browne and Gregson, 1994).

in a greater amount after a 14-day cultivation. It is known that vanadium stabilises the β-phase in which it is in solution (Castro and Séraphin, 1966). For optimisation of the mechanical properties the material is aged in the temperature range of 450–650°C, whereby the superlattice phase ω is precipitated in the transformed β-phase. Besides this isothermally formed ω an athermal ω is known which is precipitated during cooling, e.g. from the deformation temperature (Duerig et al., 1980). These ω-phases appear locally in submicroscopic sites and contain up to 22% vanadium. Although this phase may be thermodynamically stable, release of ions cannot be totally avoided (Eisenbarth et al., 1996).

Even in the region of passivity, general corrosion combined with this release of ions, which may produce undesired interaction, is observed. This release can be minimised by changing the surface composition, for example, through a surface layer of TiN produced by PVD. It was shown that the ion release of Co and Cr in a CoCr alloy was diminished and simultaneously the pitting potential was increased to 1.16 V compared with the uncoated material which had a potential of 0.83 V (Wisbey and Gregson, 1987). Using the same coating a decrease in the ionic release of titanium from the alloy Ti6Al4V was not achieved. Uncoated samples of Ti6Al4V in bovine serum showed the highest release of Ti ions. In the same investigation a TiO_2 surface layer with a higher density and better stoichiometry was produced by annealing for 45 min at 400°C, whereby the ion release was decreased, also in comparison with samples without this heat treatment (Figure 5.25). Samples consisting of cp-titanium with the same heat treatment showed the lowest corrosion rate (Browne and Gregson, 1994). A TiO_2 surface layer with a higher density and a more complete stoichiometry can be produced by the sol-gel method. Figure 5.26 shows the reaction scheme of the TiO_2 precipitation on samples of Ti5Al2.5Fe. After dip coating of the samples a mixture of an organic substance containing titanium was heated together with CH_3COCH_3 at 120–150°C in order to produce a gel. After annealing at 600°C a dense coating of TiO_2 with a high adhesion strength to the substrate was produced. A corrosion measurement (current density–potential) of the sol-gel-coated samples in a 0.9%

SURFACES, SURFACE MODIFICATION AND TAILORING

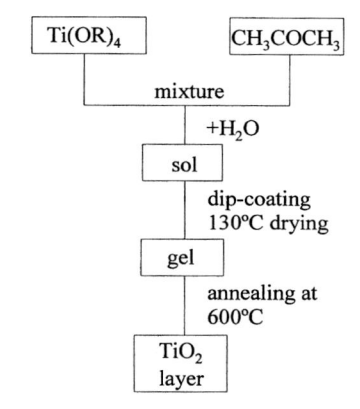

Figure 5.26 TiO$_2$ surface layer production by sol-gel (Breme, 1995).

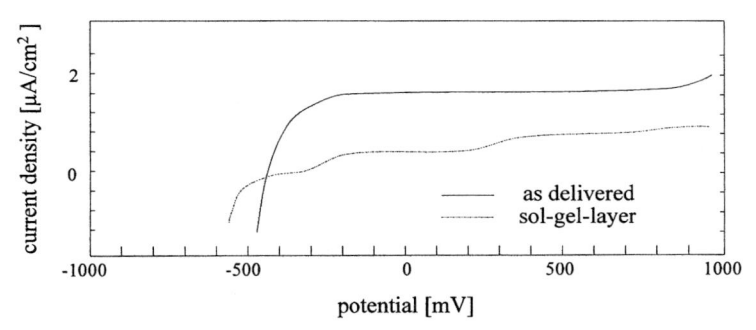

Figure 5.27 Current density–potential curves of Ti5Al2.5Fe samples with and without TiO$_2$ sol-gel surface layers (Breme, 1995).

sodium chloride solution (pH 7.4) resulted in a low current density in the passive region compared with samples without the sol-gel treatment (Figure 5.27) (Breme, 1995). The osseointegration of implants can be accelerated by a change in the surface composition using bioactive ceramics (hydroxyapatite) and/or organic substances (Chapters 6 and 8).

REFERENCES

Alberts, B. and Bray, D. (1990) *Molekularbiologie der Zelle*, VCH, Weinheim.
Barbier, L. (1995) Adaptive bone remodelling around oral implants under load-bearing conditions in the mandible of the dog, Ph.D. thesis, Katholieke Universiteit de Leuven, Leuven, Belgium.
Biehl, V., Breme, J., Wack, T., Schulte, W., d'Hoedt, B. and Donath, K. (1996) *In-vitro* and *in-vivo* study of isoelastic dental implants, in *Proceedings of the 8th World Conference on Titanium*, Institute of Materials, Cambridge, pp. 1828–35.
Bombelli, R. and Mathys, R., Jr (1982) Cementless isoelastic RM total hip prosthesis, *J. R. Soc. Med.*, **75**, 588–97.

Breme, J. (1995) Beitrag zur Oberflächenmodifikation von dentalen Implantaten für eine optimierte Osteointegration, in *Verbundwerkstoffordnung* (eds J. Bossert, N. Claussen and R. Nitsche), Expert, Renningen, pp. 217–19.
Breme, J., Biehl, V., Schulte, W., d'Hoedt, B. and Donath, K. (1992a) Prüfung der Funktionalität und In-vivo-Tests an dentalen Implantaten aus TiTa30 mit drahtförmiger Oberflächenstruktur (Schlaufenimplantat), *Z. Zahnärz. Implantol.* **8**, 174–8.
Breme, J., Biehl, V., Schulte, W., d'Hoedt, B. and Donath, K. (1993) Development and functionality of isoelastic dental implants of titanium alloys, *Biomaterials* **14**, 887–91.
Breme, J., d'Hoedt, B., Schulte, W. and Wadewitz, V. (1991) Contribution to the functional surface structure of endosseous implants, *Int. J. Oral Maxillofac. Implants* **6**, 37–41.
Breme, J., Glieden, T., Schmitt, B. and Biehl., V. (1992b) Development of dental implants isoelastic to the bone and testing their isoelastic behavior, in *Transactions of the 4th World Biomaterials Congress*, Berlin, p. 379.
Browne, M. and Gregson, P.J. (1994) Surface modification of titanium alloy implants, *Biomaterials*, **15**, 894–8.
Brunski, J.B., Moccia, A.F., Jr., Pollack, S.R., Korostoff, E. and Trachtenberg, D.I. (1979) The influence of functional use of endosseous implants on the tissue–implant interface. Histological aspects, *J. Dent. Res.* **58**, 1953–61.
Campbell, C.E. and von Recum, A.F. (1989) Microtopography and soft tissue response, *J. Invest. Surg.* **2**, 51–74.
Castro, R. and Séraphin, L. (1966) Métallographie et structure de l'alliage Ti6Al4V, *Rev. Mét.* **12**, 1025–55.
Clark, P., Connolly, P., Curtis, A.S.G. and Dow, J.A.T. (1991) Cell guidance by ultrafine topography in vitro, *J. Biomed. Mater. Res.* **99**, 73–7.
Curtis, A.S.G. and Clark, P. (1990) The effects of topographic and mechanical properties of materials on cell behavior, *Crit. Rev. Biocomp.* **5**, 343–62.
Donath, K. (1985) The diagnostic value of the new method for the study of undecalcified bones on teeth with attached soft tissue, *Path. Res. Pract.* **179**, 631–3.
Duering, T.W., Terlinde, G.T. and Williams, J.C. (1980) The ω-phase reaction in Ti alloys, in *Proceedings of the 4th International Conference on Titanium* (eds H. Kumura and P. Izumi), AIME, New York, pp. 1299–308.
Eisenbarth, E., Meyle, J., Nachtigall, W. and Breme, J. (1996) Influence of the surface structure of titanium materials on the adhesion of fibroblasts, *Biomaterials* **17**, 1399–404.
Eisenbarth, E., Wenzel, M., Breme, J., Meyle, J. and Nachtigall, W. (1997) Einfluß der Oberflächenstruktur und -zusammensetzung auf die Zellhaftung, in *Werkstoffe für die Medizintechnik*, Symposium 4, Werkstoffwoche (ed. J. Breme), DGM, Frankfurt, pp. 99–104.
Feagin, R.C. (1986) Titanium investment casting, in *20th EICF Conference on Investment Casting*, Brussels, pp. 45–53.
Fink, U. (1996) Plasmapore: a plasma sprayed microporous titanium coating to improve the long term stability, in *Actualités en Biomatériaux*, Vol. III (eds D. Mainard, M. Marie, J.P. Delagaute and J.P. Louis), Editions Romillat, Paris, pp. 97–104.
Friedlander, D.R., Hoffman, S. and Edelman, G.M. (1988) Functional mapping of cytotact in proteolytic fragments active in cell-substrated adhesion, *J. Cell Biol.* **107**, 2329–40.
Griss, P. and Heimke, G. (1976) Record of discussion on stability of joint prostheses, in *Biocompatibility of Implant Materials* (ed. D. Williams), Sector Publishing, London, pp. 52–68.
Guy, S.C., McQuade, M.J., Scheidg, M.J., McPherson, J.C., Rossmann, J.A. and Van Dyke, T.E. (1993) *In vitro* attachment of human gingival fibroblasts to endosseous implant materials, *J. Periodontol.* **64**, 524–46.
Hansson, H.A., Albrektsson, M.D. and Branemark, P.I. (1983) Structural aspects of the interface between tissue and titanium implants, *J. Prosthet. Dent.* **50**, 108–16.
Heimke, G. (1990) The aspects and modes of fixation of bone replacements, in *Osseo-Integrated Implants*, Vol. I (ed. G. Heimke), CRC Press, Boca Raton, FL, pp. 2–26.
Heimke, G., Schulte, W., d'Hoedt, B., Griss, P., Büsing, C.M. and Stock, D. (1982) The influence of fine structures on the osseointegration of implants, *Int. J. Artif. Organs* **5**, 207–12.

Heimke, G., Schulte, W., Griss, P., Jentschura, G. and Schulz, P. (1980) Generalization of biomechanical rules for fixation of bone joint and tooth replacement, *J. Biomed. Mater. Res.* **14**, 537–45.

Henssge, E.J., Dufek, P., Bensmann, G. and Ljutow, A. (1990) Surface structured implants consisting of Co-based alloys, in Osseo-Intergrated Implants, Vol. I (ed. G. Heimke), CRC Press, Boca Raton, FL, pp. 154–65.

Henssge, E.J., Grundei, H., Etspüler, R., Köller, W. and Fink, K. (1985) Die anatomisch angepaßte Endoprothese des proximalen Fermurendes, *Z. Orthrop.* **123**, 820–6.

Henssge, E.J. and Peschel, U. (1987) Anatomisch angepaßte Hüftendoprothese mit spongiösmetallischer Oberfläche, in *Zementfreie Implantation von Hüftgelenkendoprothesen* (ed. D. Refior), Teubner, Stuttgart, pp. 132–45.

Hulbot, S.F., Young, F.A., Matthews, R.S. Klawitter, J.J., Talbot, C.D. and Stelling, F.H. (1970) Potential of ceramic materials as permanently implantable skeletal prosthesis, *J. Biomed. Mat. Res.* **4**, 433–9.

Hynes, R.O. and Yamada, K.M. (1982) Fibronectins – multifunctional modular glycoproteins, *J. Cell Biol.* **95**, 369–77.

Kinzi, L., Burri, C., Mohr, W., Paull, K. and Wolter, D. (1976) Gewebeverträglichkeit der Polymere Polyäthylen, Polyester und Polyacetalharz, *Orthopädie ihre Grenzgeb.* **114**, 777–84.

Kirsch, A. (1980) Titan-spritzbeschichtetes Zahnwurzelimplantat unter physiologischer Belastung beim Menschen, *Dtsch. Zahnärtzl. Z.* **35**, 112–18.

Krekeler, G., Sotter, F. and Schilli, W. (1984) Das ITI-Implant Typ H: Technische Entwicklung; Tierexperiment und klinische Erfahrung, *Quintessenz* **35**, 2253–63.

Lotz, M., Burdsal, C., Erikson, H. and McClay, D. (1989) Cell adhesion to fibronictin and tenoxin: quantitative measurements of initial binding and subsequent strengthening response, *J. Cell Biol.* **109**, 1795–1805.

Meyle, J., Gültig, K., Wohlburg, H. and van Recum, A.F. (1993) Fibroblast anchorage to microtextured surfaces, *J. Biomed. Mater. Res.* **27**, 1553–7.

Morscher, E. Mathys, R. and Henche, H.R. (1976) Iso-elastic endoprosthesis – a new concept in artificial joint replacement, in *Advances in Artificial and Hip and Knee Joint Technology*, Springer, Berlin.

Niinimaki, T., Puranen, J. and Jalovaara, P. (1994) Total hip arthroplasty using isoelastic femoral stems. A seven- to nine-year follow-up in 108 patients, *J. Bone Joint Surg.* **76**, 413–18.

Plitz, W. and Böhme, F. (1988) Wie beeinträchtigen osteoinduktive Oberflächenstrukturen die Gestaltfestigkeit von Endoprothesenschäften, Vol. 8, *Sitzung des DVM Arbeitskreises Implantate*, DVM, Berlin, pp. 25–40.

Renpo, T., Tao, L. and Changchun, L. (1985) Development in PM HHDH-Ti6Al4V technology for aircraft application, in *Proceedings of the Fifth International Conference on Titanium* (eds G. Lütjering, U. Zwicker and W. Bunk), DGM, Oberursel, pp. 443–50.

Schädlich-Stubenrauch, J., Sahm, P.R. and Linn, H. (1988) Numerical simulation of the α-case as a quality criterion for the investment casting of small thin walled titanium parts, in *Proceedings of the 6th World Conference on Titanium* (eds P. Lacombe, R. Tricort and G. Béranger), Les Éditions de Physique, Les Ulis, pp. 649–54.

Schmitz, H.J., Gross, U., Kinne, R., Fuhrmann, G. and Strunz, V. (1988) Der Einfluß unterschiedlicher Oberflächenstrukturierung alloplastischer Implantate auf das histologische Zugfestigkeitsverhalten des Interface, Vol. 8, *Sitzung des DVM Arbeitskreises Implantate*, DVM, Berlin, pp. 163–72.

Schwickerath, H. (1976) Kaukraft-Kaudruck-Belastbarkeit, *Dtsch. Zahnärztl. Z.* **31**, 870–3.

Wack, T., Biehl, V. and Breme, J. (1997) Dauerschwingverhalten poröser Sinterwerkstoffe der Legierung TiTa30 für die Herstellung isoelastischer Implantate, in *Werkstoffe für die Medizintechnik*, Symposium 4, Werkstoffewoche (ed. J. Breme), DGM, Frankfurt, pp. 171–6.

Winkler-Gniewek, W., Fink, U. and Stallforth, H. (1991) *Biomechanische Aspekte plasmagespritzter Oberflächenbeschichtungen zur zementfreien Prothesenverankerung, Hüftnekrose* (ed. Th. Stuhler), Springer, Berlin.

Wisbey, A. and Gregson, R.J. (1987) Application of PVD TIN coating to Co-Cr-Mo based surgical implants, *Biomaterials* **96**, 477–80.

6
Special thin organic coatings

H. WORCH
Technical University of Dresden, Dresden, Germany

6.1 INTRODUCTION

To date, organic coatings have been scarcely used on metallic implants. Nevertheless, it is expected that these materials will significantly improve their market share as improved biocompatibility becomes the decisive criterion for patients and surgeons in the future (Wintermantel and Ha, 1996). This approach, which is based on the latest medical and cellular biological results, employs biopolymers (proteins) (Ebert, 1993) that have been immobilised on the surface of metallic implants. The intention is to reduce the foreign character of the implant for the body. This is accomplished by coating with substances that are normally found on the surface or in the vicinity of the tissue that has to be substituted by the implant.

It has been found that these coatings act as local mediators of cell adhesion and, in consequence, as a stimulating factor for the growth and proliferation of the cells normally found around the substituted tissue. The tight attachment at the oxide-coated surface of the metallic implant and the conservation of the biological function of the proteins involved are prerequisites for obtaining these highly desirable properties (Walton, 1980).

Since the natural environment around the implant is aqueous while the surface of the implant is either bare or oxidised metal, specific demands are imposed on the coating in order to mediate successfully between these different structural entities. The purpose of these demands is to obtain the native conformation of all proteins and cells that are in contact with the coating and to avoid all forms of aggregation and other conformational changes that might lead to protein denaturation or cell death.

In recent years new insights into the function of a special class of signal proteins have improved our understanding of this integration process. These morphogenetic proteins influence significantly the adhesion, proliferation and differentiation of cells, and are therefore capable of controlling the tissue structure in the vicinity of an implant. However, our knowledge concerning the adsorption of proteins in inorganic materials is comparatively poor (Schmidt, 1994). The mechanistic details of the process as well as the nature of the chemical bonds involved in immobilising the protein at the inorganic surface have been the subject of recent research.

Metals as Biomaterials ISBN 0 471 96935 4 Edited by J.A. Helsen and H.J. Breme. © 1998 John Wiley & Sons Ltd

Figure 6.1 Chemical structure of (a) an α-amino acid and the (b) α-imino acid proline.

6.2 COMPOSITION AND STRUCTURE OF BIOPOLYMERS

To achieve a deeper understanding of protein adsorption at surfaces it is necessary to recall some basic knowledge about the composition and structure of proteins. It is estimated that the human genomic codes contain between 50 000 and 80 000 peptides and proteins. Approximately 5000 of these polypeptides have been well characterised and another 10 000 have been at least partially characterised (Ebert, 1993). A closer look at the composition of the human polypeptides, as well as the polypeptides of all other terrestrial organisms (animals, plants, algae, yeast, fungi, bacteria and viruses) shows that these polypeptides are predominantly built by only 20 different structural elements, the α-amino acids (Voet and Voet, 1992). α-Amino acids (Figure 6.1a) usually consist of an asymmetric carbon atom (with the exception of glycine) which also contains a primary amino group (with the exception of the secondary amino group in proline; see Figure 6.1b), a carboxy group, a hydrogen atom and a variable side-chain which determines the individual character of each amino acid. Proline, strictly speaking an α-imino acid is, regardless of its deviating chemical structure, commonly referred to as one of the 20 basic α-amino acids.

A closer look at the pK_A values of the carboxy group and the α-amino group reveals a rather narrow interval (1.9–2.95) for the C-terminus and a slightly broader interval (8.84–10.78) for the N-terminus of individual amino acids. Consequently, both groups remain dissociated within the physiological pH range (around pH 7) (Figure 6.2).

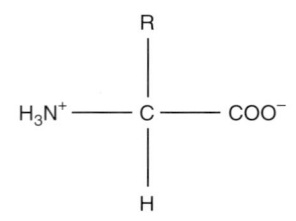

Figure 6.2 Chemical structure of a dissociated α-amino acid within the physiological pH range.

SPECIAL THIN ORGANIC COATINGS

Since all α-amino acids consist of at least one basic and one acidic group which carry opposing charges within the physiological pH range they are referred to as being dipolar or amphoteric. A classification of the 20 basic α-amino acids is obtained by categorising the properties of their side-chains (-R) (Table 6.1). They are either apolar, polar but uncharged, or polar and charged (Figure 6.3).

Along with the 20 basic α-amino acids some highly specialised amino acids exist. 3-Hydroxyproline and 4-hydroxylysine, which are found in the collagenic tissue of vertebrates, are of special importance in this respect. For the 20 basic α-amino acids as well as for 3-hydroxyproline (Hyp, O) and 4-hydroxylysine (Hyl, J) a three-letter notation and a one-letter notation are commonly used within the biochemical literature (Karlson, 1988).

Proteins (> 99 amino acids), polypeptides (10–99 amino acids) and oligopeptides (1–9 amino acids) are built by polycondensation (Figure 6.4). A -CO-NH- link, the peptide bond, is formed while water is being split off. The newly formed bond has a high double-bond character, as revealed by the work of Pauling and Corey and is also called the Pauling–Corey peptide bond. With a few exceptions, the Cα-atoms of neighbouring amino acids within a peptide chain form a trans-configuration (Figure 6.5).

Proteins are synthesised as an unbranched sequence starting at the N-terminus. The N-terminus of the first amino acid and the C-terminus of the last amino acid remain free. The C-terminus of the first amino acid is linked to the N-terminus of the second, and so on (Creighton, 1989). This arrangement reflects the striking

Table 6.1 The 20 proteinogenic amino acids

Name/side-chain	code 3/1	Apolar	Polar, uncharged	Polar, charged
Glycine	Gly/G	-H		
Alanine	Ala/A	$-CH_3$		
Valine	Val/V	$-CH(CH_3)_2$		
Leucine	Leu/L	$-CH_2CH(CH_3)_2$		
Isoleucine	Ile/I	$-CHCH_3C_2H_5$		
Phenolalanine	Phe/F	$-CH_2C_6H_5$		
Tryptophane	Trp/W	$-CH_2C_8H_6N$		
Methionine	Met/M	$-CH_2CH_2SCH_3$		
Cysteine	Cys/C	$-CH_2SH$		
Proline	Pro/P	see Figure 6.2		
Asparagine	Asn/N		$-CH_2CONH_2$	
Glutamine	Gln/Q		$-CH_2CH_2CONH_2$	
Serine	Ser/S		$-CH_2OH$	
Threonine	Thr/T		$-CHCH_3OH$	
Tyrosine	Tyr/Y		$-CH_2C_6H_4OH$	
Aspartine	Asp/D			$-CH_2COO^-$
Glutamate	Glu/E			$-CH_2CH_2COO^-$
Histidine	His/H			$-CH_2C_3H_4N_2^+$
Lysine	Lys/K			$-C_4H_8NH_3^+$
Arginine	Arg/R			$-C_3H_6NHCNH_2NH_2^+$

Glycine

```
        COO⁻
         |
  H ─── C ─── H
         |
        NH₃⁺
```

Asparagine

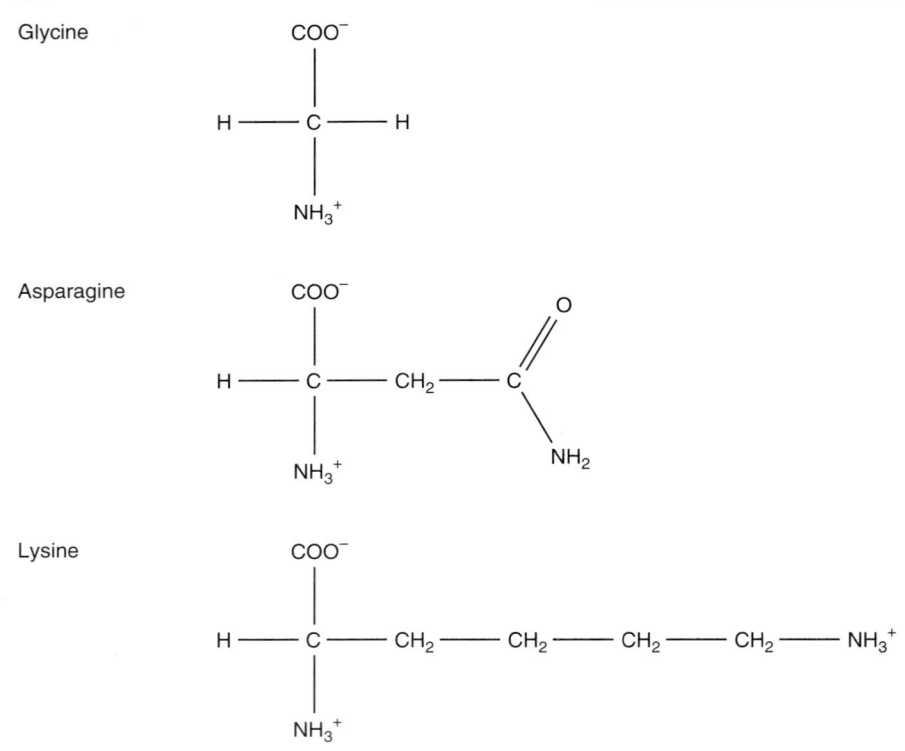

```
        COO⁻                    O
         |                      ‖
  H ─── C ─── CH₂ ─── C
         |                  \
        NH₃⁺                  NH₂
```

Lysine

```
        COO⁻
         |
  H ─── C ─── CH₂ ─── CH₂ ─── CH₂ ─── CH₂ ─── NH₃⁺
         |
        NH₃⁺
```

Figure 6.3 α-Amino acids categorised by polarity and charge.

simplicity of the formation of these macromolecules in living matter. The architecture of the proteins generated as a consequence of this build-up reaction is characterised by their primary, secondary, tertiary and quarternary structure (Figure 6.6). The primary structure describes the sequence of the amino acids, starting from the N-terminus. The secondary structure characterises local conformations of the polypeptide chain (Milner-White and Poet, 1987), such as α-helices, β-sheets, turns and random coil structures. The tertiary structure describes the three-dimensional locations of all atoms of a protein or polypeptide which is built by a single peptide chain, while the quarternary structure describes the spatial distribution of all subunits (different polypeptide chains) that form a protein complex.

The structure of polypeptides and proteins is stabilised by different binding interactions. The covalent bonds within the amino acid chain determine the primary structure. Electrostatic interaction, hydrogen bonds and disulfide bridges between cysteine residues (if present), together with weak van de Waal's and hydrophobic interactions, are responsible for the formation of the higher spatial structures.

Table 6.2 (Norde and Lyklema, 1990; Haynes and Norde, 1994) gives a survey of the relevant binding interactions and their influence on the free enthalpy, G.

SPECIAL THIN ORGANIC COATINGS

Figure 6.4 Formation of a dipeptide by polycondensation of two α-amino acids.

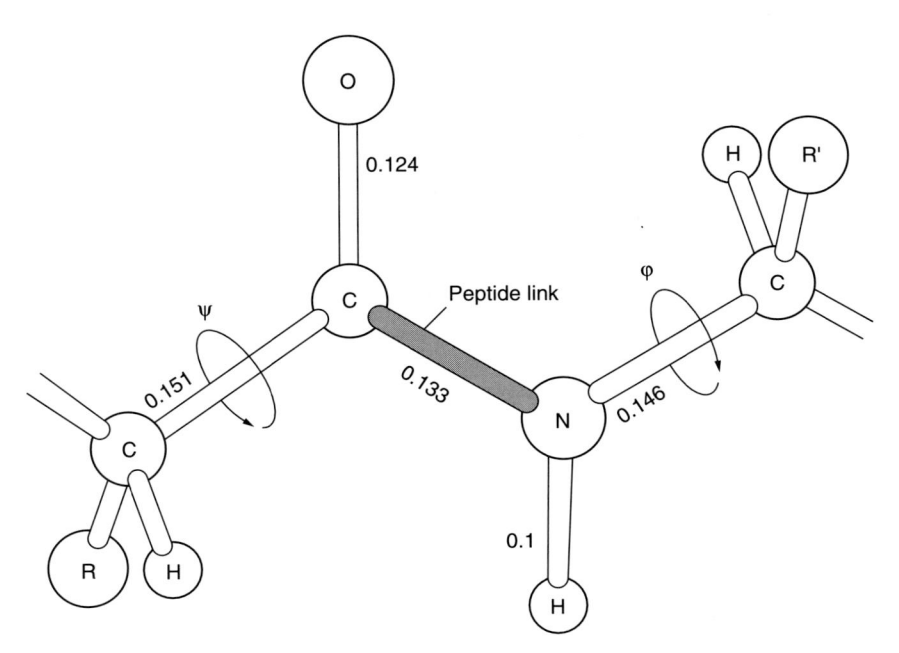

Figure 6.5 Typical dimensions of a planar trans-peptide bond (Marsh and Donohue, 1967).

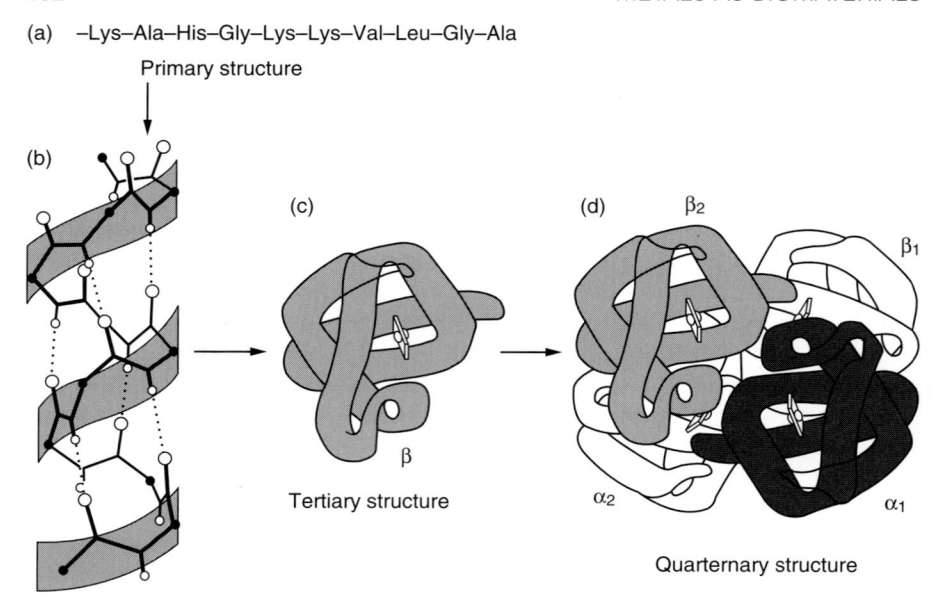

(a) –Lys–Ala–His–Gly–Lys–Lys–Val–Leu–Gly–Ala
Primary structure

(b) Secondary structure

(c) Tertiary structure

(d) Quaternary structure

Figure 6.6 Structural hierarchy of protein structures: (a) primary, (b) secondary, (c) tertiary, (d) quaternary structure (Voet and Voet, 1992).

Table 6.2 Interactions determining the three-dimensional structure of proteins in an aqueous environment

Type of interaction	$\Delta G_{compact-unfolded}$	Remarks
Coulomb	0	Depending on the pH relative to the isoelectric point
Dipole	≈ 0	Formation of bonds inside the protein molecule and between water molecules at the expense of protein–water bonds
Hydrogen bonding	≥ 0	
Dispersion	≤ 0	Atom packing density in compact protein molecules higher than in water
Hydrophobic dehydration	< 0	Entropy increase in the water released from contact with hydrophobic components
Distortion of bond lengths and angles	> 0	
Rotational freedom along the polypeptide chain	> 0	Folding, especially the formation of secondary structures such as α-helix and β-pleated sheets, reduces the conformational entropy of the polypeptide chain

SPECIAL THIN ORGANIC COATINGS

A negative enthalpy change ($\Delta G < 0$), as a consequence of a new conformation during protein folding, stabilises the newly folded structure, while a positive ΔG favours the former conformation. As a consequence, protein folding can be understood as a process of self-organisation. The protein modifies its spatial structure to achieve, together with its environment, a minimum of free enthalpy, G. The products of this complicated build-up process, i.e. the mature proteins, can be roughly catagorised as globular, soluble proteins, membrane proteins or fibre proteins. These protein categories differ significantly in their tertiary and quarternary structures. Figures 6.7 and 6.8 show the structure of collagen I, which is the dominating fibre protein in bones (approximately 90%) and therefore of special relevance within the framework of this chapter.

Membrane proteins are either membrane attached (mainly bound by electrostatic interaction) or membrane integral, i.e. anchored within the cell membrane by one to approximately seven α-helices. They frequently form protein complexes made of two or more subunits. Many of these proteins additionally bind cofactors which act

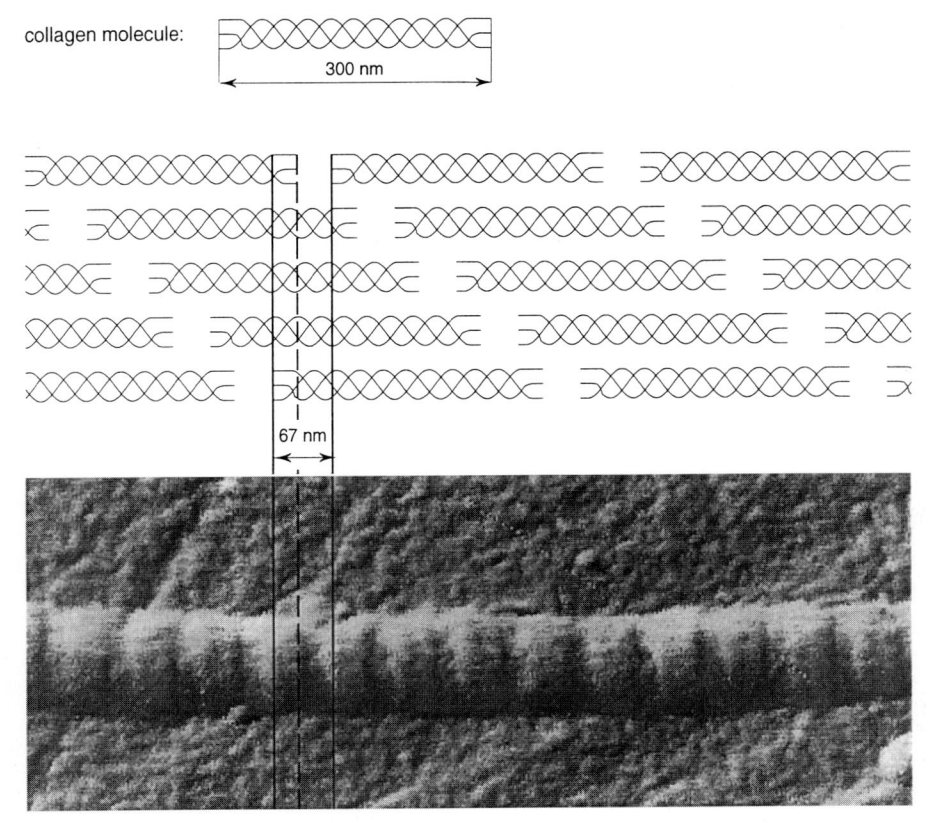

Figure 6.7 Structure of collagen I (Mertig *et al.*, 1997).

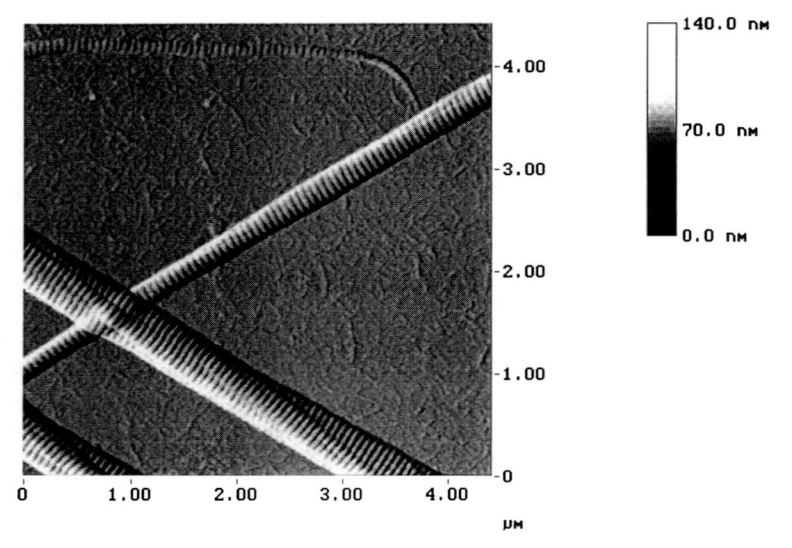

Figure 6.8 AFM image of collagen I.

either as a prosthetic group within the catalytic centre of an enzyme (e.g. transition metal clusters) or as structure-stabilising factors (e.g. lipids, sugars).

Fibre proteins such as collagens (Eyre, 1980; Jones and Miller, 1991) are molecules of extraordinary length. Like all other natural proteins, collagen is synthesised within specialised cell organelles, the ribosomes. After synthesis collagen is translocated to the extracellular space. Since it is built by fibres of high tensile strength it is capable of handling high mechanical loadings in a variety of body tissues. About 20 different types of collagen have been identified. They can be found in bone, teeth, cartilage, tendons, ligaments, and the fibrillar matrix of skin and blood vessels.

The secondary structure of a single, 300 nm long polypeptide chain of tropocollagen I is a straight, but slightly twisted thread (1.4 nm diameter) of approximately 1050 amino acids (molecular mass 95 000). These entities, which consist mainly of the structural element $(GXY)_n$ are often called α-chains. Proline is frequently found in position X, while hydroxyproline is frequently found in position Y. Like all other collagens, collagen I exhibits a characteristic amino acid composition. It consists of a high percentage of glycine (33%), proline (12%), 3-hydroxyproline and 4-hydroxyproline (10%). The content of α-imino acids varies depending on the source of collagens, while the glycine content varies only slightly among different species. The secondary structure of collagen I is similar to that of polyglycine II.

The tertiary structure of one of these α-chains, a left-handed helix, is similar to the spatial structure of one of three fibres in a stretched rope. The quarternary structure of collagen I is that of a heterotrimer consisting of two α_1-chains and one α_2-chain and resembles the complete rope. All of the glycines (i.e. every third amino

SPECIAL THIN ORGANIC COATINGS

acid) of the α-chains lie in the centre of this triple helix. This results in a close package of the collagen I molecule, with hidden hydrophobic amino acids, exposed polar amino acids and a reduction in the surface of the molecules. The driving force towards trimerisation of the collagens is the decrease in hydrophobic interactions between hydrophobic amino acids and water. The close, relatively rigid triple-helix structure of collagens is responsible for their characteristic tensile strength. The entity of one triple helix is often referred to as tropocollagen.

A bundle of tropocollagen forms a new superstructure, the collagen fibril. Electron-microscopic images of collagen fibrils reveal a staggered macrostructure with a periodicity of approximately 68 nm (see Figure 6.14). This macroscopic identity period is usually termed D. The observed macrostructure is caused by periodic variations in the thickness of the collagen fibril. This periodic variation originates from the mode of linkage between individual tropocollagen molecules. Binding occurs between the neighbouring tropocollagens, rather than between succeeding tropocollagens, and a shift of approximately a quarter of the length of a tropocollagen exists between the N-termini of neighbouring tropocollagens. Consequently, a gap area ($0.6D$) and an overlap area ($0.4D$) are formed within the collagen fibril. In electron-microscopic images these gap and overlap areas appear as transversal, periodic structures. The gap areas, which have a width of approximately 40 nm, are utilised as anchor areas for the biomineralisation of hydroxyapatite.

6.3 PROTEIN ADSORPTION AT THE SURFACE OF SOLIDS

Protein adsorption at the surface of solids is a complex interaction of reversible and irreversible sorption processes. The induced conformational changes are often large enough to denature these sensitive biomolecules. According to Chapter 7, however, adsorption is only possible if the Gibbs' energy, G, is reduced:

$$\Delta_{ads}G = \Delta_{ads}H - T\Delta_{ads}S < 0. \tag{6.1}$$

Figure 6.9 shows a schematic representation of the major processes that occur at a metal oxide surface in contact with a biosystem. The processes involved are mainly adsorption and desorption processes of cells and biomolecules. If the biomolecules undergo an irreversible conformational change as a consequence of the interaction with the metal oxide surface, major disturbance of the biological system by the desorbed species may result. Surface-induced conformational changes and chemical alterations within the desorped biomolecules are important indicators for assessing potential problems concerning the biocompatibility of a newly developed biomaterial.

Beneath the interaction of the biomaterial surface with the bare biomolecule, additional interactions with water molecules have to be considered for a deeper understanding of the adsorption process. Different possibilities have to be discussed.

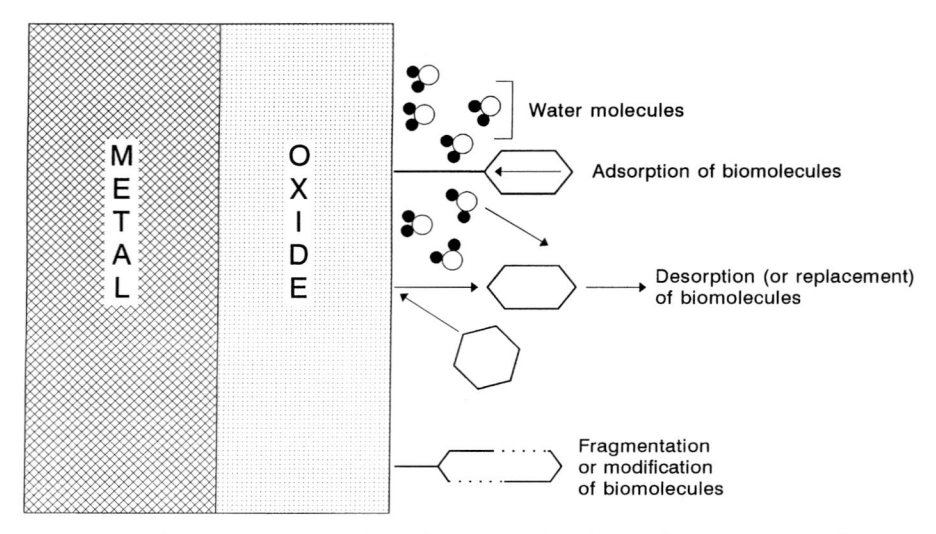

Figure 6.9 Schematic illustration of some molecular surface processes that are likely to occur at the biomaterial–tissue interface (Kasemo and Lausmaa, 1986).

If the surface of the biomaterial contains tightly bound water which does not interact with the water molecules that cover the surface of an adsorbing biomolecule, the biomaterial and the biomolecule always remain separated by a layer of water. This state frequently favours the structural integrity of the adsorbed species. However, water molecules could be repelled by hydrophobic interactions in a way that destroys the water layer between the biomaterial surface and the adsorbing biomolecule. This often leads to a rearrangement of charged groups, i.e. conformational changes. Both extremes as well as every intermediate state might occur, depending on the nature of the proteins involved (Walton, 1980). In a case where these conformational changes are not fully reversible during the desorption of the biomolecule, disturbance of the biological system may occur (Nemethy et al., 1981; Schellmann, 1987).

With respect to the coating of metallic implants by biopolymers it is important to remember from a thermodynamic point of view that, under physiological conditions, native proteins exhibit a relatively small activation energy towards denaturation. Judging from electron-microscopic measurements of the thickness of several proteins before and after adsorption (Saenger, 1987), only rather modest conformational changes were generally revealed in the work of Miller et al. (1989). It was found that only a minor portion of the side-chains was involved in the adsorption process.

Since amino acids with hydrophobic side-chains frequently promote α-helical structures, it seems possible that a loss of hydrophobic interactions, caused by the interaction with the adsorbing surface, might lead to a loss of α-helical structures. As far as globular proteins are concerned, Norde and Lyklema (1990) have shown (Figure 6.10) that the adsorption of a portion of the amino acid side-chains of an

SPECIAL THIN ORGANIC COATINGS

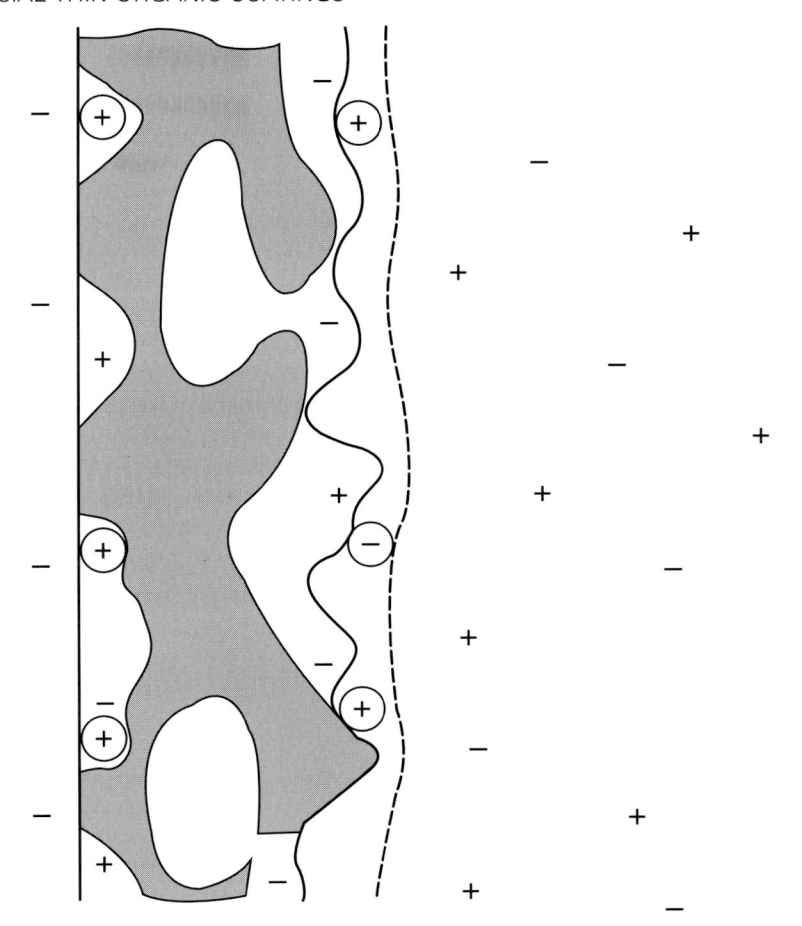

Figure 6.10 Schematic representation of a protein-covered surface (Norde and Lyklema, 1990).

α-helix or a β-sheet structure is a spontaneous process caused by the entropic part of Equation (6.1).

6.4 SOME SELECTED EXAMPLES

Most of the materials used for implants were not specifically developed for this purpose. At first noble metals were used, later CoCr alloys and high-alloy chromium nickel steel, and for a considerable time titanium and titanium alloys (Piliar, 1984; Breme, 1990, 1991; Ewers and Brockhaus, 1991). Their favourable properties, which had already been revealed in other applications, especially their resistance to corrosion (see Chapter 4), led to the expectation that these materials would be suitable as implants. Considering protein adsorption in these materials first, this choice seems to have some justification. Williams *et al.* (1985) investigated protein adsorption and desorption at selected bare metal surfaces (Table 6.3). According to this investigation, silver, copper, gold and platinum play an outstanding role. Nevertheless, a sufficient amount of adsorbed protein is a necessary requirement for obtaining a suitable coating. To achieve biocompatibility it is also necessary to avoid irreversible structural changes during the adsorption/desorption process (see Table 6.3).

The electron conductivity of the metal surface is of critical importance. Good conduction of electrons facilitates redox reactions that might interfere with cell metabolism and denature adsorbed proteins. Therefore, metals with oxide passive coatings, which exhibit no electron conduction, are expected to yield good progress towards biocompatibility. Titanium and titanium alloys are at present the best choice in this respect (Breme, 1989; Thull, 1990, 1994). CoCr alloys and high-alloy chromium nickel steel, however, show significant electron conductivity throughout their oxide passive coatings. In contrast, the oxide passive coatings of titanium and titanium alloys alone show ionic conduction, at least under physiological conditions. Therefore the succeeding sections of this chapter focus mainly on titanium-based implant materials.

Table 6.3 Amount of fibrinogen adsorbed *in vitro* at 106 h and percentages remaining on the metal surface after 5 and 19 days *in vivo*

Metal	Protein adsorbed ($\mu g\ cm^{-2}$)	Percentage remaining	
		5 days	19 days
Ag	26.0	6.6	0.8
Al	0.5	1.6	0.8
Au	20.0	11.4	5.3
Co	8.0	35.0	10.1
Cu	53.0	8.0	0.3
Fe	0.9	38.5	13.0
Mo	1.3	38.0	7.1
Nb	0.6	9.7	0.9
Ni	3.0	7.8	5.2
Pb	4.0	62.3	35.2
Pt	15.0	36.3	5.4
Ta	0.6	26.5	4.9
Ti	1.3	1.9	0.3
V	9.0	1.9	4.7
W	1.7	16.8	2.2
Zr	0.6	4.3	1.0
316 Stainless steel	0.4	10.4	1.5

6.4.1 ADSORPTION OF SINGLE AMINO ACIDS AT TITANIUM OXIDE SURFACES

Before turning to the immobilisation of macromolecules on implants it is of advantage to clarify whether monomeric amino acids are suitable for improving the properties of the surface of an implant. Experiments performed by Schmidt *et al.* (1992) revealed that amino acids can be adsorbed to titanium oxide surfaces to varying degrees. This adsorption occurs predominantly within the acidic pH range (Figure 6.11). Minor impurities are found to be of high importance since they are capable of completely suppressing adsorption. Unfortunately, no systematics concerning the influence of the amino acid side-chain (-R) can be deduced from these results. Using the argument of the amphoteric behaviour of TiO_2, the authors inferred that only the basic hydroxy groups are reacting with the deprotonated carboxy group (-COO$^-$) of an amino acid. The interaction of lysine, however, is different because of its broader adsorption range (pH 2–9). In this case, the interaction of the secondary amino group seems to be likely, at least at alkaline pH.

Insight into the spatial orientation of the adsorbed amino acids has been obtained by photoelectron spectroscopy (PES). For the relatively long lysine molecule, it has been concluded that the molecules favour a closely attached, lying position, whereas for the adsorbed homocysteine, an upright position was found to be the best explanation for a precisely evaluable set of experimental data (Figure 6.12) (Schmidt, 1992). Regardless of the details of the spatial orientation of the adsorbed

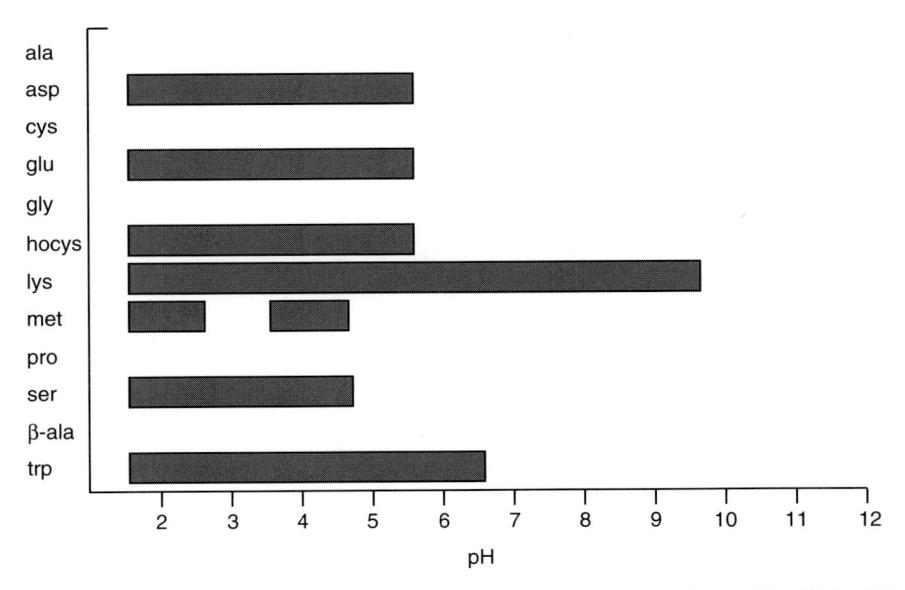

Figure 6.11 pH dependence of the adsorption of single amino acids (Schmidt, 1992).

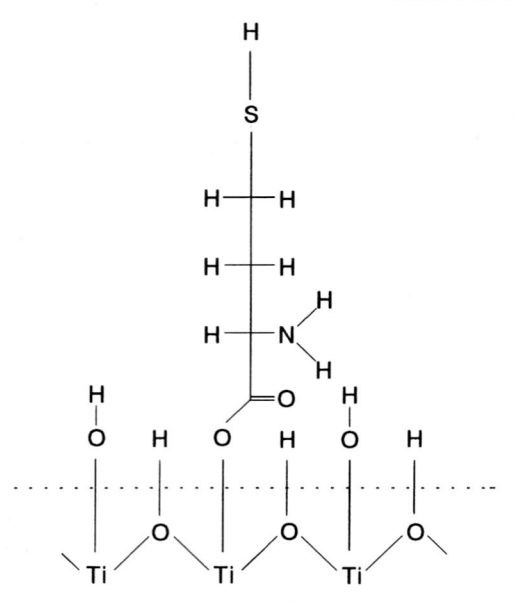

Figure 6.12 Schematic representation of homocysteine on a TiO$_2$ surface (Schmidt, 1992).

molecules, these results show that amino acids can be successfully adsorbed at oxidic titanium surfaces.

6.4.2 ADSORPTION OF GLOBULAR PROTEINS

Serum albumin, a globular protein, represents the main protein component of blood, and the adsorption of globular proteins on the surfaces of solid bodies is therefore of special relevance with respect to the integration process of implants. Serum albumins are well known for their conformative adaptability towards changes in their environment. They adsorb to most surfaces even if hydrophobic and/or electrostatic interactions are unlikely (Norde and Lyklema, 1990). As a consequence, a modification to the adsorption behaviour of serum albumin is observed depending on the state of its surface. This phenomenon might explain some of the contradictory reports on the adsorption behaviour of this protein which are found throughout the literature (van Enckevort *et al.*, 1984). Serum albumin that has been cross-linked on titanium surfaces with carbodiimide has been found to inhibit the adsorption of bacteria (An *et al.*, 1996).

These results indicate that adsorption of serum albumin on titanium implants might improve the biocompatibility. However, taking into account the high conformative adaptability of serum albumins, denaturation of this type of protein by titanium surfaces seems highly unlikely.

6.4.3 COLLAGEN I ADSORPTION ON AND INCORPORATION INTO TITANIUM OXIDE SURFACES

Taking into consideration the successful adsorption of single amino acids to titanium surfaces (see above), similar behaviour may be expected for polypeptides and proteins. This view is supported by the present author's investigations (Worch and Scharnweber, 1997; Rößler *et al.*, 1997). In the framework of these experiments freeze-dried collagen fibrils from calf skin (Figure 6.13) were solubilised by acetic acid, reassembled and adsorbed on titanium oxide surfaces (Figure 6.14). Since collagen fibrils exhibit a more or less pronounced net structure, depending on the age of the tissue, the degree of cross-linking increases with the age of the tissue. Consequently, only collagens from young tissue can be solubilised and reassembled.

Transmission electron-microscopic (TEM) images and atomic force-microscopic (AFM) images of reassembled collagen I adsorbed on titanium oxide surfaces show native-looking macrostructures (Figure 6.14). The assembly of the collagen fibrils has been carried out under near physiological conditions. Temperature, pH conditions and ionic strength have been further varied to modify the concentration, distribution and spatial organisation of collagen I on titanium oxide surfaces (Figure 6.15).

Pure titanium dioxide behaves like a ceramic material, as far as its mechanical properties are concerned. It lacks ductility and is brittle. Since the ductility of ceramic type materials can be improved by the incorporation of fibres, the idea of incorporating collagen I into the titanium dioxide surface of an implant seemed straightforward. Figure 6.16 shows that after the incorporation of collagen I fibrils

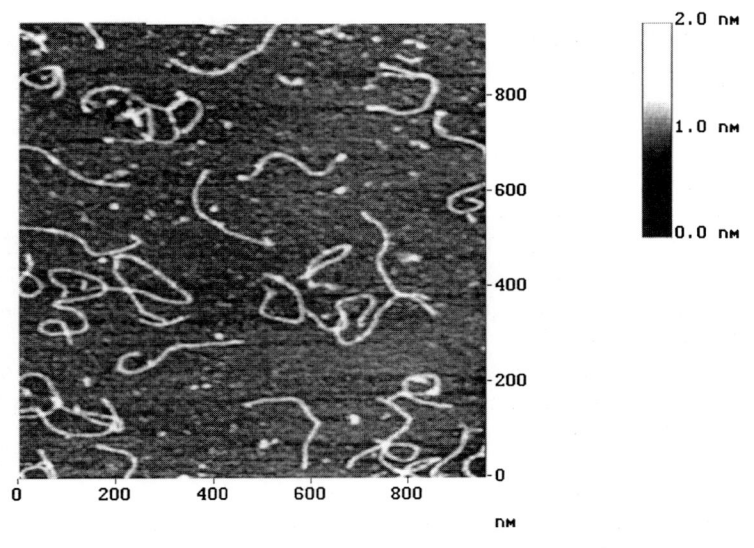

Figure 6.13 Collagen fibrils from calf skin (Bradt *et al.*, 1996).

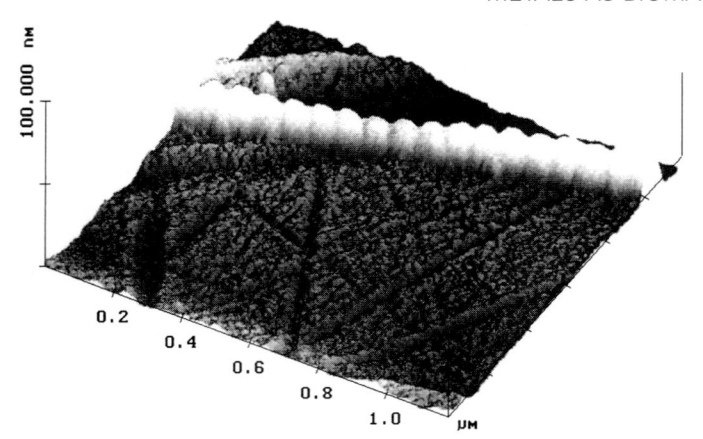

Figure 6.14 TEM and AFM images of reassembled collagen I fibrils on TiO_2.

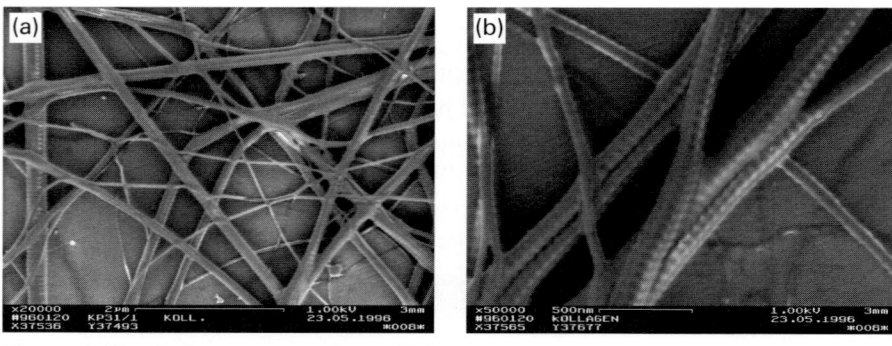

Figure 6.15 Collagen networks on TiO_2.

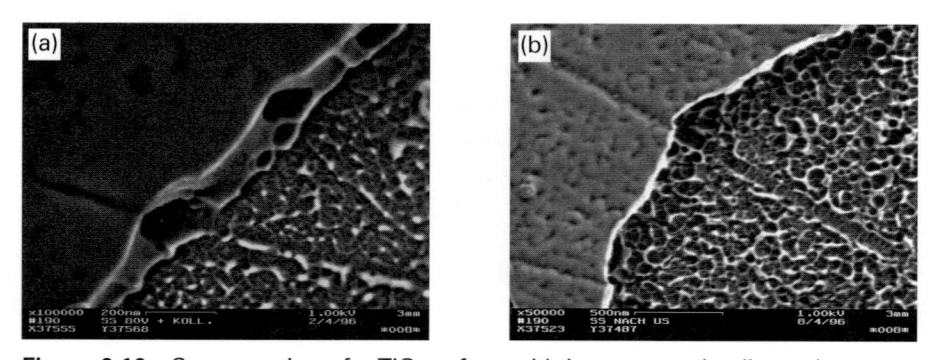

Figure 6.16 Cross-section of a TiO surface with incorporated collagen I.

into a titanium oxide surface a native-looking macrostructure can be obtained. This has been achieved by anodical oxidation of titanium in the presence of collagen I.

6.4.4 MORPHOGENETIC PROTEINS AS MEDIATORS OF THE BONE HEALING PROCESS

Experiments in cell and tissue cultures have revealed the existence of a special class of growth factors, the morphogenetic proteins (Mohen and Baylink, 1991). Growth factors can be found at the edge of wounds, and some originate from thrombocytes and have been discovered within the extravasation of bone fractures. Very low concentrations of these growth factors are capable of acting as messenger substances. They specifically bind to receptors at the surface of a target cell, thereby initiating the differentiation and growth of this cell. A varying effect on the target cell results, depending on the type, the actual differentiation state of the cell, the concentration and type of the growth factor, and the abundance of other factors and substances in the intercellular space (interstitium).

Unfortunately, it is not possible at present to systemise all types of growth factors in a simple way (Wintermantel and Mayer, 1995). Therefore only a selection of growth factors with some relevance to the bone healing process will be mentioned (Bolander, 1992).

Signal molecules for osteoinduction belong to the family of bone morphogenetic proteins (BMP) [7–11, see Ripamonti and Reddi (1997)]. They belong to the superfamily of growth and differentiation factors, which also comprise basic fibroblast growth factor (bFGF), nerve growth factor (NGF) and transforming growth factor βs (TGF-βs) (Saltzman, 1996). TGF-β2 stimulates the generation of new bone material (ossification) and the healing process of wounds, and influences some activities of the immune system.

Urist and Reddi (Urist, 1965; Reddi and Huggins, 1972) discovered that new bone material developed within 2 weeks in a devitalised and demineralised bone matrix which had been implanted into the muscles of animals. This process is comparable with the healing of a fractured bone by endochondral ossification: undifferentiated mesenchymal cells are generated and guided by chemotaxis to their target cells, and their differentiation, growth and proliferation are activated by morphogenetic proteins. They begin to secrete cartilage into the intercellular space. The cartilage is then partially mineralised and invaded by small blood vessels. Osteoprogenitor cells entering the lacuna behind the invading capillary endothelial cells differentiate into osteoblasts and secrete new bone material, which is then succeedingly mineralised. This tissue, which contains elements of both cartilage and bone matrix, then undergoes osteoclastic remodelling, i.e. the calcified cartilage is removed and replaced by bone material.

Ripamondi and Duneas (1996) reported that porous hydroxyapatite with and without collagen I can be used to immobilise BMP. Kawai *et al.* (1993) investigated the osteoinduction of BMP in the presence of pure titanium and concluded that the activity of the BMP remains unaffected by the titanium surface.

It is therefore tempting to speculate from these results that the immobilisation of morphogenetic proteins on the surface of implants might facilitate the healing process and consequently speed up the integration of implants into the body. This would be a major advance towards biocompatibility.

6.5 SUMMARY

To date, highly specialised organic coatings with promising properties for the improvement of the biocompatibility of metal implants consist solely of different proteins which are usually abundant within or around the substituted bone tissue. These protein coatings can be fixed either by adsorption or, in a more sophisticated way, by anchoring fibrillar proteins such as collagens within the oxidic passive layer of titanium. The achieved or expected improvements concerning the biocompatibility of implants are based on: (1) diminution of unwelcome interactions between the body and the implant by the coating; (2) support of the healing process by facilitating the attachment of new bone cells by a coating with a rough surface; and (3) a specific stimulation of the generation of new bone cells by coatings that additionally contain morphogenetic proteins.

REFERENCES

An, Y.H., Stuart, G.W., McDowell, S.G., McDaniel, S., Kang, Q. and Freedman, R.J. (1996) Provention of bacterial adherence to implant surfaces with a crosslinked albumin coating in vitro, *J. Orthop. Res.* **14**, 846–9.

Bolander, M.E. (1992) Redulation of fracture repair by growth factors, *Clin. Orthop. Rel. Res.* **289**, 165–70.

Bradt, J.-H., Mertig, M., Winzer, B., Thiele, U. and Pompe, W. (1996) Collagen assembly from acid solution to networks on solid surfaces and to fibrils, *Proc. SPIE*, **2779**, 78–82

Breme, J. (1989) Le titane et les alliages de titane, biomateriaux de choix, *Mem et Etudes Scient. Rév. de Métall.* **10**, 627–37.

Breme, J. (1990) Criteria for bioinertness of metals for osseointegrated implants, in *Osseointegrated Implants, I. Basics, Materials and Joint Replacements* (ed. G. Heimke), CRC Press, Boca Raton, FL, pp. 31–80.

Breme, J. (1991) Metalle als Biomaterialien, in *Biomedizinische Technik*, Fachverlag Schiele & Schön, Berlin, pp. 27–30.

Creighton, T.E. (1989) *Protein Structure: A Practical Approach*. IRL Press, Oxford.

Ebert, G. (1993) *Biopolymere*, Teubner Studienbücherei, Stuttgart.

Ewers, U. and Brockhaus, A. (1991) Metal concentrations in human body fluids and tissues, in *Metals and their Compounds in the Environment* (ed. E. Merian), VCH-Verlag, Weinheim, pp. 207–10.

Eyre, D.R. (1980) Collagen: molecular diversity in the body's protein scaffold, *Science* **207**, 1305–22.

Haynes, C.A. and Norde, W. (1994) Globular proteins at solid/liquid interfaces, in *Colloids and Surfaces, Part B: Biointerfaces*, Vol. 2, pp. 517–66.

Jones, E.Y. and Miller A. (1991) Analysis of structural design features in collagen, *J. Mol. Biol.*, **218**, 209–19.
Karlson, P. (1988) *Biochemie*, Georg Thieme, Stuttgart.
Kasemo, B. and Lausmaa, J. (1986) Surface science aspects on inorganic biomaterials, *CRC Crit. Rev. Biocomp.* **2**, 335–80.
Kawai, T., Mieki, A., Ohno, Y., Umemura, M., Kataoka, H., Kurita, S., Koie, M., Jinde, T., Hasegawa, J. and Urist, M. R. (1993) Osteoinductive activity of composites of bone morphogenetic protein and pure titanium, *Clin. Orthop. Rel. Res.* **290**, 296–305.
Marsh, R.E. and Donohue, J. (1967) Crystal structure studies of amino acids and peptides, *Adv. Prot. Chem.* **22**, 235–56.
Mertig, M., Thiele, U., Bradt, J., Leibiger, G., Pompe, W. and Wendrock, H. (1997) Scanning force microscopy and geometrical analysis of two-dimensional collagen network formation, *Surf. Interface Anal.* **25**, 514–21.
Miller, S. (1989) The structure of interfaces between subunits of dimeric and tetrameric proteins, *Protein Engng* **3**, 77–83.
Milner-White, E.J. and Poet, R. (1987) Loops, turns and hairpins in proteins, *Trends Biochem. Sci.* **12**, 189–96.
Mohen, S. and Baylink, D. (1991) Bone growth factors, *Clin. Orthop. Rel. Res.* **263**, 30–48.
Nemethy, G., Pier, W.J. and Scheraga, H.A. (1981) Effect of protein–solvent interactions on protein conformation, *A. Rev. Biochem.* **10**, 459–97.
Norde, W. and Lyklema, J. (1990) Why proteins prefer interfaces, in *The Vroman Effect* (eds C.H. Bamford, S.L. Cooper and T. Tsuruta), VSP, Utrecht, pp. 1–20.
Piliar, R.M. (1984) The processing and properties of metal implants, in *Metal and Ceramic Biomaterials*, Vol. 1 (eds P. Ducheyne and G.W. Hastings), CRC Press, Boca Raton, FL, pp. 79–105.
Reddi, A.H. and Huggins, C.B. (1972) Biochemical sequences in the transformation of normal fibroblasts in adolescent rats, *Proc. Natnl. Acad. Sci., USA* **69**, 1601.
Ripamondi, U. and Duneas, N. (1996) Tissue engineering of bone by osteoinductive biomaterials, *MRS Bull.*, 36–9.
Ripamonti, U. and Reddi, A.H. (1997) Tissue engineering, Morphogenesis, and regeneration of the peridontal tissues by bone morphogenetic proteins, *Crit. Rev. Oral Biol. Med.* **8**, 154–63.
Rößler, S., Stölzel, M., Scharnweber, D. and Worch, H. (1997) Biologisierung von Implantatoberflächen durch Immobilisierung von Biopolymeren, in *Werkstoffe für die Medizintechnik* (ed. J. Breme), DGM – Informationsgesellschaft, Frankfurt, pp. 123–6.
Saenger, W. (1987) Structure and dynamics of water surrounding biomolecules, *A. Rev. Biophys. Biophys. Chem.* **16**, 93–114.
Saltzman, W.M. (1996) Growth-factor delivery in tissue engineering, *MRS Bull.*, 62–5.
Schellmann, J.A. (1987) The thermodynamic stability of proteins, *A. Rev. Biophys. Chem.* **16**, 115–37.
Schmidt, M. (1992) Spezifische Adsorption organischer Moleküle auf oxidiertem Titan: 'Bioaktivität' auf molekularem Niveau, *Osteologie* **1**, 222–35.
Schmidt, R. (1994) *Werkstoffverhalten in biologischen Systemen*, VDI, Düsseldorf.
Thull, R. (1990) Semiconductive properties of passivated titanium and titanium based hard coatings on metals for implants – an experimental approach, *Med. Prog. Technol.* **16**, 225–34.
Thull, R. (1994) Naturwissenschaftliche Aspekte von Werkstoffen in der Medizin, *Naturwissenschaften* **8**, 481–8.
Urist, M.R. (1965) Bone: formation by autoinduction, *Science* **150**, 893–9.
Van Enckevort, H.J., Dass, D.V. and Langdon, A.G. (1984) The adsorption of bovine serum albumin at the stainless-steel/aqueous solution interface, *J. Colloid Interface Sci.* **98**, 138–43.

Voet, D. and Voet, J.G. (1992) *Biochemie* (eds A. Maelicke and W. Müller-Esterl), VCH, Weinheim.
Walton, A.G. (1980) in *Biomedical Polymers* (ed. E. Goldberg), Academic Press, New York.
Williams, D.F., Askill, I.N. and Smith, R. (1985) Protein adsorption and desorption phenomena on clean metal surfaces, *J. Biomed. Mater. Res.* **19**, 313–20.
Wintermantel, E. and Mayer, J. (1995) Anisotropic biomaterials: strategies and developments for bone implants, in *Encylopedia of Biomaterials and Bioengineering*, Part B, Vol. 1 (eds D.L. Wise, D.J. Trantolo, D.E. Altobelli, M.J. Yaszemski, J.D. Gresser and E.R. Schartz), Marcel Dekker, New York, pp. 3–42.
Wintermantel, E. and Suk-Woo Ha (1996) *Biokompatible Werkstoffe und Bauweisen – Implantate für Medizin und Umwelt*, Springer, Berlin.
Worch, H. and Scharnweber, D. (1997) Biologisierte Grenzschichten auf Titanimplantaten, in *Werkstoffe für die Medizintechnik* (ed. J. Breme), DGM-Informationsgesellschaft, Frankfurt/Main, pp. 111–15.

7
Adhesion of polymers

W. POSSART
University of the Saarland, Saarbrücken, Germany

7.1 INTRODUCTION

This chapter reviews the adhesion of polymers on other materials. Special attention is paid to the mechanisms that control the situation on the polymer side of the interface. In each particular case it is extremely difficult to probe these mechanisms experimentally and it is even much more ambitious to quantify them. This point will become obvious from the following sections and it explains why our knowledge is still fragmentary in many instances. The chapter is confined to polymer materials in the glassy and viscoelastic states, and polymer solutions are not considered in detail. The intention here is to present an introduction to the field. For detailed studies, the reader is referred to specialist textbooks (e.g. de Gennes, 1979; Doi and Edwards, 1986; Fleer *et al.*, 1993; Wool, 1995). The chapter begins with some fundamental terms concerning macromolecular behaviour in the bulk. The overview is then extended to the polymer surface and polymer–polymer interfaces and it will be shown that the surface and interfaces are indeed *interphases*. In a subsequent section, the basics of polymer adsorption are considered as the prerequisite of adhesion. Finally, the elements of relevant adhesion mechanisms are discussed in the light of examples.

7.2 IMPORTANT POLYMER FEATURES IN THE BULK

Polymer materials consist of macromolecules with a molecular mass distribution (i.e. they are polydisperse) and average masses in the range 10^4–10^6 g mol^{-1}. If all macromolecules possessed the same molecular mass a monodisperse polymer would be obtained. The macromolecular structures vary from long linear or branched chains to networks of chemically cross-linked subchains. In most cases, polymeric biomaterials consist of flexible macromolecules. Examples are polyurethanes, fluoropolymers, polysiloxanes, polyacrylates and polyethyleneoxide. Macromolecules create amorphous or partially crystalline superstructures in which the crystallites are

---

Metals as Biomaterials ISBN 0 471 96935 4 Edited by J.A. Helsen and H.J. Breme. © 1998 John Wiley & Sons Ltd

embedded in an amorphous matrix. Linear flexible macromolecules possess a coil-like shape. The coil dimension is described by the radius of gyration. It has a mean value R_g for the average coil

$$R_g = \left(\frac{C_\infty Mn}{6M_0}\right)^{1/2} b, \qquad (7.1)$$

where C_∞ is the rigidity coefficient for the given polymer, M is the mean value of the polymer molecular mass, M_0 is the monomer molecular mass, b is the bond length and n is the number of bonds per monomer unit in the backbone chain. The mean values of M and hence of R_g account for the molecular size distribution. R_g is of the order of some 10^1 nm. Despite diluted polymer solutions, flexible macromolecules always interpenetrate, similarly to spaghetti noodles in a bowl. The macromolecule must exceed a critical mass M_c to activate entanglements as constraints for the molecular dynamics. Depending on the mass of the monomer unit, M_c ranges from 10^3 to 10^4. The average distance d between the centres of gravity of two intermingled chains is estimated by

$$d = \left(\frac{M}{\rho N_L}\right)^{1/3}, \qquad (7.2)$$

where ρ is the polymer density and $N_L = 6.023 \times 10^{23}$ molecules mol^{-1}. In polymer melts and solids, the distance d has the order of 10 nm, which is considerably smaller than the mean radius of gyration R_g. The entangled coils form a transient network with an average distance ξ_c between the interchain crossings. This distance is called the correlation length. It amounts to

$$\xi_c \approx \frac{C_\infty}{6} l, \qquad (7.3)$$

where l is the segment length (see below) in amorphous viscoelastic polymers. The value of ξ_c ranges from about 2.5 to 18 nm for flexible solid polymers.

Perhaps the most characteristic feature of macromolecular systems is their dynamics. It is governed by collective motions of chain segments that should be described briefly. The macromolecular flexibility rests upon the single bonds in the chain that form the axis for a rotation (torsion) within the molecule. The chain atoms adjacent to the considered bond and the surrounding polymer chains create an interaction potential which hinders the local rotation with two main consequences. At first, the rotation around the bond prefers discrete angles of torsion corresponding to the potential minima, which are known as conformations. Secondly, the shape of the rotation potential depends considerably on the local surroundings of the chain (in terms of free space) given by the other macromolecules. In the absence of external mechanical or electric forces, conformational changes are driven only by the temperature bath inside the polymer. Under these circumstances, a single bond is not able to change conformation independently of the molecular environment. The interaction potential almost confines the motions to a rotational oscillation. A statistically accidental correlation of a certain number of these oscillating chain units is necessary for moving chain atoms from one equilibrium position to another. This number of correlated chain units is called a chain segment of length l. The statistical character of such segments is noted.

For the same reason the number of segments participating in a local mode of motion varies with the local environment of the chain (i.e. the polymer structure) and the segment length also depends on the temperature. The entanglements influence the molecular modes of motion. As a consequence, several chain motions can coexist in polymers. They create a hierarchy according to their increasing energy consumption: side-chain vibrations or rotations, and collective segmental motions that also form the base for the motion of whole macromolecules. Modes will freeze in as the temperature decreases because there is no longer sufficient thermal energy to activate collective motions. This happens in the glass transition region (characterised by the glass transition temperature T_g or, at a constant temperature, by a characteristic frequency). Here, all *collective* modes disappear and a certain amount of free volume freezes in. As the segment lengths rise with falling temperature, the polymer equilibrium structure cannot be maintained in the freezing process. The glassy state is a non-equilibrium. Only small entities such as side-groups at the chain profit from the frozen free volume and preserve some mobility.

All of this results in a spectrum of polymer chain dynamics described by the relaxation time spectrum of the material. The spectrum depends not only on the type of material but also on its structure, which in turn is determined by the temperature, the timescale (frequency) of external forces and the thermal history of the sample. Because the collective macromolecular motions are quite slow, the equilibrium in a polymer solid is easily disturbed and it takes considerable time to re-establish thermodynamic equilibrium after a change of state. Therefore, polymers exist frequently in manifold non-equilibrium states, even at temperatures above T_g.

From the thermodynamic point of view, polymers have to be considered as a mixture rather than a pure material. This can be seen from a short discussion of the free enthalpy G of a phase at a given temperature T

$$G = H - TS. \qquad (7.4)$$

The enthalpy H is independent of the individual chain length since the interaction potential between the segments is determined by the local environment but not by the properties of the whole chain. The entropy S, however, splits into a translational part due to the motion of the whole macromolecule and a configurational part. The configurational entropy becomes increasingly dominant over the translational part with rising chain length. Now, the conformational entropy contribution of any macromolecule must be smaller than the translational entropy of an equal amount of monomer molecules because the chemical bonds in the chain and the limited number of conformations reduce the thermodynamic degrees of freedom. Thus, larger macromolecules provide a smaller entropic gain to the free enthalpy of the polymer phase and the polydisperse distribution of macromolecules meets the criteria of a multicomponent mixture.

The described fundamental macromolecular features are also found in the surface or interfacial regions of polymers, but there they are modified. As a consequence one must consider an interplay of intermolecular forces and macromolecular dynamics to understand the situation in a polymer–substrate boundary (the interphase) and its contribution to material properties.

7.3 THE POLYMER SURFACE

The term polymer surface applies by convention to the interphase of a polymer in contact with a gas or vacuum. The interphases between a polymer and other condensed materials are commonly called interfaces, which may be a little confusing. Their basic features are discussed in the subsequent sections.

Several general arguments apply to all polymer interphases as any interface disturbs the isotropy of the polymer bulk structure. The consequences depend not only on whether the contacting phase interacts with the polymer or not. There is also a driving force immanent to the polymer that causes structural rearrangement at the surface. With increasing chain length, the contribution to the entropy of mixing decreases because the configurational part of entropy dominates for the large molecules, whereas the small polymer chains contribute more to the translational entropy of the polymer bulk. Hence, the small molecules would lose more entropy (strictly, more translational entropy) at the surface than the large molecules. The effect is stronger for solutions than for solids. As a result, the chains with the lower molecular mass deplete in the surface layer leaving the larger molecules at thermodynamic equilibrium. The isotropic bulk molecular weight distribution tends to fractionate at an interface. Immediately after the creation of a fresh surface, however, the small molecules will migrate there because their translational mobility is larger. This is experimentally and theoretically well documented by the relation

$$D \propto M^{-2} \tag{7.5}$$

between the self-diffusion coefficient D and the mass M of the linear macromolecule (de Gennes, 1979; Klein and Briscoe, 1979; Doi and Edwards, 1986). A complicated restructuring process has to proceed in the surface region until equilibrium is established.

The surface also influences the polymer chain conformations. All conformations that would cross the surface are forbidden. This results in a loss of configurational entropy affecting the large molecules more strongly than the smaller ones. As a consequence, the segment density should be reduced in the surface region. The forbidden conformations prevent the chains from approaching the surface more closely than the correlation length. The degree of chain interpenetration should therefore be

ADHESION OF POLYMERS

smaller. The long chains tend to direct their segments parallel to the surface in order to compensate for the depletion. This orientation may be accompanied by a density growth but the effect is more pronounced in polymer solutions than in the solid. Molecular dynamics simulations (Wattenbarger et al., 1990) on small molecules confirm these conclusions. They show flattened coils at the surface with a preference for the more compact conformations. Nuclear magnetic resonance (NMR) experiments on similar systems indicate a reduced polymer chain mobility for the interphase region. In contrast, molecular simulations (Mansfield and Theodorou, 1990, 1991) on short polypropylene chains in the glassy state (22 K *below T_g of the bulk*) provide a reduced density inside a 0.7 nm thick surface layer to the vacuum. This is accompanied by an *enhanced segment mobility* over a depth of about 1.5 nm beneath the surface, thus also involving parts of the dense region. These apparently contradictory results can be explained by the different role that the atmosphere at the polymer surface may play. Thermodynamics provide the decisive criterion: the free enthalpy of any two-phase system has to become a minimum and therefore the interfacial part of the free enthalpy is also minimised. In the literature, this criterion is often expressed (not very precisely) in terms of a minimum surface energy or of minimum surface tension. The criterion implies the following conclusions concerning the polymer surface structure and dynamics. The polymer chain segments will prefer directions parallel to the surface as long as this orientation diminishes the surface free energy. Otherwise, the segments will reduce the area of contact with the atmosphere by appropriate conformations. This case must result in a reduced density compared with the bulk.

The chain ends and side-groups introduce a further aspect. Their chemical structure differs from the rest of the macromolecule and hence they may or may not be compatible. If not, they try to segregate at an interface in principle to reduce the free enthalpy of the polymer. If the chemical nature of the chain ends or side-groups helps to reduce the surface free energy, this provides an additional driving force which increases their concentration in the surface layer.

In the literature, many results demonstrate the ability of polymers to fit their surface structure to the contacting gas phase with the help of their segmental and side-chain mobility (Lee, 1967; Baier and Zisman, 1970; de Gennes, 1988). On a polymethylmethacrylate (PMMA) surface formed in contact with air, for example, wetting experiments (Possart, W. and Kamusewitz, H., unpublished observations, 1984) with water at room temperature reveal a relatively low surface energy because the polymer conceals the hydrophilic methacrylate side-groups. During contact to a phase of high surface energy such as glass, the now compatible side-groups are directed towards the interface when the viscoelastic state (above T_g) is reached. This restructuring yields an optimum interfacial free enthalpy which corresponds to the minimum free enthalpy of the system. The different location of the side-groups was proved directly by surface spectroscopic techniques (Schmitt et al., 1985, 1986; Hook et al., 1986; Pireaux et al., 1991). The side-chain motions influence the interphase properties much more than the bulk properties.

In the case of crystallisable polymers, the more compact surface conformations can force the ordering of segments as compared with the bulk. If the segments in a flattened coil prefer an arrangement parallel to the surface, such a homogeneous nucleation can be the starting point for a crystal growth from the surface. As the c-axis in the crystallites (i.e. the chains) tend to orientate parallel to the surface, this may have an impact on the surface mechanical properties.

In binary polymer mixtures, one of the components prevails in the surface region for the same reasons of energy minimisation unless the difference in surface enthalpy per monomer between the two kinds of molecules is so small that it can be compensated by the small difference in entropy loss.

Copolymers have been less intensively studied. The behaviour at the surface should be similar to that of polymer mixtures, especially for block copolymers. The blocks are able to arrange themselves in the surface region according to interface properties.

In summary, polymer surfaces are neither rigid nor immobile in the viscoelastic state at temperatures above the glass transition. Bulk data such as glass transition temperatures, density and relaxation spectra do not apply to the polymer surface because the chain dynamics are modified by inherent thermodynamics reasons and by influences from the contacting atmosphere.

7.4 POLYMER–POLYMER INTERFACES

These interfaces deserve separate consideration because of the chain dynamics which contributes to the interphase formation when the polymer is in the viscoelastic state.

Amorphous polymer *surfaces* may consist of flattened coils with a preferred segment orientation parallel to the surface or the segment density may be reduced compared with the bulk. These are the situations from which a polymer–polymer interphase formation begins. However, the consequences on the kinetics of interphase formation are only qualitatively understood.

The final interphase structure depends on the compatibility of the two polymers, which is described by the Flory–Huggins theory (Huggins, 1942a, b; Flory, 1953). Thus, the Helmholtz free energy of mixing ΔA_{mix} for the polymers A and B is

$$\Delta A_{mix} = kT \left\{ [\chi_{AB} \varphi_A \varphi_B]_{enthalpic} + \left[\frac{\varphi_A}{N_A} \ln \varphi_A + \frac{\varphi_B}{N_B} \ln \varphi_B \right]_{entropic} \right\}, \quad (7.6)$$

where k is the Boltzmann constant, φ_A, φ_B are the volume fractions of polymer chains A and B, respectively. $\varphi_A + \varphi_B = 1$, χ_{AB} is the Flory–Huggins parameter describing the interaction between one chain moiety from A and its partner moiety from B. It depends on temperature and pressure, and N_A, N_B are the number of moieties in chains A and B, respectively.

This concept implies that the polymers interact via pairs of certain chain units or moieties. It is obvious from Equation (7.6) that the entropic contribution to ΔA_{mix} decreases quickly with growing chain length (N_A, N_B). Thus the sign for ΔA_{mix} depends

ADHESION OF POLYMERS

strongly on the interaction parameter χ_{AB}. For $\chi_{AB} \leq 0$, the ΔA_{mix} is always negative and the polymers are compatible for any mixing ratio. Further consideration of Equation (7.6) defines the critical point for demixing polymer chains of finite length

$$\chi_{AB}^{crit} = \frac{1}{2}\left(\frac{1}{\sqrt{N_A}} + \frac{1}{\sqrt{N_B}}\right)^2 \ll \frac{1}{2}. \tag{7.7}$$

Hence $\chi_{AB} \leq \chi_{AB}^{crit}$ is needed for polymer compatibility. Equation (7.7) also reveals that different chain lengths of the same type of macromolecule lead to a variation in χ_{AB}. Note in passing that the most general theory for multicomponent polymer interfaces stems from Hong and Noolandi (Hong and Noolandi, 1981a, b; Noolandi and Hong, 1982). Crystallites at interfaces between partial crystalline polymers possess no significant chain mobility. Therefore, they do not contribute to the intermixing and reduce the mechanical strength of the interphase.

7.4.1 INCOMPATIBLE POLYMER–POLYMER INTERFACES

The majority of polymers are immiscible. At the microscopic level, the contacting segments from the different polymer materials repel each other. The net interactions result in a positive free enthalpy of the system and the two contacting polymers coexist as separate phases. Whole chains do not diffuse through the interface. From the polymer surface it can be seen that an incompatible contacting phase causes an outermost region of the polymer material where the segments deplete because the conformational entropy of the chain resists densification. This corresponds to a loss of entropy which in turn results in a free enthalpy rise. With two incompatible polymers in contact, both materials will therefore intermingle somewhat in their depleted regions until an equilibrium between increasing entropy (of mixing) and rising enthalpy (chain repulsion) will result in the minimum free energy (for details, see Helfand and Tagami, 1972; Helfand and Sapse, 1975; Helfand, 1975, 1982, 1992). According to Helfand, the equilibrium thickness d_∞ of the intermingled region is estimated by

$$d_\infty = \frac{2l}{\sqrt{6\chi_{AB}}}. \tag{7.8}$$

This interphase process is called conformational relaxation. To some extent, it is hindered by the preferential segment orientation parallel to the interface. Usual values for d_∞ lie in the interval from about 3 to 10 nm.

The pair polystyrene–PMMA serves as an example for an incompatible system. Neutron reflectometry (Russell *et al.*, 1991) provided the concentration profile for the two polymers. The intermingled region is approximately 20 nm wide, much less than the radius of gyration. The value corresponds well to the theoretical estimation with Equation (7.8). The polystyrene–PMMA interphase has a mechanical strength of about 40 J m^{-2}, much lower than the virgin strength of the polymers (polystyrene has about 1000 J m^{-2}, for example) (Forster and Wool, 1991; Willet and Wool,

1993). To improve the situation for practical purposes, compatibilisers are introduced. For instance, a di-block copolymer of styrene and methylmethacrylate with medium molecular mass for each block (e.g. 50 000 g mol^{-1}) could act as a compatibiliser. The neutron reflectivity shows that each of the two blocks diffuses into its host polymer at the polystyrene–PMMA interface. These molecular bridges extend over a width of some 50 nm (Russell *et al.*, 1991) and act as anchors which improve the mechanical strength.

7.4.2 COMPATIBLE POLYMER–POLYMER INTERFACES

PMMA and polyvinylchloride (PVC) provide an example of a compatible pair of polymers. Here, the two monomers attract each other since the PMMA carbonyl group (C=O) forms a hydrogen bond with the (H–C–Cl) moiety in the PVC.

As a result of such an attraction, the macromolecules of compatible polymers diffuse through a fresh interface. The interdiffusion process and the resulting interphase structure relate to the chain mobility which in turn is determined by the chemical structure of the polymer (see Sections 7.2 and 7.3). The co-operative segment motions are most important for the diffusion which thus occurs only in the amorphous part of the material at temperatures above the glass transition region.

Five processes contribute to the macromolecular chain dynamics: short-range Fickian diffusion of monomer units, Rouse relaxation of chain sections between two entanglements, Rouse relaxation of the whole chain, reptation and long-range Fickian diffusion of whole chains. A discussion of all processes exceeds the scope of this chapter and the reader is referred to the literature for further reading (e.g. Wool, 1995, and references therein). The debate on the microscopic details of polymer dynamics in the viscoelastic state (melt) still endures. It is clear, however, that the Rouse relaxation of segments and the reptation contribute to the interphase formation and are responsible for its mechanical strength. These two processes are now considered on a qualitative level.

Rouse (1953) considered the eigenvibrations of a macromolecule under the influence of an external friction force which models the interaction between the chain atoms and the surroundings. The model provides N relaxation times associated with the normal modes of the vibrating chain, the longest of which is called the Rouse relaxation time

$$T_{\text{Rouse}} \propto M^2. \tag{7.9}$$

Chain entanglements hinder these motions and the model applies for the chain sections between two entanglement points,

$$T_{e,\text{Rouse}} \propto M_e^2, \tag{7.10}$$

where M_e is the molecular mass average of the chain section between two entanglements. At the fresh contact between two compatible polymers, the Rouse motions yield an interdiffusion of the chain sections at the interface. The corresponding penetration depth $X_{e,\text{Rouse}}$ is of the order of 1 nm.

ADHESION OF POLYMERS

The reptation model provides further essential features of the chain motion in a polymer consisting of entangled coils. The conventional diffusion equation does not apply to this type of motion. The model was developed by de Gennes (1971) for polymer melts, and by Doi and Edwards (1978a–c, 1979, 1986) with particular emphasis on polymer rheology. Wool (1995) and other authors extended it to the polymer interface. The word reptation describes well the snake-like motion of an entangled macromolecule. In brief, the constraints imposed on a chain by the entanglements with other chains confine it to a tube-like region, inside which the chain wriggles around because of the thermal fluctuations. These motions are fast but the magnitude is small compared with the radius of gyration of the coil. On a greater timescale, the statistical wriggling moves the chain forwards and backwards in the tube with a certain diffusion constant. While moving forwards or backwards, only the respective end regions of the chain have a chance of leaving the given tube. They choose their directions randomly and create new tube ends. This is a cooperative motion since the random choice also depends on the local free volume provided by the surrounding chains at a given moment. The tube is not static because the surrounding chains fluctuate thermally as well. After the reptation time, T_r, the chain has escaped from the old into a new tube. The theory provides

$$T_r \propto M^3. \tag{7.11}$$

The reptation is much slower than the Rouse motion. For example, T_r is about 1860 min and $T_{e,Rouse} \approx 10$ s in polystyrene ($M = 245\,000$ g mol^{-1}) at 118°C (Agrawal et al., 1994). The theoretical expressions for the thickness of the interdiffusion layer, the number of chains crossing the interface, etc., are omitted, and these formulae and an instructive description of the dynamics can be found in Wool (1995).

Owing to the molecular weight dependence of T_r, the short chains diffuse more quickly than the long chains. The final interphase thickness X amounts to about

$$X(t \to \infty) \approx 0.8\, R_g \propto M^{1/2}, \tag{7.12}$$

which is some 10 nm.

It is clear from the example that the reptation takes a lot of time for welding the two compatible polymers. At a time $t > T_r$, all correlation is lost and Fickian diffusion promotes the further process of intermixing until the chemical potentials are equilibrated.

Comparison with the thickness data for incompatible polymer pairs reveals that the conformational relaxation process should be a mixture of Rouse relaxation and reptation.

7.5 POLYMERS COMBINED WITH INORGANIC MATERIALS

Inorganic materials possess a dense structure of closely packed atoms or molecules. Macromolecules cannot therefore penetrate into inorganic surfaces. Additional features of interphase formation and interaction between flexible polymer chains and dense surfaces need to be considered.

7.5.1 METALLISATION OF POLYMERS

Metallisation modifies the properties of polymer surfaces with regard to their chemical, electrical, mechanical and other properties, and this deserves interest for their application as biomaterials. In the metallisation process, the metal atoms arrive as mobile individuals at a polymer surface. It is clear from the preceding sections that the metal layer formation will be influenced by the type and strength of metal–polymer interaction, the structure of the polymer (amorphous, crystalline or cross-linked) and, very importantly, the macromolecular mobility (glassy or viscoelastic state). The most common metallisation techniques are evaporation, sputtering, chemical vapour deposition and electrochemical deposition.

Transmission electron micrographs or radiotracer techniques reveal that metal atoms can diffuse considerable distances into a polymer. For titanium on polyimide, for instance (Robertson and Birnbaum, 1995), titanium atom clusters are found up to about 100 nm deep in the polymer. Similar observations are made with gold, silver, copper, tungsten, and nickel on polyimide or on polycarbonate (Ho *et al.*, 1988; Robertson and Birnbaum, 1995; Strunskus *et al.*, 1998). At a later stage, the deposition leads to a metal overlayer on the polymer and the diffusion ceases. During thermal annealing of the sample after metal deposition, the metal atoms may aggregate in clusters of about 5–50 nm (for Ag on polyimide as an example, see Mazur *et al.*, 1987; Mazur and Reich, 1986).

A number of conditions must be met for accomplishing metal penetration into polymers. The metal deposition rate must be low enough to prevent metal cluster formation at the polymer surface in an initial stage of the metallisation process. The metal bonds in such clusters immobilise the atoms. A strong interaction between the metal atom and the polymer chain reduces the diffusion for similar reasons. The metal atoms must not react with the polymer. Last but not least, the polymer substrate temperature must be well above the glass transition of the polymer surface region. The polymer segment motions have to assist the metal atom transport deep into the material.

The metal diffusion front is rough and creates mechanical interlocking, which in turn enhances the mechanical strength between metal overlayer and polymer. It also modifies the mechanical modulus of the polymer–metal interphase. The dielectric properties (dielectric constant and loss) increase in the composite region compared with the pure polymer. Electric conductivity may be affected and the thermal expansion coefficients are matched to some extent by the interphase. All of these gradient properties could have interesting application potential.

7.5.2 POLYMER ADSORPTION ON RIGID MATERIALS

In the following, the behaviour of viscoelastic polymers and polymer solutions in the interphase on flat rigid substrates is discussed briefly since polymers are often applied as a solution on solids.

In Section 7.3, the basic features of macromolecular surfaces were considered. They apply in a similar way to the polymer side of the interphase on rigid substrates. The wall restricts conformational freedom and the polymer chain tends to reduce the density of segments for entropic reasons. An additional attractive interaction between the substrate and certain chain moieties is needed to accumulate segments against the entropic force. It depends on the surface density of the attracting centres and whether or not all segments approaching the wall can find an adsorption site. A large surface density of attraction sites is mandatory for good adhesion. Section 7.6 will deal with the particular chemical and physical nature of that attraction in more detail.

In the general sense, the adsorption is defined as the concentration change at an interface with respect to the bulk. Hence a distinction must be made between an increase in polymer concentration (i.e. positive adsorption) and a decreased concentration (negative adsorption or depletion). The adsorption is characterised by the adsorbed amount Γ (positive or negative, usually in mg m^{-2}) and by the concentration as a function of the distance x from the substrate. The free energy of adsorption ΔA_{ads} rules whether the adsorption is positive or negative. Similar to the free energy of mixing in Section 7.4, ΔA_{ads} is defined by

$$\Delta A_{ads} \equiv (A_{interphase} - A_{bulk}) = \Delta U_{ads} - T\Delta S_{ads}, \tag{7.13}$$

where $A_{interphase}$ is the integral free energy of the adsorbed layer (interphase), A_{bulk} is the corresponding free energy of that interphase as it was in the bulk state (solution or solid), ΔU_{ads} is the internal energy change of the adsorbed layer with respect to the corresponding bulk value, and ΔS_{ads} is the entropy change of the adsorbed layer with respect to the corresponding bulk value.

As the segments are the mobile units of the polymer chain, their adsorption behaviour determines whether ΔA_{ads} can be negative (positive adsorption) or positive (depletion). ΔS_{ads} is always negative, even for depletion, since the conformational freedom remains restricted at the non-adsorbing rigid wall. Hence, ΔA_{ads} will be only negative if the attractive interaction between the polymer chain and the substrate is sufficiently large to produce a negative ΔU_{ads} that overcompensates the negative entropic part $T\Delta S_{ads}$. For the viscoelastic pure polymer, the result clearly depends on the interplay of the interaction strengths between segments and segment–substrate. In solutions, the solvent molecules come into play. For instance, a bad solvent will force positive adsorption, although the substrate–segment attraction may be weak. Things become even more complicated if copolymers or mixtures are considered.

The following discussion is focused on a qualitative description of the main features of homopolymer adsorption layers. For a comprehensive overview on the theoretical background, the reader is referred to Fleer et al. (1993).

Depletion is the least favourable situation from the adhesion point of view. Figure 7.1 depicts the corresponding segment concentration profile. In diluted solutions, the depleted region extends to about $2R_g$, i.e. it grows with the molecular weight. In *concentrated* systems (solutions and viscoelastic solid), the depletion zone reduces to the correlation length ξ_c.

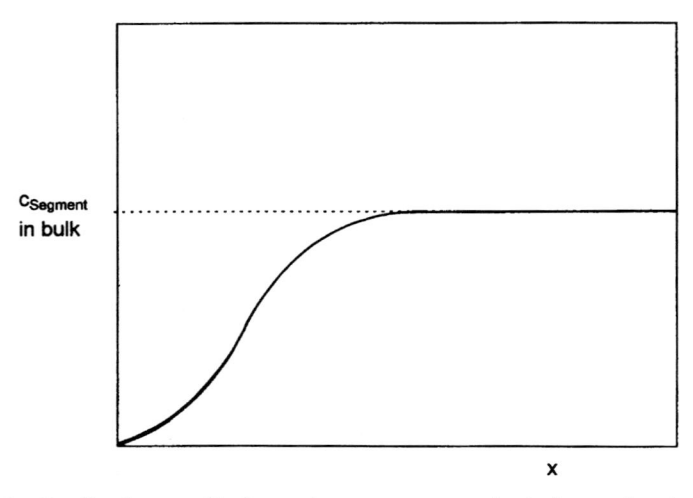

Figure 7.1 Qualitative profile for polymer segment depletion at hard substrates from the theoretical approach of Flory (1969).

$$\xi_c \approx \frac{C_\infty}{6} l\varphi^{-1} \xrightarrow{\text{melt}} \frac{C_\infty}{6} l \quad (7.14)$$

where φ is the polymer volume fraction in the bulk solution.

Accordingly, the depleted zone shrinks with increasing concentration in the bulk phase. It is very difficult to detect negative adsorption experimentally as the reductions of concentration are small.

Up to now, positive adsorption has been investigated more intensively. According to the theory, a part of the macromolecular chain adsorbs as trains of segments while the rest forms loops and tails (see Figure 7.2 for the usual intuitive picture). If side-chains are present, the chain can also form single contacts. In this way the macromolecules balance their internal energy with their entropic contribution to the free energy. The corresponding concentration profile is sketched qualitatively in Figure 7.3. Here, $c_{\text{segment}}(x)$ gives the total segment concentration while $c_{\text{free chain}}(x)$ stands for the segment concentration of those chains having no segments attached to the substrate. The adsorbed amount of polymer *in excess* to the bulk is calculated by

$$\Gamma^{\text{excess}} = \int_0^\infty [c_{\text{segment}}(x) - c_{\text{bulk}}]\,\mathrm{d}x. \quad (7.15)$$

The totally adsorbed amount is given by

$$\Gamma = \int_0^\infty [c_{\text{segment}}(x) - c_{\text{free chain}}(x)]\,\mathrm{d}x. \quad (7.16)$$

ADHESION OF POLYMERS

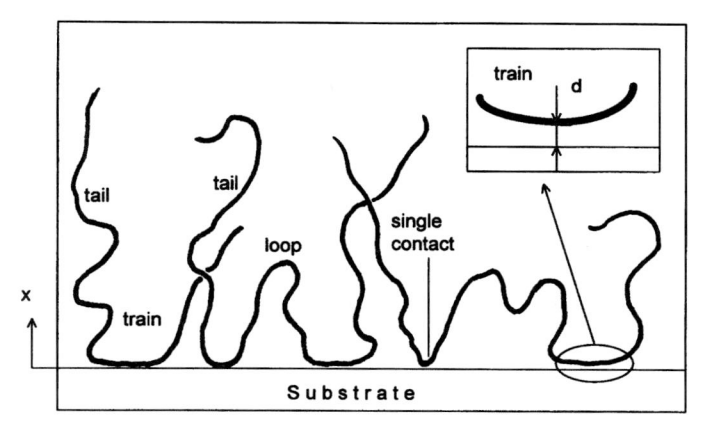

Figure 7.2 Structure elements of a polymer chain adsorbed from solution on to a rigid substrate. d = Distance between the middle of the attached segment and the substrate surface.

Since for concentrated systems

$$\lim_{c_{\text{bulk}} \to 1} c_{\text{segment}}(x) \approx c_{\text{bulk}}$$

the adsorbed amount is estimated by

$$\lim_{c_{\text{bulk}} \to 1} \Gamma \approx \int_0^\infty [c_{\text{bulk}} - c_{\text{free chain}}(x)] dx. \tag{7.17}$$

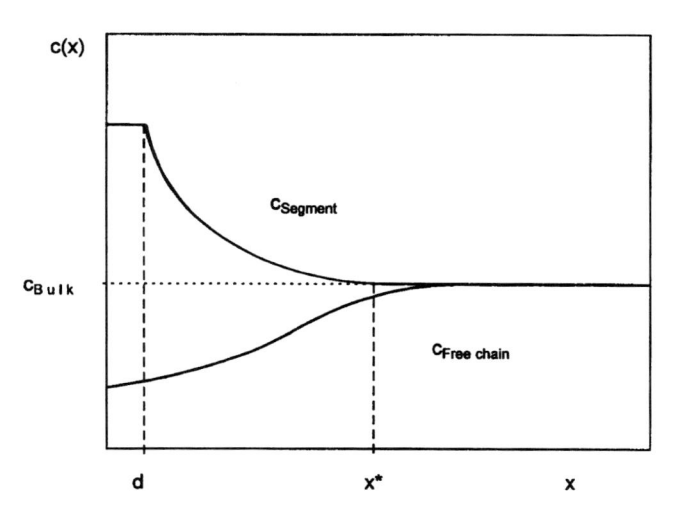

Figure 7.3 Qualitative scheme of the concentration profile for positive adsorption. The macromolecules possess equal weight.

Figure 7.4 shows Γ as a function of the bulk solution concentration for a monodisperse polymer, the adsorption isotherm. Only a small concentration range of about 10^{-6}–10^{-2} is accessible by experiments (i.e. small-angle neutron scattering). The pseudo-plateau value $\Gamma^{plateau}$ of a few mg m^{-2} is reached at a concentration of 10^{-4} by the order of magnitude. The plateau indicates the beginning overlaps of adsorbed chains where the chains have to compete for adsorption sites on the substrate. It shifts to higher values for decreasing solvent quality (that is for rising χ).

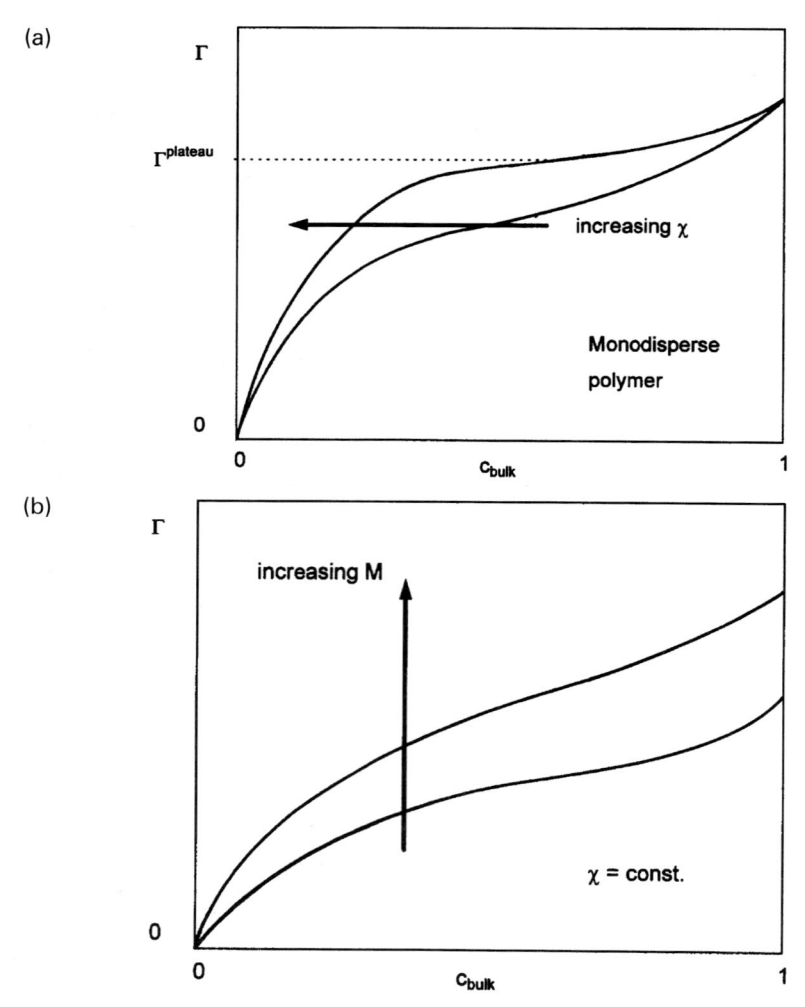

Figure 7.4 Schematic drawing for the adsorption isotherm of monodisperse polymers: (a) influence of the solvent interaction parameter χ; (b) influence of molecular weight.

ADHESION OF POLYMERS

For $c_{\text{bulk}} \to 1$ the influence of the solvent interaction parameter χ vanishes and the limiting value for the adsorption scales with

$$\lim_{c_{\text{bulk}} \to 1} \Gamma \propto M^{1/2}. \tag{7.18}$$

Γ also increases with the adsorption energy per surface site.

For polydisperse homopolymer solutions, the long chains are found to adsorb preferentially because they lose less translational entropy per molecule, while they gain almost the same adsorption energy ΔU_{ads} as short chains. In equilibrium, small molecules adsorb only at sites that the large chains cannot approach due to mutual steric hindrance. Hence the pseudo-plateau in the adsorption curve almost corresponds to the heavy weight molecules but the transition to the plateau is more rounded than with monodisperse chains. It is almost impossible to desorb adsorbed polymer chains from a substrate by dissolution.

The number of trains reflects the degree of coupling between the polymer and the substrate. Therefore trains are important for the adhesion (i.e. the gross interaction energy between the polymer and the substrate). As each train covers quite a number of adsorption sites, a weak adsorptive interaction per site can be sufficient for good adhesion. Tails and loops manage the entanglement of the adsorbed chains and the macromolecules in the polymer bulk. This entanglement contributes essentially to the mechanical strength of the compound, which is often called the adhesive strength. The concentration profile shown in Figure 7.3 decays more and more gradually with rising c_{bulk} of the polymer solution. This indicates a growing length for tails and loops. The theory reveals that the polymer fraction in trains, Γ^{train}, decreases with increasing chain length. It rises with the concentration up to an almost constant value which is reached on the pseudo-plateau. NMR and electron spin resonance experiments are capable of determining Γ^{train}. For example (van der Beek et al., 1991), a value $\Gamma^{\text{train}} \approx 0.2$ mg m^{-2} is estimated from NMR results on the pseudo-plateau ($\Gamma^{\text{plateau}} \approx 0.51$ mg m^{-2}) for polyethyleneoxide (M = 2.7 × 10^5 g mol^{-1}) adsorbed on SiO$_2$ from a solution in water. According to the theory, the tail fraction in solution is nearly independent of the chain length for chains with more than approximately 20 segments. Hence the tail length is proportional to the chain length. The tail fraction rises with the concentration. For the melt (viscoelastic state), about two-thirds of the long chains belong to tails. Since it is very difficult to distinguish in concentrated polymer systems between free and adsorbed chains, experimental information on the structure is scarce. Dynamic experiments (with NMR, for instance) revealed reduced segment mobilities in the interphase (Lipatov, 1980).

Up to now we have considered the macromolecule as a chemically homogeneous species. The structure and hence the adsorptive forces of chain ends actually differ from the rest of the chain. The consequences for the interphase structure in the case of a preferential chain end adsorption are depicted in Figure 7.5. The mushroom structure results on surfaces that are non-adsorbing for the chain segments. It develops into the brush with a rising polymer concentration in the solution. As there is just one contact per chain for both the mushroom and the brush structures, good adhesion

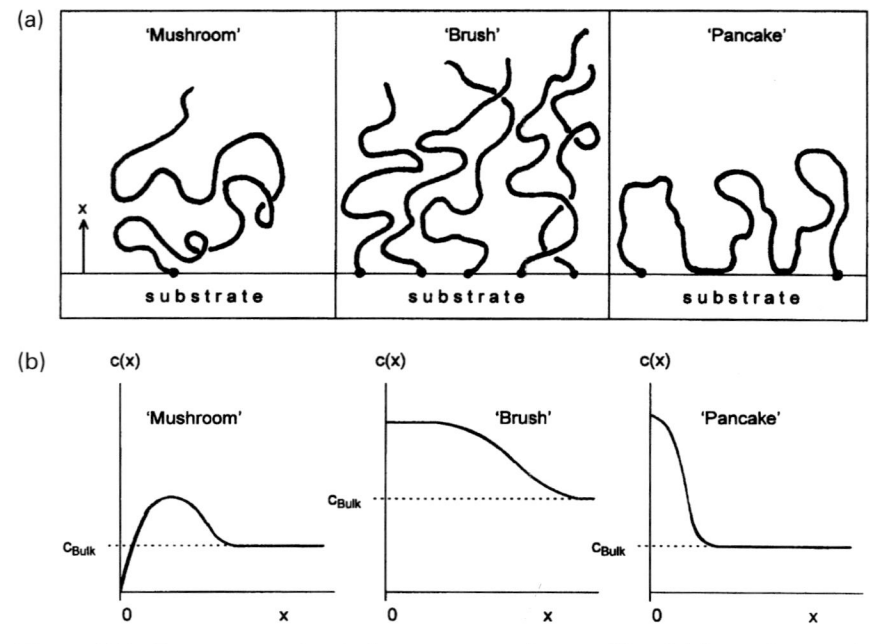

Figure 7.5 Structure and solution concentration profile $c(x)$ for polymer chains terminally attached to substrates. The mushroom and brush occur on substrates that do not adsorb chain segments. The pancake forms on substrates adsorbing both chain ends and segments.

requires very strong interaction between the chain end and the substrate. The pancake structure arises on surfaces that adsorb both the ends and the segments of the chains. The close packing reduces the probability for entanglements with other chains. Hence a weak boundary layer with low mechanical strength could result.

Other cases of preferential or competitive adsorption can occur with mixtures from polymers or from a polymer with low molecular weight organics (e.g. a solvent). Whenever a polymer competes with another polymer for adsorption sites, the one with the stronger adsorption interaction will win because the entropy loss is quite similar for the two polymers. Small molecules are also able to displace macromolecules on the adsorption sites when their adsorption interaction is considerably stronger than that between the chain unit and the adsorption site. The loss of translational entropy has to be overcompensated. The higher the concentration of the small molecules, the more easily this condition is met.

The adsorption of copolymers is even more complex and a description goes beyond the scope of this chapter.

The polymer adsorption kinetics has as yet no quantitative theoretical background. This is easy to understand since the macromolecular mobility comes into play, with all of the difficulties that were touched on briefly in Section 7.2. Experiments show that the adsorption rate $d\Gamma/dt$ is fast in the initial stage of the process but then slows down as the substrate surface saturates. In solutions, the pseudo-plateau, $\Gamma^{plateau}$, is usually reached within a few minutes. As the smaller chains diffuse more quickly to the substrate, they have to be displaced afterwards by the long chains. In the adsorption measurement with a polydisperse polymer, this can be seen by an initial steep slope of the isotherm and a Γ-value on the pseudo-plateau still rising with time.

7.6 ADHESION

The word adhesion is used in several contexts in the scientific literature and in everyday life, so that some confusion about the exact meaning may easily arise. For the present discussion, the term adhesion is restricted to the mechanisms that appear in the interphase owing to the formation of a contact between two materials (i.e. condensed phases). Such mechanisms yield a particular interaction energy and morphological structure which contribute to the resistance of the material compound to external forces. However, this resistance is not the mechanical strength itself.

The former consideration of polymer dynamics in interphases revealed two mechanisms of adhesion: the interpenetration of chains at polymer–polymer interfaces, and the interlocking between the polymer and the diffusion front of properly deposited metal overlayers. This interlocking occurs at the molecular level. It must not be confused with the classical mechanical adhesion model where macroscopic filling of a surface roughness profile was supposed to improve the compound strength. (Experiments proved the mechanical adhesion to be negligible.)

The picture can now be completed by a brief discussion of the possible interaction mechanisms between the rigid substrate and the polymer chain segments in the adsorbed trains. In principle, adsorption forces and adhesion forces are simply different names for the same thing.

The physical or van der Waals interactions occur always and everywhere between matter. They summarise the (usually attractive) forces between the *bound* electrons and the nuclei of different atoms. In more detail, the electric multipole attraction (above all the homocharges and the dipoles), the multipole induction (dominated by the induced dipoles) and the universal London forces form a physical contribution to the adhesion. These forces are distinguished by a pairwise interaction that does not saturate. The energy gain from a single interacting pair is relatively small. Hence the forces are very difficult to characterise experimentally and the resulting physical adhesion forces are often considered as being not very strong. This could be invalid for adsorbed polymer trains (compare with Section 7.5) where the sum of many interacting pairs (chain unit–surface site) may provide the decisive factor for adhesion.

Another adhesion component is provided by the electric double layer (EDL), which is tied with the *mobile* electric charge carriers in a material (electrons or ions). For instance, the systems of mobile electrons in both phases move through the contact in order to equilibrate their chemical potential. As a consequence, the electrical neutrality is disturbed both on the side losing electrons and on the side receiving them. The resulting positive and negative space charges established on each side of the contact form the EDL. This process also occurs in insulating polymers since there is always a certain number of accessible electronic states. These states are localised, however, and they therefore trap the incoming electrons. The amount and the distribution of the space charge on the polymer side was established by Possart and Röder (1984) and Possart and Müller (1988) for various materials. The attractive electrical potential between the space charges contributes to the adhesion. In the 1940s Deryaguin et al. (see Deryaguin, 1940; Deryaguin and Krotova, 1949; Deryaguin et al., 1973) had already recognized that the EDL in insulating polymers provides a contribution to the strength against the separation of the two phases. During a fast separation process such as failure, the trapped space charge cannot flow back quickly enough. Work has to be performed against the electric field in the growing gap between the separating space charges until an electric discharge process compensates the charging. The discharging dissipates the mechanical energy stored in the electric field. An estimation for polyethylene on aluminium foil shows, however, that the process amounts to just a few per cent of the gross failure energy (Possart, 1988). Hence the electrostatic adhesion component is considered to be less important for practical purposes.

The last but not least important adhesion mechanism rests on chemical interactions. Quite rarely, direct chemical conversions involving functional groups at the polymer chains and on the surface are observed without doubt. PMMA on natively oxidised aluminium may serve as an example. Investigations (Possart et al., 1985; Unger and Possart, 1989; Konstadinidis et al., 1992; Possart and Schlett, 1995; Leadley and Watts, 1996) by photoelectron spectroscopy, infrared reflection spectroscopy, thermodesorption mass spectrometry and NMR revealed that the OH-groups on the aluminium surface hydrolyse a part of the ester bond in the PMMA side-group ($-CO-O-CH_3$). Methanol is released as a byproduct. The resulting carboxylate ion [$(-CO-O)^-$] should bond ionically on the surface.

During the past few years, considerable experimental evidence was found that electron donor–acceptor interactions might play a more general role. In chemical terms this is the Lewis acid–base interaction. Whether a molecule acts as a donor or as an acceptor for another molecule depends first of all on the energetic position of its frontier orbitals [highest occupied molecular orbital (HOMO) and lowest unoccupied molecular orbital (LUMO)] relative to the energies of the frontier orbitals of the partner molecule. The spatial orientation of the two molecules relative to each other is no less important since a favourable energetic situation becomes effective only for a very short distance (a few tenths of a nanometre) between the corresponding frontier orbitals. With polymers, this condition is influenced by the modes of motion of both the main chain and the side-groups. Similarly, the donor–acceptor picture applies to molecules on solids where the frontier electronic bands (valence band and lowest virtual band) replace the frontier orbitals (e.g. Hoffmann, 1988). Several recent studies were devoted to the quantum chemical basis of this picture (Chakraborty et al., 1990; Lee, 1991a, b, 1992, 1994; Holubka et al., 1992; Drabold et al., 1993). An example is the results reported for acrylic polymers (see Chakraborty et al., 1990; Holubka et al., 1992; Drabold et al., 1993, and references therein).

Accordingly, metallic aluminium prefers to interact exclusively with the carbonyl group (–C=O) forming, for instance, an (Al–O–C) link to the polymer chains of PMMA or polyacrylic acid (PAA). The methyl group or even more bulky side-groups only hinder the carbonyls from approaching the Al atoms. The same holds for an amorphous Al_2O_3 surface (no hydroxyls). Moreover, the oxygen atoms repel the carbonyls. This picture differs completely from the reaction of these polymers with the native oxide layer on aluminium surfaces. As mentioned above, here the surface hydroxyls react with either the (–O–CH_3) groups (PMMA) or with the (–OH) groups (PAA). Thus the nature of the side-groups will also influence the adhesion interaction in this case.

7.7 SUMMARY

The chapter touched briefly on the many different aspects of the state and the microscopic dynamics of interphases in polymers. Most of them are very difficult to investigate experimentally or theoretically. Only a very small number of papers could be mentioned from the large body of literature on these topics, but it can be seen that our knowledge of adhesion mechanisms is still rather empirical. Even a qualitative correlation to macroscopic properties such as mechanics or electric conduction is very difficult to establish since many complex microscopic processes are involved both from the interphase and from the bulk sides of the contacting materials. More exact information is needed, considering both the experimental and the theoretical aspects. The measuring techniques have still to be improved. The new powerful theoretical simulation methods promise valuable support for further verification and quantification of adhesion for practical purposes.

REFERENCES

Agrawal, G., Wool, R.P., Dozier, W.D., Felcher, G.P., Russell, T.P. and Mays, J.W. (1994) Short-time interdiffusion at polymer interfaces, *Macromolecules* **27**, 4407–9.

Baier, R.E. and Zisman, W.A. (1970) The influence of polymer conformation on the surface properties of poly(γ-methyl-L-glutamate) and poly(benzy glutamate), *Macromolecules* **3**, 70–9.

Chakraborty, A.K., Davis, H.T. and Tirrell, M. (1990) A molecular orbital study of the interactions of acrylic polymers with aluminum: implications for adhesion, *J. Polymer Sci. A: Polymer Chem.* **28**, 3185–219.

de Gennes, P.G. (1971) Reptation of a polymer chain in the presence of fixed obstacles, *J. Chem. Phys.* **55**, 572–9.

de Gennes, P.G. (1979) *Scaling Concepts in Polymer Physics*, Cornell University Press, Ithaca, NY.

de Gennes, P.G. (1988) Tension superficielle des polymères fondus, *C.r. Acad. Sci. Paris* **307 II**, 1841–4.

Deryaguin, B.V. (1940) On the repulsive forces between charged colloid particles and on the theory of slow coagulation and stability of hydrophobe sols, *Trans. Faraday Soc.* **36**, 203, 203–15.

Deryaguin, B.V. and Krotova, N.A. (1949) *Adhesion*, Academy of Sciences, Moscow (in Russian).
Deryaguin, B.V., Krotova, N.A. and Smilga, V.P. (1973) *Adhesion of Solids*, Nauka, Moscow, (in Russian).
Doi, M. and Edwards, S.F. (1978a) Dynamics of concentrated polymer systems. Part 1. Brownian motion in the equilibrium state, *J. Chem. Soc., Faraday Trans. II* **74**, 1789–801.
Doi, M. and Edwards, S.F. (1978b) Dynamics of concentrated polymer systems. Part 2. Molecular motion under flow, *J. Chem. Soc., Faraday Trans. II* **74**, 1802–17.
Doi, M. and Edwards, S.F. (1978c) Dynamics of concentrated polymer systems. Part 3. The constitutive equation, *J. Chem. Soc., Faraday Trans. II* **74**, 1818–32.
Doi, M. and Edwards, S.F. (1979) Dynamics of concentrated polymer systems. Part 4. Rheological properties, *J. Chem. Soc., Faraday Trans. II* **75**, 38–54.
Doi, M. and Edwards, S.F. (1986) *The Theory of Polymer Dynamics*, Clarendon Press, Oxford.
Drabold, D.A., Adams, J.B., Anderson, D.C. and Kiefer, J. (1993) First principles study of polymer-metal–metal-oxide adhesion, *J. Adhesion* **42**, 55–63.
Fleer, G.M., Cohen Stuart, M.A., Scheutjens, J.M.H.M., Cosgrove, T. and Vincent, B. (1993) *Polymers at Interfaces*, Chapman & Hall, London.
Flory, P.J. (1953) *Principles of Polymer Chemistry*, Cornell University Press, Ithaca, NY.
Flory, P.J. (1969) *Statistical Mechanics of Chain Molecules*, Interscience, New York.
Forster, K.L. and Wool, R.P. (1991) Strength of polystyrene–poly(methyl methacrylate) interfaces, *Macromolecules* **24**, 1397–403.
Helfand, E. (1975) Theory of inhomogeneous polymers: fundamentals of the Gaussian random-walk model, *J. Chem. Phys.* **62**, 999–1005.
Helfand, E. (1982) *Polymer Interfaces*, in *Polymer Compatibility and Incompatibility; Principles and Practices* (ed. K. Solc), MMI Press Symposium Series, Harwood Academic, New York, pp. 143–63.
Helfand, E. (1992) Theory of homopolymer/binary-polymer-mixture interface, *Macromolecules* **25**, 1676–85.
Helfand, E. and Sapse, A. (1975) Theory of unsymmetric polymer–polymer interfaces, *J. Chem. Phys.* **62**, 1327–31.
Helfand, E. and Tagami, Y. (1972) Theory of the interface between immiscible polymers II, *J. Chem. Phys.* **56**, 3592–601.
Ho, P.S., Haight, R., White, R.C. and Silverman, B.D.(1988) Chemistry and microstructure at metal–polymer interfaces, *J. Phys. Colloq. (C5, Interface Sci. Engng. '87)* **C5**, 49–59.
Hoffmann, R. (1988) *Solids and Surface – A Chemist's View of Bonding in Extended Structures*, VCH, Weinheim.
Holubka, J., Dickie, R.A. and Cassatta, J.C. (1992) Molecular modeling of adhesion: the interaction of acrylate and methacrylate esters with aluminum oxide, *Adhesion Sci. Technol.* **6**, 243–52.
Hong, K.M. and Noolandi, J. (1981a) Theory of inhomogeneous multicomponent polymer systems, *Macromolecules* **14**, 727–36.
Hong, K.M. and Noolandi, J. (1981b) Conformational entropy effects in a compressible lattice fluid theory of polymers, *Macromolecules* **14**, 1229–34.
Hook, T.J., Schmitt, R.L., Gardella, J.A., Salvati, L., Jr and Chin, R.L. (1986) Analysis of polymer surface structure by low-energy ion scattering spectroscopy, *Analyt. Chem.* **58**, 1285–90.
Huggins, M. (1942a) Some properties of solutions of long-chain compounds, *J. Phys. Chem.* **46**, 151–8.
Huggins, M. (1942b) Theory of solutions of high polymers, *J. Am. Chem. Soc.* **64**, 1712–9.
Klein, J. and Briscoe, B.J. (1979) The diffusion of long-chain molecules through bulk polyethylene, *Proc. R. Soc. Lond.* **A 365**, 53–73.
Konstadinidis, K., Thakkar, B., Chakraborty, A., Potts, L.W., Tannenbaum, R. and Tirrell, M. (1992) Segment level chemistry and chain conformation in the reactive adsorption of poly(methyl methacrylate) on aluminum oxide surfaces, *Langmuir* **8**, 1307–17.

Leadley, S.R. and Watts, J.F. (1997) The use of monochromated XPS to evaluate acid–base interactions at the PMMA/oxidised metal surface, *J. Adhesion* **60**, 175–96.
Lee, L.-H. (1967) Adhesion of high polymers. II. Wettability of elastomers, *J. Polymer Sci. A-2* **5**, 1103–18.
Lee, L.-H. (1991a) Relevance of the hard–soft acid–base (HSAB) principle to solid adhesion, *J. Adhesion* **36**, 39–54.
Lee, L.-H. (1991b) Relevance of the density-functional theory to acid–base interactions and adhesion in solids, *J. Adhesion Sci. Technol.* **5**, 71–92.
Lee, L.-H. (1992) Molecular bonding mechanism for solid adhesion, *J. Adhesion* **37**, 187–204.
Lee, L.-H. (1994) Molecular bonding and adhesion at polymer–metal interphases, *J. Adhesion* **46**, 15–38.
Lipatov, Y.S. (1980) in *Adhesion and Adsorption of Polymers*, Part 12B (ed. L.-H. Lee), Plenum Press, New York, p. 601–27.
Mansfield, K.F. and Theodorou, D.N. (1990) Atomistic simulation of a glassy polymer surface, *Macromolecules* **23**, 4430–45.
Mansfield, K.F. and Theodorou, D.N. (1991) Molecular dynamics simulation of a glassy polymer surface, *Macromolecules* **24**, 6283–94.
Mazur, S., Lugg, P.S. and Yarnitzky, C. (1987) Electrochemistry of aromatic polyimides, *J. Electrochem. Soc.* **134**, 346–53.
Mazur, S. and Reich, S. (1986) Electrochemical growth of metal interlayers in polyimide films, *J. Phys. Chem.* **90**, 1365–72.
Noolandi, J. and Hong, K.M. (1982) Interfacial properties of immiscible homopolymer blends in the presence of block copolymers, *Macromolecules* **15**, 482–92.
Pireaux, J.J., Gregoire, C., Caudano, R., Rei Vilar, M., Brinkhuis, R. and Schouten, J.A. (1991) Electron-induced vibrational spectroscopy. A new and unique tool to unravel the molecular structure of polymer surfaces, *Langmuir* **7**, 2433–7.
Possart, W. (1988) Experimental and theoretical description of the electrostatic component of adhesion at polymer–metal contacts, *Int. J. Adhesion Adhesives* **8**, 77–83.
Possart, W. and Müller, I. (1988) The electric double layer at the polymer–metal contact. A phenomenological model, *Phys. Stat. Sol. (A)* **106**, 525–34.
Possart, W. and Röder, A. (1984) Measurement of electrical potential distribution in a polymer near the contact to a metal by means of SEM, *Phys. Stat. Sol. (A)* **84**, 319–25.
Possart, W. and Schlett, V. (1995) XPS of the interphase between PMMA and metals. A study of degradation and interaction, *J. Adhesion* **48**, 25–46.
Possart, W., Yudin, V.S., Redkov, B.P., Ziegler, H.-J., Pozdnyakov, O.F. and Bischof, C. (1985) The state of ultra-thin PMMA films on steel as revealed by mass spectrometry, *Acta Polymer.* **36**, 631–6.
Robertson, I.M. and Birnbaum, H. (1995) Cited in Wool, R.P., *Polymer Interfaces. Structure and Strength*, Carl Hanser, München, p. 127.
Rouse, P.E. (1953) A theory of linear viscoelastic properties of dilute solutions of coiling polymers, *J. Chem. Phys.* **21**, 1272–80.
Russell, T.P., Anastasiadis, S.H., Menelle, A., Fletcher, G.P. and Satija, S.K. (1991) Segment density distribution of symmetric diblock copolymers at the interface between two homopolymers as revealed by neutron reflectivity, *Macromolecules* **24**, 1575–82.
Schmitt, R.L., Gardella, J.A., Jr, Magill, J.H., Salvati, L., Jr and Chin, R.L. (1985) Study of surface composition and morphology of block copolymers of bisphenol A polycarbonate and poly(dimethylsiloxane) by X-ray photoelectron spectroscopy and ion scattering spectroscopy, *Macromolecules* **18**, 2675–9.
Schmitt, R.L., Gardella, J.A., Jr and Salvati, L., Jr. (1986) Studies of surface composition and morphology in polymers. 2. Bisphenol A polycarbonate and poly(dimethylsiloxane) blends, *Macromolecules* **19**, 648–51.

Strunskus, T., Kiene, M., Willecke, R., Thran, A., v. Bechtolsheim, C. and Faupel, F. (1998) Chemistry, diffusion and cluster formation at metal–polymer interfaces, *Materials and Corrosion* **49**, 180–8.

Unger, W. and Possart, W. (1989) An XPS investigation of the interface between thin polymethylmethacrylate (PMMA) and natively oxidized Al, *Phys. Stat. Sol. (A)* **114**, K175–7.

van der Beek, G.P., Cohen Stuart, M.A. and Cosgrove, T. (1991) Polymer adsorption and desorption studies via ^{1}H NMR relaxation of the solvent, *Langmuir* **7**, 327–34.

Wattenbarger, M.R., Chan, H.S., Evans, D.F., Bloomfield, V.A. and Dill, K.A. (1990) Surface-induced enhancement of internal structure in polymers and proteins, *J. Chem. Phys.* **93**, 8343–51.

Willett, J.L. and Wool, R.P. (1993) Strength of incompatible amorphous polymer interfaces, *Macromolecules* **26**, 5336–49.

Wool, R.P. (1995) *Polymer Interfaces. Structure and Strength*, Carl Hanser, München.

8
Adhesion to ceramics

H.J. BREME[1], M.A. BARBOSA[2] AND L.A. ROCHA[3]
[1]University of the Saarland, Saarbrücken, Germany
[2]INEB-Mat, Porto, Portugal
[3]University of Minho, Quirnarex, Portugal

8.1 INTRODUCTION

Compared to metals, ceramics have a number of specific mechanical, chemical, physical and biological properties that warrant their application in medical devices. However, ceramics have without exception poor mechanical properties under tensile stresses, so it is often the custom to produce composites containing the favourable properties of both materials, by means of a surface coating on the metal. However, it is also possible to incorporate bulk ceramic parts in medical devices. In these cases the bonding of a ceramic to a metal, or a ceramic to a ceramic part must be accomplished by welding or brazing. The basic requirement for the metal–ceramic component is an optimum bonding strength, which can be guaranteed only if an interdiffusion producing a chemical bonding of both materials takes place and if the residual stresses are at a minimum. Under mechanical loading, such a material fails not in the interfaces of the bond but in the ceramic, if tensile stresses are applied. Therefore, the residual stresses that may occur during the production of the composite must be as low as possible. The residual stress σ_{rs} can be estimated by the empirical equation

$$\sigma_{rs} = \overline{E} \mid (\alpha_c - \alpha_M) \mid \Delta T \tag{8.1}$$

where $\overline{E}$ is the average Young's modulus of the produced interface, α_c and α_M the thermal expansion coefficient of the ceramic and the metal, respectively, and ΔT is the difference between room temperature and the temperature at which the chemical bonding is accomplished. From this equation it is easy to understand that the difference in the thermal expansion coefficients must be as low as possible in order to avoid residual stresses. If a large difference in the α values exists, the residual stress can reach a level where it may predamage the ceramic. This effect is demonstrated in Figure 8.1, which shows the finite element calculation of a ceramic (Si_3N_4) and a metal (steel) bond. Because of the great difference in the expansion coefficients during cooling from the welding temperature, the tensile stresses at the edges of the bond are high enough to produce cracks (Suganuma and Okamoto, 1985). Therefore, in order

---

Metals as Biomaterials ISBN 0 471 96935 4 Edited by J.A. Helsen and H.J. Breme. © 1998 John Wiley & Sons Ltd

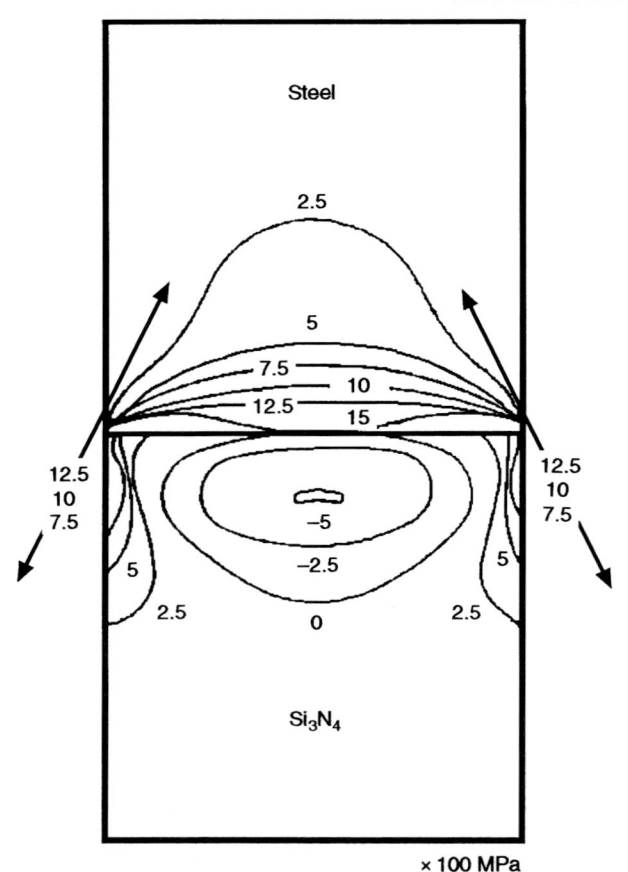

Figure 8.1 Thermal residual stress of a composite Si_3N_4–steel, finite element calculation (Suganuma and Okamoto, 1985).

to avoid any predamage and to provide an optimum bonding strength it is necessary that the thermal expansion coefficient of the metal and the ceramic must be adapted in order to avoid residual stresses. As shown in Table 8.1, which summarises the expansion coefficients of various metallic biomaterials and ceramics, the values may differ to an extreme degree. The adaptation of the coefficient of the base metal, e.g. titanium, can be attained by the metallurgical method of alloying the metal with suitable biocompatible elements. In some cases the insertion of a ductile metallic intermediate layer may help to reduce the stresses because of its ability to undergo plastic deformation.

In the following sections the different methods for the bonding of ceramics to metals, i.e. brazing, welding (diffusion bonding, fusion welding), sticking and encapsulating (sealing) by polymers (see Chapter 7), and surface coating will be discussed for various metal–ceramic composites in view of the above consideration and the essential requirement of biocompatibility. In addition, at the end of the chapter examples of medical devices made from metal–ceramic bonds are given.

Table 8.1 Thermal expansion coefficient α of metallic biomaterials and ceramics

	α (10^{-6} K^{-1})	Temperature range (°C)
X2CrNiMo1813 (316L)	15.9	70–300
Co25CrMo	12.3	300–600
Co20Cr15W110Ni	16	300–1000
cp-Ti	9	20–20
Ti6Al4V	8.6	20–30
TiO_2 (rutile)	7	300–500
TiO_2 (brookite)	11	300–500
TiO	7.6	300–500
ZrO_2	7	300–500
Ta_2O_5	3	300–600
Nb_2O_5	1	600–1000
TiC	6.5	300–1800
NbC	6	300–600
TaC	8.2	300–800

8.2 BRAZING

There are various established methods for brazing ceramics to metals and ceramics to ceramics. A process operating with glass brazing fillers has the advantage that the thermal expansion coefficient of the brazing filler can easily be adapted to that of the ceramic. Through the correct control of the crystallisation process it is possible to adjust the expansion coefficient of a glass ceramic. A glass ceramic for making matched seals with AISI 430 stainless steel (thermal expansion coefficient = 11.0×10^{-6} K^{-1}) with the composition SiO_2 67.1, LiO_2 23.7, Al_2O_3 2.8, K_2O 2.8, Be_2O_3 2.6 and P_2O_5 1.0 mol% has been reported (Loehman and Tomsia, 1988). The glass ceramic was made by nucleation heat treatment at 500°C, followed by the crystallisation stage at 750–800°C. The result was a mixture of lithium metasilicate (Li_2SiO_3), lithium disilicate ($Li_2Si_2O_5$) and residual glass. Using the same glass, its thermal expansion coefficient was raised to 14.5×10^{-6} K^{-1} by a three-stage seal cycle with successive plateaux at 1000°C (to form the seal), 650°C and 820°C. It was shown that this treatment was able to produce high-strength seals with NiCr and Ni-based alloys. According to the authors, after the three-stage heat treatment the thermal expansion coefficient of the glass–ceramic is higher because substantial amounts of cristobalite are formed in addition to the Li_2SiO_3 and $Li_2Si_2O_5$ (Kunz and Loehman, 1987). With the same system it was shown that the different phases form preferentially by expitaxial growth on specific faces of small Li_3PO_4 crystallites that precipitate during the 1000°C heat treatment. Growing the Li_3PO_4 particles by heating the glass for longer at 1000°C increased the volume fraction of cristobalite in the glass–ceramic and raised the thermal expansion coefficient (Loehman, 1989). The application of these nucleation mechanisms to other lithium silicate compositions permitted the development of glass–ceramics with thermal expansion coefficients in the order of 22.0×10^{-6} K^{-1}, which were used for producing hermetic seals with high expansion stainless steels, such as AISI 303 and AISI 316, and with Cu (Loehman and Tomsia, 1988).

Alternatively, when a direct bond technique is used, the matching of the expansion characteristics of the parent glass with those of the metal to which it is bonded can be a minor consideration (Klomp, 1986). If a larger mismatch occurs at this state, the temperature of the glass-to-metal joint should not be allowed to fall below the strain point of the glass before subjecting the assembly to the crystallisation heat treatment that will approach the thermal expansion coefficients. The strain point is the temperature derived by extrapolation of the data obtained in the tests for determining the annealing point (the temperature at which the viscosity of the glass is 10^{13} P, corresponding to a viscosity of $10^{14.5}$ P). At the strain point stresses can be relieved by viscous flow.

Several researchers studied the influence of the crystallisation process of glass ceramics on the thermal expansion behaviour. Knowledge of the nature, physical properties and proportion of the crystalline phases that can be formed in the crystallisation process is essential for these studies (Lascar, 1985).

The importance of the knowledge of the nature and physical properties of the phases present in the microstructure of the glass ceramic may be illustrated by the use of a commercially available glass ceramic with the composition SiO_2 55.5, Al_2O_3 23.5, P_2O_5 7.9, LiO_2 3.7, ZnO 1.4, MgO 1.0, TiO_2 2.3, ZrO_2 1.9, Na_2O 0.05 and As_2O3 0.5 wt%. In this glass ceramic the presence of Al_2O_3 and P_2O_5 allows the formation of an alumino-phosphate ($AlPO_4$) that decreases the melting point to below 1700°C. The titanium and zirconium oxides are nucleating agents. They are the first to crystallise, producing small-dimension particles homogeneously distributed in the glass matrix. Nucleation starts at 1500°C with the formation of aluminium titanate ($Al_2Ti_2O_7$) and aluminium zirconate ($Al_2Zr_2O_7$). These crystallites act as nuclei for the growth of mixed crystals of aluminosilicates of lithium (eucryptite β). This crystalline phase may form hybrid crystals with Li_2O, Al_2O_3, MgO, ZnO and P_2O_5. The vitreous matrix is made of SiO_2, P_2O_5 and Al_2O_3 (Campbell and Hagy, 1975).

The as-delivered glass–ceramic is constituted by 70–75% of eucryptite β and 25–30% of amorphous phase. The thermal expansion coefficient of the glass–ceramic is low and of the order of 0.1×10^{-6} K^{-1}, with the crystalline phase having a negative coefficient (-0.9×10^{-6} K^{-1}), while that of the glass matrix is of the order of 2.1×10^{-6} K^{-1}. The relative crystalline and glassy phase contents of the glass determine the global expansion characteristics of the glass–ceramic and can be controlled by heat treatment. By heating at 600°C for several hours the amount of crystalline phase was increased to 78% (Lascar, 1985).

Electrostatic bonding, also called anodic bonding or field-assisted metal–glass bonding, is a technique used to promote hermetic bonding between metallic materials and glasses. The process is carried out in the solid state, without any intermediate layers. It requires relatively high temperatures to produce ionic conductivity within the glass and high voltage to promote ion migration, which will allow bond

ADHESION TO CERAMICS

formation to take place. The equipment consists of a furnace where the parts are heated and a dc power supply to apply the potential difference between the metal and the glass parts (Barbosa et al., 1993).

The disadvantages of glass bondings are their limited strength properties under tensile stresses and their limited corrosion resistance (Klomp, 1986; Pask, 1987). In addition, it is necessary that the alumina to be bonded should contain a certain amount of silica in order to accomplish the brazing by the formation of a glassy phase. A similar problem arises with a process operating with a metallisation of the ceramic. Powders of molybdenum, manganese or tungsten are applied to the ceramic and fired in a hydrogen atmosphere with a controlled dew point. Because of the higher thermodynamic stability of the manganese, molybdenum or tungsten oxides, a reaction takes place with silica whereby the bonding is produced by the formation of a glassy phase (Hayduk, 1985; Mattox and Smith, 1985; Klomp, 1986). Because of the interaction with silica this method numbers among the active brazing processes. Other active filler metals are able to react directly with alumina. The most commonly used active metal additive is titanium (Crispin and Nicholas, 1976; Nicholas and Mortimer, 1985). Further recommended active elements are hafnium, lanthanum, niobium, tantalum, vanadium and zirconium (Barret, 1962; General Electric, 1968; Clarke and Berry, 1968). In addition to the melting point of the brazing filler, which should be as low as possible, the main requirements for good bonding strength are:

(1) a heat of formation (Gibbs enthalpy) as negative as possible in the oxide formed by the reduction of alumina
(2) high conductivity (low ionicity) of the oxide which constitutes the reaction-induced interlayer to be wetted
(3) a thermal expansion coefficient of the brazing filler as close to that of alumina as possible in order that stresses may be avoided.

Requirements (1) and (2) are fulfilled for both titanium and the titanium oxide TiO. Titanium has a high affinity to oxygen. According to the phase diagram at 1000°C the solubility amounts to about 30 at% before formation of the oxide TiO, which may have a stoichiometry ranging from $TiO_{0.88}$ to $TiO_{1.2}$ (Murray and Wiedt, 1990). On the supposition of a high titanium activity, the following reaction can take place

$$3[Ti] + Al_2O_3 \rightarrow 3TiO + 2[Al] \tag{8.2}$$

with the free energy change

$$\Delta G° = -RT \ln \frac{a_{Al}^2}{a_{Ti}^3}. \tag{8.3}$$

The titanium oxide formed has metallic conductivity and metallic interatomic bands (low ionicity), whereby the wettability and the work of adhesion are increased. The work of adhesion is a measure of the chemical bonding strength at the ceramic–metal interface, which can be expressed by the Dupré equation

$$W_{ad} = \gamma_M + \gamma_c - \gamma_{MC} \tag{8.4}$$

where W_{ad} is the work of adhesion and γ_M, γ_C and γ_{MC} are the surface energy of the metal, ceramic and metal–ceramic interface, respectively.

Using the Young equation

$$\gamma_c = \gamma_{MC} + \gamma_M \cos\theta, \tag{8.5}$$

where θ is the contact angle which stands for the wettability, the work of adhesion can be expressed as

$$W_{ad} = \gamma_M(1 + \cos\theta). \tag{8.6}$$

From Equation (8.6) it becomes clear that the work of adhesion and therefore the chemical bonding strength will be increased if the contact angle is small and $\gamma_{MC} < \gamma_c$. It was shown that the contact angle depends on the ionicity of the ceramic and/or the reaction-induced interlayer. Wetting experiments of carbides of different ionicity by copper (Figure 8.2) showed a decreasing contact angle with decreasing ionicity (Pauling, 1949; Nicholas, 1968, 1989; Naidich and Zhuravlev, 1989). Table 8.2 summarises the free energies for the formation of different oxides compared with Al_2O_3 and the dielectric constant ε for those oxides, which represent their electrical conductivity and ionicity, respectively. From this comparison it can be seen that, for example, both titanium and beryllium oxide fulfil simultaneously both requirements, i.e. high activity and conductivity. Zirconium, too, has a high activity, but the

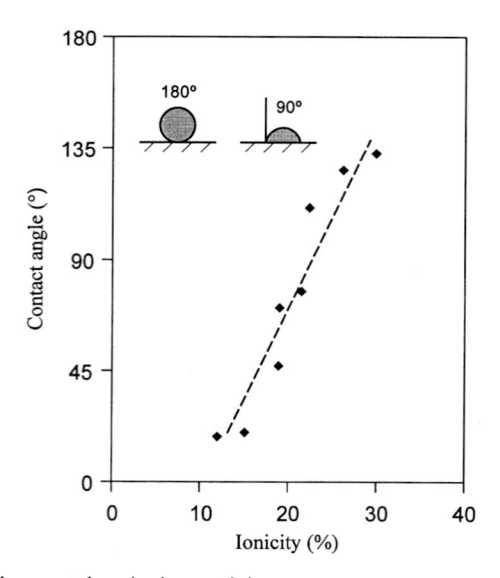

Figure 8.2 Reactive wetting (schematic).

ADHESION TO CERAMICS

Table 8.2 Gibb's free enthalpy and dielectric constant of different oxides

Oxide	$\Delta G°$ at $T=1000°C$ per mole O_2	ε
Al_2O_3	−847	5–10
BeO	−968	6.5–7.5
ZrO_2	−859	12.4
TiO	−840	–
TiO_2	−714	48–110
Ti_2O_3	−784	–
Cr_2O_3	−537	12
NiO	−248	–
CoO	−290	–
FeO	−366	–

resulting ZrO_2 has a high dielectric constant and ionicity so that only a poor wettability can be expected. Different brazing fillers containing titanium as an active additive element have been tested. The most important group consists of AgCu-based alloys containing up to 2–3 wt% titanium. This optimum concentration is accompanied by the formation of a continuous thin interlayer of TiO (Nicholas, 1987). An increase in the titanium content leads to a higher brazing temperature and to the formation of thicker layers with a lower bonding strength and/or to the formation of Ti_2O_3 which has a higher ionicity and lower wettability. The concentration of titanium in the active brazing filler can be reduced by the addition of alloying elements such as Sn and In, which decrease the solubility of titanium and increase its activity (Nicholas *et al.*, 1980).

The active brazes have an improved wetting behaviour by reacting with the substrates to change the chemistry of their surfaces (Nicholas and Peteves, 1994). This introduces a new concept known as reactive wetting, i.e. wetting in which material transfer occurs at the solid–liquid interface (Li, 1994a; Eustathopoulos, 1994; Ferro and Derby, 1995), as represented in Figure 8.3. These reactive systems

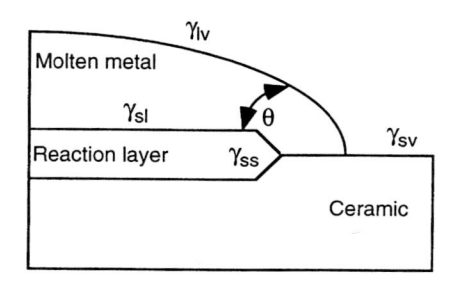

Figure 8.3 Time dependence of the contact angle of some reactive systems (Nicholas and Peteves, 1994).

are characterised by a pronounced kinetics of wetting, i.e. significant variations of θ with time, θ also being highly dependent on temperature (Li, 1994b).

At present there is no generally accepted theory capable of satisfactorily describing reactive wetting (Eustathopoulos, 1994). A reason for this is the complexity of the reactions that occur at the interface, which are almost always different from one system to another (Pask and Tomsia, 1981).

In reactive wetting Young's equation can be expressed by (Loehman, 1989):

$$(\gamma_{sv} - \gamma_{sl}) - \gamma_{ss} + A\Delta G - \gamma_{lv} \cos\theta = 0, \tag{8.7}$$

where γ_{sv} is the vapour interfacial energy, γ_{sl} is the solid–liquid interfacial energy, γ_{lv} is the liquid surface tension, γ_{ss} is the energy of the solid reaction layer interface, ΔG is the variation in free energy of the reaction and A is the constant related to the moles of product formed per unit area of the base of the drop.

As a consequence, the expression for the work of adhesion becomes

$$W_{ad} = \gamma_{lv}(1 + \cos\theta) + \gamma_{ss} - A\Delta G. \tag{8.8}$$

Thus, a thermodynamically favourable reaction (negative ΔG) increases the work of adhesion and should result in a lower contact angle, if all other conditions remain the same.

The smallest contact angle (θ_{min}) possible in a reactive system is given by:

$$\cos\theta_{min} = \cos\theta_0 - \frac{\Delta\gamma_r}{\gamma_{lv}} - \frac{\Delta G_r}{\gamma_{lv}}, \tag{8.9}$$

where θ_0 is the contact angle of the liquid on the substrate in the absence of any reaction, $\Delta\gamma_r$ is the change in the interfacial energies brought about by the interfacial reactions, and ΔG_r is the change in free energy per unit area released by the reaction of the material contained in the immediate vicinity of the metal–substrate interface (Eustathopoulos, 1994).

Because the chemical reaction is taking place in the interfacial region, it would only influence the interfacial energy γ_{sl}. Thus, the maximal lowering in interfacial energy due to the free energy released by the chemical reaction would be given by the following differential equation (Li, 1994a, c):

$$\gamma_r = \gamma_{sl}^\circ + \frac{d(\Delta G_r)}{d\Omega_{sl}} dt \quad (\text{with } \Delta G_r < 0), \tag{8.10}$$

where γ_r is the dynamic interfacial energy at time t, γ_{sl}° is the initial interfacial energy for $t = 0$, and Ω_{sl} is the interfacial area.

If the formation of a new compound occurs at the interface, then the contribution of the change in interfacial energy ($\Delta\gamma_r$), resulting from the replacement of the initial solid–liquid interface with at least one new interface after reaction, has to be included in Equation (8.10), which becomes

$$\gamma_r = \gamma_{sl}^\circ + \frac{d(\Delta G_r)}{d\Omega_{sl}} dt - \Delta\gamma_r. \tag{8.11}$$

ADHESION TO CERAMICS

The surface of the oxides is constituted by large oxygen anions (Passarone, 1986). Metallic cations, of a smaller size, are shifted towards the bulk phase, this shift being a function of the reciprocal dimensions of the two species and of the polarisability of the cations. If the reaction occurring at the interface is:

$$M_y + M_xO \leftrightarrow M_yO + M_x \qquad (8.12)$$

and n' and n'' are the number of moles of the oxide M_xO and of M_y per unit surface area, then one contribution to the work of adhesion would come from the interactions of the liquid metal with the surface oxygen anions of the oxide

$$W_{ad_{chem}} = -RT/n' \ln\left(1 - \frac{\alpha^\circ}{n'}\right) + n'' \ln\left(1 - \frac{\alpha^\circ}{n''}\right), \qquad (8.13)$$

where α°, the degree of reaction at equilibrium, can be calculated from the value of the free energy of the reaction.

The other contribution would be that arising from physical interactions, which is given by Equation (8.14) for secondary van der Waals forces between, for example, carbides and Cu (Nicholas and Mortimer, 1985)

$$W_{ad_{phys}} \approx n \frac{3}{2} \frac{\alpha_M \alpha_C}{R^6} \frac{I_M I_C}{I_M + I_C}, \qquad (8.14)$$

where n is the bond density, α_M, α_C are the polarisations of the metal and carbon, respectively, I_M, I_c are the ionisation potentials of the metal and carbon, respectively, and R is the distance between atom centres.

The total adhesion work is given by the chemical and physical contributions

$$W_{ad} = W_{ad_{chem}} + W_{ad_{phys}}. \qquad (8.15)$$

The literature contains other fundamental studies on the dynamic wetting behaviour of reactive molten alloys on ceramic surfaces (Ambrose et al., 1993), the kinetics of wetting (Nicholas and Peteves, 1994), the kinetics of liquid braze spreading and the role of bandgap energy on wettability (Li, 1992a–d, 1993, 1994a, b; Li and Hausner, 1992).

It is also a common observation that the contact angle of active metal brazes on ceramic substrates decreases exponentially with time, as can be seen in Figure 8.4, in which the time dependence of the contact angle of several reactive systems is presented. This exponential decay can be described in terms of characteristic time for spreading (τ) by the following empirical equation

$$(\theta_t - \theta_\infty) = (\theta_0 - \theta_\infty)e^{-t/\tau}, \qquad (8.16)$$

where θ_0, θ_t and θ_∞ are the contact angles after times 0, t and ∞, respectively. For the example in Figure 8.4 values of τ vary between 0.7 and 17.7 min, being lower for titanium-rich brazes (Nicholas and Peteves, 1994).

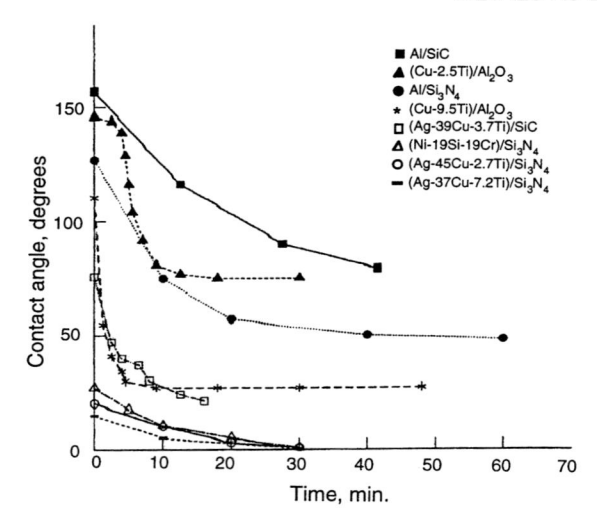

Figure 8.4 Influence of the ionicity on the wetting of carbides by copper (Pauling, 1949).

Another relatively low-melting (900–960°C) active brazing filler contains, in addition to titanium, zirconium and nickel. In the ternary system its composition appears in the neighbourhood of the eutectic ZrNi groove (Hegner *et al.*, 1994). Compared with the CuAg-based alloys, this brazing filler has an improved corrosion resistance and bonding strength. Both filler metals have the disadvantage that their

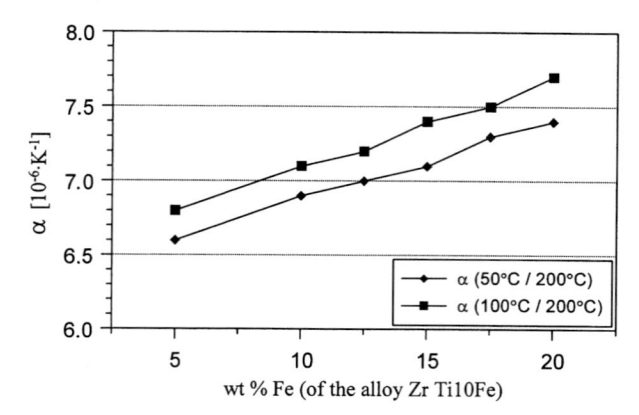

Figure 8.5 Influence of the iron content of an alloy ZrTi10FeX on the thermal expansion coefficient (Breme *et al.*, 1996).

ADHESION TO CERAMICS

thermal expansion coefficient is higher than that of the ceramic. Moreover, they both contain elements (Cu and Ni) which, from the point of view of biocompatibility, must be considered as critical elements. In a more recent development the nickel content in the ZrNi-based alloy is replaced by iron. This active brazing filler has the advantage of biocompatible behaviour. In addition, besides a low melting point which is comparable to that of ZrNi alloys, the thermal expansion coefficient can be adapted as a function of the iron content (Figure 8.5) to that of alumina (Breme *et al.*, 1996). When this ZrFeTi alloy is used, the bonding strength is so high that the fracture during testing of an Al_2O_3 bond occurs in the ceramic. These filler types can also be used for the bonding of other ceramics such as carbides and nitrides which can be even more easily reduced than oxides. This is the reason why aluminium, in addition to other active metals, is suitable for brazing nitrides and carbides (Iseki *et al.*, 1984; Suganuma *et al.*, 1985, 1987; Naka and Okamoto, 1989). A disadvantage of the presence of aluminium carbides, e.g. Al_4C_3, which are formed during brazing, is their extremely low corrosion resistance in water (Iseki *et al.*, 1984).

8.3 WELDING

8.3.1 DIFFUSION BONDING

Welding processes such as diffusion bonding are seen to be successfully carried out, i.e. with an optimum bonding strength, if after the procedure the distance between the joined parts amounts to the lattice distance a (about 10^{-8} cm). Compared with fusion welding procedures, diffusion bonding requires a relatively long time for completion. As shown schematically in Figure 8.6, it is carried out in two steps. During the first step a contact of the atoms must be made, with the aim of an approach in the region of the interaction (van der Waals bonding). During the second step, which guarantees the high bonding strength, an energetic interaction of the atoms must occur. For this purpose a creep of at least the metallic materials and an interdiffusion must take place. The diffusion bonding temperature therefore lies between the recrystallisation and melting temperature of the metal component in the range of 0.5–0.95 T_m, where T_m is the melting temperature of the metal. In addition to the welding temperature and time, the welding load plays an important role. All three parameters act together and complete each other, as can be seen schematically in Figure 8.7. At a given welding load the welding time can be decreased if the temperature is increased, owing to a higher creep rate and a better diffusivity. For the same reason, at a given welding temperature, the welding load can be diminished if the welding time is longer. Nevertheless, the welding temperature is of considerable importance. The plastic deformation of the metal caused by creep is not only sufficient to produce a full interfacial contact of the parts to be welded, but another mechanism, the vacancy diffusion in the metal along the interfaces, helps to cause the pores to disappear. The shrinkage of the pore volume is described by Equation (8.17)

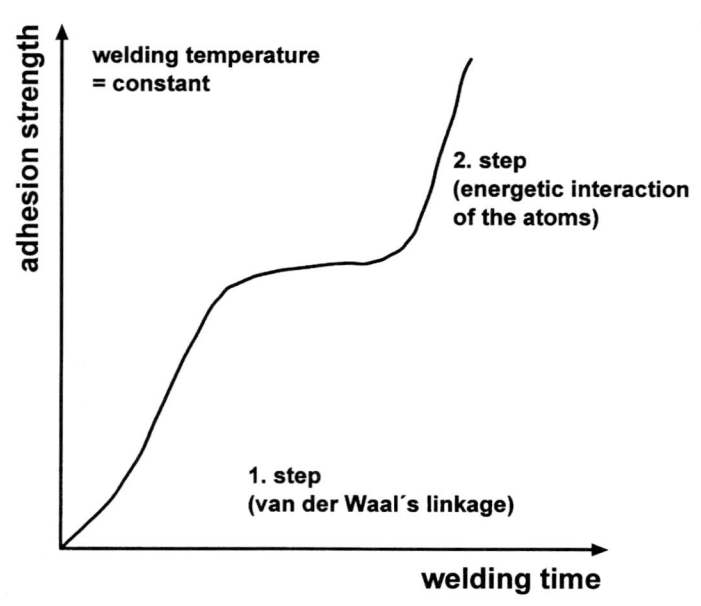

Figure 8.6 Influence of the welding time on the adhesion strength during pressure welding (schematic).

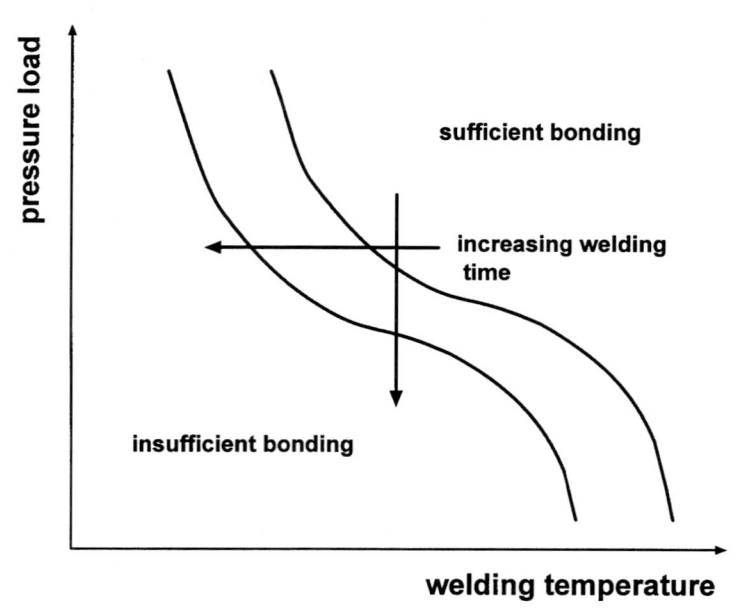

Figure 8.7 Interaction of the welding parameters (time, pressure and temperature) during pressure welding (schematic).

ADHESION TO CERAMICS

$$-\frac{dv}{dt} = 8\pi D\gamma_M \frac{\Omega}{kT} \tag{8.17}$$

where D is the coefficient of the vacancy diffusion, γ_M the surface energy of the metal, Ω the vacancy volume, k the Boltzmann constant and T the temperature (Elssner and Petzow, 1990). According to this equation the welding temperature should be as high as possible in order to guarantee a high diffusivity. However, a high temperature may produce an excessive formation of brittle interfacial layers if there is an active element present which reacts with the ceramic. Since this behaviour should be avoided, the welding temperature must be optimised for each bond. The bonding is normally performed in a controlled atmosphere (vacuum or inert gas). Since the working temperature is relatively high compared with active brazing, according to Equation (8.1), if there is a mismatch between the thermal expansion coefficients of the metal and the ceramic, the residual stresses will be high. Therefore, it may be important to use a ductile metal interlayer which can absorb the stresses by deformation, or a metal with an adapted expansion coefficient. Because of the dissimilar expansion coefficients, the method of the TiH_2 diffusion bonding of ceramics is only able to produce local bonding. During this process a slurry of hydride is introduced on to the ceramic parts to be welded. During drying and firing in a reduced vacuum the hydride decomposes and, supported by a pressure load, the diffusion bonding takes place together with a reduction of the ceramic by titanium (Bondley, 1947). It was shown that because of the misfit of the expansion coefficients of alumina and titanium during cooling after diffusion bonding, cracks occur in the edges of the welded couple (Gibbesch et al., 1992). The residual stresses at the metal–ceramic interface can be reduced by using titanium alloys containing tantalum and niobium (Breme and Wadewitz, 1989; Breme et al., 1989), which show biocompatible behaviour.

For applications such as dental implants, a bond between a titanium alloy and alumina is required to combine the advantages of the metallic material (adhesion to the bone, sufficient ductility under tensile stresses and a relatively low Young's modulus for good load transfer, stimulating new bone formation) with that of the ceramic (good contact to the gingiva in order to seal the implant post against bacteria from the oral cavity, and low plaque deposition).

This composite material, combining all of the advantages mentioned, can be formed by diffusion bonding. Initial welding tests with cp-Ti, Ti512.5Fe and several TiAl alloys showed that good weldability with alumina can be achieved. However, because of the thermal misfit between these titanium materials and Al_2O_3 during cooling, cracks were produced in the ceramic caused by tensile stresses. Therefore, it is necessary to adapt the high thermal expansion coefficient of the titanium by alloying to the lower coefficient of alumina in order to avoid the formation of cracks in the ceramic during cooling following the welding operation. Since only recognised biocompatible alloying elements should be used, tantalum and niobium were chosen, as they have relatively low thermal expansion coefficients.

The average thermal expansion coefficients of the TiTa and TiNb alloys in the

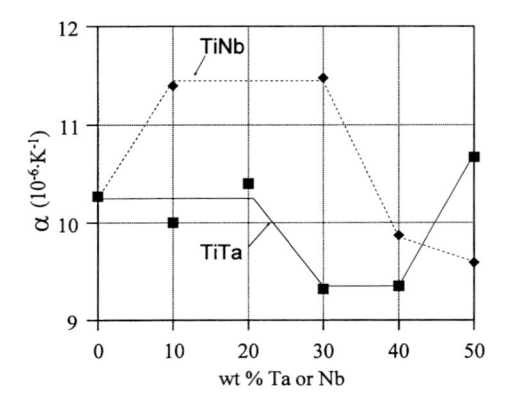

Figure 8.8 Average thermal expansion coefficient in the range of 200–1000°C of the TiTa and TiNb alloys studied (Breme and Wadewitz, 1989).

temperature range of 200–1000°C are shown in Figure 8.8. With TiTa alloys containing 30–40 wt% tantalum the thermal expansion coefficient is diminished towards the value of alumina. The increase to values of approximately 10.5×10^{-6} K^{-1} at 50 wt% tantalum is based on the occurrence of the athermal ω phase, which is connected with an increase in volume of approximately 3% (Jayaraman et al., 1963). For the TiNb alloys a decrease in the thermal expansion coefficient is observed only in those alloys with more than 40 wt%. In the binary system TiNb the athermal ω phase occurs at about 20 wt% (Collings, 1984). The influence of temperature on the thermal expansion coefficient of those alloys studied, compared with that of cp-Ti

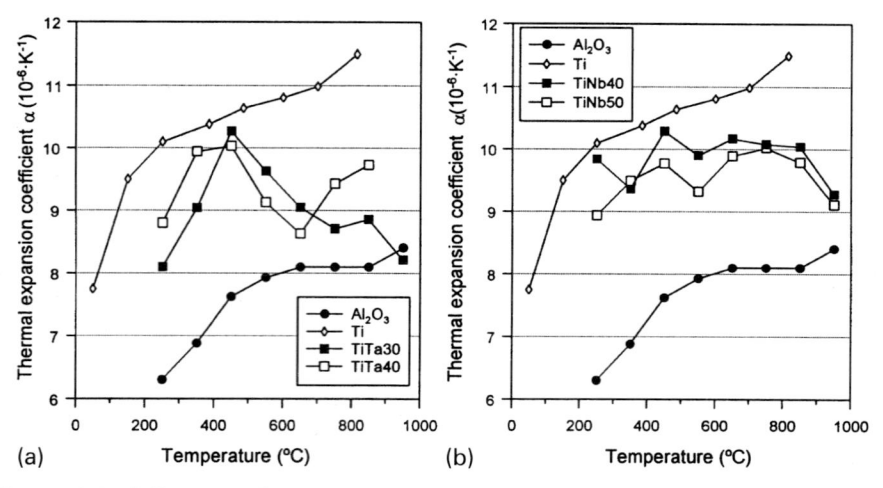

Figure 8.9 Influence of temperature on the thermal expansion coefficient of (a) TiTa and (b) TiNb40 and TiNb50 compared with cp-titanium and alumina (Breme and Wadewitz, 1989).

ADHESION TO CERAMICS

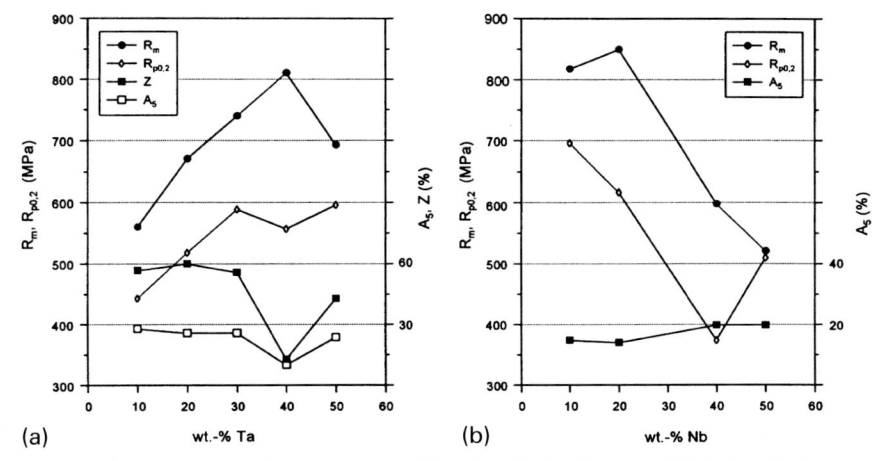

Figure 8.10 Mechanical properties of (a) the TiTa alloys and (b) the TiNb alloys. R_m, ultimate tensile strength; $R_{p0.2}$, yield strength; A_5, elongation at fracture (Breme and Wadewitz, 1989).

and an Al_2O_3 ceramic, is shown in Figures 8.9. It can be seen that alloying titanium with 30–40 wt% tantalum shifts the thermal expansion coefficient of the metal towards that of alumina in the whole temperature range of 200–1000°C.

The mechanical properties of the alloys studied are shown in Figure 8.10. For TiTa alloys the strength properties have their maximum values at 40 wt% tantalum. This effect is related to the increasing portion of the body-centred cubic β phase which generates a decrease in the grain size of the material. At 50 wt% tantalum the structure consists mainly of the β phase, whereby the grain size of the material becomes coarse and the tensile strength decreases. The minimum elongation at fracture (A_5) and the reduction in area (Z) at 40 wt% tantalum correspond to the start of precipitation of the athermal ω phase. The values of the rotating–bending fatigue strength increase with increasing tantalum content from 375 (Ti10Ta) to 425 N mm^{-2} (Ti40Ta).

The TiNb alloys have a maximum tensile strength at a niobium content of 20 wt%. The alloy Ti20Nb is comparable to the alloy Ti40Ta because the β stabilising effect of niobium is twice as high as that of tantalum. The minimum Young's modulus and the yield strength at 40 wt% niobium are probably caused by a martensitic transformation during the rolling operation carried out after forging at 750°C. The elongation at fracture increased slightly with increasing niobium content. Because of their superior mechanical properties, the TiTa alloys were chosen for the welding experiments which were performed in the temperature range of 1200–1300°C. Bonding between Ti30Ta and Al_2O_3 was possible without any crack formation.

A reduction of the thermal stresses is also obtained by using intermediate layers of niobium or tantalum between the ceramic and the metal to be welded. Niobium, in particular, shows a negligible deviation in its thermal expansion coefficient compared to that of alumina. In addition, the affinity of niobium to oxygen is extremely high, so that a reduction of Al_2O_3 appears, whereby both aluminium and oxygen will be dissolved in niobium (Gibbesch et al., 1992). Possibly because of this effect, the bonding strength between niobium and Al_2O_3 depends on the orientation of the interface planes and directions of the materials. From ultra-high vacuum welded pieces (1 h at 1300°C), produced from niobium and single sapphire crystals of different crystallographic orientations, four-point bending test specimens were cut and notched at the ceramic–metal interface, and the fracture energy G_c (Suga and Elssner, 1985) was measured. (110) Nb parallel to (11$\bar{2}$0) Al_2O_3 and [001] Nb parallel to [0001] Al_2O_3 welded samples showed with $G_c = 2330$ J m^{-2} the highest value, while (100) Nb parallel to (0001) Al_2O_3 and [001] Nb parallel to [11$\bar{2}$0] Al_2O_3 welded samples had the lowest value ($G_c = 68$ J mm^{-2}) (Gibbesch et al., 1989c). It is clear that the G_c values of bonded polycrystalline materials must lie within these limits.

Ti30Ta–Al_2O_3, Ti/Ta–Al_2O_3 and Ti/Nb–Al_2O_3 joints were vacuum welded (2×10^{-5} mbar) for 1 h in the temperature range of 900–1500°C under a pressure of 4 MPa. Figure 8.11 shows the results of the fracture energy G_c measured in the four-point bending test. The fracture energy of Ti30Ta–Al_2O_3 bonds depends on both the welding temperature and the thickness of the reaction layer formed. A G_c maximum is observed after bonding at 1300°C. For good adhesion a critical reaction layer is necessary (optimum at 1300°C). The layer thickness increases linearly as a function of the temperature from 2.5 μm at 1000°C to 12 μm at 1400°C. Since the reaction zone consists of the intermetallic compounds TiAl and Ti_3Al, which have a thermal expansion coefficient of about 10.5×10^{-6} K^{-1} (40% higher than that of Al_2O_3), high residual stresses arise. Compared with Ti30Ta the residual stresses in joints with intermediate layers of tantalum or niobium should be lower (Gibbesch et al., 1989a,b, 1992). The insertion of metal foils as intermediate layers between the metal and the ceramic parts prior to welding has proved to be a suitable tool for reducing the residual stresses and also for limiting excessive chemical reactions causing new phases such as brittle intermetallic compounds at the metal–ceramic interface, whereby the bonding strength can be improved. Metallic foils have also been

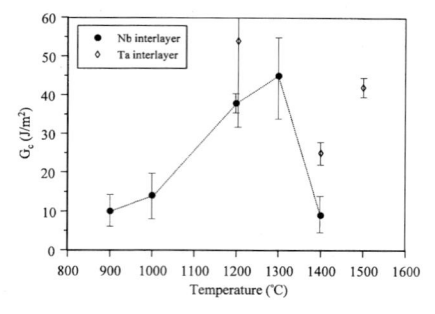

Figure 8.11 Fracture energy G_c of Ti30Ta–Al_2O_3 bonds as a function of the welding temperature (Gibbesch et al., 1992).

successfully used for welding other ceramics such as carbides and nitrides (Iino and Tagushi, 1988; Schiepers *et al.*, 1988; Gibbesch *et al.*, 1989a, c; Miura *et al.*, 1989; Gottselig *et al.*, 1989).

8.3.2 FUSION WELDING

Electron beam, laser and imaging arc welding techniques have been studied in order to evaluate their ability for metal–ceramic joining (Nicholas and Mortimer, 1985). Although some success was achieved (bond strengths up to 210 MPa were obtained) (Nicholas, 1990), the applicability of welding to ceramic–metal systems is very limited. For successful welding the melting points and thermal contraction characteristics of the materials to be joined should be closely matched. In addition, the thermal contraction characteristics of the material formed in the welding pool must match those of the pieces to be joined. Additional problems may arise if the ceramics sublime or decompose instead of melting, or if solid-state phase transformations occur in either material.

Studies on the systems Mo–Al_2O_3, Nb–Al_2O_3, W–Al_2O_3, FeNiCo–Al_2O_3 (Nicholas and Mortimer, 1985), Ta–Al_2O_3 Mo–ZrO_2, Nb–ZrO_2 and Ta–ZrO_2 (Nicholas, 1990) are reported in the literature.

8.4 SURFACE COATING

Surface coating is performed for many different applications and functions. Tailored composite materials consisting of a structural metallic and a functional ceramic component are often developed for special uses. In these cases the metallic part is covered by a ceramic layer which improves the metallic properties (e.g. corrosion or fretting resistance), or provides specific biological properties (e.g. an acceleration of bone adhesion by means of hydroxyapatite coatings or antithrombogenic layers of amorphous SiC) or physical properties (e.g. increased electrical conductivity by means of TiN layers on heart pacemaker leads). For the surface coating produced by the different layers, various procedures are applied, e.g. plasma spraying, physical (PVD) or chemical vapour deposition (CVD) and ion implantation. As in brazing and welding, a high bonding strength of the layer to the substrate is required. In addition to their functionality, the coatings must provide a complete density. If, for example, a corrosion-resistant surface layer consisting of a ceramic on a metallic implant is damaged by cracks or fissures, the beneficial behaviour of the coating will be reversed because the current density of the metallic material will be multiplied owing to the small surface area set free by the fissure. Considering these facts and the most important requirement of biocompatibility being absolutely necessary, the following subsections discuss examples of the coating of metals with hydroxyapatite, wear-resistant ceramics and ceramics with high electrical conductivity.

8.4.1 TITANIUM–HYDROXYAPATITE COMPOSITES

Implants consisting of titanium materials possess an adhesion with a high shear strength to the bone. This adhesion has a mainly mechanical character because the bone grows in close contact with the implant and penetrates cavities and grooves on the implant surface (Schmitz et al., 1987), owing to the inert behaviour of the titanium materials caused by the constant presence of an oxide layer, which has an isolating effect because of its high dielectric constant ($\varepsilon = 78$) corresponding to that of water. Because of this fact and in order to provide a high shear strength between the bone and the implant during the healing period, any perceptible relative implant–bone motion must be avoided (Pilliar et al., 1986). Therefore, during this period, which takes about 100 days (Eulenberger et al., 1983), implants such as hip prostheses should be loaded only to a slight degree.

By the use of hydroxyapatite, with its osteoconductive properties, the healing period can be decreased to about 20 days and the bone is able to bridge the gap to the implant by the formation of a chemical bonding to the hydroxyapatite. The favourable behaviour of hydroxyapatite has been verified in many medical investigations, including *in vivo* and *in vitro* experiments, as well as studies of components retrieved during autopsy (Bauer et al., 1991; Frayssinet et al., 1992, 1993; Hardy et al., 1994; Moroni et al., 1994; Block and Kent, 1994; Marinoni et al., 1995). Since hydroxyapatite has inadequate mechanical properties, it is only of advantage if it is used as a coating for a composite material based on a metallic material, i.e. a titanium alloy. The problem of the implant anchorage is thus shifted to the metal–ceramic interface.

Various procedures for the coating of metallic materials with hydroxyapatite have been studied. In addition to plasma spraying, which until now has been the only process that has found industrial application, ion implantation and electrophoretic deposition have been investigated. For ion implantation the target consisted of a disc which was hot pressed and sintered at 1150°C. Prior to sputtering fluoroapatite powders were applied to the surface of the target disc. The deposition was performed in a vacuum chamber after sputter cleaning of the titanium substrate with argon of 99.999% purity. The sputter process itself was accomplished under a presssure of 4×10^{-4} Torr and with an energy of 1000 eV and 41 mA. The sputter rate was 0.15 μm h^{-1} (Ong et al., 1992; Ong and Lucas, 1994). Electrophoretic deposition has been performed from a 3% suspension powder in isopropanol. The cathodic substrate of Ti6Al4V and porous titanium were at a distance of about 10 mm from the lead anode. The electrical field amounted to 100 V cm^{-1} for a deposition time of 10–600 s (Ducheyne et al., 1990). In order to achieve an optimum bonding strength to the substrate by chemical bonding for all deposition procedures including plasma spraying, subsequent annealing was carried out in the temperature range of 40–1100°C (Ducheyne et al., 1990; Ong et al., 1992; Filiaggi et al., 1993; Ji and Marquis, 1993; Ong and Lucas, 1994). The bonding strength measured in various investigations revealed a large scatter, depending on the testing method, the Ca:P ratio of hydroxyapatite, exposure of the sample to humidity (e.g. sodium chloride solution) and whether the test was performed with *in vivo* or *in vitro* samples or

ADHESION TO CERAMICS

whether interlayers (e.g. bioglass) were used. The most critical testing method seems to be the pull-off test. For this *in vivo* test the end faces of cylinders (diameter 5 mm) were coated with hydroxyapatite of variable composition and roughness by plasma spraying. The cylinder was encased in a plastic ring so that only the coated area came into contact with the animal bone. The contact was made by a surgical tightening of the implant with a surgical wire inserted through a drill hole in the metallic material against the flattened bone. After a defined exposure time of 12 and 24 weeks, respectively, the bone was pulled off the implant. Fracture always occurred between the coating and the substrate (Kangasniemi *et al.*, 1994). After an implantation period of 4 weeks, Ti6Al4V and CoCrMo samples with a smooth polished surface, which had been plasma coated without subsequent annealing, showed in the push-out test a shear strength amounting to only 0.4 and 0.3 MPa, respectively (Nimb *et al.*, 1993). After 24 weeks polished hydroxyapatite had a higher tensile strength (1.86 MPa) than hydroxyapatite with a surface roughness of about 10 µm (1.17 MPa). The tensile strength of uncoated titanium after the same period was not measurable (Kangasniemi *et al.*, 1994).

In other investigations the Ca:P ratio was varied using pure hydroxyapatite, tetracalcium (TETRA) and tricalcium phosphate (TCP) as a plasma-sprayed coating on Ti6Al4V. The roughness of the coatings amounted to 11–12 µm, while the roughness of a control sample of uncoated Ti was only about 4 µm. Figure 8.12 shows the influence on the shear strength of the exposure time after implantation in

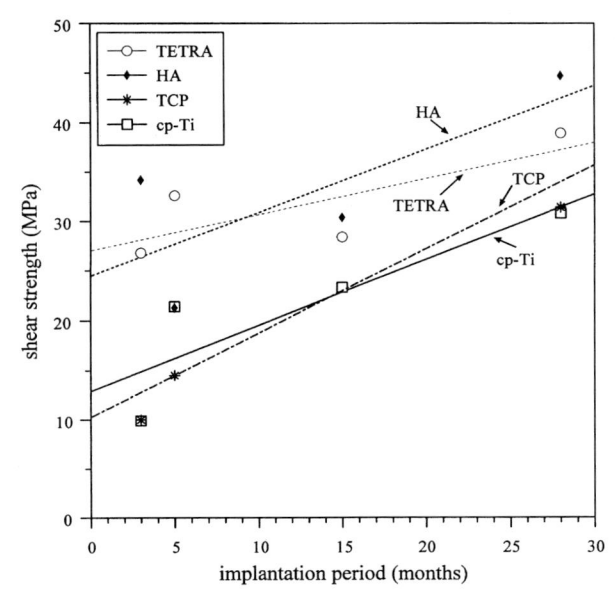

Figure 8.12 Shear strength of hydroxyapatite with different compositions to the bone as a function of the implantation period (Klein *et al.*, 1994).

the legs of dogs. The highest shear strength was achieved with pure hydroxyapatite (Klein *et al.*, 1991, 1994).

The influence of humidity (>95% and 30% at room temperature) on the bonding strength of plasma-sprayed hydroxyapatite to Ti6Al4V was tested and compared with bioglass and bioglass coating. The bioglass had a composition of SiO_2, CaO, P_2O_5 and Na_2O in a ratio of 10:5:2:3. Figure 8.13 shows the results. In a humidity of >95% and after an exposure time of 30 days the bioglass–hydroxyapatite layer shows the highest bonding strength (Chern Lin *et al.*, 1993).

The structure of hydroxyapatite also has an influence on the solubility in a solution. With hydroxyapatite sputtered on titanium the amorphous structure has a higher solubility than the crystalline structure (Ong *et al.*, 1992). By comparison, an extended interlayer of TiO_2 between the titanium substrate and hydroxyapatite has a negative influence on the bonding strength. This was shown by the coating rate after diffusion annealing of an ion-beam-sputtered hydroxyapatite layer. Furnace cooling leading to a relatively thick TiO_2 layer, compared with water quenching, produced a comparatively lower bonding strength (Ong *et al.*, 1992). Subsequent annealing and cooling cause predamage by cracks or fissures in the layer, as shown in many investigations (Filiaggi *et al.*, 1991; Ong *et al.*, 1992; Ji and Marquis, 1993; Ong and Lucas, 1994). Among the various factors mentioned above, these cracks may be the reason for the large scattering in the measured bonding strengths. Despite annealing after plasma spraying of hydroxyapatite on the surface of Ti6Al4V samples, the

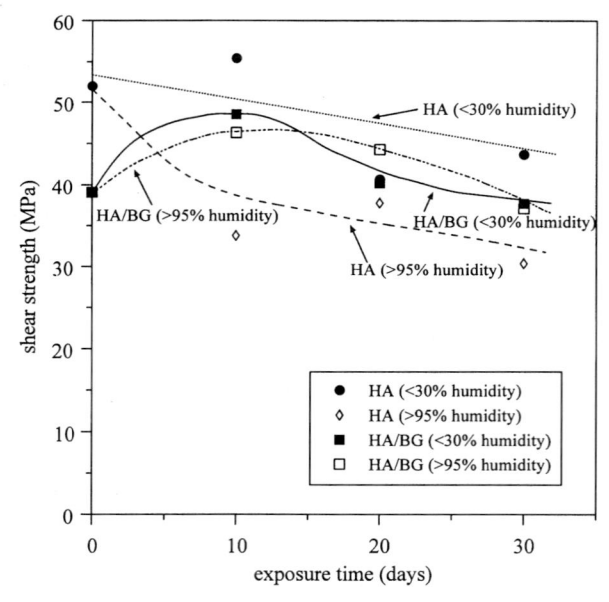

Figure 8.13 Influence of humidity on the shear strength of hydroxyapatite to Ti6Al4V (Chern Lin *et al.*, 1993).

fracture toughness values K_{IC} measured for the coated material were extremely low, about 1–5 MPa m$^{1/2}$ (Ong et al., 1992; Filiaggi et al., 1993). Similar results were obtained when the bonding strength was tested. In the as-sprayed condition the bonding strength was extremely low (6.7 MPa) compared with the strength (>50.2 MPa) of samples heat treated after plasma spraying (24 h at 960°C), which were tested immediately after the annealing operation. After exposing the coated samples for a period of 14 days, followed by heat treatment to normal laboratory atmosphere, the bonding strength amounted to only 22.1 MPa. This effect was explained by a delamination because of moisture (Filiaggi et al., 1993) and can also explain other phenomena. The release of metal ions observed in Hanks solution, especially of Al ions with a Ti6Al4V sample coated with hydroxyapatite (Ducheyne et al., 1992), may have its source in the predamaged coating. Because of the small metal surface in a crack, in combination with a drop in the pH value, metal ions can be more easily set free. Also, the increased solution observed for hydroxyapatite itself can be caused for the same reason (Ducheyne et al., 1990). By the use of characterisation methods such as Auger, ESCA and scanning electron microscopy, it was shown that the chemical bonding produced by annealing at higher temperatures is achieved by the diffusion of phosphorous from hydroxyapatite in the titanium lattice, whereby the intermetallic compound Ti$_3$P can be formed (Ji and Marquis, 1993). Owing to this effect the Ca:P ratio of hydroxyapatite is changed, with a resulting increase in solubility. Because of the cracks the saline solution has access to the phosphorous depleted hydroxyapatite.

The difficulty of the production of a dense of hydroxyapatite coating on titanium arises from the thermal expansion coefficient α of titanium, which amounts to only 60% of that of hydroxyapatite.

Therefore, in order to overcome this problem causing predamage to the ceramic after diffusion bonding, the aim was to develop a corrosion-resistant biocompatible titanium alloy with adequate mechanical properties (similar to those of standard alloys) and a thermal expansion coefficient adapted to that of hydroxyapatite. However, in accordance with theoretical considerations, the hydroxyapatite coating layer should be as thin as possible because, in the case of implants such as hip prostheses, which are loaded by bending, the maximum bending strength (tension) is found on the lateral side in the surface fibre which consists of the hydroxyapatite ceramic. Therefore, thick hydroxyapatite layers in particular risk being damaged.

Manganese has an extremely high thermal expansion coefficient compared with titanium ($\alpha = 22 \times 10^{-6}$ K^{-1} and $\alpha = 8.4 \times 10^{-6}$ K^{-1}, respectively, between 20 and 100°C) and like Fe, it is an important trace element in the human organism (Geldmacher et al., 1984). Therefore, it has been chosen as an alloying element in order to adapt the expansion coefficient of titanium to that of hydroxyapatite. Alloys with varying contents of manganese (2–8 wt%) were produced by melting from cp-Ti grade 1 and manganese of 99.99% purity in an electric arc furnace in an argon atmosphere (pressure ≈ 600 mbar). Before hot deformation the cigar-shaped samples, weighing about 200 g, were homogenised in a vacuum for 4 h at 1000°C. Hot deformation of about 80% was performed with grooved rolls at 750°C in the $\alpha + \beta$

Table 8.3 Mechanical properties of TiMn(Al) alloys, as-rolled and aged

	Yield strength (N mm^{-2})	Tensile strength (N mm^{-2})	Elongation at fracture (%)	Reduction in area (%)
Ti5Mn	835	919	14	18
Ti5Mn1Al	834	960	13	11
Ti5Mn3Al	960	1052	6	3
Ti6Mn	1019	1072	10	12
Ti6Mn1Al	1109	1130	3	2
Ti6Mn3Al	1132	1177	3	2
Ti8Mn[a]	827	1000	15	24

[a] As-rolled, not aged.

phase field. The bulk material was used for the investigation of the microstructure, mechanical properties and corrosion behaviour, and for the performance of the coating tests. The thermal expansion coefficient was determined with a dilatometer in a temperature range of 20–950°C and compared with that of cp-Ti and hydroxyapatite.

The mechanical properties of the various alloys are summarised in Table 8.3 as a function of the manganese content. The strength properties increased directly in proportion to the manganese content, while the elongation at fracture and the reduc-

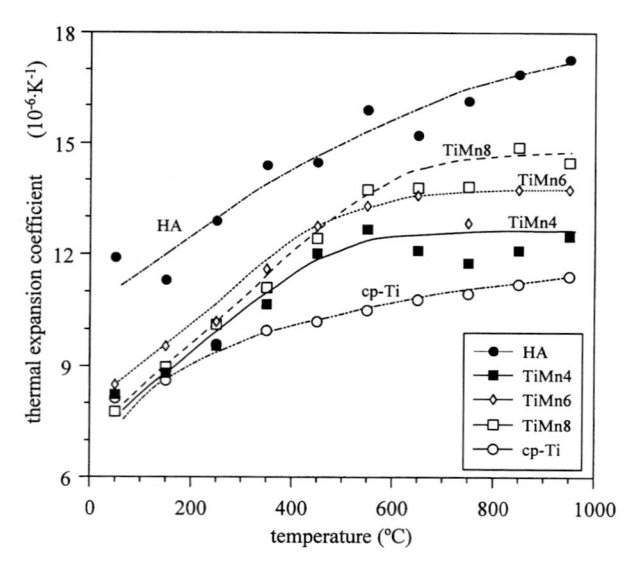

Figure 8.14 Thermal coefficient of TiMn alloys compared with those of cp-titanium and hydroxyapatite. (●) titanium, (◇) Ti4Mn, (■) Ti6Mn, Ti8Mn, (+) hydroxyapatite (Breme et al., 1995a).

ADHESION TO CERAMICS

tion in area were diminished. Figure 8.14 gives the results of the measurement of the thermal expansion coefficient of the various alloys compared with the coefficients of cp-Ti and hydroxyapatite. With increasing manganese content the misfit between titanium and hydroxyapatite is reduced. For a content of 6% manganese the difference between the metallic alloys and the ceramic is less than 20%.

Since the alloy Ti6Mn proved to have satisfactory mechanical properties, including sufficient ductility, together with a thermal expansion coefficient similar to that of hydroxyapatite and a corrosion-resistant and biocompatible behaviour, this alloy was selected for coating tests with hydroxyapatite (Breme et al., 1995b).

In order to produce the thin coating layers of hydroxyapatite on the titanium materials two methods were studied. The first method was a direct sintering of hydroxyapatite on the surface of the titanium samples with and without a bonding agent. The bonding agent consisted of a suspension containing 10% phosphoric acid (1 ml), butyl alcohol (9 ml) and hydroxyapatite. The dip-coated suspension was dried at room temperature and at 60°C (15 min) and burnt in at 600°C (15 min). Finally, the hydroxyapatite layer was produced by annealing commercially pure hydroxyapatite together with the bonding agent at 1200°C (Breme and Groh, 1993).

The second coating method consisted of a sol-gel procedure as shown schematically in Figure 8.15. The starting materials were a solution of CaO and an organic compound, either triethylphospate, $PO(OC_2H_5)_3$, or trimethylphosphate, $PO(OCH_3)_3$. The samples were dip coated with a mixture of the starting materials.

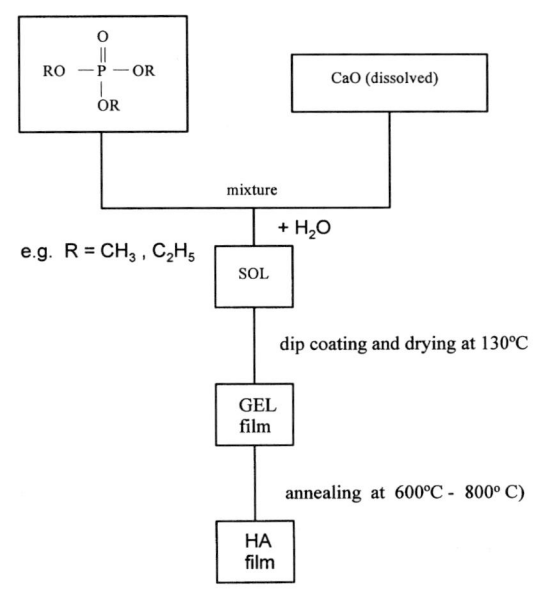

Figure 8.15 Schematic representation of the production of hydroxyapatite by the sol-gel process (Breme and Zhou, 1994).

The dip coating was followed by drying for 1 h at 130°C, leading to the production of a gel. Finally, by annealing at 600–800°C (5–15 min) the coating was developed. With both methods cylindrical samples were coated so that traction adhesive strength tests could be performed. The resulting hydroxyapatite coatings were characterised by X-ray studies.

Figures 8.16 and 8.17 show scanning electron micrographs (SEM) of samples of cp-Ti and of Ti6Mn which were coated with hydroxyapatite at 1200°C using a bonding agent and cp-hydroxyapatite. In the case of the hydroxyapatite layer on cp-Ti (Figure 8.16) many cracks were observed owing to the high misfit in the thermal expansion coefficient of the metal and the ceramic, whereas the layer on the Ti6Mn alloy was practically free of cracks (Figure 8.17). Consequently, there is a significant difference in the shear stress of the two coatings (Table 8.4). The shear strength of the hydroxyapatite layer on TiMn6 was about twice as high as that of the layer on cp-Ti.

Figure 8.18 shows line scans of the various elements over the diffusion metal–ceramic interface after annealing at 1200°C. A diffusion zone of about 10 μm thickness was formed, especially in the case of the diffusion of calcium and phosphorous into the metallic material. Owing to a smaller atomic radius the diffusion distance of phosphorous is greater than that of calcium. The layer itself has a thickness of about 50 μm (Breme and Zhou, 1994).

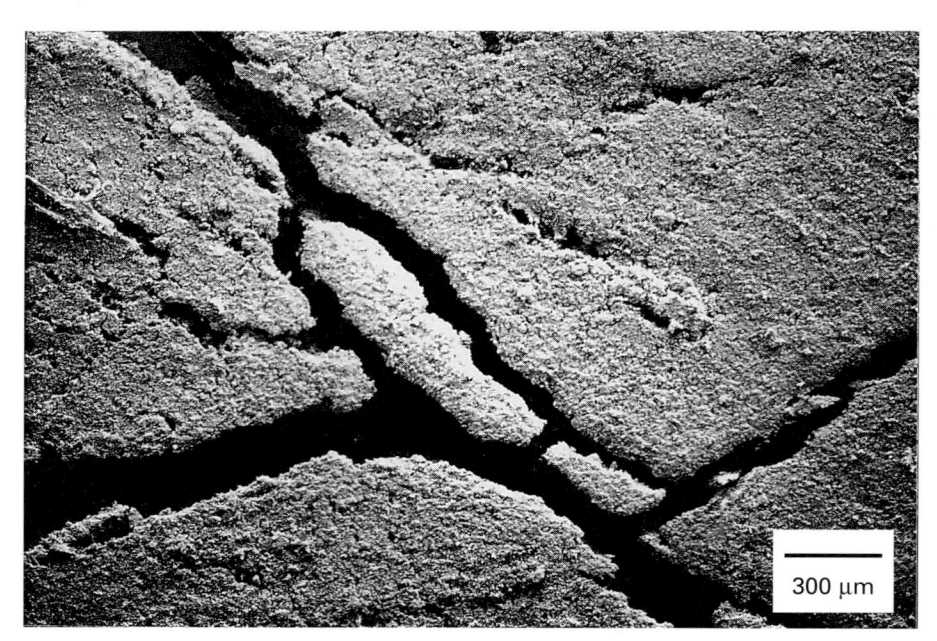

Figure 8.16 SEM of a hydroxyapatite coating on cp-titanium produced by annealing together with a bonding agent at 1200°C (Breme and Zhou, 1994).

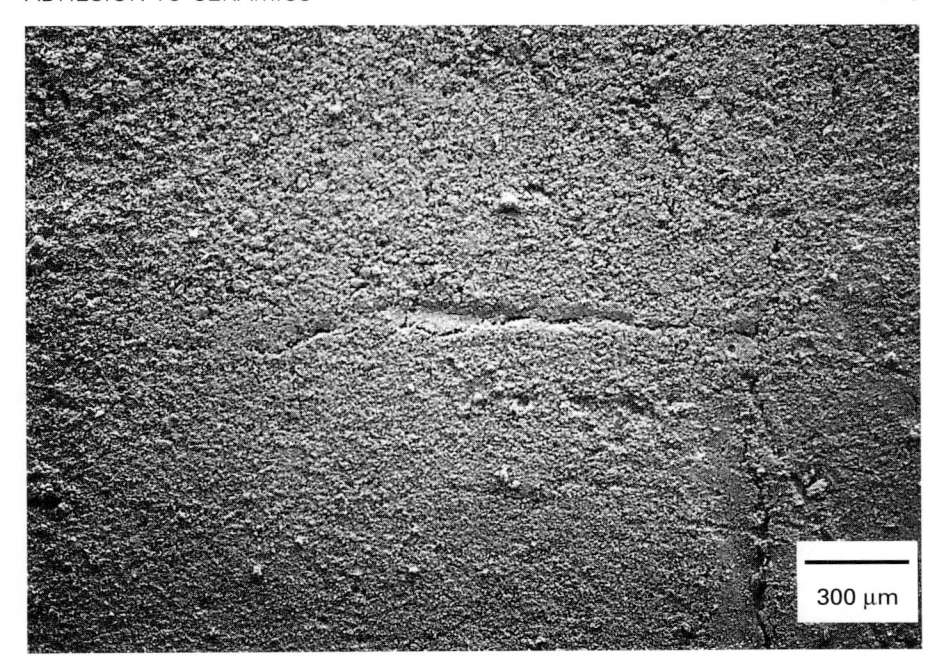

Figure 8.17 SEM of a hydroxyapatite coating on Ti6Mn produced by annealing together with a bonding agent at 1200°C (Breme and Zhou, 1994)

Extremely thin coatings of hydroxyapatite with a thickness of about 1 µm were produced using the sol-gel method. Hydroxyapatite powders developed from CaO and $PO(OC_2H_5)_3$ by annealing at 600°C and 800°C, respectively, were characterised. By means of X-ray diffraction investigations of the hydroxyapatite powder produced by annealing at 600°C and 800°C it was possible to observe the diffraction pattern of pure hydroxyapatite according to ASTM-JCPS 9-432 (Figure 8.19). The only difference was in the crystallinity. The hydroxyapatite produced at 600°C was seen to be more amorphous than the material produced at 800°C. From the (002), (211),

Table 8.4 Shear strength ($N\ mm^{-2}$) of hydroxyapatite coatings produced by annealing at 1200°C and by annealing using a bonding agent and cp-hydroxyapatite

	cp-Ti	TiMn6
One HA layer	9.7	18.8
Two HA layers	10.2	21.5

HA, hydroxyapatite.

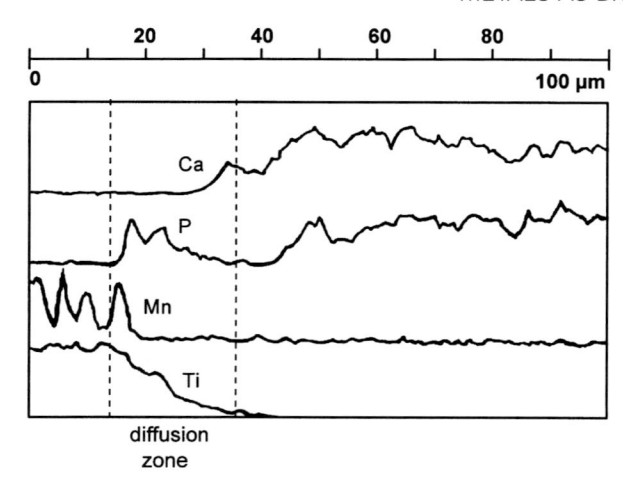

Figure 8.18 Line-scans of the diffusion zone at the Ti6Mn–hydroxyapatite interface (Breme and Zhou, 1994).

(112), (300), (222) and (213) reflexes the lattice parameters of hydroxyapatite (800°C) were calculated to be $a = 9.423$ Å and $c = 6.884$ Å. The average grain size of this powder amounted to about 36 nm. An X-ray diffraction diagram of the coating at 800°C on the Ti6Mn alloy shows, in addition to the hydroxyapatite peaks, peaks of Ti and TiO_2 (Figure 8.20).

The investigation of the traction adhesive strength of the layers produced at 600 and 800°C showed that no real value could be determined because the rupture

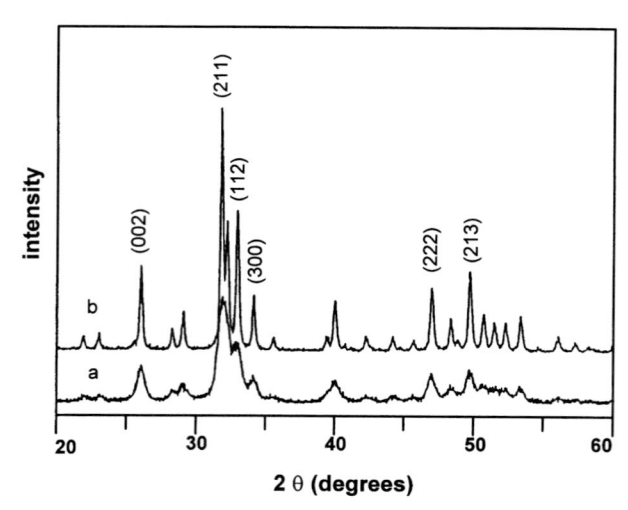

Figure 8.19 X-ray diffraction of hydroxyapatite powder produced by the sol-gel method at (a) 600°C and (b) 800°C (Breme et al., 1995b).

ADHESION TO CERAMICS

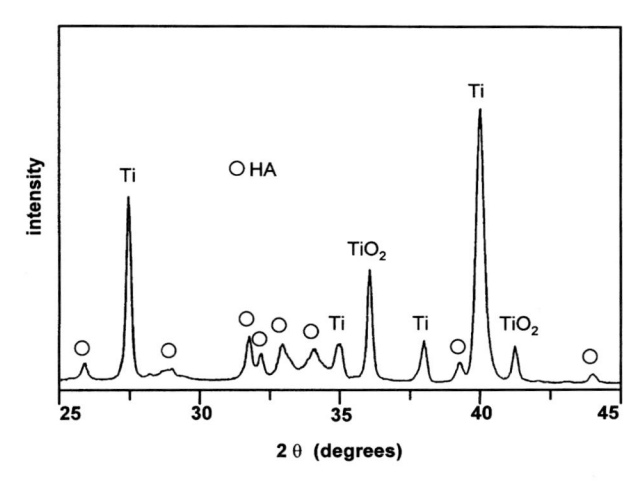

Figure 8.20 X-ray diffraction of a composite material Ti6Mn–hydroxyapatite produced by the sol-gel method at 800°C (Breme et al., 1995b).

always occurred in the glue. Since the tensile strength of the applied glue was indicated and also measured to be about 70 N mm^{-2}, the value of the adhesion strength of hydroxyapatite applied by the sol-gel process to the TiMn6 alloy must be even higher than 70 N mm^{-2} (Table 8.5) (Breme and Zhou, 1994; Breme et al., 1995a, b; Breme, 1996).

A further advantage of the sol-gel method is the possibility of changing the Ca:P ratio within close limits. The interaction of hydroxyapatite with differing calcium contents and with cells was studied in proliferation tests. After γ sterilisation of titanium samples coated with different Ca:P ratios, L132 cells were cultured on the surface of these samples. After an exposure time of 72 h the survival rate of the cells was determined by counting and then comparing the result with a standard sample

Table 8.5 Adhesion strength of hydroxyapatite to Ti6Mn as produced by the sol-gel procedure

Depth (μm)	Sol and average roughness viscosity (Pa s)	Heat treatment (min)	(°C)	Adhesion strength (N mm^{-2})	Fracture
0.043	TMeP^a 0.0035	30	400	>70	In the glue
		15	600		
		5	800		
	TBuP^b 0.0047	30	400	>70	In the glue
	TBuP 0.0071	30	400	35^{+3}_{-4}	In the interlayer
		15	600	>70	In the glue
		5	800		
0.097		30	400	41^{+1}_{-3}	In the interlayer

^{a}Trimethyl PO(OCH$_3$)$_3$; ^{b}tributyl PO(OC$_4$H$_9$)$_3$.

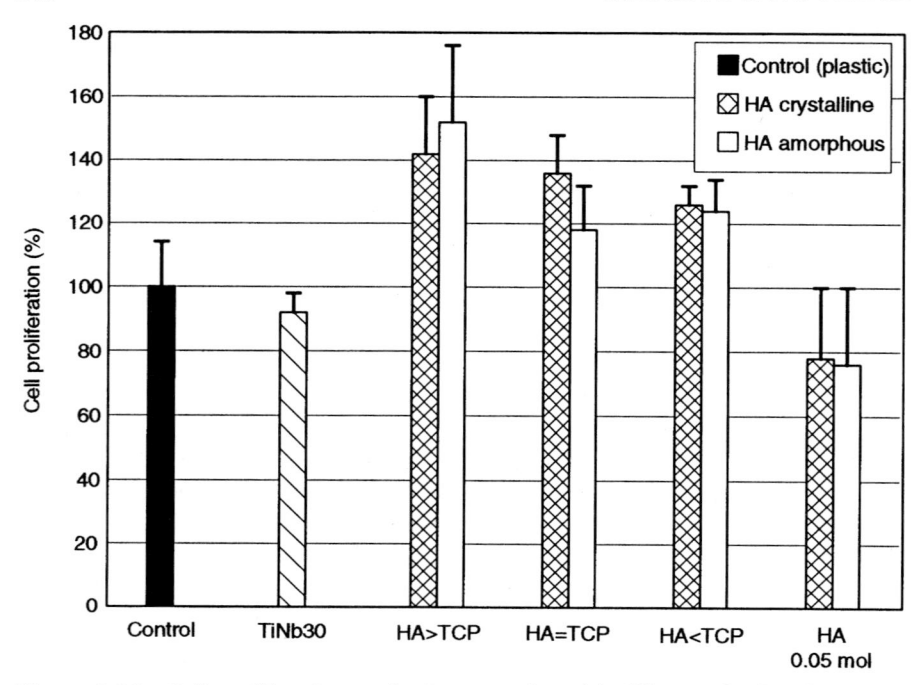

Figure 8.21 Cell proliferation on hydroxyapatite with different Ca:P ratios.

of polysterene. The percentage of proliferation was calculated as the ratio to the number of initially cultured cells on polysterene. Figure 8.21 shows the proliferation on the different coatings. There is no significant difference between the crystalline and amorphous coatings. Nevertheless, a certain content of tricalcium phosphate seems to stimulate the proliferation of the cells (Floquet et al., 1997).

8.4.2 TITANIUM–CERAMIC COATINGS WITH SPECIAL PHYSICAL AND BIOLOGICAL PROPERTIES

For artificial stimulation of the heart an electric field is required which is determined by the electrical potential and current of the pacing electrode. Inside the electrode the current is carried by electron mobility, whereas outside a flux of ions is the main contributor to the current distribution. The coupling takes place at the electrode surface predominantly by the formation of an electrical double layer. The properties of the electrode–tissue interface are of major importance for the pacing leads as they must serve two main functions: (1) to conduct the electrical pulses from the pacemaker to the heart, and (2) to sense intracardiac signals and transmit them to the pulse generator. Pacing and sensing performance may be improved by adjusting the electrochemical and physical parameters to the interface without disturbing the biological equilibrium. For long-term stability it is essential to avoid chemical

ADHESION TO CERAMICS

reactions that decrease irreversibly the signal amplitude and increase the threshold. The behaviour of the phase boundary can be explained by the structure of the double layer. A simplified equivalent circuit of the electrode–myocardium interface demonstrates that the potential distribution is determined by the Helmholtz capacity and the Faraday impedance. If the double-layer capacity is large, the pacing losses will be low and the amplitudes of the depolarisation signals will be high. This behaviour explains in general the advantage of porous over smooth electrode surfaces (Schaldach et al., 1989). The surface influence of the double-layer capacity can be described qualitatively by the relation

$$C = \varepsilon\varepsilon_0 \frac{A}{d}, \qquad (8.18)$$

where C is the capacity, ε is the dielectric constant of the electrolyte, ε_0 is the dielectric constant of the vacuum, A is the surface area and d is the thickness of the layer. It is therefore clear that an increase in the surface A causes the observed favourable behaviour of porous titanium electrodes. TiN-Thornton surface layers produced by PVD or CVD are able to improve the electrical conductivity of the electrode surface (Table 8.6). TiN is also known to have a biocompatibility similar to that of TiO_2.

According to these considerations porous-sintered electrodes of titanium materials with a TiN surface layer can have the following advantages:

- safe fixation to the myocardium owing to a possible ingrowth of the tissue
- long-term stability of the electrode owing to the well-known corrosion resistance and biocompatibility of titanium materials
- relatively high electrical conductivity owing to a TiN surface layer
- high capacity and therefore lower losses and a longer battery lifetime.

For the sintering of the hemispherical shape of the electrode tip, which is shown schematically in Figure 8.22, powder of the alloy Ti5Al2.5Fe was used. The pulverisation was accomplished by HDH. Bulk material was treated with pure hydrogen under a pressure of 1.6 bar at 750°C. Owing to the pick-up of the gas the material was embrittled and could be reduced to powder. After screening and separating a grain size fraction of 40–60 μm the electrodes were sintered in an argon

Table 8.6 Electrical resistance of various coating materials

Material	Specific electrical resistance ρ (μΩ cm)
Ti	41.8
TiO_2	10^{16}
Ir	5.3
IrO_2	49
TiB_2	14.4
TiN	25

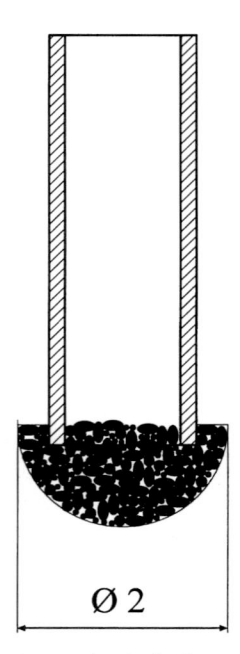

Figure 8.22 Porous-sintered electrode tip (schematic).

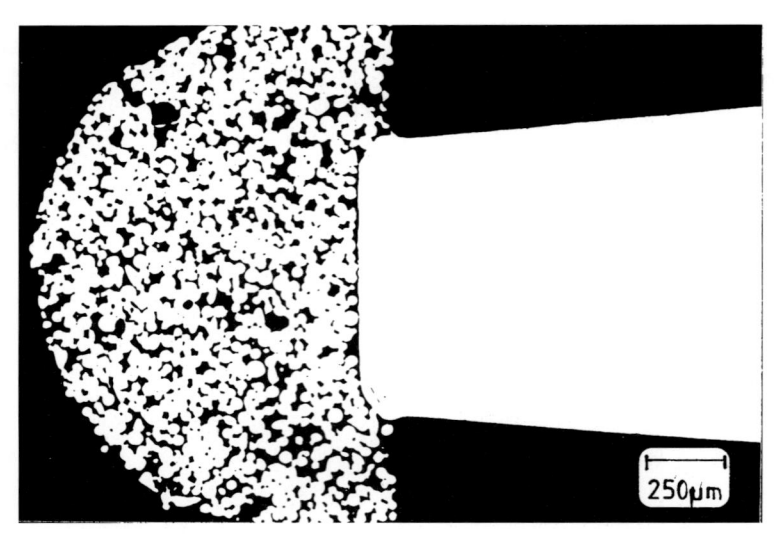

Figure 8.23 Cross-section of a porous-sintered electrode tip (Schaldach and Breme, 1990).

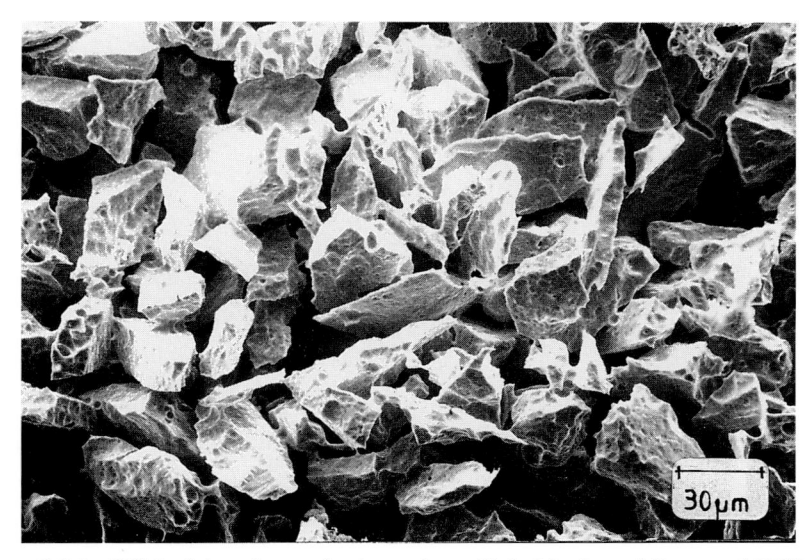

Figure 8.24 SEM of the electrode tip surface (Schaldach and Breme, 1990).

atmosphere at 950°C. Simultaneously with the sintering operation, a contact supplying tube of commercially pure titanium was diffusion bonded to the head of the electrode tip. The temperature of 950°C was chosen in order to guarantee sufficient bonding strength of the tube to the head and the highest possible porosity. Figure 8.23 shows a cross-section of such an electrode prepared by grinding and polishing. The average porosity amounted to about 70% and the pore size to about

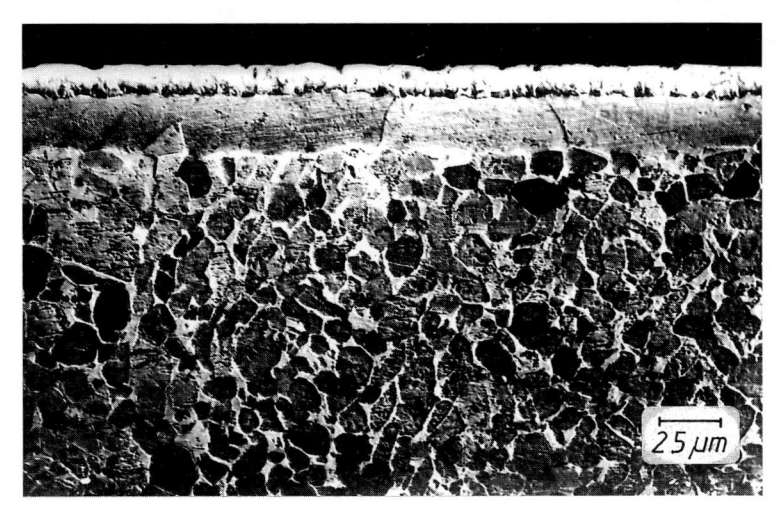

Figure 8.25 Sample of Ti5Al2.5Fe nitrided for 76 h at 900°C (Schaldach and Breme, 1990).

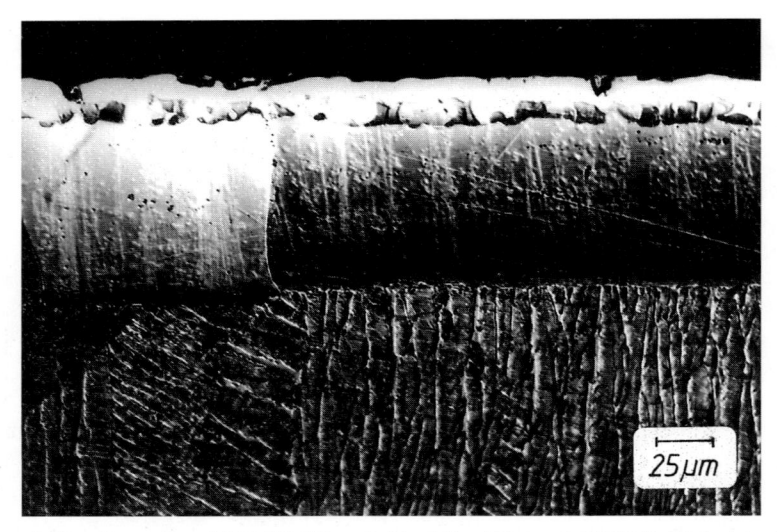

Figure 8.26 Sample of Ti5Al2.5Fe nitrided for 76 h at 1000°C (Schaldach and Breme, 1990).

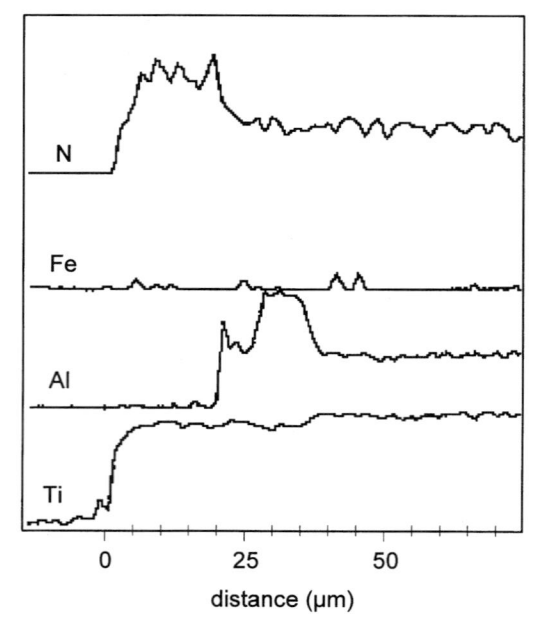

Figure 8.27 Electron microprobe analysis (wavelength dispersive) of the layers, element distribution (Schaldach and Breme, 1990).

ADHESION TO CERAMICS

50 μm, as can be seen in Figure 8.24, which shows the surface of the electrode by means of scanning electron microscopy.

Thermal nitriding was performed at 900–1000°C for periods between 1 and 76 h with bulk material in order to investigate the optimum gas nitriding parameters. Figures 8.25 and 8.26 show two examples of the microstructure of samples nitrided for 76 h at 900 and 1000°C, respectively. Figure 8.27 shows the line-scan of the element distribution measured by wavelength dispersive electron microprobe analysis. Except for the thickness of the different layers and the microstructure of the bulk matrix material, which had, after annealing at 900°C, an ($\alpha + \beta$) structure and, after annealing at 1000°C, a β structure, no differences in the structure of the various layers could be observed. The third film, about 50 μm thick (sample of 900°C), consists of the α phase of titanium which is stabilised by nitrogen. In this layer the iron content is extremely low. Figure 8.28 shows the different layer thicknesses of Ti5Al2.5Fe samples as a function of the annealing temperature and time compared with samples of commercially pure titanium. The increase in thickness follows a characteristic parabolic time law. Ti5Al2.5Fe shows a behaviour similar to commercially pure titanium. In addition, porous-sintered electrodes were nitrided by PVD.

Figure 8.29 shows the results of the impedance measurement as a function of the frequency and the calculated capacities of various thermally nitrided and PVD coated porous electrode tips compared with non-porous and non-nitrided electrodes. The non-porous solid electrode tips showed, as expected, a lower capacity than the porous-sintered tips. By means of surface nitriding it was possible to decrease the impedance because of the superior electrical conductivity over that of the non-nitrided electrodes, where the surface consisted of an oxide layer with low

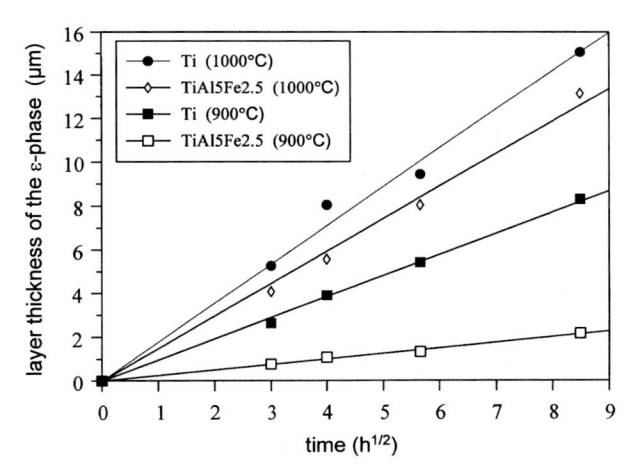

Figure 8.28 Thickness of the ε and α layers dependent on nitriding time and temperature (Schaldach and Breme, 1990).

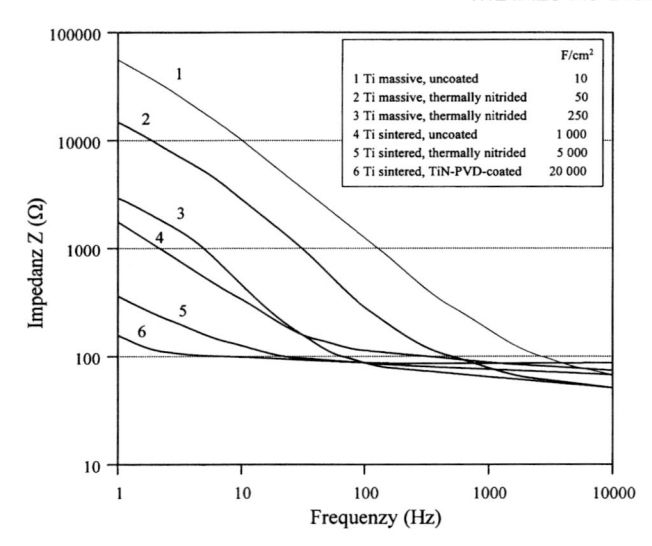

Figure 8.29 Impedance measurement and capacity of different electrode tips (Schaldach and Breme, 1990).

	F/cm²
1 Ti massive, uncoated	10
2 Ti massive, thermally nitrided	50
3 Ti massive, thermally nitrided	250
4 Ti sintered, uncoated	1 000
5 Ti sintered, thermally nitrided	5 000
6 Ti sintered, TiN-PVD-coated	20 000

conductivity. Because of the large surface area even a non-nitrided porous electrode had an increased capacity, with 1000 µF cm^{-2} compared to a solid, but surface-nitrided electrode (250 F cm^{-2}). Because of the stem-like columnar microstructure of a TiN-Thornton layer, the PVD coated porous electrode had the highest capacity of 20 000 µF cm^{-2} (Bolz et al., 1990b; Schaldach and Breme, 1990; Schaldach and Bolz, 1991; Schaldach et al., 1991a).

An alternative as a conductive ceramic surface layer could be TiB_2 which has an even lower specific electrical resistance than TiN (14.4 and 25 µΩ cm, respectively) (Table 8.6). TiB_2 coatings on titanium electrodes can easily be produced at an increased temperature, e.g. 950°C. For this purpose the electrodes were embedded in an oxygen-free boron powder. The boriding was performed in an argon atmosphere (1 h). The results of the impedance measurements of TiB_2-coated porous titanium electrodes are given in Figure 8.30. Compared with TiN-coated samples, there is no significant difference in the results. Both types of layer (TiN and TiB_2) have the crucial disadvantage of a lower thermodynamic stability than TiO_2 (Table 8.7). Therefore, if anodic loading takes place, the formation of electroactive oxides, which have the disadvantage of a low electrical conductivity (Table 8.6), is inevitable. This problem can be overcome by the use of iridium coatings (Riedmüller et al., 1995) which provide not only a metallic layer and an oxide layer (after anodic loading), but also high conductivity and impedance (Table 8.6 and Figure 8.30). The Ir layers can be produced by different methods such as PVD and CVD. For the latter process metallorganic precursors such as iridium tri-acetyl-acetonate ($CH_3COCHCOCH_3$)Ir, can also be used (Gelfond et al., 1992).

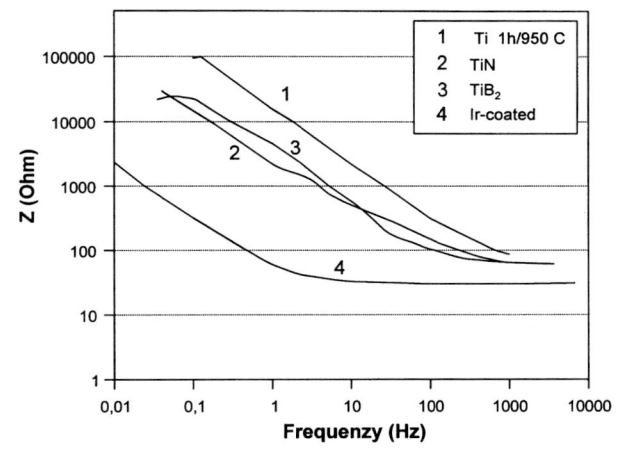

Figure 8.30 Impedance measurement of differently coated Ti electrode tips.

For an understanding of the interaction between blood and the implants a microscopic model of thrombogenesis at alloplastic surfaces was developed. According to this model, the electronic requirements for a high haemocompatibility are a low band-gap density of states and a high surface conductivity (Bolz and Schaldach, 1993). Coatings that seem to be able to fulfil these requirements are amorphous hydrogenated silicon carbides deposited by plasma-enhanced CVD (Bolz et al., 1990a) and TiN deposited by PVD (Dion, 1993). Amorphous layers are thought to be advantageous because they do not obey stoichiometric rules, so that they allow a continuous adjustment of the electronic parameters without a fundamental change in their remaining properties. Layers of a-SiC:H on tantalum have already be used for the production of stents in the therapy of coronary vasculopathy (Amon, 1995).

8.4.3 WEAR-RESISTANT CERAMIC COATINGS

Of all metallic biomaterials, only the cast CoCr alloys show sufficient wear resistance, owing to the precipitation of carbides. All other materials, including titanium and its alloys, when used for the construction of articulating parts of medical

Table 8.7 Standard heat of formation of various coatings

Material	$-\Delta H$ (kJ mol^{-1})
TiO_2	889.41
TiN	309.15
TiB_2	319.61
IrO_2	188.39

devices, must be surface coated to improve their friction behaviour. Since maximum values of the acceleration tension are achieved by ion implantation, the best reaction and binding can be expected with this procedure. By ion implantation of TiN on wrought CoCr, not only the fretting behaviour, but also the corrosion resistance of the material tested in 0.17 M saline solution was improved. The pitting of the surface-treated material amounted to 1.16 V (Higham, 1986). Any cracks and fissures in the surface layer will lead to an accelerated corrosion rate because of the lower pH value in these crevices. Experiments with ion implantation of nitrogen in titanium surfaces showed good results with regard to fretting behaviour. Even the fatigue strength of the alloy Ti6Al4V, which was surface treated by nitrogen ion implantation, is reported to be increased by compression stresses generated by the high acceleration tension of the nitrogen ions (Williams et al., 1985). CVD or PVD layers consisting of TiN often have the disadvantage of a low adhesion strength because of unfavourable residual tension stresses. Better behaviour seems to be found in Ti/Nb oxinitrides or Ti/Zr oxides (Thull and Repenning, 1990; Hennig and Repenning, 1995).

A simple method for surface hardening Ti is oxidation of the surface. In order to investigate the influence of oxide layers on the friction behaviour, cylindrical samples of Ti5Al2.5Fe were oxidised by induction heating and quenched in paraffin oil. These samples, with a radius corresponding to the head of a hip prosthesis, were tested in a pin-on-disc apparatus. The disc material used was a plate of ultra-high molecular weight (UHMW) polyethylene in a 0.9% NaCl solution. The direction of the cylinder of the pin was the rolling direction. Therefore the microstructure of the tip of the pin was the same as that of the heads produced for hip prostheses. The rod material was produced by hot rolling and annealing at 850, 900 and 950°C. The results of the pin-on-disc tests are shown in Table 8.8. By oxidising and quenching in paraffin oil the depth of the grooves on the polyethylene disc was diminished by nearly half the amount of non-oxidised samples. The difference decreases with increasing rolling temperature. One can also see that the increase in the peak to valley height of the Ti5Al2.5Fe pins of samples is lower in the oxidised condition

Table 8.8 Results of pin-on-disc tests of TiAl5Fe2.5 pins (diameter 9.6 mm, radius 16 mm) against UHMW polyethylene discs (55 mm diameter) in a 0.9% NaCl solution (39°C, 7 h, 50 N)

Rolling temperature (°C)	Treatment	Peak to valley height (μm)		Depth of grooves on disc (μm)
		Before testing	After testing	
850	Polished and oxidised	0.70	2.92	44
850	Polished and oxidised	0.86	1.89	24
900	Polished	0.41	2.83	18
900	Polished and oxidised	0.78	1.88	12
950	Polished	0.61	1.86	23
950	Polished and oxidised	0.54	1.79	21

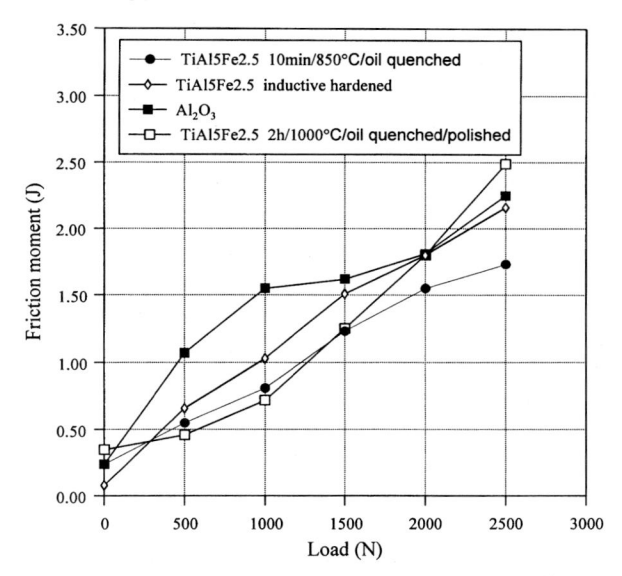

Figure 8.31 Influence of the load on the friction moment of Ti5Al2.5Fe and Al_2O_3 heads against a UHMW polyethylene cup (Zwicker and Breme, 1984).

than in the polished condition. As the microstructure of the material rolled at 850 and 900°C showed better friction properties, this material was used for further experiments. For the measurement of the friction forces between the head of a hip prosthesis and a UHMW polyethylene cup a testing apparatus was used which measured the torque moment of the head as a function of the load. The heads were rotated in a 0.9% NaCl solution at 39°C to simulate conditions in the human body. The results of such torque measurements of Ti5Al2.5Fe heads with different treatments and of one aluminium oxide head of the same dimensions are presented in Figure 8.31. All data show the difference of two measurements of the friction between the third and fifth minute of testing. In this range of time the friction moment showed an almost constant value. The torque of the inductive hardened Ti5Al2.5Fe head and of the two oxidised Ti5Al2.5Fe heads (10 min at 850°C, oil-quenched; and 2 h at 1000°C, oil-quenched and polished) is similar at loads from 1500 to 2500 N. At a load of 1000 N and lower, the head oxidised for 30 min at 850°C had the highest friction moment (Zwicker and Breme, 1984; Zwicker et al., 1984).

8.5 EXAMPLES OF MEDICAL DEVICES CONSISTING OF METAL–CERAMIC BONDS

Figure 8.32 shows an instrumented hip prosthesis aimed at monitoring the stresses exerted on the implant. This three-dimensional force-measurement system would

METALS AS BIOMATERIALS

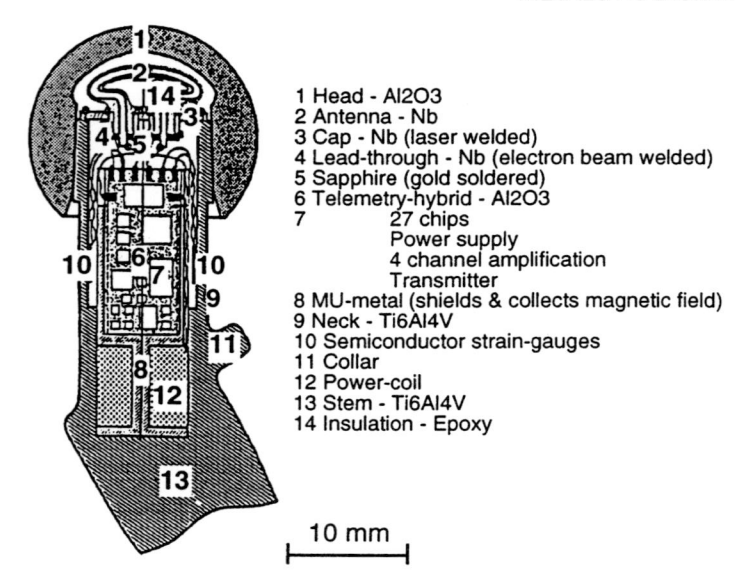

1 Head - Al2O3
2 Antenna - Nb
3 Cap - Nb (laser welded)
4 Lead-through - Nb (electron beam welded)
5 Sapphire (gold soldered)
6 Telemetry-hybrid - Al2O3
7   27 chips
      Power supply
      4 channel amplification
      Transmitter
8 MU-metal (shields & collects magnetic field)
9 Neck - Ti6Al4V
10 Semiconductor strain-gauges
11 Collar
12 Power-coil
13 Stem - Ti6Al4V
14 Insulation - Epoxy

Figure 8.32 Instrumented hip prosthesis (Bergmann and Graichen, 1987).

allow follow-up of the mechanical properties and anatomical variations occurring in bones as a function of time. All the electronics were placed inside the neck of the Ti6Al4V prosthesis, with the exception of the antenna, which was inside the Al$_2$O$_3$ head. The antenna was made of niobium and was electron-beam welded directly to the lid of the neck, which was also made of niobium. The hermetic sealing of the neck of the prosthesis was achieved by laser welding the niobium lid to the Ti6Al4V neck of the prosthesis. As the ceramic head of the prosthesis forms a compression seal with the Ti6Al4V neck, a second moisture barrier, to protect the antenna, was introduced by means of an epoxy layer (Bergmann and Graichen, 1987).

Another example of the application of hermetic metal–ceramic bonding in orthopaedics is the development of a protective encapsulation system for the instrumentation of an ostheosynthesis plate (Paiva, 1994). An electronic telemetric strain-measurement passive system was developed and integrated in a fixation nail-plate, as shown in Figure 8.33. The aim of the system was the evaluation of the bone healing process by the measurement of the plate deformation, which can be related to the stress to which the plate is subjected (Puers, 1993). The *in vivo* measurement of the deformation of the implant helps in understanding the mechanical characteristics of the bone–callus–implant system, and is a tool for reducing the failure rate of high-risk ostheosynthesis and the clinical complications associated with these failures (Burny *et al.*, 1993).

An encapsulation system was developed to protect the complex telemetric electronics from mechanical and chemical degradation (Paiva, 1994). It consisted of a lid that was specially designed to close the cavity of the plate where the electronics were placed (see transverse section of Figure 8.33). This lid consisted of a

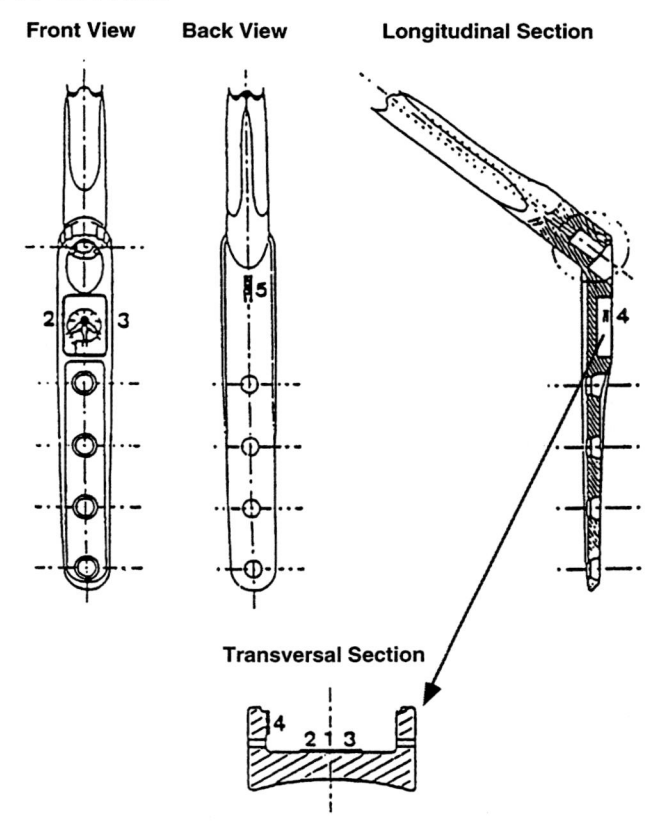

Figure 8.33 Instrumented nail-plate (Paiva, 1994). Numbers refer to the position of strain gauges.

metallic material (AISI 316L stainless steel, the same material as the plate) and a ceramic (alumina, Al_2O_3), which were hermetically bonded together by an active metal brazing technique. The aim of the metallic part was to assure mechanical strength, while the ceramic acted as a window transparent to radio-frequency sig-nals. The hermetic sealing of the cavity in the plate where the electronics were enclosed was achieved by laser welding the external metallic part of the lid to the plate.

Other examples of the use of metal–ceramic chemical bonds come from the field of dentistry, where metal–ceramic interfaces were developed for dental restoration (Kawahara, 1987; Saha, 1989). Typical examples are those related to the fabrication of crowns and bridges. Porcelain is the material commonly used for these applications (Winkler and Wongthai, 1986; Bagnall, 1989; Hegdahl, 1991). For instance, in crowns several porcelain layers with different optical properties are built up to reproduce the various layers of tooth dentine, enamel, etc. As porcelain is brittle and crowns are subjected to severe compressive stresses up to 850 N (Park, 1984) and cyclic mechanical loads, it is common practice to use a metallic substrate to support the porcelain layers. A thin metal shell is cast and porcelain pastes with different compositions are built up on the metal and fused to it by firing. The final product may be regarded as a laminate in which the adhesion of porcelain to metal is critical in preventing crack propagation into the porcelain (Winkler and Wongthai, 1986; Bagnall, 1989).

NOMENCLATURE

a	activity
A	surface area
C	capacity
d	thickness
D	coefficient of diffusion
E	Young's modulus
G_c	fracture energy
I	ionisation potential
k	Boltzmann's constant
n'	number of moles of the oxide M_xO
n''	number of moles of M_y
n	bond density
R	distance between atom centres
T	temperature
T	time for spreading
T_m	melting temperature
W_{ad}	work of adhesion
α	thermal expansion coefficient
$\alpha°$	degree of reaction at equilibrium
α_M	polarisation of the metal
$\Delta G°$	variation in frequency of the reaction per mole (Gibbs free energy per mole)
ε	dielectric angle
ε_0	dielectric constant of the vacuum
γ	surface energy
γ_{sv}	vapour interfacial energy
γ_{sl}	solid–liquid interfacial energy
γ_{lv}	liquid surface tension
γ_{ss}	energy of the solid reaction layer interface
γ_r	dynamic interfacial energy at time t
$\gamma_{sl}°$	initial interfacial energy for $t = 0$
Ω	vacancy volume
Ω_{sl}	interfacial area
σ_{P5}	residual stress
θ	contact angle

REFERENCES

Ambrose, J.C., Nicholas, M.G., and Stoneham, A.M. (1993) Dynamics of liquid drop spreading in metal–metal systems, *Acta Metall. Mater.* **41**, 2395–401.
Amon, M., Winkler, S., Bolz, A. and Schaldach, M. (1995) Beschichtung von Tantal-Stents mit amorphem Siliziumkarbid und deren Charakterisierung, *Biomed. Technik* **40**, 39–42.
Bagnall, R.D. (1989) Adhesion in dentistry. Part 1: Critical overview, *Mater. Sci. Technol.* **5**, 621–6.
Barbosa, M.A., Rocha, L.A. and Puers, S. (1993) Biomaterials in orthopedic implant monitoring, in *Monitoring of Orthopedic Implants: A Biomaterials–Microelectronics Challenge*, (eds F. Burny and R. Puers), European Materials Research Society Monography, Vol. 7, Elsevier Science, Amsterdam, pp. 222–40.
Barrett, P.C. (1962) UK Patent 891705.
Bauer, T.W., Geesink, R.C.T., Zimmerman, R. and McMahon, J.T. (1991) Hydroxyapatite-coated femoral stems, *J. Bone and Surg.* **73-A**, (10), 1439–52.
Bergman, G. and Graichen, F. (1987) Telemetry for long term orthopaedic implants, in *Biotelemetry IX* (eds H.P. Kimmich and M.R. Neumann), pp. 295–302.
Block, M.S. and Kent, J.N. (1994) Long-term follow-up on hydroxyapatite-coated cylindrical dental implants, *J. Oral Maxillofac. Surg.* **52**, 937–43.
Bolz, A., Brem, B. and Schaldach, M. (1990a) The electrochemical corrosion behavior of antithrombogenic coatings of amorphous silicon carbide, *Biomed. Tech. Berl.* **35**, 21–4.
Bolz, A., Matlok, H., Still, M., Schaldach, M., Hubmann, M. and Hardt, R. (1990b) Langzeitstabilität des Detektions- und Reizschwellenverhaltens von Titannitrid-Herzschrittmacher-Elektroden, *Biomed. Technik* **35** (Erg.-Band), 131–3.
Bolz, A. and Schaldach, M. (1993) Haemocompatibility optimisation of implants by hybrid structuring, *Med. Biol. Engng Comput.* **31**, 123–30.
Bondley, R.J. (1947) Metal–ceramic brazed seals, *Electronics* **20**, 97–103.
Breme, J. (1996) Titanlegierungen in der Medizintechnik, in *Titan und Titanlegierungen, DGM-Fortbildungsseminar, Köln* (eds M. Peters, C. Leyens and J. Kumpfert), DGM, Oberursel, pp. 205–27.
Breme, J. and Groh, L. (1993) Möglichkeiten der Verbesserung der Beschichtung von Titanimplantaten mit Hydroxylapatit-Keramik, in *Verbundwerkstoffe und Werkstoffverbunde* (eds G. Leonhardt and G. Ondracek), DGM, Oberursel, pp. 377–84.
Breme, J., Müller, H., Turnsek, J., Hegner, F., Schmidt, E., Güther, S. and Otto, W. (1996) US Patent 9611 1902.2.
Breme, J. and Wadewitz V. (1989) Comparison of Ti–Ta and Ti–Nb alloys for the application of dental implants, *J. Oral Maxillofac. Implants* **4**, 113–18.
Breme, J., Wadewitz V. and Burger K. (1989) Verbund Titanlegierung/Al_2O_3–Keramik für dentale Implantate – Entwicklung geeigneter Legierungen, in *Verbundwerkstoffe in Technik und Medizin*, Vol. 2, DGM, Oberusel, pp. 123–31.
Breme, J. and Zhou, Y. (1994) Metall/Keramik-Verbundwerkstoffe für die Medizintechnik, insbesondere für die Endoprothetik, in *Orthopädie und orthopädische Grenzgebiete*, Vol. 15, Met. Lit. Verlagsgesellschaft, Uelzen, pp. 77–85.
Breme, J., Zhou, Y. and Groh, L. (1995a) Development of a titanium alloy suitable for an optimized coating with hydroxyapatite, *Biomaterials*, **16**, 239–44.
Breme, J., Zhou, Y. and Hildebrand, H.F. (1995b) Herstellung und Eigenschaften optimierter Hydroxylapatitschichten auf Titanwerkstoffen, *Biomed. Technik*, **40** (Erg.-Band), 42–4.
Burny, F., Donkerwolcke, M. and Moulart, F. (1993) Clinical application of the monitoring of orthopaedic implants, in *Monitoring of Orthopedic Implants: A Biomaterials–Microelectronics Challange* (eds F. Burny and R. Puers), European Materials Research Society Monographs, Vol. 7, Elsevier Science, Amsterdam, pp. 138–46.
Campbell, D.E. and Hagy, H.E. (1975) Glasses and glass–ceramics, in *Handbook of Materials Science*, Vol. 22, *Metals, Composites and Refractory Materials* (ed. C.T. Lynch), CRC Press, Cleveland, OH.

Chern Lin, J.H., Lin, M.L. and Ju, C.P. (1993) Environmental effect on bond strength of plasma sprayed hydroxyapatite/bioactive glass composite coatings, *Dent. Mater.* **9**, 286–90.
Clarke, C.A. and Berry, R.D. (1968) UK Patent 1109108.
Collings, E.W. (1984) *The Physical Metallurgy of Titanium Alloys*, ASM, Metals Park, OH, pp. 78–85.
Crispin, R.M. and Nicholas, M. (1976) The wetting and bonding behaviour of some nickel alloy-aluminia systems, *J. Mater. Sci.* **11**, 17–22.
Dion, I., Roques, X., More, N., Labrousse, L., Caix, J., Lefebvre, F., Rouais, F., Gautreau, J. and Baquey, C. (1993) *Ex vivo* leucocyte adhesion and protein adsorption on TiN, *Biomaterials* **14**, 712–19.
Ducheyne, P., Bianco, P.D. and Kim, C. (1992) Bone tissue growth enhancement by calcium phosphate coatings on porous titanium alloys: the effect of shielding metal dissolution product, *Biomaterials* **13**, 617–24.
Ducheyne, P., Radin, S., Heughebaert, M. and Heughebaert, J.C. (1990) Calcium phosphate ceramic coatings on porous titanium: effect of structure and composition on electrophoretic deposition, vacuum sintering and *in vitro* dissolution, *Biomaterials* **11**, 244–50.
Elssner, G. and Petzow, G. (1990) Metal/ceramic joining, *ISIJ Int.* **30**, 1011–32.
Eulenberger, J., Kelle, F., Schroeder, A. and Steinemann, S.G. (1983) Haftung zwischen Knochen und Titan, Vol. 4, DVM, *Vortragsreihe des Arbeitskreises Implantate*, pp. 131–40.
Eustathopoulos, N. (1994) Influence of interfacial reactions on wettability and bonding in metal/oxide systems, in *Reviewed Proceedings of the 1st International Conference on High Temperature Capillarity* (ed. N. Eustathopoulos), Smolenice Castle, 8–11 May 1994, Bratislava, Slovakia, pp. 11–17.
Ferro, A.C. and Derby, B. (1995) Development of a micro-droplet technique for wettability studies: application to the Al–Si/SiC system, *Scripta Metall. Mater.* **33**, 837–42.
Filiaggi, M.J., Coombs, N.A. and Pilliar, R.M. (1991) Characterization of the interface in the plasma-sprayed HA coating/Ti–6AL–4V implant system, *J. Biomed. Mater. Res.* **25**, 1211–29.
Filiaggi, M.J., Pilliar, R.M. and Coombs, N.A. (1993) Post-plasma-spraying heat treatment of the HA coating/Ti–6Al–4V implant system, *J. Biomed. Mater. Res.* **27**, 191–8.
Floquet, J., Ralison, A., Eisenbarth, E., Jost, A., Breme, J. and Hildebrand, H.F. (1997) Le comportement biologique in vitro d'un alliage TiNb30 traité avec hydroxyapatite et phosphates tricalciques, *Rév. Stomatol. Chir. maxilofac.* **98**, Supp. 1, 47–9.
Frayssinet, P., Hardy, D., Conte, P., Delince, P., Guilhem, A. and Bonel, G. (1993) Analyse histologique de l'interface os/prothèse après implantation humaine de prothèses de hanche revêtues d'hydroxyapatite par projection plasma, *Rev. Chirur. Orthop.* **79**, 177–84.
Frayssinet, P., Hardy, D., Rouquet, N., Giammara, B., Guilhem, A. and Hanker, J. (1992) New observations on middle term hydroxyapatite-coated titanium alloy hip prostheses, *Biomaterials* **13**, 668–74.
Geldmacher, V., Mallinckrodt, M., Machata, G., Nürnberg, H.W., Schlipköter, H.W. and Stumm, W. (1984) in *Metalle in der Umwelt* (ed. E. Merian), pp. 471–7.
Gelfond, N.V., Igumenov, I.K., Boronin, A.I., Bukhtiyarov, V.I., Smirnov, M.Yu., Prosvirin, I.P. and Kwon, R.I. (1992) An XPS study of the composition of iridium films obtained by MO CVD, *Surf. Sci.* **275**, 323–31.
General Electric Co. (1968) UK Patent 1128228.
Gibbesch, B., Elssner, G., Bischoff, E. and Petzow, G. (1989a) *Z. Zahnärztl. Implantol.* **5**, 108–13.
Gibbesch, B., Elssner, G. and Petzow, G. (1992) Investigation of Ti/Al$_2$O$_3$ joints with intermediate tantalum and niobium layers, *Biomaterials* **13**, 455–61.
Gibbesch, B., Elssner, G., Mader, W. and Fischmeister, H.F. (1989b) Ultrahigh vacuum diffusion bonding of Nb and Cu single crystals to sapphire; joining of ceramics, in *Glass and Metal* (ed. W. Kraft), DGM, Oberursel, pp. 65–74.
Gibbesch, B., Elssner, G. and Petzow, G. (1989c) *Int. J. Oral Maxilofac. Implants* **4**, 131–4.

Gottselig, B., Gyarmati, E., Naoumidis, A. and Nickel, H. (1989) Development of methods for joining non-oxide silicon ceramics; joining of ceramics, in *Glass and Metal* (ed. W. Kraft), DGM, Oberursel, pp. 191–8.

Hardy, D.C.R., Frayssinet, P., Bonel, G., Authom, T., Le Naelou, S.A. and Delince, P.E. (1994) Two-year outcome of hydroxyapatite-coated prostheses, *Acta Orthop. Scand.* **65**, 253–7.

Hayduk, E.A. (1985) Effect of atmosphere composition on metallizing Al_2O_3 substrates with Mo-Mn paste, *Solid State Technol.* **28**, 321–8.

Hegdahl, T. (1991) The evaluation of materials for dentistry and dental surgery, in *Biomaterials Degradation: Fundamental Aspects and Related Clinical Phenomena* (eds M.A. Barbosa, F. Burny, J. Cordey, E. Dorre, G.W. Hastings, D. Muster and P. Tranquilli-Leali), European Materials Research Society Monographs, Vol. 1, Elsevier, Amsterdam, pp. 13–22.

Hegner, F., Schmidt, E., Klähn, T., Reimann, P., Breitenstein, H. and Messmer, S. (1994) US Patent 5334344.

Hennig, F.F. and Repenning, D. (1995) PE-verschleißmindernde Keramik-Metallverbund-Hüftgelenkkugeln, *Unfallchirurg* **98**, 526–9.

Higham, R.A. (1986) *Proceedings of the Conference on Biomedical Materials*, Boston, p. 237.

Iino, Y. and Tagushi, N. (1988) Ultrahigh vacuum diffusion bonding of Nb and Cu single crystals to sapphire, *J. Mater. Sci. Lett.* **4**, 981–6.

Iseki, T., Maruyama, T. and Kameda, T. (1984) *Proc. Br. Ceram. Soc.* **34**, 241–6.

Iseki, T., Yano, T. and Chung, Y.S. (1989) *J. Ceram. Soc. Jpn. Int. Ed.* **97**, 697–703.

Jayaraman, A., Klement, W. and Kennedy, G.C. (1963) Solid solution transitions in titanium and zirconium at high pressure, *Phys. Rev.* **131**, 644–50.

Ji, H. and Marquis, P.M. (1993) Effect of heat treatment on the microstructure of plasma-sprayed hydroxyapatite coating, in *Biomaterials*, Vol. 14 (1) (ed. M.B. Bever), Pergamon Press, New York, pp. 64–8.

Kangasniemi, I.M.O., Verheyen, C.C.P.M., Van der Velde, E.A. and De Groot, K. (1994) In vivo tensile testing of fluorapatite and hydroxyapatite plasma-sprayed coatings, *J. Biomed. Mater. Res.* **28**, 563–72.

Kawahara, H. (1987) Bioceramics for hard tissue replacements, *Clin. Mater.* **2**, 181–206.

Klein, C.P.A.T., Patka, P., Van der Lubbe, H.B.M., Wolke, J.G.C. and De Groot, K. (1991) Plasma-sprayed coatings of tetracalciumphosphate, hydroxylapatite and α-TCP on titanium alloy: an interface study, *J. Biomed. Mater. Res.* **25**, 53–65.

Klein, C.P.A.T., Patka, P., Wolke, J.G.C., De Blieck-Hogervorst, J.M.A. and De Groot, K. (1994) Long-term in vivo study of plasma-sprayed coatings on titanium alloys of tetra-calcium phosphate, hydroxyapatite and α-tricalcium phosphate, *Biomaterials* **15**, 146–50.

Klomp, J.T. (1986) Glass bonding in advanced ceramics, in *Encyclopedia of Material Science and Engineering*, M.B. Bauer, New York, p. 1958.

Kunz, S.C. and Loeham, R.E. (1987) Thermal expansion mismatch produced by interfacial reactions in glass-ceramic to metal seals, *Adv. Ceram. Mater.* **2**, 69–73.

Lascar, G. (1985) Étude des liaisons entre méteaux et une céramique. Application à la réalisation d'ensembles electro-optiques, *Verres Réfract.* **39**, 569–85.

Li, J.G. (1992a) Kinetics of wetting and spreading of Cu–Ti alloys on alumina and glassy carbon substrates, *J. Mater. Sci. Lett.* **11**, 1551–4.

Li, J.G. (1992b) Role of bandgaps on some interfacial phenomena with ionocovalent oxides, *Rare Metals* **11**, 81–5.

Li, J.G. (1992c) Ion beam enhanced adhesion of metal/ceramic systems, *Rare Metals* **11**, 1–5.

Li, J.G. (1992d) Role of electron density of liquid metals and bandgap energy of solid ceramics on the work of adhesion and wettability of metal–ceramic systems, *Mater. Sci. Lett.* **11**, 903–5.

Li, J.G. (1993) Influence of oxygen partial pressure on the wetting behaviour of titanium carbide by molten copper and other metals, *Mater. Lett.* **17**, 74–8.

Li, J.G. (1994a) Wettability of solid inorganic materials by gold, *Scripta Metall. Mater.* **30**, 337–42.

Li, J.G. (1994b) A comparative study between energetics of metal/ceramic interfaces and metal–semiconductor Schottky contacts, in *Reviewed Proceedings of the 1st International Conference on High Temperature Capillarity* (ed. N. Eustathopoulos), Smolenice Castle, 8–11 May 1994, Bratislava, Slovakia, pp. 70–9.

Li, J.-G. (1994c) Wetting of ceramic materials by liquid silicon, aluminium and metallic melts containing titanium and other reactive elements: a review, *Ceram. Int.* **10**, 391–412.

Li, J.-G. and Hausner, H. (1992) Wetting and adhesion in liquid silicon/ceramic systems, *Mater. Lett.* **14**, 329–32.

Loehman, R.E. (1989) Interfacial reactions in ceramic–metal systems, *Ceram. Bull.* **68**, 891–6.

Loehman, R.E. and Tomsia, A.P. (1988) Joining of ceramics, *Ceram. Bull.* **67**, 375–80.

Marinoni, E.C., Fontana, A. and Castellano, S. (1995) Osteointegration of 96 cementless hip prostheses with hydroxyapatite coating; 5 years follow-up, *Chir. Organ. Mov.* **LXXX**, 147–55.

Mattox, D.M. and Smith, H.D. (1985) Role of manganese in the metalization of high alumina ceramics, *Am. Ceram. Bull.* **64**, 1363–8.

Miura, K., Narita, T. and Ishikawa, T. (1989) in Proceedings of MRS International Meeting on Advanced Materials, Vol 8, *Metal–Ceramic Joints*, MRS, Pittsburgh, PA, pp. 29–36.

Moroni, A., Caja, V.L., Egger, E.L., Trinchese, L. and Chao, E.Y.S. (1994) Histomorphometry of hydroxyapatite coated and uncoated porous titanium bone implants, *Biomaterials* **15**, 926–30.

Murray, J.L. and Wiedt, H.A. (1990) in Massalski, T.B., *et al. Binary Alloy Phase Diagrams*, 2nd edn, ASM, Materials Park, OH.

Naidich, Y.V. and Zhuravlev, V.S. (1989) Wettability and adhesion of metallic melts in contact with non-metallic materials in soldering processes, joining of ceramics, in *Glass and Metal* (ed. W. Kraft), DGM, Oberursel, pp. 17–24.

Naka, M. and Okamoto, T. (1989) in *Proceedings of MRS International Meeting on Advanced Materials*, Vol. 8, *Metal-Ceramic Joints*, MRS, Pittsburgh, pp. 61–7.

Nicholas, M. (1968) The strength of metal/alumina interfaces, Ceramic–metal interfaces, Fundamentals of diffusion bonding *J. Mater. Sci.* **3**, 571–8.

Nicholas, M.G. (1987) Ceramic-Metal Interfaces, in *Fundamentals of Diffusion Bonding* (ed. Y. Ishida), Elsevier, Amsterdam, pp. 25–31.

Nicholas, M.G. (1989) Reactive brazing of ceramics, in *Joining of Ceramics, Glass and Metal* (ed. W. Kraft), DGM, Oberursel, pp. 49–59.

Nicholas, M.G. (1990) Overview, in *Joining of Ceramics* (ed. M.G. Nicholas), Chapman and Hall, London, pp. 1–6.

Nicholas, M.G. and Mortimer, D.A. (1985) Ceramic/metal joining for structural applications, *Mater. Sci. Technol.* **1**, 657–68.

Nicholas, M.G. and Peteves, S.D. (1994) The kinetics of liquid braze spreading, in *Reviewed Proceedings of the 1st International Conference on High Temperature Capillarity* (ed. N. Eustathopoulos), Smolenice Castle, 8–11 May 1994, Bratislava, Slovakia, pp. 18–27.

Nicholas, M.G., Valentine, T.M. and Waite, J.M. (1980) The wetting of alumina by copper alloyed with titanium and other elements, *J. Mater. Sci.* **15**, 2197–202.

Nimb, L., Gotfredsen, K. and Jensen, J.S. (1993) Mechanical failure of hydroxyapatite-coated titanium and cobalt–chromium–molybdenum alloy implants, an animal study, *Acta Orthopaed. Belgica* **59**, 333–7.

Ong, J.L. and Lucas, L.C. (1994) Post-deposition heat treatment for ion beam sputter deposited calcium phosphate coatings, *Biomaterials* **15**, 337–41.

Ong, J.L., Lucas, L.C., Lacefield, W.R. and Rigney, E.D. (1992) Structure, solubility and bond strength of thin calcium phosphate coatings produced by ion beam sputter deposition, *Biomaterials* **13**, 249–54.

Paiva, O.C. (1994) Desenvolvimento de interfaces estanques para proteçao de dispositivos telemétricos usados em placas orthpédicas, Nsc. Thesis, Faculdade de Engenharia da Universidade do Porto.

Park, J.B. (1984) *Biomaterials Science and Engineering*, Plenum Press, New York.

Pask, J.A. (1987) From technology to the science of glass/metal and ceramic/metal sealing, *Am. Ceram. Bull.* **66**, 1587–94.

Pask, J.A. and Tomsia, A. (1981) Wetting, spreading and reactions at liquid/solid interfaces, in *Surfaces and Interfaces in Ceramic and Ceramic–Metal Systems* (eds J. Pask and A. Evans), Plenum Press, New York.

Passerone, A. (1986) Interfacial phenomena in metal–ceramic systems, *Mater. Chem. Phys.* **15**, 263–79.

Pauling, L. (1949) *The Nature of the Chemical Bond*, 2nd edn, Cornell University Press, Cornell, pp. 69–421.

Pilliar, R.M., Lee, J.M. and Mamatopoulos, C. (1986) Observations on the effect of movement on bone implants into porous-surface implants, *Clin. Othop. Rel. Res.* **20B**, 108–15.

Puers, R. (1993) Conversing stress into strain: basic techniques, in *Monitoring of Orthopedic Implants: A Biomaterials–Microelectronics Challenge* (eds F. Burny and R. Puers), European Materials Research Society Monographs, Vol. 7, Elsevier Science, Amsterdam, pp. 33–53.

Riedmüller, J., Rzany, A., Fröhlich, R., Bolz, A. and Schaldach, M. (1995) Langzeitstabilität bei elektrischer Belastung von galvanisch abgeschiedenem Iridiumnoxid, *Biomed. Tech.* **40**, 37–9.

Saha, S. (1989) Ceramics for orthopaedic and dental applications, *IEEE Engng Med. Biol. Mag.* **8**, 37–9.

Schaldach, M. and Bolz, A. (1991) Longterm stability of TiN, in *Proceedings of the Conference on Bioceramics and the Human Body (IRTEC-CNR)*, Faenza, 40–4.

Schaldach, M., Bolz, A. and Breme, J. (1991a) Porous heart pacemaker electrodes of TiAl5Fe2.5 and TiN, in *Proceedings of the 1st European Conference on Biomedical Engineering*, Nice, 312–13.

Schaldach, M., Bolz, A., Breme, J., Hubmann, M. and Hardt, R. (1991b) Acute and long-term sensing and pacing performance of pacemaker leads having titanium nitride electrode tips, *Pacemaker Leads* 441–50.

Schaldach, M. and Breme, J. (1990) Porous heart pacemaker electrodes of TiAl5Fe2.5 Alloy, in *Titanium 1990 – Products and Applications, Proceedings of the Technical Program*, Vol. II, pp. 604–11.

Schaldach, M., Hubmann, M., Hardt, M., Weikl, R. and Weikl, A. (1989) Titannitrid-Herzschrittmacher-Elektroden, *Biomed. Techn.* **34**, 185–90.

Schiepers, R.G.J., van Loo, F.J.J. and de With, G. (1988) Reactions between α-silicon carbide ceramic and nickel or iron, *J. Am. Ceram. Soc.* **71**, C-284–90.

Schmitz, H.J., Gross, U., Kinne, R., Fuhrmann, G. and Strunz, V. (1987) Der Einfluß unterschiedlicher Oberflächenstrukturierung alloplastischer Implantate auf das histologische und Zugfestigkeitsverhalten des Interface, in *DVM-Vortragsreihe des Arbeitskreises Implantate*, Vol. 8, DVM, Berlin, pp. 163–72.

Suga, T. and Elssner, G. (1985) Determination of the fracture energy and the fracture resistance of interfaces, *J. Phys.* **46**, C634–57.

Suganuma, K. and Okamoto, T. (1985) Interlayer bonding methods for ceramic/metal-systems with thermal expansion mismatches, in *Seiken Symposium 1, Interface Structure, Chemistry, Mechanical Properties and Diffusion Bonding*, Tokyo.

Suganuma, K. Okamoto, T. and Koizumi, M. (1985) Method of preventing metal expansion mismatch effect in ceramic metal joining, *J. Mater. Sci. Lett.* **4**, 648–54.

Suganuma, K., Okamoto, T. and Koizumi, M. (1987) *J. Mater. Sci. Lett.* **22**, 2702–9.

Thull, R. and Repening, D. (1990) Funktionelle Beschichtungen für Implantate in Orthopädie und Zahnheilkunde, *Z. Biom. Technik.* **25**, 56–61.

Williams, J.M. and Buchanan, R.A. (1985) *Mater. Sci. Engng.* **69**, 237–41.

Winkler, S. and Wongthai, P. (1986) Increasing the bond strength of metal–ceramic restorations, *J. Prosthet. Dent.* **56**, 396–401.

Zwicker, U. and Breme, J. (1984) Investigations on the friction behaviour of oxidized TiAl5Fe2.5 surface layers of implant material, *J. Less Common Metals* **100**, 371–5.

Zwicker, U., Etzold, U. and Moser, Th. (1984) Abrasive properties of oxide layers on TiAl5Fe2.5 in contact with high density polyethylene, in *Proceedings of the Fifth International Conference on Titanium* (eds G. Lütjering, U. Zwicker and W. Bunk), Munich, pp 1343–8.

9
Biological response and biocompatibility

H.F. HILDEBRAND AND J.-C. HORNEZ
University of Lille, Lille, France

9.1 INTRODUCTION

Metals have complex effects on the human organism and four different forms of biological reaction can be distinguished, depending on the concentration, the exposure time and the administration route.

- At very low concentrations, some elements such as cobalt, copper, iron, manganese, zinc and even nickel are **essential or trace elements** (Anke *et al.*, 1980).
- At high or excessive concentrations, the same substances can induce **toxic reactions** in humans and other animals, which are well known for arsenic, cobalt, nickel, lead and many others (Haguenoer and Furon, 1982; Merian, 1984). Cytotoxic effects of metal ions have also been demonstrated in cell-culture systems (Frazier and Andrews, 1979).
- Metals also have an **allergenic potency**. Nickel, cobalt and chromium are recognised to be redoubtable sensitising agents, whereas only very few cases are known of allergic contact dermatitis to gold, palladium, platinum, titanium, etc. (Marcussen, 1957; Dooms-Gossens *et al.*, 1980; Wall and Calnan, 1980).
- Finally, numerous metals and their compounds are considered, at least in experimental animals, to be strong **carcinogenic agents**. At present, little is known of the carcinogenic action of these metals, but recent research investigations suggest that the induction of free radicals by metal compounds is one of the primary factors in the mechanism of metal carcinogenesis (Sunderman, 1988, 1989a, b; Shirali *et al.*, 1994).

An increasing source of metals and metal ions in humans is the use of metallic biomaterials for dental and orthopaedic implants and prostheses, which are made of a large variety of alloys containing between two and eight different metals. A total of more than 30 elements including boron, carbon and nitrogen may be contained in different classes of alloys, which are used for external contact with the skin (maintaining exoprostheses), for fixed or mobile medical devices in orifices (mouth,

---

Metals as Biomaterials ISBN 0 471 96935 4 Edited by J.A. Helsen and H.J. Breme. © 1998 John Wiley & Sons Ltd

nose, ear and vagina) in contact with mucosal epithelia, and for implantable devices in hard and soft tissues to replace organ functions (total joint prostheses and dental implants), to consolidate failures (orbital floor, rachis and osteosynthesis) and to maintain grafts (trellis membranes and grids).

9.2 ALLOYS

9.2.1 ALLOYS USED FOR SURGICAL IMPLANTS

The implants used in stomatology and modern orthopaedic surgery are manufactured from three different alloy systems, each presenting main characteristic components (see Chapter 2):

- Fe–base alloys with a high chromium content are summarised as **stainless steel**.
- Co–base alloys with 25–30% chromium, 5–7% molybdenum and low amounts of other metals such as nickel, manganese, zirconium and tin are called **CoCr alloys**, those with about 20% chromium, 10% nickel and up to 15% tungsten are called **wrong CoCr alloys**.
- **Ti–base alloys** with 70–90% or more titanium are increasingly being used for surgical implants. They contain low amounts of other metals such as aluminium, vanadium, niobium, tantalum, manganese, zirconium and tin. The only pure metals used for medical devices are titanium and tantalum. The only binary alloys applied for biomaterials are Ti–base alloys, e.g. Ti30Nb, Ti30Ta Ti(n)Mn, and memory super alloys, e.g. NiTi (Breme and Wadewitz, 1989; Bradley, 1994; Breme, 1994).

All of these alloys can also be integrated in medical devices for neurosurgery and cardiovascular, maxillofacial, otological and visceral surgery, etc. Their most frequent application, however, is in osteosynthesis and partial and total arthroplasties.

For several decades, stainless steel was the most frequently used alloy for joint replacements. Co–base alloys have since been used and about 70% of all orthopaedic implants are made from CoCr alloys. Titanium and its alloys have become more important since the late 1970s owing to their excellent biological behaviour.

9.2.2 DENTAL ALLOYS

Many more variations exist for use as dental alloys and they can be classified according to their multiple use in dentistry:

- crown and bridge casting alloys (conventional alloys)
- porcelain fused to metal alloys (ceramometallic alloys)
- wires
- partial denture alloys
- implant alloys
- solders
- dental amalgams.

BIOLOGICAL RESPONSE AND BIOCOMPATIBILITY

A range of more than 1100 alloys is available on the European Market. According to their chemical composition they can be classified into five families:

- dental amalgams (mercury, silver, zinc, tin and copper)
- precious alloys (gold, platinum, silver, copper and low amounts of other metals of the platinum group)
- semiprecious, low-gold and Pd–base alloys (palladium, silver, gold and lower amounts of platinum and copper)
- non-precious alloys, i.e. stainless steel, CoCr and NiCr alloys, some of which may also contain cadmium and beryllium
- Ti–base alloys.

Progressive dental reconstructions within the lifetime of a patient, and in particular the use of different alloys for total or partial dentures, for dental fillings, porcelain fused restorations, transcutaneous implants, etc., generate unavoidable oral polymetallism. Indeed, two alloys of different composition have different electric potentials and inevitably induce corrosion and subsequently the release of metal ions into the human body (Bundy, 1994).

9.2.3 METALS USED FOR BIOMEDICAL ALLOYS

The variation in biomedical alloys is determined by their application. More than 30 different elements are currently used for dental materials and surgical implants. Other metals (cerium, caesium, selenium, etc.) are added in alloys for needles and tools applied in acupuncture and hair transplantation:

- orthopaedic and stomatological implants and prostheses (Al, Co, Cr, Fe, Mn, Mo, Nb, Ni, Sn, Ta, Ti, V, W, Zr, etc.)
- dental alloys: non-precious (Al, B, Be, Cd, Co, Cr, Fe, Mn, Mo, Ni, Si, Ti, V, W, etc.); precious and semi-precious (Ag, Au, Cu, Fe, Ga, In, Ir, Pd, Pt, Rh, Ru, Sn, Ti, Zn, etc.); dental amalgams (Ag, Cu, Hg, Sn, Zn, etc.)

9.3 METAL TOXICITY

This section will give a short overview of the toxicity in humans of the most frequently used metals and their compounds. As most of these effects have been known for a long time and multiple monographs have been published (Haguenoer and Furon, 1982; Brown and Savory, 1983; Merian, 1984; Aitio et al., 1991), only the most important characteristics are emphasised and called to mind. It must be stressed that the pure metals are rarely toxic, that the toxic, allergenic and carcinogenic effects depend on the concentration and the nature of compounds (oxides, simple or complex salts) that two compounds of the same metal may induce strongly different responses and that the toxic potency of different ions or compounds varies by two to three orders of magnitude. Thus the speciation of compounds is of primary importance, e.g. $NiCl_2$ is toxic with no evident carcinogenic effect, whereas Ni_3S_2 is highly carcinogenic.

9.3.1 ALUMINIUM

Intoxications with metallic aluminium are recognised in occupational medicine and in patients submitted to renal dialysis. The main penetration route, however, is the respiratory tract via inhalation. Aluminium compounds are absorbed slowly. The target organ is the brain and Alzheimer-like encephalopathies are the most frequently reported diseases due to continued occupational exposure (Haguenoer and Furon, 1982; Merian, 1984). Since the disease has been linked to a genetic defect, aluminium is considered to play a minor role (if any) in the onset of Alzheimer's disease.

The interference with phosphate absorption explains the influence of aluminium on bone metabolism. It inhibits the phosphorylation process and ATP synthesis, and subsequently reduces the intracellular energy reserve (Undreicka *et al*., 1966; Arsalane *et al*., 1992). The amount of aluminum increases in bone with subsequent alteration of mineralisation and reduction in the rapidity of the bone turnover, which may lead to pathological fractures (Bradley, 1981; Williams, 1981; Toth *et al*., 1985). The low solubility of Al_2O_3 is the reason for the very low toxic effect of this compound, which even favours cell proliferation (Labat and Chamson, 1995).

9.3.2 BERYLLIUM

The principal penetration routes of beryllium into the organism are the skin, lungs and digestive tract. Soluble compounds are rapidly transformed into insoluble orthophosphates and accumulate in the lung with a retention level of 80%.

Beryllium and its compounds are carcinogenic in experimental animals (Reeves and Vorwald, 1967; Reeves *et al*., 1967) and in occupationally exposed workers (Mancuso, 1970; Hasan and Kazemi, 1974). Several cases of pneumoconiosis and berylliosis in dental technicians have been reported in the past (Lob and Hugonnaud 1977; Choudat, 1982; Choudat *et al*., 1983). In 1975 NIOSH proposed $0.5\ \mu g\ m^{-3}$ as the maximum admissible air concentration at the worksite. As industrial and laboratory hygiene have since been strictly respected, the occurrence of beryllium-induced pneumopathies has been reduced considerably.

Beryllium is a highly sensitising agent and its presence in allergic standard test batteries was prohibited long ago. A single application of beryllium in an allergic epicutaneous test can induce pulmonary berylliosis (Haguenoer and Furon, 1982).

9.3.3 CADMIUM

The respiratory tract is the main route of introduction, by smoking and occupational exposure to cadmium and its compounds. The lung is the target organ after inhalation of cadmium oxides and sulfides, leading to bronchitis, bronchopneumonia and lung oedema (Haguenoer and Furon, 1982; Merian, 1984).

The cadmium metabolites are stored in the liver and the kidney where cadmium is bound to metallothionein, a specific low molecular weight (6800) protein with 33% cysteine as the main amino acid. The clearance of cadmium is directly dependent on

BIOLOGICAL RESPONSE AND BIOCOMPATIBILITY

the synthesis of metallothionein. There is a suspicion but no evidence for cancer induction by cadmium in humans.

Cadmium is found in some semiprecious dental alloys, in particular in solders (Bundy, 1994).

9.3.4 COBALT

The absorption of cobalt occurs via the digestive, cutaneous and pulmonary routes. It is compound dependent: 0.5% for CoO, 18% for $CoCl_2$ and 70% for vitamin B_{12}. Cobalt is considered to be an essential element.

Cobalt is stored in the kidney, liver and pancreas. Within a few days, 20% of the absorbed cobalt is cleared out of the system, mostly by the urinary route. It is stored in the organism by binding to a specific cobalt metallothionein in the liver and kidneys. One of the most well-known complexes is vitamin B_{12} (Haguenoer and Furon, 1982; Merian, 1984).

Cobalt is the main cause of hard metal-induced pulmonary fibrosis. It takes third place, after nickel and chromium, among the metallic allergens (Hildebrand *et al.*, 1989a, b). Its carcinogenic potency is not evident for humans.

9.3.5 CHROMIUM

Chromium belongs to the group of essential elements. Its toxicity depends on its oxidation state, with hexavalent chromium being more toxic than trivalent chromium. Cr(VI) is a potent mutagenic and carcinogenic agent (IARC, 1973).

It is essentially absorbed by the gastrointestinal tract and in addition by the respiratory tract and skin. Cr(III) compounds do not pass through the tegument or through the cellular membrane, where they are bound to stable protein complexes.

In contrast, Cr(VI) compounds have a high oxidation potency for organic molecules. They pass easily through the cellular membrane, and are reduced to the stable form Cr(III), which penetrates the nucleus and induces mutations by interaction with DNA (Ziats *et al.*, 1988).

Chromium accumulates in the liver, uterus, kidney and bones (Hildebrand *et al.*, 1986b). The retention is stronger for Cr(VI) than for Cr(III). In humans, the amount of chromium decreases with age except in the lung. It is eliminated by renal clearance and also has a highly allergenic action (Hildebrand *et al.*, 1989a, b).

9.3.6 COPPER

Copper is an essential element and is a component of some essential enzyme systems such as tyrosinase and cytochrome oxidase. Copper deficiency induces Menke's disease, a metabolic disease with too rapid copper clearance. In contrast, Wilson's disease is the accumulation of copper in the liver and in the nuclei of grey cells. It is a hereditary disease with recessive autosomal transmission. Its antagonist is zinc (Haguenoer and Furon, 1982; Merian, 1984).

Copper is essentially absorbed by the digestive and pulmonary route. It is totally bound to cellular proteins, and in the blood to coeruloplasmin (90%) and to serum albumin (2%) (Giroux and Henkin, 1973). Copper increases the synthesis of coeruloplasmin and a specific metallothionein in the liver.

Copper is rapidly cleared by the bile where it is bound to at least two proteins of different molecular weights. On the clinical level, copper intoxication may lead to granulomatous fibrosis in the lung, micronodular cirrhosis or haemangiosarcoma in the liver, cellular necrosis in the proximal tube of the kidney and cell lysis of mucosal epithelia (Haguenoer and Furon, 1982; Merian, 1984).

9.3.7 IRON

Iron is a biologically omnipresent essential element. It plays a central role in the haem molecule and has a key position in the transport of oxygen and electrons. Human tissues contain 50 ppm iron, bound in particular to haemoglobin, myoglobin and different cytochromic enzyme systems. Iron is toxic only after extremely high levels of exposure. Iron released by the oxidation process does not accumulate in tissues and is immediately metabolised (Haguenoer and Furon, 1982). In contrast, iron issuing from haemoglobin degradation in a haematoma, e.g. after surgical intervention, can be recovered even after several years (Hildebrand *et al.*, 1988).

9.3.8 MANGANESE

Manganese has no toxic effect except after extreme occupational exposure. It is an essential element and plays a primary role in the activation of multiple enzyme systems, i.e. hydrolases, kinases, transferases, decarboxylases and mitochondrial respiration. Manganese is the antagonist of iron and its excess decreases iron absorption and subsequently the amount of haemoglobin (Haguenoer and Furon, 1982; Merian, 1984).

In addition, a manganese excess may substitute magnesium in the DNA polymerase and thus lead to miscoding of DNA replication by incorporating ribonucleotides instead of deoxyribonucleotides (Zakour *et al.*, 1979).

9.3.9 MOLYBDENUM

Molybdenum is considered to be essential element and humans need a daily amount of 0.1 mg. It maintains the equilibrium of multiple enzyme activities, e.g. xanthine oxidase, aldehyde oxidase, nitrate reductase and nitrogenase (Merian, 1984). The LD_{50} (oral absorption) is 101 mg kg^{-1} for calcium molybdate, 125 mg kg^{-1} for MoO_3 and 333 mg kg^{-1} for ammonium molybdate (Haguenoer and Furon, 1982).

Ingestion of higher amounts of molybdenum than those mentioned above disturbs the copper and sulfate metabolism in experimental animals and humans. Pulmonary emaciation and gout symptoms were observed in occupationally exposed workers

BIOLOGICAL RESPONSE AND BIOCOMPATIBILITY

after inhalation of high amounts of metallic molybdenum particles. Under these conditions, molybdenum compounds can produce higher toxic effects than lead and mercury (Merian, 1984).

9.3.10 NICKEL

Nickel, together with chromium, is one of the most widely studied elements with respect to its biological behaviour. Several thousand papers have dealt with treating the toxic, allergenic, mutagenic and carcinogenic effects of nickel and its compounds (Anonymous, 1990). It is omnipresent in our environment and is principally absorbed via the digestive, pulmonary and cutaneous routes. The amount of nickel in urine and blood is a precise criterion for estimating nickel intoxication (Haguenoer and Furon, 1982; Merian, 1984). The target organ is the lung for any kind of exposure, i.e. inhalation, oral absorption, intraperitoneal, intramuscular and intravenous injections (Parker and Sunderman, 1974; Herlant-Peers *et al.*, 1982) and metallic implants (Bergman *et al.*, 1980).

Nickel has a high affinity to proteins of the mitochondrial and microsomal fractions of lung cells (Herlant-Peers *et al.*, 1983). These fractions are the most important sites of cellular energy reserve and multiple enzyme systems. Nickel compounds such as nickel hydroxycarbonates and nickel sulfides activate interleukin synthesis and lipid peroxidation, thus generating free radicals, which are essential factors in carcinogenesis (Arsalane *et al.*, 1992; Shirali *et al.*, 1994). Nickel oxides and sulfides have a redoubtable carcinogenic potency in experimental animals and humans (Anonymous, 1990).

Nickel is the most sensitising metallic agent for allergic contact dermatitis (Barrière et al., 1979; Hildebrand *et al.*, 1989a, b). It produces more allergic reactions than all other metals together.

9.3.11 PLATINUM GROUP ELEMENTS

The metals platinum, iridium, palladium, rhodium and ruthenium and their mineral salts have low toxic effects in humans. Sensitisation to these metals is known after occupational exposure in platinum refineries (Hildebrand *et al.*, 1996a). Holbrook *et al.* (1975) revealed some hepatotoxic effects in experimental animals treated with different soluble platinum and palladium salts. This study clearly shows that complex salts such as chloroplatinate and chloropalladosamine have a higher toxic effect than simple chlorides. The toxic action of $PdCl_2$ has also been assessed in mice and rats. The median lethal dose (LD_{50}) values for $PdCl_2$ exposure in mice were determined to be 87 mg kg^{-1} and more than 1000 mg kg^{-1} for intraperitoneal and oral exposure, respectively (Phielepeit *et al.*, 1989). Similar results were obtained on rats after exposure by different methods of administration (Moore *et al.*, 1975). This confirms a higher tolerance of $PdCl_2$ after ingestion than after injection. The low oral toxicity of palladium is comparable to that of molybdenum and this fact is important for the use of palladium in dental alloys.

9.3.12 SILVER

Silver is absorbed by the digestive, cutaneous and mucosal routes, and is retained in the reticuloendothelial system (Haguenoer and Furon, 1982; Merian, 1984). It is preferentially bound to collagen and other fibrillar structures such as the basal lamina of epithelia, endothelia and the sheaths of muscle, tendon and nerves. This was demonstrated by tissue analyses of gingival amalgam tattoos generated by dental amalgams (Eley, 1982; Eley and Garret, 1983; Véron et al., 1984, 1985).

The most evident clinical symptom of silver intoxication is argyrism giving rise to a grey–blue colour of the skin and mucosa. It may be accompanied by gastrointestinal problems, anorexia, anaemia, hepatic deficiency and respiratory insufficiency. The most toxic reactions are found with silver chloride and sulfate. Metallic silver alloyed with other metals, in particular with certain amounts of gold, does not show significant toxic effects.

9.3.13 TITANIUM

Titanium is not considered to be an essential element. Its normal tissue concentration in humans is 0.2 ppm. No clinical tissular toxicity has been observed, even at local concentrations higher than 2000 ppm (Toth et al., 1985). Schroeder et al. (1981) showed that titanium is biologically inert and it induces neither toxic nor inflammatory reactions in connective or epithelial tissues (Breme, 1989). Titanium is bacteriostatic (Elagli et al., 1992) and does not significantly activate or inhibit different enzyme systems specific for toxic reactions, e.g. β-glucuronidase, lactate dehydrogenase, glucose-6-phosphate dehyrogenase and acid phosphatase (Elagli et al., 1995). The real biological actions of titanium, if any, have not yet been established.

The excellent biological behaviour, the remarkable corrosion resistance (Bundy, 1994) and the bone-like elasticity of titanium justify its increasing use for biomaterials and as a component of medical and dental devices.

9.3.14 VANADIUM

The level of vanadium in the human organism is very low and normal values do not exceed 0.1 ppm. For some authors, vanadium has a positive effect on some physiological processes, e.g. growth, lipidic metabolism, bone and tooth mineralisation (Toth et al., 1985; Lagerkvist et al., 1986).

Other authors report strongly toxic effects of vanadium: it decreases coenzyme A and Q by liberating oxidative phosphorylation. Its interference with multiple enzyme systems may induce irreversible physiological perturbations (Macara, 1980). Its high solubility certainly contributes to its toxicity, which is estimated to be ten times higher than that of the Ni–Co–Cu group. The presence of low concentrations of vanadium (1–4%) in surgical alloys, e.g. Ti6Al4V, does not seem to induce major toxic or other unwanted biological reactions.

This controversy should stimulate more fundamental research in this field in order to assess the biological behaviour of vanadium. In *in vitro* cell-culture systems,

BIOLOGICAL RESPONSE AND BIOCOMPATIBILITY

titanium has been reported to be tolerated well (Cahoon and Regalbuto, 1975), but this is not so for vanadium, one of its main alloying elements (Yamage and Perren, 1983).

9.3.15 OTHER METALS

The physiological and biological behaviour of other metals, i.e. gallium, indium, niobium, selenium and tantalum, used in low concentrations in some alloys, is not well known. The few experiments performed and clinical and occupational observations have shown that they induce very low and insignificant toxic effects (Haguenoer and Furon, 1982; Merian, 1984).

The biocompatibility of gold no longer needs be emphasised (Hildebrand *et al.*, 1987). It is currently used as an immunological marker with reversible enzyme inhibition. Phagocytosed colloidal gold particles have no influence on cell metabolism and are easily extruded or rejected after the completion of *in vitro* experiments. Only some synthetic organic compounds, formerly applied for rheumatoid polyarthritis therapy, may produce some secondary effects. These compounds have almost totally disappeared from the pharmaceutical market (Sharp *et al.*, 1982).

Zinc is recognised as a highly essential element (Haguenoer and Furon, 1982; Merian, 1984). In zinc deficiency, nearly all physiological functions are strongly perturbed. Nevertheless, metallic zinc, owing to its reductive power, some salts and ZnO may generate *in vitro* toxic effects. Extremely high concentrations produce unwanted biological reactions in humans, i.e. zinc-fever during occupational inhalation of ZnO and metallic powder. This disease is reversible (Haguenoer and Furon, 1982).

ZnO favours wound healing and is therefore contained in multiple pharmaceutical ointments.

9.4 PRESENT KNOWLEDGE OF RISKS

The harm caused by the use of metallic alloys are essentially due to the release of ions resulting from the corrosion of these alloys. This concerns principally nickel, chromium and cobalt for any application, beryllium, cadmium, palladium, silver and copper for dental alloys, and titanium for stomatological and orthopaedic implants (Hildebrand *et al.*, 1995).

The second risk factor is wear, in particular produced by articular prostheses and mobile, non-stabilised implants generating wear particles by abrasion.

9.4.1 ION RELEASE

The ion release of ions from metallic prostheses and implants is the main origin of any unwanted primary or secondary reaction (Black, 1988), except for the electrogalvanic phenomena occurring in the oral cavity due to the presence of different dental alloys. In this case, the primary factor may be an electrochemically induced galvanoelectric current used by the saliva as a favourable saline electrolyte (Bundy, 1994).

9.4.1.1 Alloys for Surgical Implants

For several years increasing interest has been shown in the effects and reactions produced by ion release. Nevertheless, thoroughly conducted investigations of these phenomena are rare, and no systematic epidemiological and statistical study exists on this subject, although the high release of nickel, chromium and cobalt ions has generally been recognised. In some cases, 200–300-fold concentrations of maximum normal values could be demonstrated in body fluids and implants surrounding tissue (Hildebrand *et al.*, 1988, 1996b).

Cobalt seems to produce similar effects to those of nickel and chromium. Most authors agree that secondary harmful reactions are generated not directly by the presence of ions, but by their still scarcely known metabolites. The degree of oxidation and the formation of metallo-organic complexes may play an essential role, in particular for chromium, the primary ionic form of which after liberation is the trivalent ion. Its active toxic, allergenic and carcinogenic form, however, is the hexavalent ion (Bartolozzi and Black, 1985).

The alloy composition is less important than the physicochemical structure and characteristics, and the amount of ions released from CoCr alloys is similar to that liberated from stainless steel (Pazaglia *et al.*, 1987).

9.4.1.2 Dental Alloys

Regarding dental alloys, other metals have to be considered:

- cadmium, the toxic effects of which are generally recognised, in particular those of sulfides, oxides and metallo-organic compounds
- beryllium, unfortunately still contained in some dental alloys because mechanical qualities are improved by its presence. This metal is highly allergenic and toxic, and several cases of lung berylliosis have been reported in dental technicians working with alloys containing beryllium (Lob and Hugonnaud, 1977; Choudat, 1982; Choudat *et al.*, 1983)
- palladium, contained in semiprecious alloys, has provoked strong controversy concerning its innoxiousness or harmfulness. At present, there is no serious criterion justifying the anxiety concerning this metal (Hildebrand *et al.*, 1996a), except that it may induce a nickel concomitant allergic sensitisation. Very few cases of clinical manifestations such as allergic contact dermatitis or stomatitis have been reported.

9.4.2 WEAR PARTICLES

Wear particles produced by abrasion appear essentially in the vicinity of articular prostheses and of implants with a certain mobility, e.g. uncemented total hip replacements. These particles may induce multiple tissue reactions, including osteolysis, degradation of normal bone structure, severe macrophagic reactions, granuloma, fibrotic capsules, inflammatory and immune reactions, which may cause destabilisation and loosening of prostheses and implants (Sarmiento and Gruen, 1985; Dorr *et al.*, 1990; McKellop *et al.*, 1990; Weissman *et al.*, 1991).

An arthroplasty with different compounds may subsequently produce different wear particles, i.e. metallic, ceramic and polymeric. Generally, it seems to be admitted that:

- polymers and ceramics give rise to fewer problems than metals (Pazaglia et al., 1987)
- the size and form of the particles play an important role, with small or irregular particles being more active than larger or regular ones (Black, 1988; Dorr et al., 1990)
- alloys containing Co–Cr–Ni raise more concern than titanium alloys (Sarmiento and Gruen, 1985; McCutchen et al., 1990).

These differences are due to the physicochemical characteristics of alloys and their particles. The particles from Co–Cr–Ni alloys are continuously dissolved in the organism and undergo chemical modifications by the formation of precipitates or metallo-organic complexes, which have been demonstrated to bind calcium and, in particular, phosphorus or phosphates (Black, 1988; Hildebrand et al., 1988; Dorr et al., 1990).

Particles from titanium alloys, however, arise from the passivation layer of the implant and are not titanium ions, but mostly insoluble titanium oxides or suboxides, which are recognised to be biologically inert. Indeed, the passivation layer is immediately reformed after abrasion because of the high oxidability of titanium (some microseconds). This behaviour protects the alloy and prevents the formation of chemical compounds other than oxides. Some authors, however, do not believe in the innoxiousness of vanadium and aluminium contained in some titanium alloys with widespread application, e.g. Ti6Al4V (Hildebrand et al., 1988, Breme, 1989).

9.4.3 TISSULAR REACTIONS

Multiple investigations have been published reporting one or more tissular reactions in the vicinity of implants or prostheses. No systematic study exists allowing a statistical or epidemiological evaluation of these reactions relative to primary and/or secondary unwanted effects of metallic implants.

The most frequent injuries are certainly granulomas (particularly around Co–Cr–Ni alloys). These are characterised by a high density of collagen fibres and the presence of multinucleated giant cells (MGC, i.e. severe macrophage reaction), fibroblasts, plasmocytes, histocytes, etc. Benign granulomas generally contain precipitates conferring a black colour to the tissue. The evolution of granulomas may sometimes lead to the blockage of an articular prosthesis that requires surgical reintervention (Griffith et al., 1987; Nasser et al., 1990).

Some granulomas related to titanium implants have also been reported. The tissue contains multiple intracellular and extracellular particles, but very few inflammatory cells have been observed and most of the tissue reactions to titanium have no clinical consequences (Griffith et al., 1987; Nasser et al., 1990).

Another type of injury is the structural modification of bone. Osteosynthesis plates have been observed to be totally recovered by newly formed bone tissue after an exposure period of 3–4 years. The retrieval of such implants becomes particularly difficult (Hildebrand et al., 1988).

Numerous authors reported osteolysis, induced in most cases by non-cemented arthroplasties which always gain a certain mobility by mechanical solicitation during movement. The same phenomenon may arise for craniofacial (after resection of tumours) and unattached otological prostheses, which may potentially be mobilised.

Osteonecrosis is also observed, producing in some cases sclerosis of the bone–implant interface, known as metallosis. Two characteristics have to be emphasised with respect to metallosis:

- the frequency and the importance of necrosis, which in some cases may be total
- the simultaneous existence of a lymphocyte reaction. In some cases a real lymphoid islet beginning with a clear centre may appear inside the bone.

Thus different criteria have to be observed in order to improve the performance of metallic implants and cranofacial, otological and orthopaedic prostheses (Bischoff et al., 1994):

- unattached implants must remain immobile
- articular prostheses should be cemented
- tissue reactions must be lower than 5%
- the performance of an implant must be characterised by the absence of persistent or irreversible symptoms such as pain, infection and neuropathies.

Regarding dental non-precious alloys, multiple papers report lingual lesions, injuries to the oral mucosa in the form of stomatitis, cheilitis, tissular hypertrophy, oral redness, dryness, angular stomatitis, etc., without precisely identifying the aetiology of these pathologies as mechanical, bacterial, inflammatory, immunological, toxic or electrogalvanic (Hildebrand et al., 1989a, b, 1995; Bundy, 1994).

9.4.4 INFLAMMATORY REACTIONS

The majority of tissue reactions are of inflammatory origin. Most granulomas are provided with different inflammatory cell types, i.e. MGC, histiocytes, plasmocytes, mast cells and lymphocytes (Griffith et al., 1987; Nasser et al., 1990). In addition, neutrophilic polymorphonuclear cells frequently exhibit degranulation (Shanbhag et al., 1992).

The density, activity and function of these cells are controlled by endogenous mediators of inflammation, including histamine, prostaglandins, derivatives of the complement, lymphokines, cytokines and leukotrienes. This problem has been approached in very few investigations. Initial studies revealed the stimulation of prostaglandin E_2, interleukin-1 and collagenase (Dorr et al., 1990; Cook et al., 1991). These investigations are the first studies to consider the general effects induced by metals.

9.4.5 IMMUNOLOGICAL REACTIONS

The inflammatory and immunological symptomatologies are often very closely connected. Certain metals, especially iron, nickel and cobalt, have a well-known

BIOLOGICAL RESPONSE AND BIOCOMPATIBILITY

effect on lymphocyte proliferation as they stimulate the direct complements DC_2 and DC_3, which are implicated in this process. These rare studies provide precise and highly specific indications on metal action (Choudat et al., 1983; Bjurholm et al., 1990; Bravo et al., 1990).

9.4.5.1 Sensitisation and Allergy

Allergy was first defined as a pronounced reaction of an individual to a substance when that substance is reintroduced into the organism. This definition has been modified as immunological research has progressed. The sensitising substance, called the antigen, is a molecule or a cell which, once introduced into the organism, induces the formation of antibodies or specific defence cells. Coombs and Gell (1975) defined four different classes of allergy.

The allergic reactions caused by stainless steel or alloys containing Ni–Co–Cr are called contact dermatitis and belong to type IV of the classification cited above. For this form of allergy, the allergen or hapten is a substance with a low allergenic power (Dupuis and Benezra, 1982). It is at first strongly bound to certain endogenous proteins to form a stronger antigenic macromolecule. By a very simplified mechanism, the newly formed antigen is captured by macrophages and memorised by certain T-lymphocytes (Dupuis and Benezra, 1982).

After renewed contact the formerly sensitised lymphocytes produce different substances, e.g. lymphokines, which they liberate into the organism, thus provoking certain tissue reactions. The hypersensitive effect in contact dermatitis generally appears on the skin as eczema. Mucosal reactions and especially stomatitis are possible.

Allergies of type IV thus appear after cellular mediation and without the production of antibodies. For this reason desensitisation is not possible (Dooms-Gossens et al., 1980; Dupuis and Benezra, 1982; Hildebrand et al., 1989a, b). The immunological feature is called sensitisation or hypersensitisation, and one speaks of an allergy when clinical manifestations appear.

A large number of statistical and epidemiological investigations of contact dermatitis was performed to establish the frequency of allergies. Tables 9.1 and 9.2 summarise the data of a previous paper, in which more than 20 statistical studies of allergy in a consultant population (Table 9.1) and five statistical studies of the general population were reviewed (Table 9.2) (Hildebrand et al., 1989a).

9.4.5.2 Alloys for Surgical Implants

Scientific opinion is still divided on the allergic sensitisation of metals in patients with implants and endoprostheses. Several authors have demonstrated a direct relationship between metals contained in medical devices (Ni, Cr and Co) and allergic sensitisation, and draw particular attention to this concerning the use of these materials as implants in patients with prior sensitisation to these metals (Merrit and Brown, 1981; Rostoker et al., 1986; Black, 1988). Other authors, however, still repudiate any such relationship (Carlsson and Moller, 1989; Gawkrodger, 1993). By

Table 9.1 Statistical assessment of sensitisation to nickel, chromium and cobalt in the consultant population (%) (Hildebrand et al., 1989a)

Allergen	Reported cases	Male (%)	Female (%)	Total (%)
Nickel	37 849	3.1	12.9	9.6
Chromium	36 914	12.7	7.1	9.3
Cobalt	31 330	4.7	5.3	6.0

analysing the references cited by these authors, one can easily observe tendencious and unscientific behaviour regarding this problem. This becomes even more evident from the fact that in the literature several hundred cases are cited demonstrating a clear relationship between allergy and orthopaedic implants.

9.4.5.3 Dental Alloys

The relationship between allergy and metallic biomaterials has also been confirmed for alloys used in dentistry, i.e. nickel, chromium and cobalt in non-precious alloys (Hildebrand *et al.*, 1989a, b), and mercury and silver in dental amalgams (Vron *et al.*, 1986). The sensitising potency of palladium was long an unexplained phenomenon. Most investigations suggested a crossed hypersensitivity between nickel and palladium, i.e. a patient sensitised to nickel may react positively in a palladium allergy test. This would represent an extremely rare case of non-recognition of an antigen by a healthy and immunologically intact organism (Hildebrand *et al.*, 1996a).

Very recent studies have shown that palladium has its own sensitising potency, but the cross-reaction between nickel and palladium is still not excluded. In contrast to nickel sensitisation, it seems that sensitisation to palladium very rarely leads to clinical symptoms. Only a dozen cases of palladium hypersensitivity related to dental alloys have been described to date.

Table 9.2 Statistical assessment of sensitisation to nickel, chromium and cobalt in the general population (Hildebrand et al., 1989a)

Allergen	Reported cases	Male (%)	Female (%)	Total (%)
Nickel	3207	1.5	8.9	4.2
Chromium	822	2.0	1.5	1.7
Cobalt	758	1.0	1.6	1.4

9.4.6 CANCER INDUCEMENT

Although different cases of cancer in relation to orthopaedic implants and endoprostheses have been reported, there exists no statistical or epidemiological evidence of cancer caused by metals contained in implants (Laffargue *et al.*, 1997). Some cases were reported of malignant fibrous histiocytoma of bone arising at the site of metallic implants, plate and screws, hip prostheses, metallic foreign bodies from shrapnel fragments, etc. The causal relationship between metal implants in humans with this kind of tumour and other types such as Ewing's sarcoma, osteosarcoma, chondrosarcoma, fibrosarcoma, rhabdomyosarcoma, haemangiosarcoma and immunoblastic lymphoma is difficult to assess (Lee *et al.*, 1984; Sunderman, 1988, 1989b; Goodfellow, 1992; Jacobs *et al.*, 1992; Laffargue *et al.*, 1997). The observation of new cases has led in the last few years to an interest in establishing whether the association between orthopaedic implants and local malignancy is purely coincidental or represents real carcinogenic risks.

The carcinogenic feature of some metals is well known. Tumours arising at the site of metal implants were observed in experimental animals. Heath *et al.* (1971) showed that wear particles from prostheses made in CoCr alloys were carcinogenic for rat muscles. Sinibaldi *et al.* (1976) reported eight cases of bone sarcomas originating in close proximity to various metallic surgical implants used in the treatment of common canine and feline fractures.

In 1988, Sunderman reviewed the clinical and experimental evidence and appraised the carcinogenic hazards from implanted metal alloys containing nickel, chromium or cobalt. In the same paper, the author gives general background information on epidemiological evidence that certain occupational and environmental exposures to metal compounds are associated with excess cancer risks in both humans and experimental animals.

In addition, 24 cases have been reported of sarcomas developing in dogs around implanted orthopaedic pins, nails, plates and screws, mostly fabricated from stainless steel. Furthermore, local sarcomas have been observed in rodents after parenteral injection of metallic nickel or cobalt powders, but not after injection of metallic chromium powder. Since the metal powders release ions which undergo biological metabolism and oxidation, different nickel, cobalt and chromium compounds can be formed which have genotoxic and mutagenic effects. This has largely been demonstrated in *in vitro* tests and summarised in several review papers (Sunderman, 1988, 1989a, b; Anonymous, 1990).

The most frequently reported tumours in humans at the sites of metal implants are malignant fibrous histiocytoma, fibrosarcoma, osteosarcoma and rhabdomyosarcoma, with a description of at least 20 cases for each type (Mathiesen *et al.*, 1995). The same number (80–100 cases) can be estimated as the total of the other tumour types cited above (Laffargue *et al.*, 1997). Epidemiological studies (Anonymous, 1990) have shown that latent periods of less than 5 years cannot be associated with chemically induced tumours in humans. In the case of lower exposure periods, the association between malignancy and metal implants was probably coincidental. Longer periods of 7–44 years are consistent with a possible aetiological relationship between the metal implant and subsequent tumour development.

9.5 *IN VITRO* TOXICITY ASSESSMENT

Biological testing of medical and dental devices is necessary in order to evaluate the biological behaviour of biomaterials. Biocompatibility testing includes numerous methods starting with mechanical, physicochemical and electrochemical investigations, i.e. corrosion tests, from *in vitro* and *in vivo* tests such as implantation in animals and preclinical evaluation in humans to final clinical use in patients. Cytocompatibility is the *in vitro* adequate behaviour of cells in the presence of biomaterials, whereas cytotoxicity is the harmful or noxious unwanted effect induced by a biomaterial in cell-culture systems.

A scheme for *in vitro* cytotoxicity testing is defined by the International and European standards ISO 10993-5 (Standards, 1992) and EN 30993-5 (Standards, 1994), which make available a battery of tests, the choice of which depends on the nature of the sample to be evaluated, the potential site of use and the nature of use.

The numerous methods applied and the endpoints measured in cytotoxicity determination can be performed by either qualitative or quantitative means. The following examples and results on the cytotoxicity of metals and implantable alloys correspond to Section 8.5.1.b, Quantitative evaluation, of the above-mentioned standards:

> Measure cell death, inhibition of cell growth, cell proliferation or colony formation. The number of cells, amount of protein, release of enzyme, release of vital dye, reduction of vital dye or other measurable parameters may be quantified by objective means. The objective measure and response is recorded in the test report.

In the authors' laboratory, *in vitro* tests have been conducted on numerous alloys and pure metals to determine their effect on cell viability and their capacity to induce inflammatory reactions (Table 9.3).

9.5.1 CELL VIABILITY

Viability tests consisted of the establishment of the relative plating efficiency (RPE) and subsequently, the 50% lethal concentration LC_{50} (or RPE_{50}) by using the colony-forming method on human epithelial cells in culture (L132 cell-line). This test measures quantitatively only one criterion of toxicity, i.e. cell death or cell survival, and is subsequently specific, reliable and easily reproducible. It makes it possible to rank the cytotoxic effect of any chemical substance by comparison of the LC_{50} (Puck and Marcus, 1955; Frazier and Andrews, 1979).

9.5.1.1 Liability of Tests

The LC_{50} is the concentration, expressed in $\mu g\ ml^{-1}$ or $mg\ l^{-1}$, which produces 50% cell death in *in vitro* tests on different cell-culture systems. It should not be confused with the LD_{50}, which is the lethal dose of a substance inducing a 50% death rate of experimental animals or humans exposed to this substance by oral administration.

Table 9.3 Cytotoxic effects of pure metal and alloy powders on cell cultures of L132 cells

Pure metal or alloy	LC_{50} (µg ml^{-1})	Survival rates (%±SD) at 400 µg ml^{-1}	Multinucleated giant cells (%±SD)
Control	NO	100 ± 5	2.6 ± 0.7
Pt	NO	99 ± 3	ND
Sn	NO	91 ± 4	ND
In	NO	88 ± 4	ND
Ti	NO	81 ± 4	2.7 ± 0.7
Au	NO	78 ± 4*	2.7 ± 0.7
Pd	NO	68 ± 7*	2.8 ± 0.5
Cr	600	62 ± 3***	7.8 ± 1.9**
Cu	450	58 ± 6***	ND
Ag	75	32 ± 8***	16.0 ± 2.8***
Zn	25	NO	ND
Ni	25	NO	15.9 ± 2.6***
Co	20	NO	20.3 ± 4.9^a***
Al$_2$O$_3$	NO	95 ± 2	ND
Stainless steel	NO	72 ± 7*	9.1 ± 1.8**
NiCrCo	100	23 ± 8***	16.6 ± 3.3***
NiCrMo	75	14 ± 2***	15.7 ± 2.9***
Dental amalgam	20	NO	17.1 ± 2.1***
TiAl6V4	NO	98 ± 5	2.5 ± 0.8
TiAl5Fe2.5	NO	91 ± 6	2.5 ± 0.7
TiNb30	NO	60 ± 4***	2.6 ± 0.7
Pd79Au10	NO	95 ± 7	2.8 ± 0.5
Au75Pd19	NO	82 ± 3	2.9 ± 0.7
Au61Pd29	NO	82 ± 3	2.8 ± 0.6
Au32Ag31Pd8	NO	77 ± 5*	2.6 ± 0.6
Au50Ag27Pd14	NO	76 ± 4*	2.9 ± 0.7
Au36Pd50	NO	75 ± 9*	2.7 ± 0.5
Au6Ag51Pd18	200	41 ± 8***	2.9 ± 0.6
Ag32Pd57	200	38 ± 10***	14.4 ± 2.1***

LC_{50}, survival rates ($n = 8$) and frequency of multinucleated giant cells in cultures exposed to metal and alloy powders (100 µg ml^{-1}) for 8 days ($n = 5 \times 500$ cells) are given
^{a}25 µg ml^{-1}.
*$p < 0.05$, **$p < 0.01$, ***$p < 0.001$ with respect to controls.
NO, Not obtained; ND, not determined.

The LD_{50} is expressed in mg kg^{-1} or g kg^{-1} of a living organism and generally has higher values than the LC_{50}. The reason for this is the capacity of natural defence in a living organism by the interaction with different cell types in an organ and the active immune system primarily preventing cell injury and organ damage.

In cell-culture systems only one cell type normally exists, precluding any natural defence by an active immune system or the interaction with other cell types. There is a lack of systemic interaction and no provision for circulation. In addition, laboratories mostly use established cell lines which have reduced physiological responses, i.e. decreased enzymatic activities and energy production, and may under certain circumstances be considered as 'ghost cells'.

This problem can be avoided by the use of primary cultures obtained from the *in vitro* outgrowth of cells from a fresh biopsy. In these cultures, the physiological response is much more realistic, but they have the disadvantage that they rarely contain only one cell type and thus the biological response cannot be attributed to a specific cell. Moreover, the reproducibility of results is less reliable, since the physiological state of fresh primary cells may be different from that of their origin and depends on gender, age and other individual parameters. With this in mind, the choice of experiments requires good qualification and long experience on the part of the person responsible for making decisions, and it is sometimes necessary to perform different experiments to obtain better correlation of the results.

9.5.1.2 Influence of Metals on Cell Survival

Pure powders of platinum, tin, indium, gold and palladium exhibit an identical, excellent biological behaviour, and at extremely high concentrations (400 µg ml^{-1}) they still have a survival rate of 99–70% (Figure 9.1). Chromium, copper and silver have a medium cytotoxic effect, with a survival rate at the same high concentration of 60–30% (Figures 9.1 and 9.2), whereas cobalt, nickel and zinc induce rapid cell death, as expressed by a very low LC$_{50}$ (Figure 9.2). The survival rate at the highest concentration could not be obtained, since total cell death occurred for significantly lower concentrations.

Precious and semiprecious alloys, most Pd–base alloys, Ti–base alloys and stainless steel also produce excellent biological responses, with a survival rate of 98–70% at the highest concentration. Two semiprecious alloys with a high silver content reflect the cytotoxic effect of pure silver (Figure 9.1). NiCr alloys (14% and 23%) induce a strong cytotoxic action and dental amalgams produce total cell death at very low concentrations. The compound Al$_2$O$_3$ was added to these test series for comparative purposes in order to emphasise its excellent cytocompatibility (Figure 9.1).

9.5.1.3 Influence of Metals on the Inflammatory Response

MGC normally appear in cultures of macrophages through the fusion of individual cells. Established cell-lines generally exhibit a low percentage of 2–5% binucleated or multinucleated cells. MGC may appear not only in cellular or organotypic cultures (Ziats *et al.*, 1988), but also *in vivo* in patients with amalgam tattoos (Buchner and Hansen, 1980; Véron *et al.*, 1985, 1986) or orthopaedic implants (Hildebrand *et al.*, 1988). They are characteristic constituents of granulomas in the vicinity of implants and their presence is generally considered to be a specific inflammatory response (Buchner and Hansen, 1980; Veron *et al.*, 1986; Hildebrand *et al.*, 1988; Ziats *et al.*, 1988).

The test of inflammatory reactions consisted of quantifying the MGC in monolayer cell cultures of L132 cells. This test reveals morphological modifications in a cell culture by the appearance of MGC, which are directly related to physiological, i.e. functional, alterations to the cells.

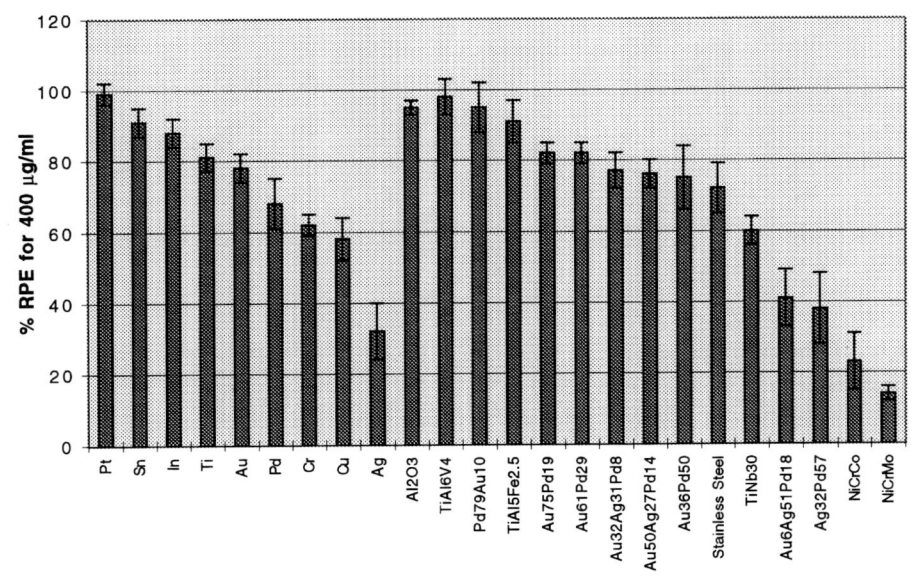

Figure 9.1 Survival rates (RPE %±SD) of L132 cells cloned in the continuous presence of an extremely high powder concentration (400 µg ml^{-1}) of pure metals and multiple dental and orthopaedic alloys. Al$_2$O$_3$ was added to this series for comparative purposes. The control culture is 100%.

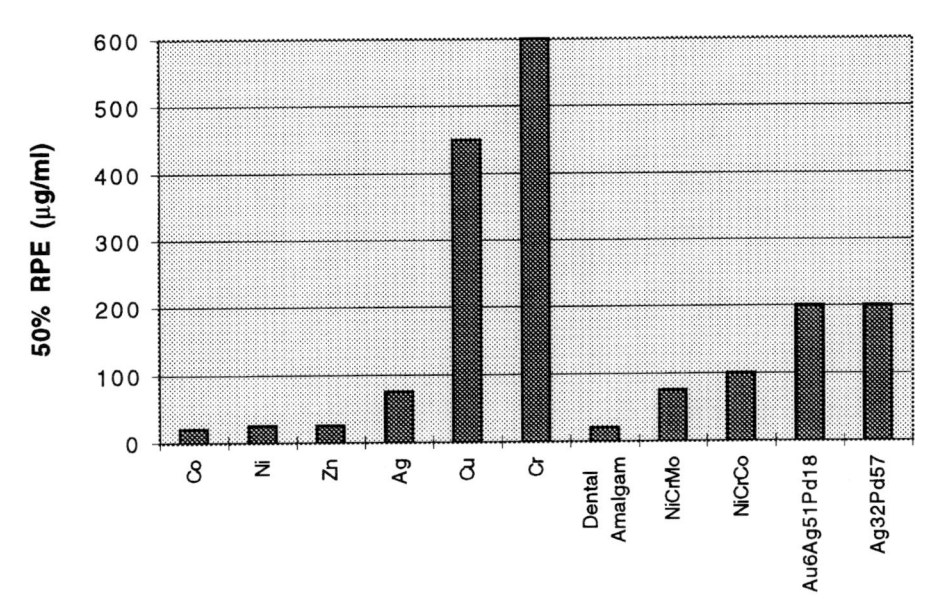

Figure 9.2 Fifty per cent lethal concentrations (RPE$_{50}$) determined for pure metals and alloys.

The MGC test confirmed the quasi-perfect cytocompatibility of the palladium, gold and titanium powders and of alloys containing these metals, since the number of MGC in exposed cultures was identical to that in control cultures (Table 9.3; Figures 9.3 and 9.4). However, cultures exposed to pure nickel, cobalt, silver, and to nickel-rich alloys and dental amalgams developed eight- to 10-fold increases in MGC compared with control cultures (Table 9.3; Figures 9.3 and 9.5). The inflammatory effect of silver is confirmed in the Ag32Pd57 alloy. Stainless steel without a major influence on cell viability induces inflammatory reactions comparable to those produced by chromium.

9.6 CONCLUSIONS

Wear particles and metal ions released from dental and surgical alloys can be recovered in the human organism, i.e. in urine, blood, plasma, nails, hair and tissues surrounding an implant, and they may induce not only allergic reactions, but also immune and inflammatory reactions, the strength of which remains underestimated. This has been demonstrated by numerous investigations.

Precious and semiprecious dental alloys, with rare exceptions, are generally recognised to be harmless and perfectly biocompatible. Ti–base alloys seem to fulfil all mechanical, clinical and biological requirements.

There is no evidence for the inducement of cancer by dental alloys, but

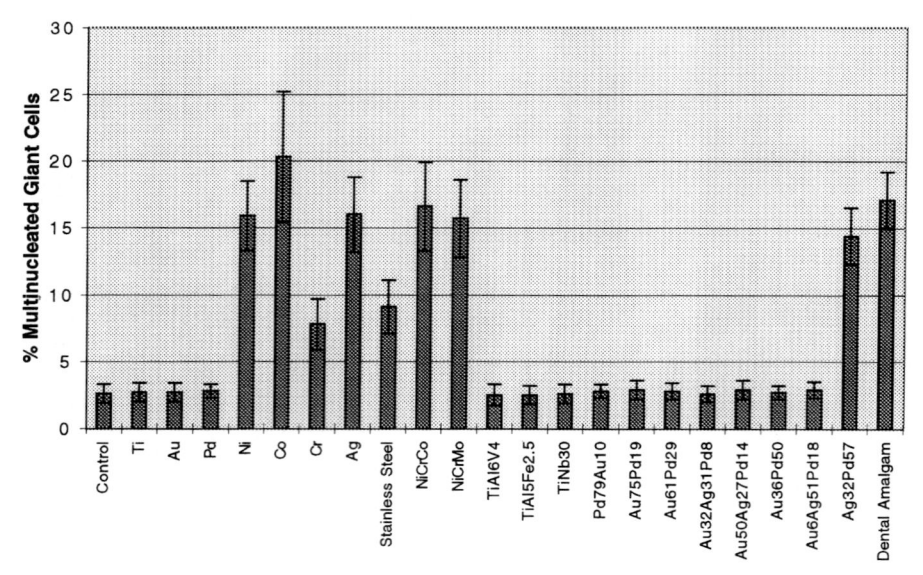

Figure 9.3 Frequency (% ± SD) of MGC induced in L132 cells exposed to pure metals and alloy powders (100 μg ml^{-1}) for 8 days. The values were established by counting 500-cell areas in five different experiments.

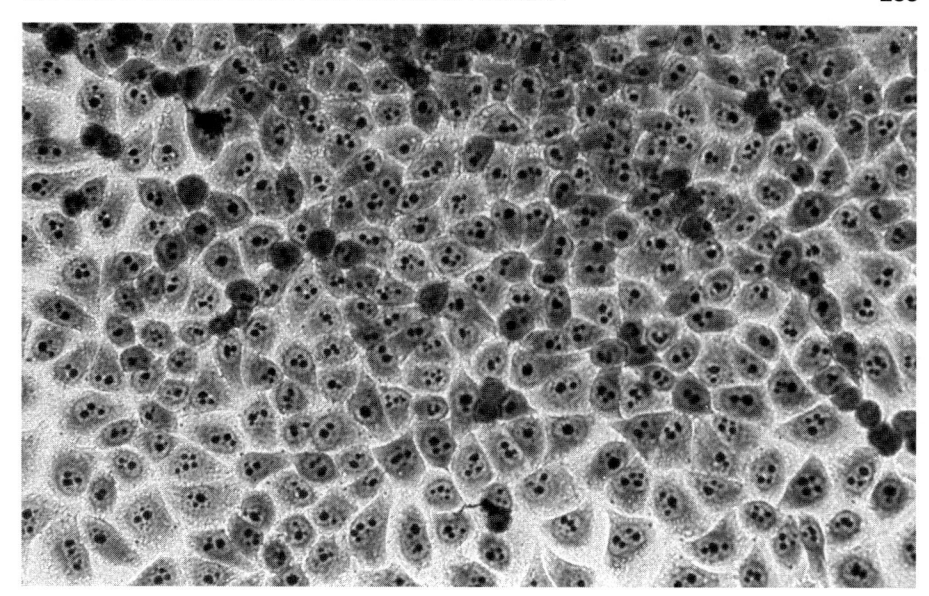

BIOLOGICAL RESPONSE AND BIOCOMPATIBILITY 285

Figure 9.4 Typical feature of L132 cells corresponding to either control cultures, cultures exposed to gold, palladium or titanium, or precious, semiprecious and Ti–base alloys.

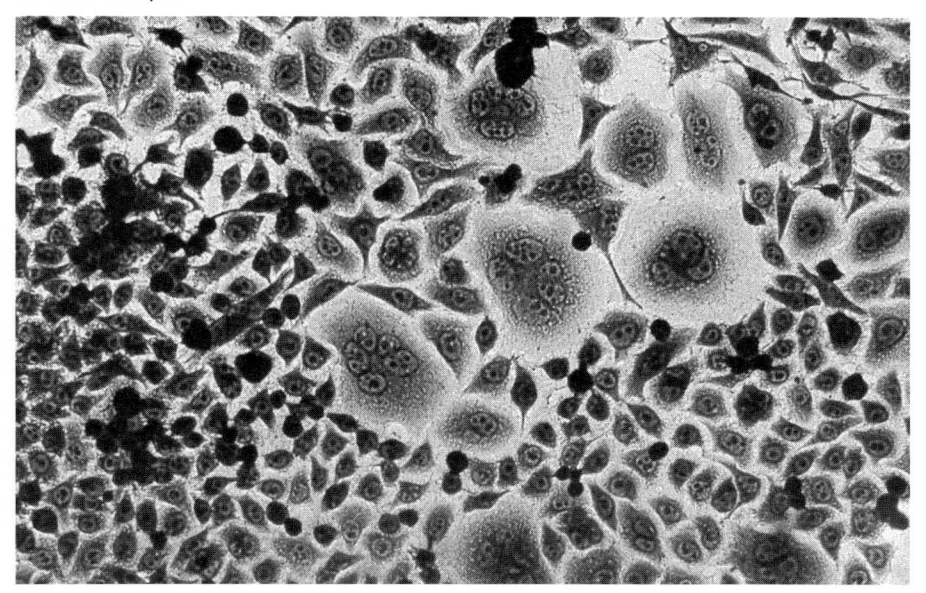

Figure 9.5 Typical feature of L132 cells grown in the presence of powders of pure nickel or cobalt, dental amalgam, NiCr-containing alloys or alloys with high amounts of silver. Note the presence of a large number of MGC, indicating an inflammatory reaction.

orthopaedic implants and endoprostheses with evidently higher metal release may cause different types of tumours, as is reported in several hundred cases.

Some metals should definitely be prohibited. These are beryllium, which is still used in some dental alloys, and nickel, which appears to be one of the worst metals used in biomaterials.

When considering metal-induced pathologies, one should be careful not to confuse the metallic element in its chemical zero state with its salts, oxides and organic complexes, as these may induce strongly different responses and the toxic potency of different ions or compounds varies by two to three orders of magnitude. Vanadium chloride is extremely toxic, but low amounts of metallic vanadium do not seem to induce major unwanted biological effects. Metals such as silver and zinc, in the zero state, no longer exhibit a toxic action in an alloyed state. A low zinc release may even be used favourably by the human body.

Particular attention must be given to any metallic biomaterial or medical device. Both known and new devices should be submitted to continuous medical survey in order to avoid potential unfavourable tissue reaction as early as possible.

REFERENCES

Aitio, A., Aro, A., Järvisalo, J. and Vainio, H. (1991) *Trace Elements in Health and Disease*, Royal Society of Chemistry, London.

Anke, M., Kronemann, H., Groppel, B., Henning, A., Meissner, D. and Schneider, H.J. (1980) The influence of nickel deficiency on growth, reproduction, longevity and different biochemical parameters of goats, in *3-Spurenelement Symposium, Nickel* (eds M. Anke, H.J. Schneider and C. Bruckner), Wiss. Beitr. Karl-Marx-Univ., Leipzig and Friedr-Schiller-Univ., Jena, pp. 3–10.

Anonymous (1990) Report of the International Committee on Nickel Carcinogenesis in Man, *Scand. J. Work Environ. Hlth* **16**, 1–82

Arsalane, K., Aerts, C., Wallaert, B., Voisin, C. and Hildebrand, H.F. (1992) Effects of nickelhydroxycarbonate on alveolar macrophage functions, *J. Appl. Toxicol.* **12**, 285–90.

Barrière, H., Boiteau, H.L., Geraut, C. and Metayer, C. (1979) Allergie aux détergents et allergie au nickel, *Ann. Derm. Vener.* **106**, 33–7.

Bartolozzi, A. and Black, J. (1985) Chromium concentrations in serum, blood clot and urine from patients following total hip arthroplasty, *Biomaterials* **6**, 2–8.

Bergman, M., Bergman, B. and Söremark, R. (1980) Tissue accumulation of nickel released due to electrochemical corrosion of non-precious dental alloys, *J. Oral Rehab.* **7**, 325–30.

Bischoff, U.W., Freeman, M.A.R., Smith, D., Tuke, M.A. and Gregson, P.J. (1994) Wear induced by motion between bone and titanium or cobalt–chrome alloys, *J. Bone Joint Surg.* **76-B**, 713–16.

Bjurholm, A., Al-Tawil, N.A., Marcusson, J.A. and Netz, P. (1990) The lymphocyte response to nickel salt in patients with orthopedic implants, *Acta Orthop. Scand.* **61**, 248–50.

Black, J. (1988) *In vivo* corrosion of a cobalt–base alloy and its biological consequences, in *Biocompatibility of Co–Cr–Ni Alloys,* Vol. 158 (eds H.F. Hildebrand and M. Champy), NATO-ASI Series A, Plenum, New York, pp. 83–100.

Bradley, C.A. (1981) Biological properties of aluminium, in *Systemic Aspects of Biocompatibility* (ed. D.F. Williams), CRC Press, Boca Raton, FL, pp. 187–209.

Bradley, E. (1994) Ti-8Mn, in *Material Properties Handbook: Titanium Alloys*, ASM International, Materials Park, OH, pp. 755–63.

Bravo, I., Carvalho, G.S., Barbosa, M.A. and De Sousa, M. (1990) Differential effects of eight metal ions on lymphocyte differentiation antigens *in vitro*, *J. Biomed. Mater. Res.* **24**, 1059–68.

Breme, J. (1989) Titanium and titanium alloys, biomaterials of preference, Mémoires et Études Scientifiques, *Rev. Métall.* Octobre, 625–38.

Breme, J. (1994) Ti–5Al–2,5Fe, in *Material Properties Handbook: Titanium Alloys*, ASM International, Materials Park, OH, pp. 737–46.

Breme, J., and Wadewitz, V. (1989) Comparison of titanium–tantalum and titanium–niobium alloys for application as dental implants, *Int. J. Maxillo-Fac. Implant.* **4**, 113–18.

Brown, S.S. and Savory, J. (1983) *Chemical Toxicology and Clinical Chemistry of Metals*, Academic Press, New York.

Buchner, A. and Hansen, L.S. (1980) Amalgam pigmentation (amalgam tattoo) of the oral mucosa: a clinico-pathologic study of 268 cases, *Oral Surg.* **49**, 139–47.

Bundy, K.J. (1994) Corrosion and other electrochemical aspects of biomaterials, *Crit. Rev. Biomed. Engng* **22**, 139–251.

Cahoon, J.R. and Regalbuto, C. (1975) Electrochemical behaviour of some commercial dental amalgams in artificial saliva, *Biomater. Med. Dev. Artif. Org.* **3**, 411–23.

Carlsson, A. and Moller, H. (1989) Implantation of orthopaedic devices in patients with metal allergy, *Acta Deratol. Venerol. (Stockh.)* **69**, 62–6.

Choudat, D. (1982) Pathologie pulmonaire et prothésistes dentaires, *Inform. Dent.* **64**, 4157–60.

Choudat, D., Brochard, P., Lebas, F.X., Marsac, J. and Philibert, H. (1983) Sarcoïdose ou pneumoconiose? Coincidence ou relation, *Arch. Mal. Prof.* **44**, 339–44.

Cook, S.D., Mccluskey, L.C., Martin, P.C. and Haddad, R.J. (1991) Inflammatory response in retrieved noncemented porous-coated implants. *Clin. Orthoped. Relat. Res.* **264**, 209–22.

Coombs, R.R. and Gell, P.H.G. (1975) Classification of allergic reactions responsible for clinical hypersensitivity and diseases, in *Clinical Aspects of Immunology* (eds P.H.G. Gell, R.R. Coombs and P.J. Lachman), Blackwell Scientific Publications, Oxford, p. 761.

Dooms-Gossens, A., Ceuterick, A., Vanmaele, N. and Degreef, H. (1980) Follow-up study of patients with contact dermatitis caused by chromates, nickel and cobalt, *Dermatologica (Basel)* **160**, 249–60.

Dorr, L.D., Bloebaum, R., Emmanual, J. and Meldrum, R. (1990) Histologic, biochemical and ion analysis of tissue and fluids retrieved during total hip arthroplasty, *Clin. Orthoped. Relat. Res.* **261**, 82–95.

Dupuis, G. and Benezra, C. (1982) *Allergic Contact Dermatitis to Simple Chemicals*, Marcel Decker, New York.

Elagli, K., Neut, C., Romond, C. and Hildebrand, H.F. (1992) *In vitro* effects of titanium powder on oral bacteria, *Biomaterials* **13**, 25–7.

Elagli, K., Veron, C. and Hildebrand, H.F. (1995) Titanium induced enzyme activation on murine peritoneal macrophages in primary culture, *Biomaterials* **16**, 1345–51.

Eley, B.M. (1982) Tissue reactions to implanted dental amalgam including assessment by energy dispersive X-ray microanalysis, *J. Pathol.* **18**, 251–72.

Eley, B.M. and Garret, J.R. (1983) Tissue reactions to the separate implantation of individual constituent phases of dental amalgam including assessment by energy dispersive X-ray microanalysis, *Biomaterials* **4**, 73–80.

Frazier, M.E. and Andrews, T.K. (1979) *In vitro* clonal growth assay for evaluating toxicity of metal salts, in *Trace Metals in Health and Disease* (ed. N. Kharasch), Raven Press, New York, pp. 71–81.

Gawkrodger, D.J. (1993) Nickel sensitivity and the implantation of orthopaedic prostheses, *Contact Derm.* **28**, 257–9.

Giroux, E.L. and Henkin, R.I. (1973) Macromolecular ligands of exchangeable copper, zinc and cadmium in human serum, *Bioinorg. Chem.* **2**, 125–33.

Goodfellow, J. (1992) Editorial: Malignancy and joint replacements, *J. Bone Joint Surg.* **74B**, 645.
Griffith, H.J., Burke, J. and Bonfiglio, T.A. (1987) Granulomatous pseudotumors in total joint replacement, *Skel. Radiol.* **16**, 146–52.
Haguenoer, J.M. and Furon, D. (1982) *Toxicologie et Hygiéne Industrielle, Les Dérivés Minéraux*, Vols I and II, Technique et Documentation, Paris.
Hasan, F.M. and Kazemi, H. (1974) Chronic beryllium disease: a continuing epidemiological hazard, *Chest* **65**, 289–93.
Heath, J.C., Freeman, M.A.M.R. and Swanson, S.A.V. (1971) Carcinogenic properties of wear particles from prostheses made in cobalt–chromium alloy, *Lancet* 564–566.
Herlant-Peers, M.C., Hildebrand, H.F. and Biserte, G. (1982) ^{63}Ni(II)-incorporation into lung and liver cytosol of Balb/C mouse. An *in vitro* and *in vivo* study, *Zbl. Bakt. Hyg.*, *I Abt. Orig.* **B176**, 368–82.
Herlant-Peers, M.C., Hildebrand, H.F. and Kerckaert, J.P. (1983) *In vitro* and *in vivo* incorporation of Ni(II) into lung and liver subcellular fractions of Balb/C mice, *Carcinogenesis* **4**, 387–92.
Hildebrand, H.F., Decaestecker, A.M. and Véron, C. (1987) L'or: mise au point sur sa tolérance et sa biocompatibilité, *Rev. Franç. Prothés. Dent.* **90**, 50–60.
Hildebrand, H.F., Floquet, I., Lefèvre, A. and Véron, C. (1996a) Biological and hepatotoxic effects of palladium. An overview on experimental investigations and personal studies, *Int. J. Risk Safety Med.* **8**, 149–67.
Hildebrand, H.F., Laffargue, P., Decoulx, J., Duquennoy, A. and Mestdagh, H. (1996b) Retrieval analyses of total hip replacements, *Int. J. Risk Safety Med.* **8**, 125–34.
Hildebrand, H.F., Mercier, J.F., Herlant-Peers, M.C. and Haguenoer, J.M. (1986a) *In vivo* and *in vitro* incorporation of Ni and Cr in lung and liver, in *Proceedings of the International Conference on Health Hazards and Biological Effects of Welding Fumes*, Elsevier, Amsterdam, pp. 341–4.
Hildebrand, H.F., Ostapczuk, P., Mercier, J.F., Stoeppler, M., Roumazeille, B. and Decoulx, J. (1988) Orthopaedic implants and corrosion products, in *Biocompatibility of CoCr–Ni Alloys*, Vol. 158 (eds H.F. Hildebrand and M. Champy), NATO-ASI Series A, Plenum, New York, pp. 133–53.
Hildebrand, H.F., Véron, C., Elagli, K. and Donazzan, M. (1995) Réactions tissulaires au port des appareils de prothèse dentaire partielle ou totale, *Encycl. Méd. Chir. (Paris), Stomatol.-Odontol II*, 23-325-P-10, 7 pp.
Hildebrand, H.F., Véron, C. and Martin, P. (1986b) Amalgames dentaires et allergie, *J. Biol. Buccale.* **14**, 83–100.
Hildebrand, H.F., Véron, C. and Martin, P. (1989a) Nickel, chromium, cobalt dental alloys and allergic reactions: an overview, *Biomaterials* **10**, 545–8.
Hildebrand, H.F., Véron, C. and Martin, P. (1989b) Les alliages dentaires en métaux non précieux et l'allergie, *J. Biol. Buccale.* **17**, 227–43.
Holbrook, D.J., Jr, Washington, M.E., Leake, H.B. and Brubaker P.E. (1975) Studies on the evaluation of the toxicity of various salts of lead, manganese, platinum and palladium, *Environ. Hlth Persp.* **10**, 95–101.
IARC (1973) *Monographs on the Evaluation of Carcinogenic Risk of Chemicals to Man*, Vol. 2, IARC, Lyon.
Jacobs, J.J., Rosenbaum, D.H., Hay, R.M., Gitelis, S. and Black, J. (1992) Early sarcomatous degeneration near a cementless hip replacement. A case report and review, *J. Bone Joint Surg.* **74B**, 740–4.
Labat, B. and Chamson, F.J. (1995) Effects of alpha-alumina and hyroxiapatite coatings on the growth and metabolism of human osteoblasts, *J. Biomed. Mater. Res.* **29**, 1397–401.
Laffargue, P., Hildebrand, H.F., Lecomte-Houcke, M., Biehl, V., Breme, J. and Decoulx, J. (1998) Malignant fibrous histiocytoma in association with a metal implant: analysis of corrosion products and their possible role in malignancy, *Int. J. Risk Safety Med.* (in press)

Lagerkvist, B., Nordberg, G.F. and Vouk, V. (1986) Vanadium, in *Handbook on the Toxicology of Metals* (eds L. Friberg, G.F. Nordberg and V. Vouk), Elsevier Science, Amsterdam, pp. 638–63.
Lee, Y.S., Pho, R.W.H. and Nather, A. (1984) Malignant fibrous histiocytoma at site of metal implant, *Cancer* **54**, 2286–9.
Lob, M. and Hugonnaud, C. (1977) Pathologie pulmonaire, *Arch. Mal. Prof.* **38**, 543–9.
Macara, I.G. (1980) Vanadium, an element in search of a role, *Trends Biochem. Sci.* **5**, 92–5.
Mancuso, T.F. (1970) Relation of duration of employment and prior respiratory illness to respiratory cancer among beryllium workers, *Environ. Res.* **3**, 251–75.
Mathiesen, E.B., Ahlbom, A., Berman, G. and Lindgren, J.U. (1995) Total hip replacements and cancer: a cohort study, *J. Bone Joint Surg.* **77B**, 345–50.
Marcussen, P.V. (1957) Occupational nickel dermatitis. Rise in incidence and prevention. *Acta Derm. Venereol. (Stockh.)* **2**, 289–95.
McCutchen, J.W., Collier, J.P. and Mayor, M.B. (1990) Osseointegration of titanium implants in total hip arthroplasty *Clin. Orthoped. Relat. Res.* **261**, 114–25.
McKellop, H.A., Sarmiento, A., Schwinn, C.P. and Ebramzadeh, E. (1990) In vivo wear of titanium-alloy hip prostheses, *J. Bone Joint Surg.* **72A**, 512–17.
Merian, E. (1984) *Metalle in der Umwelt: Verteilung, Analytik und biologische Relevanz*, Verlag Chemie, Weinheim.
Merrit, K. and Brown, S.A. (1981) Metal sensitivity reactions to orthopedic implants, *Int. J. Dermatol.* **20**, 89–94.
Moore, W., Hysell, D., Hall, L., Campbell, K. and Stara, J. (1975) Preliminary studies on the toxicity and metabolism of palladium and platinum. *Environ. Hlth Persp.* **10**, 63–71.
Nasser, S., Campbell, P.A., Kilgus, D., Kossovsky, N. and Amstutz, H.C. (1990) Cementless total joint arthroplasty prostheses with titanium-alloy articular surfaces: a human retrieval analysis, *Clin. Orthped. Relat. Res.* **261**, 171–85.
Parker, K. and Sunderman, F.W., Jr (1974) Distribution of ^{63}Ni in rabbit tissues following intravenous injection of ^{63}NiCl$_2$, *Res. Commun. Chem. Path. Pharmac.* **7**, 755–62.
Pazaglia, U.E., Dell'orbo, C. and Wilkinson, M.J. (1987) The foreign body reaction in total hip arthroplasties: a correlated light-microscopy, SEM, and TEM study, *Arch. Orthop. Trauma Surg.* **106**, 209–19.
Phielepeit, T., Legrum, W., Netter, K.J., and Klotzer W.T. (1989) Different effects of intraperitoneally and orally administered palladium chloride on the hepatic monooxygenase system of male mice *Arch. Toxicol.* Suppl. 13, 357–62.
Puck, T.T. and Marcus, P.I. (1955) A rapid method for viable cell titration and clone production with HeLa cells in tissue culture: the use of X irradiated cells to supply conditioning factors, *Proc. Natn. Acad. Sci. USA* **41**, 432–7.
Reeves, A.L. and Vorwald, A.J. (1967) Beryllium carcinogenesis II – pulmonary deposition and clearance of inhaled beryllium sulfate in the rat, *Cancer Res.* **27**, 446–541.
Reeves, A.L., Deitch, D. and Vorwald, A.J. (1967) Beryllium carcinogenesis I – inhalation exposure of rats to beryllium sulfate aerosol, *Cancer Res.* **27**, 439–45.
Rostoker, G., Robin, J., Binet, O. and Paupe, J. (1986) Dermatoses d'intolérance aux métaux des matériaux d'ostéosynthése et des prothèses (nickel–chrome–cobalt), *Ann. Dermatol. Venerol.* **113**, 1097–108.
Sarmiento, A. and Gruen, T.A. (1985) Radiographic analysis of a low-modulus titanium-alloy femoral total hip component. Two to six year follow up, *J. Bone Joint Surg.* **67A**, 48–56.
Schroeder, A., van der Zypen, E., Stoch, H. and Sutter, F. (1981) The reaction of bone connective tissue and epithelium to endosteal implants with titanium sprayed surfaces, *J. Maxillofac. Surg.* **9**, 15–25.
Shanbhag, A., Yang, J., Lilien, J. and Black, J. (1992) Decreased neutrophil respiratory burst on exposure to cobalt–chrome alloy and polystyrene *in vitro*, *J. Biomed. Mater. Res.* **26**, 185–95.
Sharp, J.T., Lidsky, M.D. and Duffy, J. (1982) Clinical response during gold therapy for rheumatoid arthritis, *Arthrit. Rheum.* **25**, 540–9.

Shirali, P., Teissier, E., Marez, T., Hildebrand, H.F. and Haguenoer, J.M. (1994) Effect of Ni_3S_2 on arachidonic acid metabolites in cultured human lung cells, *Carcinogenesis* **15**, 759–62.
Sinibaldi, K., Rosen, H., Liu, S.K. and Deangelis, M. (1976) Tumors associated with metallic implants in animals, *Clin. Orthop.* **118**, 257–66.
Standards ISO 10993-5 (1992) and EN 30993-5 (1994) Biological testing of medical and dental devices. Tests for cytotoxicity: *in vitro* methods.
Sunderman, F.W., Jr (1988) Carcinogenic risks of metal implant and prostheses, in *Biocompatibility of Co–Cr–Ni Alloys*, Vol. 158 (eds H.F. Hildebrand and M. Champy), NATO-ASI Series A, Plenum, New York, pp. 11–19.
Sunderman, F.W., Jr (1989a) Mechanisms of nickel carcinogenesis, *Scand. T. Work Environ. Hlth* **15**, 1–2.
Sunderman, F.W., Jr (1989b) Carcinogenicity of metal alloys in orthopedic prostheses: clinical and experimental studies, *Fund. Appl. Toxicol.* **13**, 20–216.
Toth, R.W., Parr, G.R. and Gardner, L.K. (1985) Soft tissue response to endosseous titanium oral implants, *J. Prosth. Dent.* **54**, 546–67.
Undreicka, R., Ginter, E. and Kortus, J. (1966) Chronic toxicity of aluminium in rats and mice and its effects on phosphorus metabolism, *Br. J. Ind. Med.* **23**, 305–11.
Véron, C., Hildebrand, H.F. and Fernandez, J.P. (1984) Les pigmentations gingivales par l'amalgame dentaire: étude ultrastructurale, *J. Biol. Buccale.* **12**, 273–86.
Véron, C., Hildebrand, H.F., and Fernandez, J.P. (1985) Les pigmentations gingivales par l'amalgame dentaire: étude ultrastructurale et microanalyse, *J. Biomat. Dent.* **1**, 47–52.
Véron, C., Hildebrand, H.F. and Martin, P. (1986) Les amalgames dentaires et l'allergie, *J. Biol. Buccale.* **14**, 83–100.
Wall, L. and Calnan, C.D. (1980) Occupational nickel dermatitis in the electroforming industry, *Contact Derm.* **6**, 414–20.
Weissman, B.N., Scott, R.D., Bridk, G.W. and Corson, J.M. (1991) Radiographic detection of metal-induced synovitis as a complication of arthroplasty of the knee, *J. Bone Joint Surg.* **73A**, 1002–7.
Williams, D.F. (1981) Toxicology of implanted metals, in *Fundamental Aspects of Biocompatibility*, Vol. II (ed. D.F. Williams), CRC Press, Boca Raton, FL, pp. 1–10.
Yamage, M. and Perren, S.M. (1983) Influence of metal chlorides on DNA synthesis of human blood lymphocytes, in *Transactions of the 9th Annual Meeting of the Society for Biomaterials*, Society for Biomaterials, Minneapolis, p. 72.
Zakour, R.A., Loeb, L.A., Kunkel, T.A. and Koplitz, R.M. (1979) Metals, DNA polymerization, and genetic miscoding, in *Trace Metals in Health and Disease* (ed. N. Kharasch), Raven Press, New York, pp.135–5.
Ziats, N.P., Miller, K.M. and Anderson, J.M. (1988) *In vitro* and *in vivo* interactions of cells with biomaterials, *Biomaterials* **9**, 5–13.

10
Tissue–implant interaction

R. THULL
University of Würzburg, Würzburg, Germany

10.1 INTRODUCTION

Some materials in dental and orthopaedic implants, in particular spontaneously passivating metals of groups 4b and 5b of the periodic table of elements show a close connection to the force-transmitting tissue and are virtually free of reactions with recognition cells of the immunological system. This behaviour, sometimes indicated as integration, is based on the oxide layer arising spontaneously on the surfaces of passivating metals within the extracellular fluid. This property and some other physicochemical properties are important sources of biocompatibility. Causes of tissue reactions around alloplastic materials are identified as cell-mediated hypersensitivity to an implant component and tissue modifications due to the presence of wear particles, debris and corrosion products of the prostheses used. Refractory metals used for implants, such as titanium, zirconium, niobium, tantalum and their alloys, as well as ceramic materials, are characterised by very low disintegration rates and prompt and justify the question of how physicochemical communication between material surfaces and the extracellular matrix actually occurs (Figure 10.1).

The interaction between the surface of the implant and the body's electrolytes begins with the adsorption of charged ions and polarisable molecules, such as water molecules or biological macromolecules. Through forces of attraction and repulsion and the exchange of charge carriers, as electrons for metals or electrons and holes for semiconducting coatings, reactive and reversible or irreversible and structural changes to adsorbed substances can take place. In particular, in organic macromolecules intramolecular and intermolecular bonds, together with oxygen bridge bonds, may break down, giving rise to structural or conformational changes, or both. The degree to which this process is reversible will depend on, for example, in the case of proteins, whether the peptide chains are destroyed, or whether disulfide bridges have detached to form cysteinyl residues.

Conformational changes may arise as a result of an exchange of charge carriers between the surface of the biomaterial and the biological macromolecules. However, changes can also be initiated by high field strengths, such as occur as a result of the

---

Metals as Biomaterials ISBN 0 471 96935 4 Edited by J.A. Helsen and H.J. Breme. © 1998 John Wiley & Sons Ltd

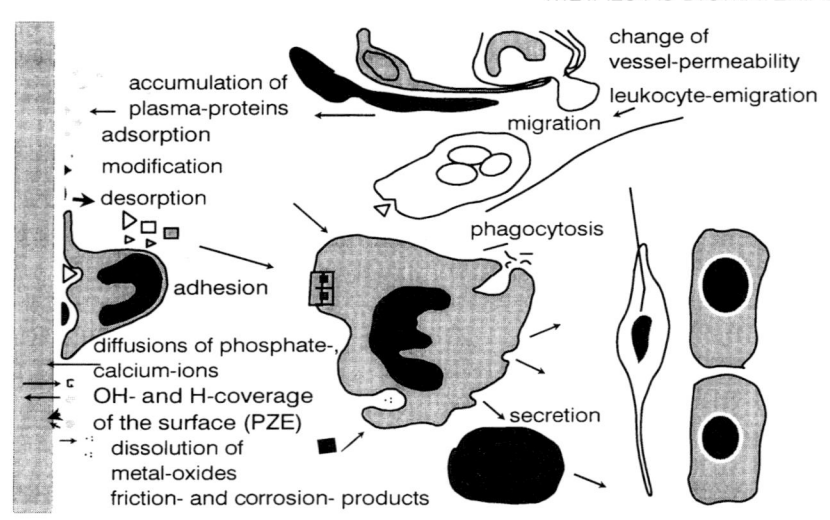

Figure 10.1 Overview of the complex reactions at the surface of passivated metal biomaterials (Thomsen *et al.*, 1991). The initial adsorption pattern and conformational changes to constituents of the formed biofilm will be influenced by the physicochemical properties of the implant surface.

presence of local elements, in particular semiconductive or non-conductive surfaces layers.

A conception for the actual changes in the protein molecule during the adsorption process is not yet available, but these changes could be similar to those occurring if the pH value of the surrounding electrolyte is changing. The adsorption of hydrogen ions or hydroxyl groups leads to changed potential gradients at the surface of the protein comparable with the potential gradient within the biomaterial–electrolyte interface and may result in:

- hydrogen binding of the protein (pH 3.6–3.9), expansion of the molecule (Tanford, 1952), N–F transition (Foster and Aoki, 1957) and masking of the carboxylate groups in the N-state. Masking occurs as ion pairs (Vijai and Foster, 1967). It seems safe to conclude that the N–F transition involves the rupture of a number of ion-pair bonds
- hydroxyl-ion binding of the protein (pH 7–9), minor anomalies in the titration of hystidyl residues (Decker and Foster, 1967) and demasking of imidazolium residues in histidyl titration (Harmsen *et al.*, 1971). Calcium ions favour the N–B transition (Zurawski and Foster, 1974) and B binds more calcium than does the N form (Pedersen, 1972).

The equilibrium state of the material surface in the biological environment is characterised by identical rates of adsorption and desorption of ions and constituents of, for instance, the extracellular matrix. The adjustment of equilibrium overlaps with the beginning of the interaction between tissue cells and the surface of the material.

TISSUE–IMPLANT INTERACTION

Cell adhesion involves contact and spreading of cells over the surface, followed by the subsequent differentiation and growth of cells. Cells attach to proteins adsorbed on the surface through specific transmembrane adhesion molecules and to specific sites on these proteins.

In chronological order, the interaction runs in the following steps:

(1) The implant surface builds an interface according to the properties of the solid state and the surrounding liquid phase.
(2) A protein layer adsorbs and is structured in response to the physicochemical properties of the surface in the equilibrium state.
(3) Cells recognise the protein film and react.
(4) Tissue is structured according to the properties of the protein and cell layer on the surface.

The passivated surface of titanium has been shown by morphological studies to favour osteointegration. This applies in particular to dental implants (Abrektsson *et al.*, 1983), which are inserted in such a manner that the passivated layer on the surface remains fully mechanically unloaded during the first few weeks after implantation.

A criterion for the suitability of materials as a biomaterial for close tissue contact is the physicochemical reactivity of the surface. Bulks and surfaces have properties as either a metal, a semiconductor or an insulator. The differences are caused by the electronic structure of the materials described by the density of electronic states and their occupation by charge carriers.

10.1.1 SURFACE PROPERTIES DETERMINE BIOCOMPATIBILITY

When a biomaterial (solid) and the extracellular fluid (liquid) come into contact with each other, an interface between them occurs. The region that includes the surface and the immediate adjacent anisotropic boundary is called the interface. The molecules making up a surface are different from those of the bulk phase because they are not surrounded by bulk phase molecules. The bonding energy of the surface molecule is less than that associated with a bulk phase molecule, and the energy of the surface molecule is therefore higher than that of molecules in the bulk phase. The force in the surface that attempts to keep the surface area at a minimum is called the surface tension and is usually given in mJ m^{-2}.

Indications in the literature show that the critical surface tension should be in the region of 60–120 mJ m^{-2} for good tissue adhesion (Figure 10.2). The adhesion energy is measured via the contact angle of a sessile drop of a liquid lying on a solid substrate (Figure 10.3). This yields:

$$\gamma_{SL} = -\gamma_{SV} - \gamma_{LV} \cos \theta \qquad (10.1)$$

where θ is the contact angle. The general relation that correlates wetting and bonding behaviour at the interface of a solid–liquid–vapour system in thermodynamic equilibrium is:

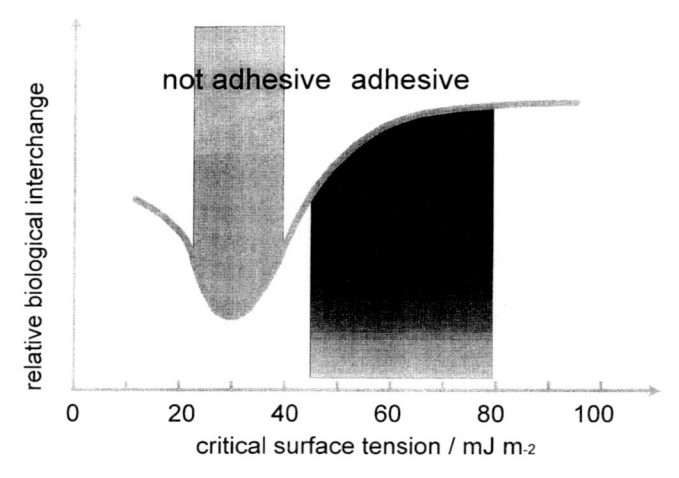

Figure 10.2 Critical surface tension leading to adhesion or non-adhesion of the adjacent tissue.

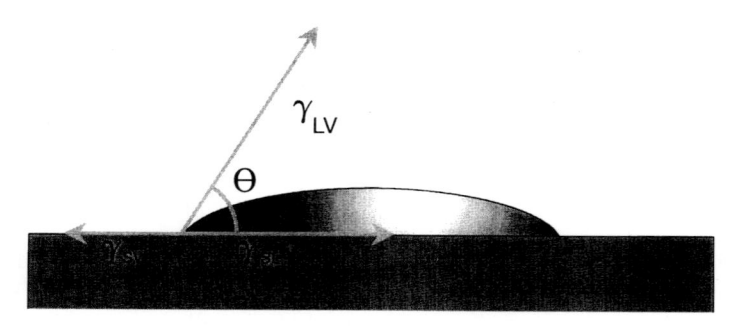

Figure 10.3 Contact angle of a drop placed on the surface is a measure for the adhesion energy.

$$W_a = \gamma_{SV} + \gamma_{LV} - \gamma_{SL} = \gamma_{LV}(1 + \cos\theta), \qquad (10.2)$$

where γ_{SV} and γ_{LV} are the surface energies of the solid and liquid phases, respectively, γ_{SL} is the interfacial energy of solid–liquid and W_a is the work of adhesion. $\gamma = \gamma^d + \gamma^p$, dispersion and polar interactions, respectively, results from a variety of intermolecular forces (Fowkes, 1964), the contribution of which to the total surface energy is additive. It yields:

$$\cos\theta = -1 + \frac{2(\gamma_{SV}^d \gamma_{LV}^d)^{1/2}}{\gamma_{LV}} + \frac{2(\gamma_{SV}^p \gamma_{LV}^p)^{1/2}}{\gamma_{LV}}. \qquad (10.3)$$

For metals in contact with polar liquids as the extracellular fluid the interfacial interactions are due almost entirely to the dispersion, γ^d, and therefore, the metal-bond–dipole interactions can be neglected. This means that the second term in the equation for $\cos\theta$ vanishes for simplification. For water, $\gamma_{LV} = 71.4$ mJ m^{-2} as the sum of $\gamma_{LV}^d = 21.8$ mJ m^{-2} and $\gamma_{LV}^p = 49.6$ mJ m^{-2}, the work of adhesion is calculated and leads to the results shown in Figure 10.4a and b for titanium and a (TiZr)O coating on titanium. The biocompatible coating is used, for instance, as a shear and fretting corrosion-resistant surface modification of an endosteal implant system. For serum, plasma and blood as contacting fluids, values for the work of adhesion which are 20% lower can be taken into account (Agathopoulos and Nikolopoulos, 1995). These values would agree with the requirements for good tissue adhesion.

The concentration of solute molecules at a surface is different to that in the bulk. The surface excess concentration, denoted by the symbol Γ, represents the quantity of solute adsorbed to the surface. The surface excess can be quantified through the Gibb's adsorption isotherm:

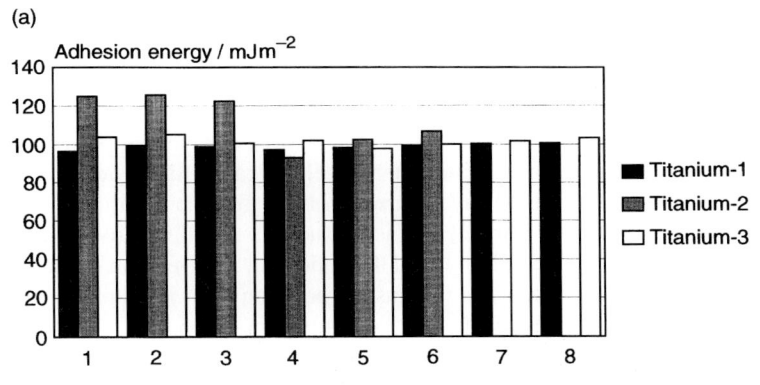

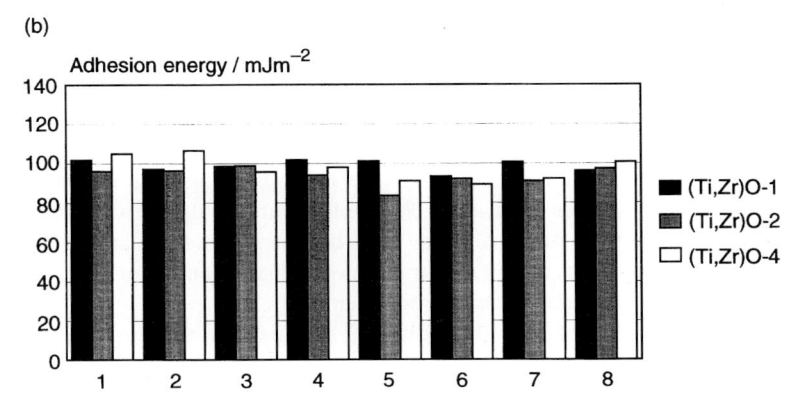

Figure 10.4 Adhesion energy, determined via the contact angle at chemically cleaned (a) titanium and (b) (TiZr)O-coated titanium surfaces. The contact angle was measured eight times for each of the eight specimens.

$$\Gamma_i = \frac{-1}{RT} \frac{\delta\gamma}{\delta \ln a_i}. \tag{10.4}$$

Γ_i has the units of mol m^{-2}. The surface tension is γ and the activity of the solute, i, in solution is a_i. This expression indicates that a solute that decreases the surface tension will concentrate at the surface, since the sign of the excess concentration is opposite that of the change in surface tension.

Some of the most important surface-active compounds in biological systems are the amphiphilic long-chain fatty acids. Their hydrophilic –COOH groups will preferentially attract to water molecules. For biomaterials this fact leads to the idea of functionalising surfaces with active chemical groups, for example prepared by a modified sol-gel procedure. The modification should improve the selectivity of absorption for distinct biomacromolecules that promote close cell adhesion for better fixation of mechanically loaded implants in hard tissue.

10.1.2 ELECTRIFIED BIOMATERIAL SURFACE

When a material is immersed in an aqueous electrolyte space–charge layers are formed, leading to electrical double layers. They consist of layers of positive charge, layers of negative charge and regions of high electrical field between, or within, the charged layers. The double layers are dominant for the control of electrical and chemical properties of implant surfaces, such as reactions involving charge exchange between ions of the solution and the solid and, in case of an implant within the body, the charge exchange or transfer between the implant surface and biomacromolecules being adsorbed after the adsorption of ions.

The description of the structure of the double-layer region has to consider the role of water and its dielectric properties. Building on the pictures of the Helmholtz model, which considers solely the electrostatic type of interactions between ions of the electrolyte and the surface of the solid body, and the Stern model, which takes into account the finite size of ions and adsorption properties, a more complete description combines the two models and starts from the space charge region of the material. The surface will be hydrated in an analogous to that known for an ion. Unlike an ion, however, the charge within the space charge region of the material can be changed, for instance, by a change in pH value. In this case the direction of the water dipole can also be induced to change to a varying degree with the surface charge. The arrangement of the dipoles and the energy of their attraction to the electrode play an important role in the strength of influence of different materials on the conformational structure of biomacromolecules.

The rigidly hydrated surface will be followed by the Gouy–Chapman layer, which consists primarily of hydrated ions of appropriate countercharge. In the case of a positive charged surface, this layer shows excess anions, which are not usually hydrated, and for a negatively charged surface, excess hydrated cations. The possibility of storing charge in the space charge layer of the material surface and the Helmholtz planes is always related to electrical capacitances, which characterise important properties of the solid body, influencing their suitability as a biomaterial.

10.2 ZETA POTENTIAL AND SURFACE CHARGE

Investigations on interfaces between different types of biomaterials and the biological environment are still in their early stages. There is no doubt that more knowledge of the physical chemistry of the interface is the key to an improved understanding of the interaction of materials with elements of the extracellular matrix, and determining implant properties concerning their integration and their durability. The interface plays an important role, for instance in the transfer of charge in the electron transport chain, the behaviour of the cell–material interaction, and the adsorption of proteins and other chemical messengers on the material surface.

In addition, the structure of the double-layer region gives rise to a number of important effects associated with motion relative to the double layer, called electrokinetic effects.

Charge located in the Helmholtz region is bound tightly and is an essential part of the same kinetic entity as the interface. The Helmholtz layer will move locked with the movement of the interface. In contrast to that excess charge in the diffuse layer is not held as tightly to the surface. In a sense, the ions making up the countercharge in the Gouy–Chapman diffuse layer have split loyalties to the interphase region and the bulk solution. When the solution phase and interphase are at rest relative to one another, the ions making up the diffuse layer are held by the forces from the electrified interface, which are moderated by thermal randomising forces.

However, if either the solution or the surface moves relative to the other, the ions located in the diffuse layer can move from the interphase region in direction to the bulk phase. When charge is separated, the result is a potential difference. The motion of the bulk phase with respect to the surface therefore has resulted in a new potential field, the electrokinetic potential called the zeta potential, ζ. The magnitude of ζ is found by measuring the potential difference between the portion of the diffuse layer that can be removed by a shearing force and the bulk of the solution, representing the reference zero. The entire diffuse layer is generally considered to be removable under a kinetic shearing force, so the shear plane is considered to be located within the Gouy–Chapman region close to the rigid Helmholtz layer. Knowledge of ζ can be used to indirectly infer some information about the surface charge excess and the compact layer.

The zeta potential is measurable via the streaming potential, which arises when a pressure difference is applied to an electrolyte in, for instance, a gap between two plates of which one is made from the material of interest, and the electrolyte has to be moved through the gap with laminar flow (Van Wagenen and Andrade, 1989). As the electrolyte begins to flow, its motion is opposed by the viscous force of the solution. The velocity of flow will increase until the force exerted by the pressure gradient is opposed equally by the viscous force. The movement of the bulk elements that contain Gouy–Chapman charge leads to the condition where the flowing lamina of electrolyte carries a charge. A separation and accumulation of charge occurs and, as a result, an electrical potential is generated, known as the streaming potential. If the amount of charge drawn away from the double layer is measured as it moves through a plane normal to the surface, then a streaming current can be found.

The streaming potential, V_s, is found to depend on the viscosity η and conductivity κ of the fluid, the pressure gradient Δp in the gap in direction of the flow, and the zeta potential ζ

$$V_s = \frac{\zeta \varepsilon_0 \varepsilon \Delta p}{\eta \kappa}. \tag{10.5}$$

10.3 EQUIVALENT CIRCUIT REPRESENTATION FOR THE BIOMATERIAL INTERFACE

As outlined in the description of the double layer, the interphase can in some respect be represented in terms of capacitance. Also, the extracellular fluid and the bulk of the biomaterial have finite resistances that must be taken into account. Thus, a half cell with the material of interest in contact with the electrolyte can be represented by an equivalent circuit consisting of at least the double-layer capacitance C_H.

In addition to its capacitive impedance, each double layer has a resistive impedance associated with a dc flow and the surface is polarisable. If there is no resistive impedance through the double layer the surface is perfectly polarisable, as a change in voltage results in a transient current that charges the double layer capacitance. For metals in implants, the intermediate case is usually present, i.e. a polarisable implant surface with some current if a voltage is applied. The combination of the double-layer capacitance C_H and the faradic resistance R_p parallel connected represents the interface. The difference between polarisable and non-polarisable interphases can be easily understood in terms of this equivalent circuit. A high value of R_p is associated with a polarisable interphase, whereas a low value of R_p represents a non-polarisable interphase.

The simple equivalent circuit does not take into account factors such as mass transport, heterogeneity of the surface and the occurrence of reaction intermediates adsorbed at the surface. Even in the simplest cases, in which this circuit represents the response of the interphase to an electrical perturbation reasonably well, C_H and R_p depend on potential and, in fact, R_p depends on potential exponentially over a wide range.

As is commonly known, an electrolytic cell always consists of at least two electrodes, the working electrode (WE) and the counter electrode (CE). However, only the part of the circuit representing the material under investigation, the WE, is usually considered, since the experiment is set up in such a way that only one of the electrodes is studied at a time. For this purpose, a third electrode, the reference electrode (RE), is placed close to the surface of the WE and measures and controls the potential at this point that its potential is at any time equal to an adjusted value. The potential control begins with the measurement of the actual voltage between the working and the reference electrode. The measured value is subtracted from the actual true voltage, and the difference between the two should be zero. Any

TISSUE–IMPLANT INTERACTION

difference arising is amplified as a control voltage with inverse sign and applied to the CE to bring the difference to zero.

Suitable equivalent circuits can be used for the description of the physicochemical behaviour of biomaterials, for instance the corrosion resistance of metals. The determination of the interphase impedance spectrum keeps the biomaterial surface almost in the thermodynamical equilibrium state because of the very small perturbation given by the small applied ac signal amplitude. The evaluation of R_p from the impedance spectrum renders possible corrosion resistance measurements close to the thermal equilibrium.

If the equivalent circuit indeed represents the interphase, then the evaluated capacitance is independent of frequency and is the electrical equivalent for the double-layer capacitance. However, the equivalent circuit is often much more complicated. For example, for passivated metal surfaces in contact with the physiological environment, one must consider not only a charge transfer across the interface, but also an impedance representing the diffusion of charge carriers inside the semiconducting oxide, as well as an equivalent due to surface states at the interface. Under favourable circumstances, each of the charge transport processes exhibits a characteristic relaxation time which is sufficiently separate from those of other processes so that, on an impedance–log frequency graph, a maximum is observed at a different frequency for each individual process (Randles, 1947) (see also Chapters 4 and 14).

10.4 CHARGED BIOMATERIAL SURFACES

For an implant made of a self-passivating metal, placed in a physiological environment, the charge densities on the surface and the Helmholtz plane are much higher than the charge density of any other charged layers. The interface can then be described with the aid of an equivalent circuit diagram with at least two capacitances in series, which stand for the space charge region within the surface oxide C_{sc} and the Helmholtz layer C_H. In most cases $C_{sc} < C_H$ is filled, so that C_H can be neglected in the evaluation of the impedance measurement. In this case the circuit consists of C_{sc} and R_p, parallel connected, and R as line resistance (Figure 10.5).

A numerical example hints on the importance of the double-layer structure for the communication between an implant and the surrounding extracellular fluid including, beside ions, complex structured proteins such as biomacromolecules. Considering a constant Helmholtz capacitance with voltage as a permitted simplification, the electrical field strength can be estimated as

$$E = \frac{V_H}{d} = \frac{nq}{\varepsilon \varepsilon_0}, \qquad (10.6)$$

where d is the thickness of the Helmholtz layer, q is the elementary charge, ε is the permittivity of water near a solid surface and ε_0 is the permittivity of free space.

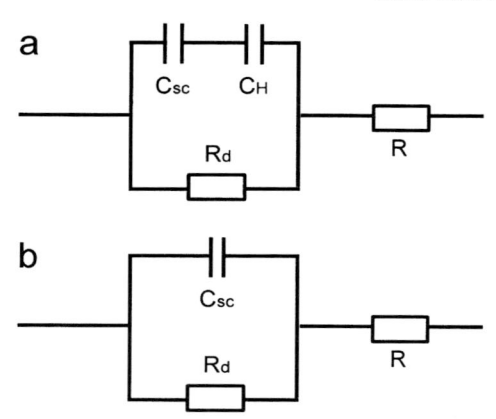

Figure 10.5 (a) Equivalent circuit of a Randles' cell, with a semiconducting material such as a passivated titanium surface under investigation; (b) simplified circuit $C_H \gg C_{sc}$.

If 10^{17}–10^{18} m^{-2} excess ions are adsorbed on the surface of the implant, OH$^-$ or H$^+$, and $\varepsilon = 5$, as commonly applied for the permittivity of water near the surface, the electrical field strength is 3.6×10^8 V m^{-1}. With a thickness of 10^{-9} m the result is $V_H = 0.36$ V.

10.4.1 INSULATORS

The charge on surfaces of insulators cannot stem from free charges such as electrons in a metal, and must be due to adsorbed charges such as ions or dipoles, in particular OH$^-$ or H$^+$. The relative adsorption of the latter depends on the pH of the electrolyte and varying the pH can change the kind of excess ions. If other ions or dipoles are adsorbed beside OH$^-$ or H$^+$ they can contribute to the voltage drop across the Helmholtz double layer. With insulators the Helmholtz potential adjusts itself so the rate of adsorption equals the rate of desorption of ions. [H^+_s] represents the concentration of adsorbed H$^+$ in excess over the charge-free surface.

According to the law of mass action the equilibrium leads to

$$\frac{[H^+_s]}{[H_3O^+]} = \exp\left(-\frac{\Delta G}{kT}\right) = A \exp\left(\frac{-qV_H}{kT}\right), \tag{10.7}$$

where ΔG is the free enthalpy, k is the Boltzmann constant, T is the temperature in kelvin and A is a constant. The double-layer potential V_H, in turn, is proportional to the charge adsorbed, if the approximation is made that C_H, the capacity per unit area of the Helmholtz double layer, is independent of V_H

$$q[H^+_s] = C_H H_H. \tag{10.8}$$

TISSUE–IMPLANT INTERACTION

$[H_s^+]$ will vary slowly with $[H_3O^+]$ and to the approximation of the analysis the Helmholtz potential V_H is

$$V_H = \frac{B}{q} + \frac{kT}{q}\ln[H_3O^+] = \frac{B}{q} - 2.3\frac{kT}{q}(\text{pH}), \qquad (10.9)$$

where B is a constant. Because $V_H = 0$ if pH = the point of zero charge (pzc) B/q can be calculated as

$$\frac{B}{q} = 2.3\frac{kT}{q}(\text{pzc}). \qquad (10.10)$$

Introduced into the equation for the Helmholtz potential, this gives

$$V_H = 2.3\frac{kT}{q}(\text{pzc} - \text{pH}). \qquad (10.11)$$

Transcribed for the pzc it follows that

$$(\text{pzc}) = \frac{qV_H}{2.3kT} + (\text{pH}). \qquad (10.12)$$

10.4.2 METALS

The Helmholtz potential is determined by electron exchange between ions in solution and the metal. Compared with the charge exchange, the charge that stems from adsorbed ions can be neglected. When a metal is immersed in an electrolyte, the Helmholtz potential adjusts itself to a value such that the exchange current from the solid into the electrolyte is equal to that from the electrolyte into the solid.

10.4.3 SEMICONDUCTORS

Depending on the band-gap energy semiconductors behave with respect to the adjustment of the equilibrium either as a metal for narrow-band, highly covalent semiconductors with clean surfaces, or as an insulator or a semiconductor with a wide band gap between valence and conduction band. This means that the Helmholtz potential is controlled either by charge transfer or adsorption/desorption of ions. The adsorption/desorption mechanism is particularly clear where the semiconductor is an oxide or is oxidised as TiO_2 on Ti. The relationship between pH and Helmholtz potential could be verified experimentally with measurements of the interface impedance.

A degenerate semiconductor, as realised in some oxide films on iron- or cobalt-based alloys, has properties between those of a semiconductor and a metal. The

Helmholtz potential is expected to become more associated with charge transfer reactions such as redox processes the more degenerate the material is.

Depending on the electronic structure of the surface of the implant material, its isoelectric point (IEP) and the composition of the surface coating and the extracellular fluid a characteristic potential distribution across the interface arises during adjustment of equilibrium. The potential within the solid body increases or decreases exponentially in semiconductors and linearly in insulators. In the double layer of 10–50 nm of the surface-adjacent electrolyte the potential increases or decreases linearly and finally returns exponentially to the value within the electrolyte.

The potential drop varies. Generally, the potential gradient within the double layer at the surface is smaller for semiconducting or insulating surface films than for metal conducting surfaces.

It is imaginable that adsorbed polar biomacromolecules, e.g. proteins, changes the conformational structure owing to high field strengths in the double layer. In this model the hazard for conformational changes of proteins is smaller for semiconducting surfaces than for metals. The latter is true also for insulators if the density of local charges is low.

10.5 POINT OF ZERO CHARGE OF PASSIVATED METAL BIOMATERIALS

At the solid–electrolyte interface two of the several types of electrical potential stand out as being relatively important: the potential describing the interface in the equilibrium state, and the pzc describing the potential that has to be applied to adjust a charge-free surface. Related to the pzc is the IEP or the point of zero zeta potential (PZZP).

When a metal biomaterial is placed in physiological saline, H^+ and OH^- ions are adsorbed to the metal oxide forming during passivation. Figure 10.6 demonstrates the situation for a titanium surface covered with a thin titanium dioxide film. The OH^- ions are attracted to the polarised titanium atoms at the surface, the Lewis acid sites of the solid, whereas the H^+ ions are attracted to the polarised oxygen atoms, the Lewis base sites. The first reaction leads to a net negative charge on the surface, while the second leads to a net positive charge. The resulting net charge will depend on the pH value of the solution.

In most cases the description of the charged surface is more complex. Stronger adsorption of water or ions other than H^+ or OH^- can occur. These are associated with sites of extra chemical activity on the oxide surface or sites of active ionic surface states. Both possibilities will be neglected to simplify the model without limitation of general validity.

The charge and potential distribution across a non-conducting or semiconducting surface oxide are dominated by the charge in the space charge layer and by the charge associated with the adsorbants at the surface. The close to the surface potential distribution within the electrolyte is described by the Helmholtz potential

TISSUE–IMPLANT INTERACTION

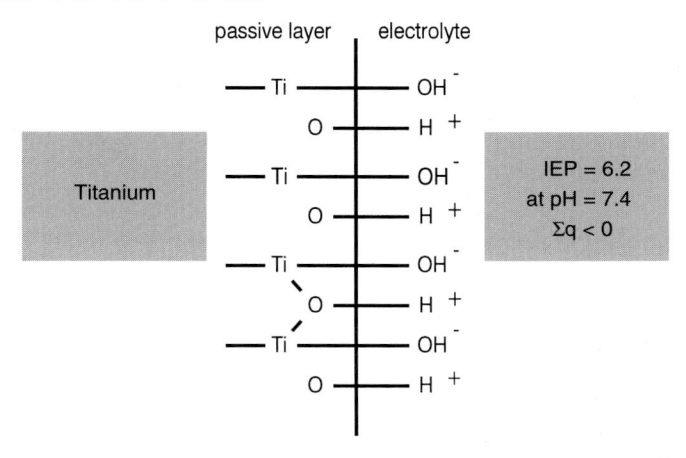

Figure 10.6 Interface forming between passivated titanium and PBS solution.

V_H. $V_H = 0$ results for the Helmholtz layer with no excess charge on the surface. The corresponding pH is termed the IEP or the PZZP. If H⁺ and OH⁻ are adsorbed in equal amounts the pH is called the pzc. If other ions are present leading to additional surface charge, the pzc and IEP are different. The presence of excess adsorbed cations raises the IEP, while the presence of anions lowers the IEP.

Evaluation of the pzc for a solid body, in particular for an implant surface, is not straightforward. Different experimental methods can be applied. The most widely used methods are the radiotracer (Balashowa and Kazarinov, 1969) and the differential capacity minimum in dilute electrolyte method (Bockris and Kahn, 1993).

In principle, the evaluation of impedance spectroscopy data with respect to the space charge capacity C_{sc} from the equivalent circuit diagram is suitable for determining the pzc, but only for semiconducting passive layers. Those surface oxides are realised with elements of groups 4b and 5b and their alloys. Applying the Mott–Schottky analysis the flat band potential can be determined which, after some calculations, leads to the pzc.

10.5.1 MOTT–SCHOTTKY ANALYSIS

A Mott–Schottky plot is based on the squared reciprocal capacitance versus the applied dc potential V_E. The well-known relation is

$$c_{sc}^{-2} = \left(\frac{1}{2}q\varepsilon\varepsilon_0 N_D\right)^{-1}\left(V_E - V_{fb} - \frac{kT}{q}\right), \tag{10.13}$$

where q is the electron charge, ε is the dielectric constant of the oxide film, N_D is the doping level and kT/q is 0.0267 V at 37°C. A Mott–Schottky plot gives a straight line with the intercept:

$$V = V_{fb} - \frac{kT}{e}. \tag{10.14}$$

N_D can be obtained from the slope of the line, provided that the surface area is accurately known, but is of no interest in connection with the determination of excess ions on the surface of passivated metals for implants.

10.5.2 CALCULATION OF THE POINT OF CHARGE

The pzc can be calculated if the flat band potential of the oxide in contact with the electrolyte is determined and some semiconductor properties are known. The connection between the flat band potential and the pzc is given by the equation

$$V_{fb}(SCE) = EA + (E_{CB} - E_F) + qV_H - E_{Redox-H^+/H}. \tag{10.15}$$

The energy scale for electrons in a solid is generally referred to as the energy of the vacuum $E = 0$, whereas the energy scale for electrons in an electrolyte is referred to as the redox system H^+/H_2 under standard conditions, i.e. the pressure of H_2 $p = 10^5$ Pa, the concentration of H^+ comply with pH = 0 and the temperature is $T = 298$ K. If all energies are referred to this scale an energy of $E_{Redox-H+/H} = 4.5$ eV as average value derived from literature is needed to transfer an electron from the redox-energy level of the H^+/H_2 couple under standard conditions to the vacuum.

With (see above)

$$V_H = 2.3 \frac{kT}{q}(pzc - pH) \tag{10.16}$$

it follows that

$$qV_{fb}(SCE) = EA + (E_{CB} - E_F) + 2.3kT(pzc - pH) - E_{Redox-H^+/H} \tag{10.17}$$

and finally

$$(pzc) = \frac{q}{2.3kT}V_{fb}(SCE) - \frac{EA}{2.3kT} - \frac{E_{CB} - E_F}{2.3kT} + (pH) + \frac{E_{Redox-H^+/H}}{2.3kT} \tag{10.18}$$

$$(pzc) = 16.28\left[\frac{V_{fb}(SCE)[V]}{[V]} - \frac{EA[eV]}{[eV]} - \frac{E_{CB} - E_F[eV]}{[eV]} + \frac{(pH)}{16.28} + \frac{E_{Redox-H^+/H}[eV]}{[eV]}\right]. \tag{10.19}$$

V_H is determined mainly by the amount of excess charge resulting for simple aqueous electrolytes from the difference between $[H^+]_s$ and $[OH^-]_s$.

The electron affinity is given by

$$EA = \phi - \frac{1}{2}E_g, \tag{10.20}$$

TISSUE–IMPLANT INTERACTION

where ϕ, the intrinsic Fermi energy of the solid, is best calculated as the arithmetic mean of the atomic values of the constituents (Frese, 1979). It was shown that a plot of experimental work functions of 42 elements as a function of their Pauling electronegativity fits to a linear relationship

$$\phi = 1.794\chi_p + 1.11, \tag{10.21}$$

where ϕ is the Fermi energy and χ_p is the Pauling electronegativity. The correlation coefficient was 0.90. Using this linear relationship, the atomic Fermi energy of elements, e.g. oxygen, was calculated in which work functions cannot be made but Pauling electronegativities are known. It was found that for AB, AB$_2$ and A$_2$B$_3$ types of compound, e.g. GaAs, TiO$_2$, and In$_2$O$_3$, the intrinsic Fermi energy of the solid could thus be calculated and agreed well with the experimental findings. The electron affinity calculation for TiO$_2$ results in 4.04 eV.

Another procedure for the determination of the electron affinity uses the Mulliken definition of electronegativity of an atom, the arithmetic mean of the atomic electron affinity (EA) and the ionisation potential (IP)

$$\chi_M = \frac{1}{2}(\text{IP} + \text{EA}), \tag{10.22}$$

where χ_M is the Mulliken electronegativity (Butler and Ginley, 1978). In accordance to the calculation of electronegativity of compounds, the geometric mean of ground-state Mulliken electronegativities was used to obtain the intrinsic level. This calculation yielded a value of EA = 4.33 eV for TiO$_2$.

$E_{CB} - E_F$ is the energy difference between the bottom of the conduction band and the Fermi energy level and can be assumed to be 0.2 eV for oxides on valve metals such as Ti, Zr, Nb and Ta.

10.5.3 EXPERIMENTAL PROCEDURE

The measurement is performed in a three-electrode set-up. The material under test is placed in an electrolytic cell, together with a counter and a saturated calomel electrode (SCE) as reference. The electrolyte simulating the physiological environment is physiological phosphate-buffered saline (PBS) solution, thermostatically heated to 37°C and aerated with oxygen gas to saturation. The determination of $C_{sc} = f(V)$ requires: (1) measurement of impedance spectra in dependence of increasing electrode potentials V, starting at equilibrium potential V_0; (2) evaluation of C_{sc} according to the Randles' equivalent circuit (Randles, 1947): the evaluation can be performed as long as $R_p > 1/(\omega C_{sc}) > R$ is fulfilled; (3) calculation of a the Mott–Schottky plot and evaluation of the flat band potential V_{fb} of the semiconducting oxide film; and (4) determination of the pzc.

A good-quality of the analysis performed by fitting needs accuracy to get systematic error-free experimental results. The investigated surfaces has to be cleaned thoroughly and pre-aged reproducibly for passivation.

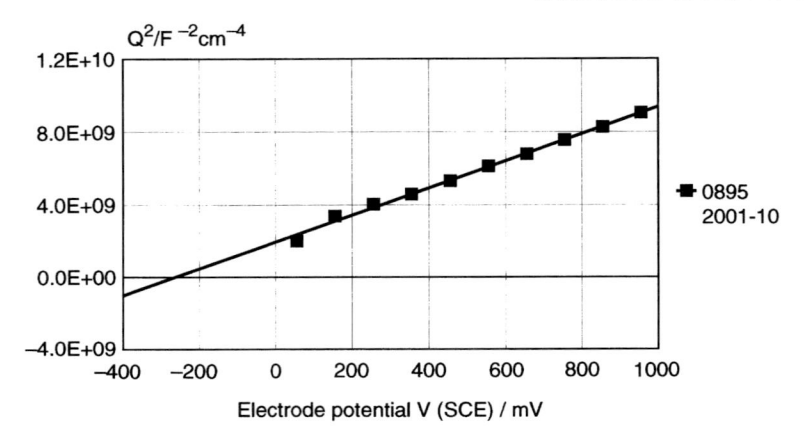

Figure 10.7 Schottky–Mott evaluation of the potential related space charge capacity of the electron depletion layer of an anodised titanium surface for the determination of the flat band potential.

10.5.4 DATA ANALYSIS

The analysis of the impedance spectroscopic data can be performed with suitable computer-aided software programs. In the example the evaluation software Equivalent Circuit (Equivcrt.pas) (Boukamp, 1989) is used. Applying the non-linear least-squares fit technique all components in the equivalent model are adjusted simultaneously, thus obtaining the optimum fit to the measured dispersion data.

10.5.5 RESULTS

The intercept of the Mott–Schottky plot with the x-axis (Figure 10.7) delivers for titanium the flat band potential $V_{fb} = -0.350$ V and with the derived relation the pzc (EA = 4.04 eV) = 5.7. The pzc is in agreement with data from the literature, with pzc = 5.8 (Watanabe et al., 1974; Bolts and Wrighton, 1976), and is close to the physiological pH value. The consequence is a small amount of negative excess charge mainly consisting of OH^- groups because pzc < pH.

10.6 ELECTROCHEMISTRY OF METAL BIOMATERIALS AND CORROSION

The Tafel equation has the same importance for the description of electrochemical reactions at metal-conducting material surfaces as the Arrhenius equation does for chemical kinetics. The Tafel equation connects the overpotential with the log of the current density:

$$\eta = a \pm b \log i \qquad (10.23)$$

TISSUE–IMPLANT INTERACTION

where a and b are independent constants of the current density. Rewriting and the introduction of some general used constants leads to

$$i_c = i_0 \exp\frac{-\alpha\eta F}{RT} \qquad (10.24)$$

where F is the Faraday constant, i_0 is exchange current density and α is a constant, known as transfer coefficient [cf. Equation (4.5) in Chapter 4]. This is the expression for a partial cathodic reaction, completed by the anodic partial current density, it follows the Butler–Volmer equation for exchange reactions at metal-conducting surfaces

$$i = i_0\left(\exp\frac{(1-\alpha)\eta_a F}{RT} - \exp\frac{(-\alpha)\eta_c F}{RT}\right), \qquad (10.25)$$

where η may be either cathodic η_c or anodic η_a. For small values of the overpotential, progressive development and the frequent assumption that $\alpha = 1/2$ lead to a linear relationship between i and η

$$i_{\eta<kT/e} = \frac{i_0\eta F}{RT}. \qquad (10.26)$$

If the values of η becomes sufficiently large and one of the exponential terms becomes 10 times greater than the other the Butler–Volmer equation is reduced to

$$i_a = i_0\left(\exp\frac{(1-\alpha)\eta_a F}{RT}\right) \qquad (10.27)$$

and

$$i_c = i_0\left(\exp\frac{(-\alpha)\eta_c F}{RT}\right). \qquad (10.28)$$

A comparison leads to the conclusion that the Tafel equation is identically to the partial Butler–Volmer equations for large overpotentials, either anodic or cathodic.

The Butler–Volmer equation or the exponential dependence of current and potential covers most charge transfer reactions through the interface at biomaterials, including the oxidation or reduction of ions or biomacromolecules of the extracellular fluid or the corrosion of the biomaterial itself.

The Butler–Volmer mechanism is not allowed to be applied if the transport of ions from the fluid or charge carriers from the material side limits the electrochemical reaction, which is characterised by the limiting current. An example of a transport-controlled reaction is the anodic oxidation of titanium in the passive region. In biological situations, charge transport within the insulator protein may control the rate of the reaction.

The transport can be controlled by complex factors. In solutions it may involve turbulence or some kind of convection process. The simplest model is the limitation by diffusion of reaction-consumed ions, molecules, or charge carriers at the surface of biomaterials.

Hence, with diffusion control, the transport flux is given by

$$\frac{i}{nF} = -D\left(\frac{dc}{dx}\right)_{x=0}, \qquad (10.29)$$

where D is the diffusion coefficient of ions in solution. The distance $x = 0$ refers to the distance at which the concentration gradient, dc/dx, is measured from the electrode, where c is the concentration of ion in the electrolyte near the electrode. The equation tells the proportionality between the rate of the reaction i/nF and the diffusion gradient.

An assumption always used is that the concentration gradients of reaction-consumed reactants or charge carriers near the surface is linear

$$\frac{i}{nF} = -D\frac{c_0 - c_{x=0}}{\delta}, \qquad (10.30)$$

where c_0 is the concentration of the rate-limiting reactant or charge carrier in the bulk of the solution or material, $c_{x=0}$ is the concentration near the surface and δ is the thickness of the diffusion layer.

10.7 CORROSION OF METAL BIOMATERIALS

Since corrosion is a process involving electrochemical oxidation and reduction reactions, it makes sense that electrochemical methods are applied to study and measure corroding systems. More specifically, when a metal biomaterial is immersed in either the extracellular body fluid or the fluid of the oral cavity, interface-specific electrochemical reactions occur, causing the metal to corrode. These reactions create an electrochemical potential, the corrosion potential V_c. V_c is a characteristic of the specific biomaterial metal–solution system and is measured with respect to a known reference system. The SCE is usually used as the reference system.

The corrosion potential of a given biomaterial in a given physiological solution is defined by the condition that the anodic oxidation (corrosion) current density is equal to the cathodic reduction current to maintain electronic neutrality, $i = i_r + i_O = 0$. Oxygen serves as a reducible species in physiological solutions, where it is reduced with a limiting current of approximately 10^{-4}–10^{-5} A cm^{-2}. Another reducible species is the hydrogen ion, the concentration of which is dependent on the pH value, which for the extracellular body fluid is pH = 7.4. At V_c the rate of the oxidation process or, if the corrosion of the material is the unique oxidation process, the corrosion rate, is exactly equal to that of the reduction process. Therefore, at V_c the system is electronically neutral and is said to be in equilibrium.

TISSUE–IMPLANT INTERACTION

The term i_r is associated with the electron flow due to the reduction process. Similarly, the oxidation current i_o, is associated with the electron flow due to the oxidation process. Neutrality at V_c requires $|i_r| = i_o = i_0$. The measurable current is $i = 0$ as a total current, and therefore the partial corrosion current can be measured only indirectly via electrical polarisation of the surface of the material.

Most corrosion measurements involve a scan of the WE potential and a measurement of the resulting current. This is referred to as a potentiodynamic scan, since the applied potential changes continuously. The corrosion rate can be determined via the polarisation resistance R_p which is evaluated from the slope of the current density–potential graph at V_c and the evaluation of the Tafel constants β_a and β_c from the potential–log current plot. Attention has to be paid to applying as small as possible a polarisation voltage to keep the surface as close to the equilibrium state as possible

$$i_c = \frac{1}{R_p} \frac{\beta_a \beta_c}{2.3 i_c (\beta_a + \beta_c)}. \tag{10.31}$$

In addition to yielding quantitative information, R_p values can help to rank different metallic materials with respect to their corrosion resistance because R_p is inversely proportional to the corrosion current.

10.8 BIOCOMPATIBILITY AND ELECTRONIC STRUCTURE OF BIOMATERIALS

Nearly all metals used in implants are pure or composed of transition elements forming spontaneously passive layers on the surface in electrolytes in a wide pH region. To describe electron transfer through a passivated or more general expressed coated surface the energy level model can be used. The problem is discussed in approximation for polycrystalline semiconducting or metal-conducting oxide layers instead of those that are amorphous.

Metals consisting of transition elements are separated from the interfaces between metal and oxide film and between the film and the fluid, as well as by the film itself, which is a metal conductor or semiconductor. Electrochemical reactions occur at the metal–film interface by oxidation, i.e. corrosion, and reduction of oxygen to oxygen ions. If oxygen is not available hydrogen ions will be reduced instead. Low conductivity reduces the possibilities for charge transfer reactions through the interface. Figure 10.8 shows the electrochemical reactions at metal-conducting, and semiconducting or non-conducting, surfaces.

The situation changes for semiconducting or non-conducting films. Because the film does not transport charge carriers, and the diffusion coefficients of titanium from the bulk to the surface or of oxygen along concentration gradients have low values, the reactions take place slowly connected with a low rate of corrosion of the metal bulk, provided that the film is tight. Redox reactions at the film–electrolyte

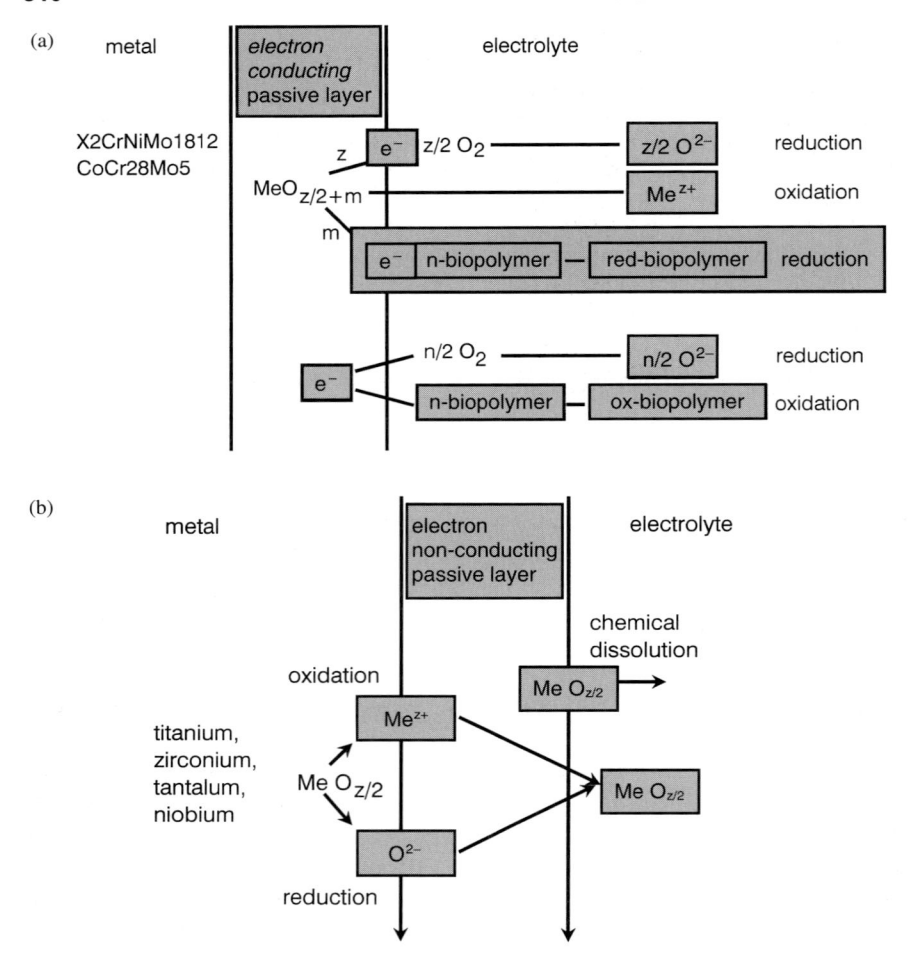

Figure 10.8 View over the possible exchange reaction at passivated metal surfaces forming (a) electron-conducting surface oxides; (b) semiconducting or non-conducting surface oxide.

interface that are charge transfer reactions are nearly inhibited potential barriers for charge carrier tunnelling. This is true for all biocompatible passivated refractory metals.

At metal-conducting passive layers, redox reactions with biomacromolecules can occur, leading to immunological reactions: (1) by the reduction of biomacromolecules, or (2) by forming haptens by binding of metal ions through corrosion to proteins. Figure 10.9 shows schematically the change of a native protein to an antigen, giving information to the immunological system to recognise an artificial material as a foreign body. This is true for all metals forming electron-conducting

TISSUE–IMPLANT INTERACTION

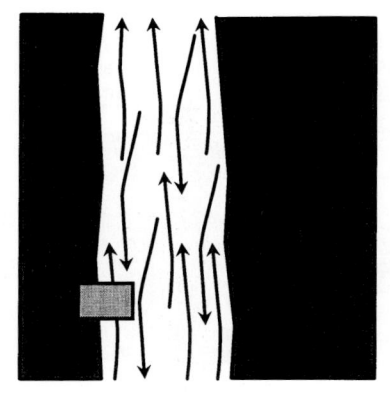

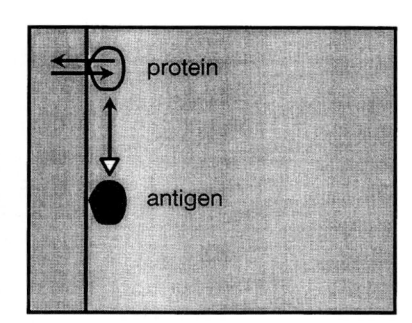

Implant   connective   bone
          tissue

Figure 10.9 Model of the recognition mechanism. The immunological system identifies the artificial material via the conformational changed biomacromolecules adsorbed at the surface of the material. Conformational changes occur owing to either electrochemical reactions between material and adsorbed biomacromolecules or the high potential gradient electrical field strength across the interface.

oxides and for refractory metals that repassivate only to non-stoichiometric oxides after mechanical destruction of the original passive layer.

The semiconductivity of refractory metal oxides is due to the electronic band structure. Semiconductivity is characterised by the position of the Fermi energy level within the energy gap between the conduction band and the valence band. The Fermi level describes the electronic state that is occupied by one electron out of two that could be on the state with reference to Pauly's principle. The conduction band is, in case of body temperature, almost carrier free, whereas the valence band is almost occupied by electrons.

The conductivity of the surface film depends on the number of charge carriers in the conduction band. If the gap is large, as for anatase, only a few carriers exist to contribute to the conductivity. The relationship between electronic structure and biocompatibility is essential for the application in dental or orthopaedic implants, as well as in applications in contact to blood.

Titanium monoxide is metal conducting. The Fermi level is a sign of metal conductivity within the conduction band. Metals or metal-conducting surface films advance the charge transfer through the interface with inorganic and organic substances of the extracellular fluid.

In summary, the following can be stated: biocompatibility depends on the electronic structure of the material. The conductivity of the surface film controls reactions across the interface with biomacromolecules of the biological environment. Conformationally unchanged macromolecules are the prior condition

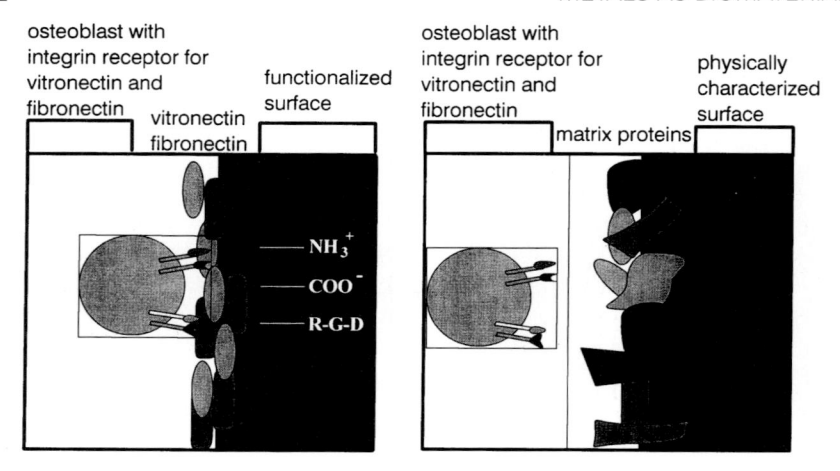

Figure 10.10 Biomaterials are, strictly speaking, materials that adsorb selectively distinct adhesive biomacromolecules with the task to attach cells to the surface. The selectivity can be prepared by surface modifications with distinct electronic properties modifications or by functionalising via localised chemical groups.

for biocompatibility and control the attachment and probably also the degree of attachment via adhesion proteins (Figure 10.10). Later on, when the cells develop tension through the cytoskeleton on these attachment sites, the strength of the integrin adhesion protein–matrix protein interaction might prove decisive in differentiation state of the cell (Möller *et al.*, 1995). For example, it has been proved by molecular biological methods that an undestroyed oxide layer of anatase on titanium through passivation leaves albumin conformational unchanged.

10.9 SURFACE ENGINEERING TO IMPROVE WEAR RESISTANCE AND BIOCOMPATIBILITY

Because of the low shearing resistance, the implant should be provided with one or, if functionally indicated, several wear-resistant osteophilic, wear-resistant or similar *in situ* working coatings. Based on the required properties, the possibilities are oxides and oxynitrides, carbides and carbo-nitrides, and nitrides of the transition metals of the fourth and fifth subgroups of the periodic system.

Several methods for surface modification are technical available and are applied in implant technology. Criteria for the quality of a suitable surface modification are: (1) biocompatibility similar to that of the stoichiometrically passivated titanium surface or a 'functional' biocompatibility, implant site dependent; (2) high mechanical stability against shearing forces; and (3) long-term chemical stability.

Application can be accomplished by various processes, including precipitations from the chemical vapour phase, i.e. chemical vapour deposition (CVD) or physical vapour deposition (PVD). Anatas and rutile films can be pyrolysed from isoprophyltitanites (iso-PrO)Ti by spraying on the surface. Disadvantages of this procedure are the relatively high substrata temperatures and low adhesive strength. Adhesive layers can be produced at low substrata temperatures after the building of a metal interface by ion implantation or by the precipitation of oxide or oxynitride from plasma (Thull and Reuther, 1991).

An example of osteophilic coating is semiconductive titanium–zirconium–oxide (TiZr)O and an example of a wear-resistant coating is titanium–niobium–oxynitride (TiNb)ON. The addition of niobium and zirconium is advantageous because of the high formation enthalpies of the oxides, which are higher for niobium and zirconium than for titanium and contribute to the chemical long-term stability of the coating material.

The process synthesis to an oxide or oxynitride takes place in a vacuum directly on the surface. Base materials are the purest metal alloys, (TiNb) or (TiZr), introduced in targets, as well as oxygen and nitrogen as pure reaction gases. Zirconium in the (TiZr) target used for the PVD coating is produced from the zirconium foam, following a complicated manufacturing process and its composition is defined according to ASTM (1993). (TiNb)ON and (TiZr)O coatings are applied to implants using plasma-aided electric arc PVD. The procedures were developed almost simultaneously in Russia and the USA.

The electrochemical and biological properties of the coating materials (TiNb)ON and (TiZr)O were examined on sheets of titanium in contact to cells and in animal experiments according to ISO 10993. (TiZr)O-coated titanium looks dark blue, whereas (TiNb)ON-coated titanium is gold-coloured. The typical thickness of coatings is in the region of 4–5 µm. The Vicker's hardness of (TiZr)O is 2200, whereas that of (TiNb)ON is even higher, at 3000.

NOMENCLATURE

a_i	activity of ion i in solution
c	ion concentration
C_H	double-layer capacitance
C_{SC}	space charge capacitance
d	double-layer thickness
D	diffusion coefficient of ions in solution
dc/dx	ion concentration gradient
E	electrical field strength
E	energy
E_{CB}	conduction-band energy
E_f	Fermi energy
E_g	energy gap
F	Faraday constant, F = 9.648456 C mol^{-1}
i	current density
i_0	exchange current density

i_a	anodic current density
i_c	cathodic current density
i_O	oxygen current density
i_r	electron flow
k	Bolzmann constant, $k = 1.380662 \times 10^{-23}$ J K^{-1}
N_D	doping level
p	pressure
q	elementary charge, $q = 1.60219 \times 10^{-19}$ C
R	resistance
R	gas constant, $R = 8.31441$ J mol^{-1} K^{-1}
R_p	polarisation resistance
T	temperature
V	electrode potential
V_0	equilibrium potential
V_c	corrosion potential
V_E	electrode dc potential
V_{fb}	flat band potential
V_H	Helmholtz potential
V_s	streaming potential
W_a	work of adhesion
α	transfer coefficient
β_a, β_c	Tafel constants
χ_p	Mulliken electronegativity
χ_p	Pauling electronegativity
δ	diffusion layer thickness
η	overpotential
η	viscosity
η_a	anodic overpotential
η_c	cathodic overpotential
ΔG	free enthalpy
γ	surface tension
γ_d	tension related to dispersion interaction
γ_{LV}	surface tension of the liquid versus vacuum
γ^p	tension related to polar interaction
γ_{SL}	tension of the solid–liquid phase
γ_{SV}	surface tension of the solid versus vacuum
Γ	surface excess concentration
κ	conductivity
ω	frequency
ϕ	intrinsic Fermi energy
θ	contact angle
ε	permittivity number of medium
ε_0	electric field constant $\varepsilon_0 = 8.854 \times 10^{-12}$ C V^{-1} m^{-1}
ζ	zeta potential

REFERENCES

Albrektsson, T., Branemark, P.J. and Hausson, H.-A. (1983) The interface zone of inorganic implants *in vivo*: titanium implants in bone, *An. Biomed. Engng* **11**, 1.

Agathopoulos, S. and Nikolopoulos, P. (1995) Wettability and interfacial interactions in bioceramic–body–liquid system, *J. Biomed. Mater. Res.* **29**, 421–9.

ASTM (1983) *Annual Book of ASTM Standards, Nuclear Energy (1) Standard Specification for Zirconium and Zirconium Alloy Sheet, Strip, and Plate for Nuclear Application*, American Society for Testing and Materials, Vol. 12.01, Philadelphia, PA.

Balashowa, N. and Kazarinov, V. (1969) Use of radioactive-tracer method for the investigation of the electric double-layer structure, in *Electroanalytical Chemistry 3* (ed. A.J. Bard), Marcel Dekker, New York, pp. 135–97.

Bockris, J.O'M. and Khan, S.U.M. (1993) *Surface Electrochemistry*, Plenum Press, New York.

Bolts, J.M. and Wrighton, M.S. (1976) *J. Phys. Chem.* **80**, 2641.

Boukamp, B.B.A. (1989) University of Twente, Department of Chemical Technology, Report CT88/265/128-CT89/214/128.

Butler, M.A. and Ginley, D.S. (1978) *J. Electrochem. Soc.* **125**, 228.

Frese, K.W., Jr (1979) Simple method for estimating energy levels of solids, *J. Vac. Sci. Technol.* **16**, 1042.

Fowkes, F.M. (1964) Attractive forces at interfaces, *Ind. Engng. Chem.* **56**, 12, 40–52.

Möller, K., Meyer, U., Szulczewski, D.H., Heide, H., Priessnitz, B. and Jones, D.B. (1995) The influence of zeta potential and interfacial tension on osteoblast-like cells, *Cells Mater.* **4**, 263–74.

Randles, J.E.B. (1947) Kinetics of rapid electrode reactions, *Faraday Soc.* **1**, 11.

Thomsen, P., Eriksen, A.S., Sennerby, L. and Erikson, L.E. (1991) Cellular reactions in the implant tissue interface, in *Metals and their Alloys in Orthopaedic Surgery* (eds G.H. Buchhorn and H.-G. Willert), Hogrefe & Huber, Seattle, WA.

Thull, R. and Reuther, J. (1991) *Enossales Zahnimplant.*, Europäisches Patentamt, Veröffentlichungsnummer: EP 0 445 667 A2.

van Wagenen, R.A. and Andrade, J.D. (1989) Flat plate streaming potential investigations: hydrodynamics and electrokinetic equivalency. *J. Coll. Sci.* **76**, 305–14.

Watanabe, T., Fujishima, A. and Honda, K. (1974) *Chem. Lett.* 897–900.

11
Cells and metals

D.B. JONES
Philipps University, Marburg, Germany

11.1 INTRODUCTION

Metals form about 75% of all elements. A few play important physiological roles in the cell (e.g. Fe, Cu, Zn, Se, Ca, Cr, K, Na, Mg and Mn) and concentrations are regulated by sophisticated pathways (e.g. Powis, 1994; Pufahl et al., 1997). Others are rarely present environmentally and can also enter the cell by these transport pathways. These often interfere with cellular processes by substituting for normal ions, by forming pathological complexes or by taking part in inappropriate oxidation reactions. Both stimulatory and inhibitory effects can occur. In some cases such as in calcium ion effects, Ba, Ni and other ions can both inhibit certain classes of calcium ion channels and at the same time, bind and activate calcium-dependent proteins in the cell. During the period of surface atomic weapons testing it became appreciated that certain metals could become concentrated in the bones of children, for example Sr and Cd, which are examples of metal ions capable of clandestinely entering metal transport pathways. An example of a complex metal transporter is that recently described for Cu by Pufahl et al. (1997). Other metals can occur in our industrialised environment, for instance Hg, As, Al and Pb. Many non-physiological metal ions in low concentrations might not obviously interfere with cellular processes but closer observation shows subtle effects, the larger significance of which is not yet fully understood. In certain concentrations and in certain compounds, metals can be used therapeutically (Salversan is one famous example), but at a different concentration or form become poisons – the first orally administered poisons were metal compounds (many famous poisoners have favoured arsenic for example). Some metals, such as bismuth, are used in treating some intestinal problems but can also have acute side-effects (Slikkerveer and de Wolff, 1996). There is an abundance of information about the **toxicity** of metals (see for instance Chang, 1996) but this is not within the scope of this chapter. There are very few metal ions which do not display physiological action at some concentration. However, since no metal is pure, very small traces of impurities can occur which, although not having an immediate toxic effect, can have a pharmacological effect. Many of these effects are not fully

---

Metals as Biomaterials ISBN 0 471 96935 4 Edited by J.A. Helsen and H.J. Breme. © 1998 John Wiley & Sons Ltd

appreciated by many investigators in the field of biomaterials and a brief overview of some of these pharmacological effects is presented in the following sections. Some of the mechanisms for these effects are also discussed elsewhere in the book.

A common source of metal ions in the body are joint prostheses. A few metals, mostly alloys, have some good properties for use as parts of prostheses. However, no prosthesis lasts a lifetime and there are numerous ideas on how to improve the survival time. Some of the perceived mechanisms of failure have included a lack of good mechanical integration of bone into the metal interface of uncemented stems. This has led to ideas for changing the interface and has also led to a number of modifications. One of the basic problems is that no material, including any metal alloy, is known that has similar mechanical properties to bone. One of the major differences is that bone displays viscoelastic behaviour whereas metals do not. This mechanical mismatch may lead to direct cellular reactions through mechano-sensors (Jones *et al.*, 1994). The mechanical mismatch will also lead to fretting and several investigations into many aspects of this problem have been carried out (Kowalec *et al.*, 1995; Merritt and Brown, 1995, 1996; Lacy *et al.* 1996).

Many modifications are based on concepts and ideas of how cells and tissues react with surfaces but often these ideas are not based on an accurate knowledge of the basic mechanisms of cellular pathways. For instance, it is widely assumed that a hydroxyapatite surface will be biocompatable since it is found in bone. However, osteoblasts are never in direct contact with hydroxyapatite, so why this material should be assumed to be better than any other is not clear. During wear or due to cellular activity, ions will be released from the implant into the surrounding tissue and many studies have been performed to determine the significance of this. Sun *et al.* (1997) investigated Al, Co, Cr, Ti, Ni and V on expression of alkaline phosphatase, osteopontin, cell division and *in vitro* culture calcification at cytotoxic and subcytotoxic levels. This work indicates significant effects of all these ions on osteoblast growth and differentiation but the concentrations at which these effects occur are not yet clear.

11.2 INTERACTIONS WITH THE SURFACE

Since cells do not possess free electrons, the electrical-conducting property of metals appears not to be an important factor. Electrochemical effects on the surface are important and the most suitable metals and alloys for implantation are self-passivating (see Chapter 5). However, cells are very reactive, producing superoxides, nitrous oxide and protons so that some direct chemical reaction is possible. Many cells such as macrophages, giant cells and osteoclasts are extremely active in this respect. In addition, hydroxyapatite is very hard, much a harder than most metals, and surface abrasion can also occur due to surface shear.

Much of our knowledge of cellular interactions comes from cell culture studies. However, there are many complications to do with the artefact of cell culture and some aspects of cellular reactions might not be relevant to the problem of performance of implants. For instance, it is not really understood what type of cells populate the surface of an implant. Are stem cells important in populating the implant surface? Or is outgrowth from the tissue important? In the marrow cavity, the first might be important and in areas in direct contact with the cortical bone the latter might be more significant. The following sections deal first with some potentially important artefacts of cell culture.

11.3 SURFACE BINDING OF PROTEINS

Cells do not simply react with pure surfaces. In general cells in culture or in the body are in a proteinaceous medium. The type of proteins present and the physicochemical properties of the surface strongly influences the subsequent attachment properties of the cells including the kinetics and strength of attachment and the selection of proteins, etc. Many of these aspects are covered elsewhere in the book and are also studied by many investigators continuing the work of Vroman and his colleagues (Vroman, 1987; Vroman and Adams, 1987). However, since cells are dynamic, many of the original surface proteins are quickly removed by enzymatic activity and new ones synthesised. Many reactive compounds such as nitric oxide and superoxides are produced by most cells and cause reactions at the surface. Most surfaces will bind proteins but the type and amount of protein-binding depends on the physicochemical nature of the surface. Aspects of this are dealt with in Chapter 10. It has been suggested that shape-changes induced by the surface in proteins bound onto surfaces may have a biological effect but there is little direct evidence to support this. Most active biological proteins need to be free to change conformation, in order to be active, and they can be released from surfaces with high protein-binding capacity such as hydroxyapatite. Clearly the quality of the protein-containing nutrient medium will have a strong effect on the outcome of a parameter (e.g. total protein or soluble alkaline phosphatase) measured at a single point in a culture. Our laboratory has measured soluble alkaline phosphatase (AP), osteocalcin, cell number and collagen type I in primary bovine osteoblasts grown on pure mirror-smooth titanium, in the presence of 15 different batches of foetal calf serum (FCS). (The composition of the thousands of factors present in serum is known to vary widely from batch to batch. Hyclone, a company in the USA, has tried to assay all major factors in each batch of serum they sell. We test each batch of serum for growth rate and cellular differentiation, and stock enough FCS to last for 18 months. It should also be recognised that serum proteins contain metal ions and that they will bind metal ions differentially, and the amount of specific binding will vary with each different batch.) All of these parameters were different in each batch of serum. In addition, the growth rate and the degree of homogeneity was also affected by the the actual basis salt medium used. There are many different nutrient media available for mammalian cell culture, usually named after the researcher who developed it, for example Ham's, Dulbecco's, or Eagle's medium. A large number of possibilities exist due to various small differences in glutamine, vitamin C, sodium bicarbonate and glucose or fructose content, for example. (Some media, or media additives, also add µM amounts of selenium, a trace element in glutathione peroxidase which is important for scavenging peroxides). While each salt solution is based on the composition of blood, and the ionic strength of each one is very similar, there are quite marked differences in the growth rate and rate of differentiation between each salt solution. Changing the type of salt solution (e.g. using FCS 1 with Ham's F10, BGJ, αMEM, etc.) also changed many of these parameters, indicating complex interactions of the cells with their nutrient medium and the response to metal surfaces. Table 11.1 shows that a complex interaction is taking place – a good FCS for plastic is not necessarily a good FCS on titanium, and that changing the salt mixture can completely change the results. Over 5 days the amounts of osteocalcin and alkaline phosphatase did not correlate with each other. This shows how difficult it is to obtain basic data and how extremely complex the whole problem is.

In order to test these conditions animal tests should also be made in parallel. A correlation with some histological parameters of an animal test could be found by choosing the 'right' FCS and medium conditions in one large set of experiments, but not in all animal experiments. One way to reduce this complexity is to use serum free media but the 'right' mixture of growth factors and other factors is not yet clear. Hence, while differences in cell growth and differentiation can be demonstrated on any metal surface, what this actually means cannot be correlated with any basic mechanism.

11.4 CONDITIONS OF CELL PLATING

Cells seem to have a particular affinity for different surfaces. This is stochastic as very poor surfaces for cell adhesion, such as regenerated methyl cellulose, still have about 1% of the cells attaching to the surface. In general, all the biomaterial surfaces we have tested, e.g. titanium alloys, steel alloys, ceramics and cements, all have a high variance when compared to standard culture plastic (treated polystyrol).

Table 11.1 Relative production of collagen on surfaces by cells on different surfaces with regard to FCS batch and medium composition

	HA	Ti	TiAl	CCP
F10	***	**	*	***
αMEM	**	**	***	*
BGJ	*	***	**	*

F10, αMEM and BGJ refer to the basal nutrient salt solution (Ham's F10); HA, is high-density hydroxyapatite (Dr Heide, Batelle Institute, Frankfurt); Ti, is pure titanium; TiAl, a titanium aluminium alloy, supplied by Aesculap; and CCP is cell-culture plastic.

Very simple kinetic data can show that rate of cell settling is a function of the relative hydrophobicity of the surface and the cell surface (Meyer *et al.* 1993). This is presumably because most proteins bind initially by their hydrophobic groups. The actual rate again is variable between experiments as the surface characteristics of the cells change between experiments, as would be expected.

A correlation between the surface charge (ζ potential) and cell growth can be found (Möller *et al.*, 1994), which is also dependent on the medium for the actual value. This means that it is impossible to obtain absolute numbers in these types of experiments, everything is relative. Once cells have settled on a surface in culture, the division kinetics show density-dependence. Hence, comparison of surfaces needs to be adjusted for cell densities, in order to provide a valid means of comparison. This might not be significant *in vivo* as outgrowth onto surfaces from tissues might be expected, rather than colonisation of the surface by single cells.

In general many biomaterial surfaces, including metals, show patchy cell growth and are assumed not to be homogenous.

11.5 CELL DENSITY

The number of cells per unit area profoundly influences the rate of cell division and the state of differentiation. Too few cells – the exact number of which varies with the medium, the foetal calf serum batch, the surface and the type of cell, but in all cases is less than 7000 per cm^2 – do not divide or differentiate. In our conditions, the starting cell density from 45 000 to 80 000 cells per cm^2 results in increasing rates of cell division and differences in ultimate cell densities. In cell culture therefore materials with poor plating efficiencies will have at the outset fewer cells on the surface, and the analysis will reflect this rather than any other property of the surface. Presumably *in vivo* the outgrowth from tissue will be more or less constant, irrespective of the plating efficiency of the material. Testing of materials should be carried out as far as possible with the same number of cells per unit area and the plating efficiency yield must be compensated for.

11.6 PLATING EFFICIENCY

Different cultures and different surfaces can plate-out at different efficiencies. Plating efficiency is defined as the percentage of live cells that are attached after 24 h. Viability testing and cell counting are not as precise as we would hope for. We usually use the Trypan Blue exclusion test. Recently, dual fluorescent stains for dead/live cells which are a little more accurate have been developed (e.g. calcein AM/ethidium bromide homodimer). In this case, the calcein enters live cells and the ethidium bromide enters dead cells. Cell counting can be done with a Coulter counter and, more recently, using automated image analysis for DNA-stained cells (ethidium bromide) directly on the surface profile. Clearly, different plating efficiencies will lead to different cell densities and different growth rates as mentioned above.

11.7 'FOREIGN BODY' RESPONSE

A lot of interest has been directed towards inflammatory cells including macrophages. Macrophages can also resorb bone directly (Athanasou and Path, 1996). Many researchers have assumed that macrophages have the ability to sense foreign bodies and have related macrophage-activation by this 'foreign' surface to fibrous capsule formation. While it is clear that macrophages can induce granulomas by TNFα, the relationship to fibrous capsule formation has never been proven. On the contrary, large shear strains have been shown to transform osteoblasts and pre-osteoblasts into fibroblastic cells and *in vivo* the shear amplitude has been shown to cause fibrous capsule formation, and fibrous capsule formation is not a result of any property of the material itself. Macrophages themselves do not appear to be able to detect foreign surfaces *per se* (Jones *et al.*, 1994). Realisation of this fact should aid design of the implant and suggest the types of materials to use. Macrophages are activated by small particles which are also often formed at the shear interface, hence the confusion. A further proof of the lack of a distinct 'foreign body' response is that macrophages are just as reactive to phagocytose bone particles derived from the host as to similarly sized particles of any other material.

11.8 OSMOTIC EFFECTS

These effects are expected to be unimportant in considerations of metal surfaces but they are important in cell culture and in preparing tests. Very small increases in the osmotic pressure is toxic to cells since most cells are living at their physiological limit. Some media, such as the Fitton–Jackson modified Bigger's medium used by some bone investigators, should not be used for biocompatability testing due to its very high osmotic pressure which is higher than considered physiologically advantageous. Additives, when not prepared with regard to their osmotic effects, can easily appear to affect cells purely because of this osmotic effect.

The osmotic pressure is given by the van't Hoff equation:

$$\Pi = RT \times (C_1 + C_2 + C_3 \ldots + C_n)$$

where Π is the osmotic pressure in units of atmospheres, R is the gas constant, T the absolute temperature and C_n are the molar concentrations of all the solutes, ions or molecules in solution.

An alternative method is to work out the osmotic pressure in milli osmoles (mos) where the mM concentration of each of the solutes, e.g. 100 mM NaCl gives 200 mos, are calculated. The physiological range is from 270 to 295 mos, and the usual range of media lies between 290 and 295 mos. Testing soluble materials such as octa-calcium phosphate and tri-calcium phosphate invariably leads to cell death due to the increase in salts in solution over the physiological ability of cells to cope. This effect does not occur in the body since the solubility products diffuse away and can be dealt with in the kidneys for example. It might be, however, that local effects occur. With some products such as corals made of calcium carbonate, some of which are transformed into hydroxyapatite, soluble calcium phosphate salts can cause problems. Hence, testing soluble materials can be impossible in normal cell culture. We have combined TCP with polylactic acid, which does not show such toxic effects, for cell-culture testing (Möller *et al.*, 1994), but interpretation of the results is difficult until the exact amount of TCP released into the medium can be measured. It is recommended that the osmotic pressure of the medium is measured after some days in culture to look for this effect.

It is not clearly understood which component of cellular colonisation is the most important: colonisation by cells or ingrowth from tissue. In the latter case many aspects of the surface, such as surface profile for example, might not be influential on the performance of a biomaterial.

11.9 MORE SOURCES OF VARIABILITY

There are a multitude of reasons for variability in cell cultures. First, the cell populations used vary from animal to animal and also within the same animal from batch to batch. Cell cultures are composed of many millions of individuals who are at different stages of differentiation and it is extremely difficult to produce cultures at exactly the same degree of differentiation, and the same percentages of cells in each stage. The cells are treated with various agents (e.g. proteases, collagenase, EDTA, etc.) to release them from the surface. The amount of digestion that takes place – which also affects receptors – will be variable. The variability of activity between batches of protease and collagenase can also be large. We can see that just the mere treatment of cells can induce large variations in the culture. Oxygen supply to cells in culture is also a significant variable. Oxygen is supplied by diffusion through the medium. At about 30 000 cells per cm^2 cells will use oxygen faster than it can be diffused and the culture becomes anaerobic. This is where lactic acid production comes from in most cell cultures. The cells switch to lactic acid production and stop using oxygen. The oxygen tension builds up in the culture over 2–3 min to about 20% (equilibrates with the gas mixture) because the cells cannot quickly switch back. The oxygen tension then cycles between 20% (toxic) and 0% (growth inhibition) (Werrlein and Clines, 1974). Factors that protect against oxygen such as mercapto-ethanol, vitamin C and vitamin E, all cause an increase in cell number. Changing the medium depth can also affect cell division by optimising the rate of oxygen diffusion, with quite complex implications. In the first instance oxygen tensions at the surface will vary between 0 and 20%, and in the second an acidic micro-environment around the cells is expected to develop. This phenomenon is not expected to be encountered *in vivo*. (However, *in vivo* we could expect to encounter highly reactive oxygen-containing molecules in some phases of the healing.) Some cell modification of the metal surface is thus to be expected in culture and *in vivo*.

Chaotic growth is a feature of cell culture. It is possible to plate-out cells of 99% viability and over 90% plating efficiency (ratio of live cells in suspension to cells plated-out after 24 h – different materials can have different plating efficiencies), with reproducibility of ±1.5%. However, the variance between the replicates grows from day-to-day until by day 5 the cultures differ in cell number by about 12–15%.

11.10 CELLULAR INTERACTIONS

There are many methods for investigating aspects of cellular interaction with the surface. We have found that the rate of cell-settling out of suspension correlates with the hydrophobicity of the surface (Meyer *et al.*, 1994) Differentiation, on the other hand, appears to correlate with the fixed charges on the surface (Möller *et al.*, 1994). Once the cells are on the surface they form attachments of different types, some of which are cell-specific. For instance, irrespective of the surface, osteoclasts form a specialised attachment in the form of a ring which appears to seal off the surface from the outside and the dissolved material is pumped through the cell to the outside.

Our present knowledge of cellular interactions with surfaces is based on the result of inadequate observations of complex non-linear phenomena at a few points in time. Since cellular activities are so complex much of our data are derived from phenomenological results. We do x and y in an experiment, then measure A and B some time later under conditions i and n. It might be possible to reproduce some but not all of the variables x and y and some but not all of the initial conditions. With luck we can measure to a certain degree of accuracy (cell cultures can vary by as much as 15% over 5 days) some of the parameters of A and B. Since A and B are the results of a non-linear process the results might appear to correlate with some changes in x and y but this does not necessarily follow.

11.11 CELL ATTACHMENT

The mechanisms by which cells attach to metal surfaces are important in understanding metal–cell interactions. Most normal (untransformed) cells do not attach to surfaces directly but through the proteins mentioned above. A transformed cell such as most osteosarcoma cell lines is defined as a cell that can undergo anchorage-independent growth, typically tested in an agarose gel, for this reason they are unsuitable for biomaterial investigations. This attachment appears to be a requirement for untransformed cultured cells as is explained in more detail below. In certain conditions such as in wound-healing, in a fibroma or in cell culture, these attachment proteins are fibronectin-type proteins while more physiological attachments are to matrix proteins such as collagen or lamnin. Specialised adhesion structures called focal adhesions (not present or not so well defined in normal tissue) appear, these are condensates of a large number of mechanical and signalling molecules in these sites (Figure 11.1). The attachment proteins are present in plasma and culture serum and are also quickly synthesised by the cell. There is a high turnover of these proteins which can have a half-life of about of 15 min. Embedded in the structure of fibronectin are epidermal growth factor-like sequences which will stimulate cell division when released by proteolytic degradation. After spreading onto a non-colonised surface *in vitro*, cells become contact-inhibited (when they touch they stop dividing or slowly divide and differentiate). During differentiation, cultured osteoblast-like cells will produce a collagenous matrix to which they preferentially attach using a different subset of attachment proteins. In culture, cells usually remain as a monolayer but under some circumstances can form nodules. Formation of small three-dimensional structures appears to correlate with the appearance of cell–cell adhesion molecules called cadherins. In culture the appearance of a collagenous matrix on the cell culture plastic correlates with a rolling up of this cell–collagen layer. This is because the cells exert tension through the actin cytoskeleton system and the collagen does not form a good mechanical bond with the substrate. Hence, the second and perhaps most important feature of tissue–material interface is not the initial cell–fibronectin colonisation phase but in forming a good mechanical bond with the matrix formed by the cells. Titanium reacts in much the same way as cell culture plastic in this second phase, there does not seem to be any mechanical strength between the collagen formed by the cells and the surface. This has also been noticed by many investigators measuring pull-out force in smooth titanium cylinders (e.g. Gross, 1989; Breme, see Chapter 5). Cells, on the other hand, attach and grow very well on these surfaces. The forces that cells exert on the surface (active actin–myosin contraction as in muscle and transmitted to the surface through the intergrins) are in fact less than the forces required to take them off (cells can exert forces of around 1 nN on their substrate). On a 'sticky' surface the adhesion interaction is much stronger than the mechanical integrity of the cell, and cells will pull part and disintegrate before they let go. It is not known if there are varying degrees of surface stickiness as cells either attach and exert force or do not attach at all. There are currently no reliable data for the mechanical properties of many cellular components *in vivo*. Dogterum and Yurke (1997) recently measured the forces exerted by microtubules during polymerisation as 3–4 piconewtons. Not all of the signalling pathways at the focal adhesion sites are understood. Recent studies have demystified one of these complex pathways and the mechanisms behind anchorage-dependent growth (Gilmore and Burridge, 1996; Chrzanowska-Wodnicka *et al.*, 1996; Lyman *et al.*, 1997). A sequence of phosphorylations, protein–protein interactions through these phosphorylated sites, results in the cell being able to react to a growth factor (perhaps released from fibronectin). The sequence starts with binding of the α-chain of an intergrin to the substrate, the binding of this to a β-intergrin chain, which then binds a number of other sequencing molecules including the phosphorylated focal adhesion site kinase ppFAK125 (**P**hospho**P**rotein **F**ocal **A**dhesion **K**inase 125 kDa molecular weight). Figure 11.1 shows a scheme of this binding. These attachment sites are very dynamic and can move several nm in a few minutes. It is thought that proteins such as tensin possibly provide a mechanical connection to the actin cytoskeleton. Vinculin was also thought to be a mechanical connector between the adhesion sites and actin but this is no longer believed to be the case (Meyer *et al.*, 1997). Vinculin might play a role in guiding the formation of the focal adhesion site and is released from the focal adhesion site by slight mechanical forces. The actin cytoskeleton is tensed by myosin as in muscle. The tension formed by these actin cables is also thought to be a reason why cells orient along surface profiles as small as 100 nm deep.

11.12 CELL–MATERIAL INTERACTIONS

The major interaction of a cell with a surface is through the specific adhesion proteins above. However, the first interaction with a surface is non-specific and is probably regulated through hydrophobic interactions. The surface binds soluble proteins through hydrophobic and fixed charge interactions, and some of these proteins can promote specific cell ligand binding. Typical adhesion proteins are fibronectin, vitronectin and osteopontin. The strength of this specific binding is very high, and often either the cell cytoskeleton and membrane will break or, less often, the adhesion proteins will rip away from the surface. The ligands the cells attach to are the intergrins which are hetrodimers, composed of an α- and a β-chain, as shown in Figure 11.1.

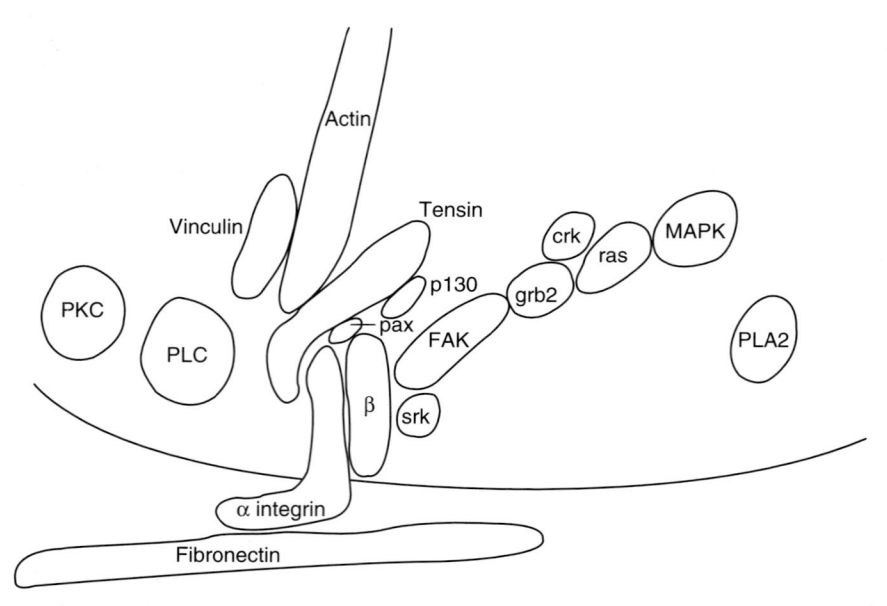

Figure 11.1 A model of cell attachment. Intergrins and cadherins (not shown, but responsible for cell–cell attachment) are linked through the membrane to complex intracellular pathways. The attachment Ca ion, dependent in both cases, and can be inhibited by other metal ions.

At least nine different α-chains are known and they can confer specificity and recognise only certain adhesion or matrix proteins. In culture and in some pathological cases (where a lot of fibrin and fibronectin is present), the attachment sites are clustered together into focal adhesion sites. This does not occur *in vivo*, so this is probably one of the few real 'foreign body' responses. At these sites many signalling molecules gather as shown in Figure 11.1. The condensation of the signalling molecules and their influence on one another provides a good explanation for the mechanism of adhesion-dependance growth. However, *in vivo* most cells attach to each other by a different set of adhesion molecules, the cadherins, and slightly different signalling pathways exist. Such large condensations of intergrins, as shown in Figure 11.1, are not found in normal tissue.

11.13 QUANTITATIVE MEASUREMENT OF CELL AND MATRIX ATTACHMENT FORCE

In the case of titanium surfaces we have found that at high cell densities the cells grow and produce a lot of matrix but this matrix does not attach to the surface. Many surfaces promote the attachment of cells but not the matrix they produce. It is possible to measure the attachment forces by the use of a fluid shear force device. There are several types described elsewhere in the book. The rotating cone does not appear to give homogenous shear forces. The parallel plate system, if the gap between the plates is less than 1 mm, does. Van Kooten *et al.* (1992) have used such chambers for investigating the role of surface hydrophobicity on cell attachment. An interesting linear gradient shear flow device is described by Usami *et al.* (1993) and is shown in Figure 11.2.

11.14 PHARMACOLOGICAL EFFECTS OF TRACE AMOUNTS OF METAL IONS

Trace amounts of metal ions can cause a number of physiological effects. In some cases the exact mechanisms of the effects are unknown. These are:

- membrane potential changes (either through concentration effects, indirectly through channel inhibition or stimulation)
- tumour promotion
- long-term toxic effects
- growth stimulation.

Sometimes an exact analysis of a material is not carried out because the composition of trace elements is assumed not to be of importance. Recently developed methods such as Time Of Flight Secondary Ion Mass Spectrometry (TOFSIMS) can detect very small amounts of all elements at a resolution of less than 1 μm. Using TOFSIMS we have detected small (6 μm) inclusions of lithium in an ionomeric cement which had escaped detection by other methods, see for instance Figure 11.3.

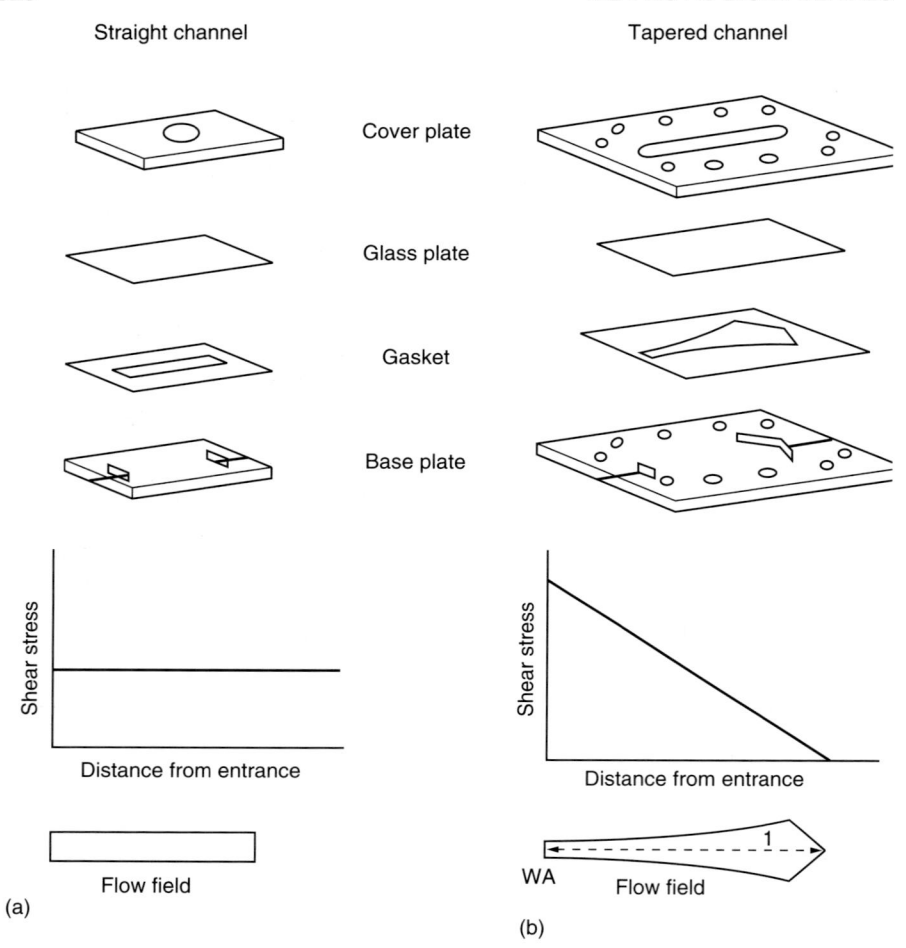

Figure 11.2 Diagram of a gradient shear flow channel (Usami et al., 1993).

As previously mentioned the cell uses certain metal ions for physiological purposes and is not usually exposed to other ions. Some introduced ions have the ability to be transported into the cell using normal physiological pathways and may interfere with cellular processes. Sometimes these effects can be measured at a concentration of ppb. These ions may enter through ion channels via transporter systems such as the transferrin system or through the proton coupled metal ion transporter, which has recently been reported and cloned, and which can transport at least Zn^{2+}, Mn^{2+}, Co^{2+}, Cd^{2+}, Cu^{2+}, Ni^{2+} and Pb^{2+} (Gunshin et al., 1997). Aluminium might enter the cell through the Fe transporter and be stored intracellularly while the concentration builds up. In the presence of silicate, the insoluble aluminium silicates might be less toxic. (Meyer et al., 1994). The recently described copper transport pathway might also be a mechanism for entry of other metals into the cell (Pufahl et al., 1997).

CELLS AND METALS

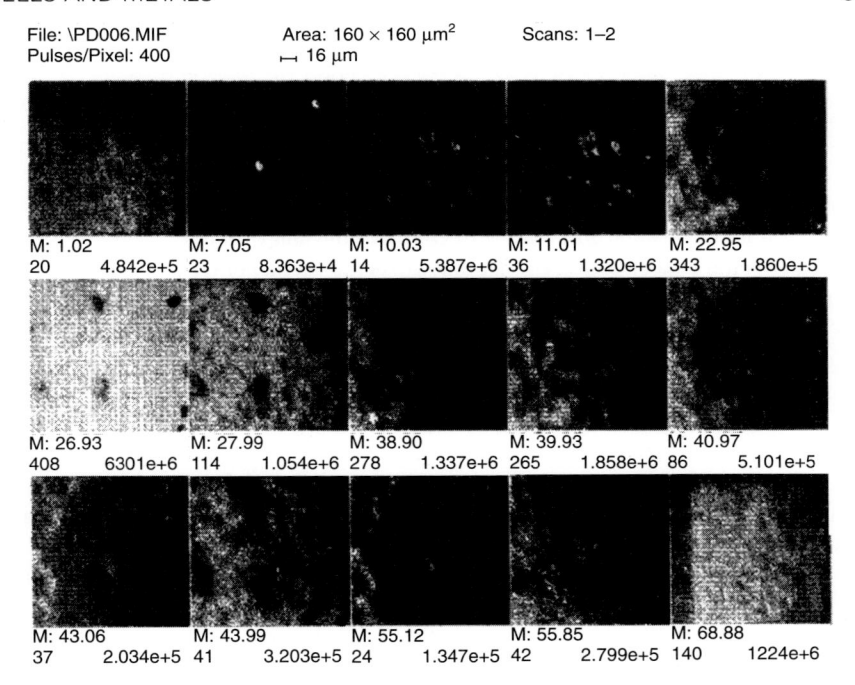

File: \PD006.MIF Area: 160 × 160 µm² Scans: 1–2
Pulses/Pixel: 400 ⊢ 16 µm

M: 1.02	M: 7.05	M: 10.03	M: 11.01	M: 22.95
20 4.842e+5	23 8.363e+4	14 5.387e+6	36 1.320e+6	343 1.860e+5
M: 26.93	M: 27.99	M: 38.90	M: 39.93	M: 40.97
408 6301e+6	114 1.054e+6	278 1.337e+6	265 1.858e+6	86 5.101e+5
M: 43.06	M: 43.99	M: 55.12	M: 55.85	M: 68.88
37 2.034e+5	41 3.203e+5	24 1.347e+5	42 2.799e+5	140 1224e+6

Figure 11.3 A TOFSIMS scan of an ionomeric cement showing other elements such as small inclusions of lithium. Local inclusions of lithium could be expected to have large local effects on cells.

11.15 MEMBRANE POTENTIAL

Cells closely control the internal concentrations of many metals especially Ca, Na and K. These ions also play a role in control of membrane potential. Cells spend a great deal of energy, perhaps as much as 30% of the cellular energy budget, in maintaining a high intracellular potassium and low sodium. Calcium is stored in specialised organelles in the cell and free cytoplasmic calcium is very low (c. 70 nM). To maintain the differential adenosine triphosphate – the 'fuel' of the cell – is used by special pumps. There are Na/K exchangers and Na/Ca exchangers to maintain the differentials. When channels are opened specific ions will pass down the gradient (either in or out). Hence when a K channel opens, K leaves the cell and the inside becomes negatively charged with respect to the outside – hyperpolarisation. When a Ca channel opens Ca flows into the cell and the cell becomes depolarised. Very many factors and hormones, for instance prostaglandins, parathyroid hormone, insulin-like growth factor, fibroblast growth factor, epidermal growth factor and so on, cause an increase in calcium either through direct action on the channel or through release from one of the many types of intracellular calcium stores. The frequency of calcium oscillations is also important information for the cell. Hence any disturbance of this system will affect cell behaviour.

Changing the proportion of ions in the extracellular solution can affect the membrane potential of cells as given by the Goldman equation below:

$$\mathrm{MP} = \frac{RT}{zF} \ln \frac{(pI_1 \cdot cI_1)+(pI_2 \cdot cI_2 \ldots)}{(pO_1 \cdot cO_1)+(pO_2 \cdot cO_2 \ldots)}$$

where R is the gas constant, T is the absolute temperature, z is the charge of the ion, F is the Faraday constant, pI is the permeability constant of the ion on the inside of the cell, cI is the concentration of that ion, pO is the permeability constant of the ion on the outside of the cell and cO is the outside concentration.

We can calculate that increasing potassium ion concentration on the outside will reduce the membrane potential. This has the effect of increasing the chance of the calcium channel opening (voltage-dependent gating) which can eventually have the effect of raising the rate of mitosis as well as causing other physiological effects. There are many enzymes which are affected by calcium. Inhibiting calcium signalling can result in cell death, and modification of the concentration of this vital metal ion will result in profound effects on the cell. Even small changes in calcium ion concentration are very important (see Figure 11.4).

Increasing calcium ion concentration in the medium or extracellular space, although theoretically increasing membrane potential, can sometimes activate the calcium channel through a positive feedback mechanism and also increase cell division. However, very high calcium concentrations are toxic. An exact measurement of the ionic composition of the extracellular medium can therefore give a good idea of the biological activity due to the membrane potential effects.

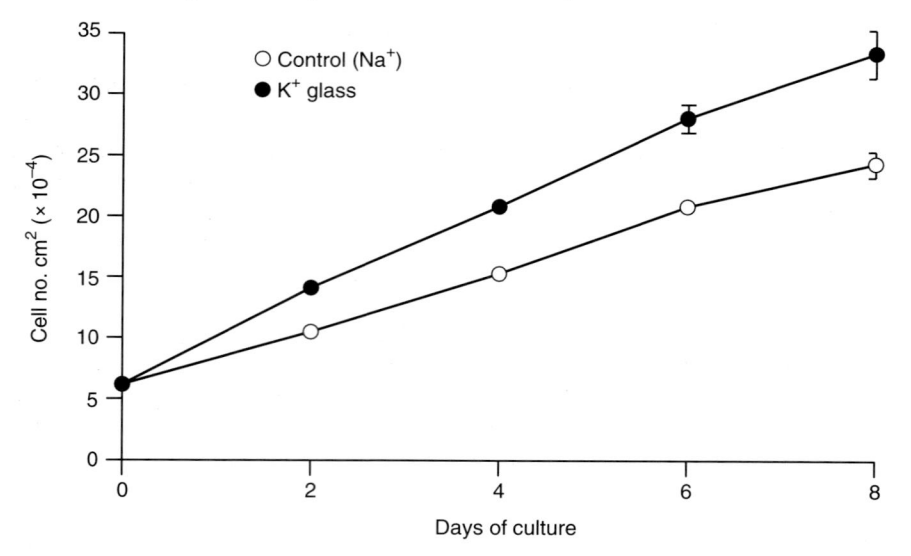

Figure 11.4 Growth of primary bovine osteoblasts on sodium borosilicate glass and on the same glass that had been hardened by ion exchange with potassium. A significant increase in the rate of division is seen.

Many metals at low concentrations of around 1 µM, can inhibit different types of calcium channels, these metals include Pb, Zn, Ni, Ba, Co, Cr, Cd and B. Many dozens of different calcium channel types exist and the effects of different metal ions seem to be channel-specific, see for example a recent review by Audesirk (1993). Manganese ions, whilst having no effect on the channel itself, can be transported through Ca^{2+} channels and interfere with some Ca^{2+}-dependent processes. Clearly lower concentrations will proportionally affect the dynamics of the channel. Some heavy metals, such as Pb above, will proportionally affect K channels. This seems to be due to these metals substituting for Ca (Vijverberg et al., 1994).

Busselberg (1995) has shown that Pb ions interact with voltage-activated and receptor-activated ion channels at µM concentrations. Al and Cd also affect both small and large Ca-activated K channels. Rengel (1994) has investigated Al, Gd, Cr and La effects on Ca^{2+} influx with some complex interactions occurring between Al and La with Al reversing the La effect. This finding together with that of Zatta et al. (1994), that Al can activate acetylcholinesterase, might account for some of the mechanisms of long-term Al toxicity.

Benders et al. (1994) have investigated the inhibitory action of Cu ions on the Na/K ATPase and the Na/Ca exchanger. This will result in altered membrane potential dynamics and direct interference with calcium signalling.

Ceramics and some other materials can contain trace amounts of metallic ions such as lithium. We have detected small lithium inclusions by TOFSIMS. Lithium, used therapeutically as an antidepressant, interferes with inositol phosphate metabolism, a vital cellular second messenger system (Dixon and Hokin, 1997).

11.16 METAL RESPONSIVE ELEMENTS

Most cells respond to heavy metal ions with a stress response. Stress proteins, also known as heat shock proteins, of the hsp 70 and hsp 90 group are induced by heavy metal ions as are many metallothionein genes. Metal response elements are parts of these gene promoter regions. One metal responsive element (MRE) is a *cis*-acting DNA motif located in the upstream region of vertebrate metallothionein genes which can confer metal responsiveness on downstream heterologous promoters. Several proteins exist that can bind MRE sequences. Physiologically, many of these use Zn ions (zinc regulatory factor: ZRF). Downstream regulation of genes by these gene products may account for many biological effects of non-physiological metal ions. Takeda et al. (1994) have described a Cd-activated *cis*-acting element inducing the haem oxygenase gene. Some effects on cell differentiation can perhaps be ascribed to similar activation of genes although metallothionein induction is generally assumed to be a protection mechanism through metal ion binding.

11.17 ONCOGENIC EFFECTS

Ni and Ti have been implicated in some studies as having a carcinogenic effect. The case for Ti is circumstantial, but more is known about Ni. Ni itself may play a physiological role in the cell. That Ni is implicated in some forms of cancer has been known for over 50 years (IARC, 1990). It has been proposed that Ni^{2+} can be oxidised to Ni^{2+} (for example by H_2O_2), and thus takes part in oxidative damage to proteins and to DNA. The mechanism of damage would then be similar to the 3^+ oxidative states of other metal ions (Fenton chemistry). Pb in pM concentrations has been suggested to have tumour-promoter activity through its activation of protein kinase C (Markovac and Goldstein, 1988). These signalling pathways have been discussed by Smith *et al.* (1994) as a mechanism for carcinogenic effects of some metals. Lead certainly activates PKC and causes phosphorylations of membranes (e.g. Belloniolivi *et al.*, 1996). It would expected that the incidence of bone tumours would be high in roman graves since lead acetate was used to sweeten wine by the romans. However, no archaeologist has reported this.

11.18 METAL ALLERGIES

Contact metal allergies are well documented. However patients with a well-defined contact allergy to nickel do not seem to react to implants containing nickel (Griss, personal communication). However, the mechanisms behind contact allergies are not that well understood. Hernandez and Macia (1996) have reported on the enhancement polymorphonuclear leukocyte adherence by cadmium and nickel (10–100 nM) which seemed to be mediated via external sulfydryl groups. Bigazzi (1994) has reviewed the effect of heavy metals on autoimmunity. Several investigators have studied some aspects of metal ions in skin and have shown that one of the effects could be entrapment of metal ions in different layers of the skin and also higher uptake by keratinocytes as opposed to fibroblasts (Merritt and Brown, 1995, 1996; Lacy *et al.*, 1996).

11.19 CONCLUSIONS

The interactions of small concentrations of metal ions released from surfaces is not well understood because of the lack of appropriate analytical tools. Non-physiological metals will, with rare exceptions, interfere with a large number of cellular pathways by a number of different mechanisms. These effects will be concentration-dependent and can affect cells at doses much less than those required for toxic effects. Long-term toxicity of aluminium seems to be related to storage of the ion in intracellular stores, possibly interfering in the long term with Fe^{2+} metabolism and also perhaps having an effect on acetylcholinesterase. Recent developments in many fields such as, for instance, various atomic probe microscopes and TOFSIMS should prove useful in investigating subtle effects of cells on metal surfaces.

REFERENCES

Athansou, N.A. and Path, F.R. (1996) Current concepts review of the cell biology of bone resorbing cells, *J. Bone Joint Surg.* **78–A**, 1096–112.
Audesirk, G. (1993) Electrophysiology of lead-intoxication – effects on voltage-sensitive ion channels, *Neurotoxicology* **14**, 137–48.
Belloniolivi, L., Annadata, M., Golstein, G.W. and Bressler, J.P. (1996) Phosphorylation of membrane proteins in erythrocytes treated with lead, *J. Biochem.* **315**, 401–6.
Benders, A.A.G.M., Li, J., Lock, R.A.C., Bindels, R.J.M., Bonga, S.E.W. and Veerkamp, J.H. (1994) Copper toxicity in cultured human skeletal muscle cells. Involvement of Na^+/K^+- ATPase and the Na^+/Ca^{2+} exchanger, *Pflugers Archive – Eur. J. Physiol.* **428**, 461–7.
Bigazzi, P.E. (1994) Autoimmunity and heavy-metals, *Lupus* **3**, 449–53.
Busselberg, D. (1995) Calcium channels as target sites of heavy metals, *Toxicol. Lett.* **82**, 255–61.
Chang, L.W. (ed.) (1996) *Toxicology of Metals*, CRC Press, Boca Raton, FL.
Chrzanowska-Wodnicka, M. and Burridge, K. (1996) Rho-stimulated contractility drives the formation of stress fibers and focal adhesions, *J. Cell Biol.* **133**, 1403–15.
Dixon, J.F. and Hokin, L.E. (1997) The antibipolar drug valproate mimics lithium in stimulating glutamate release and inositol 1,4,5-trisphosphate accumulation in brain cortex slices but not accumulation of inositol monophosphates and bisphosphates, *Proc. natn. Acad. Sci, USA* **94**, 4757–760.
Dogterom, M. and Yurke, B. (1997) Measurement of the force-velocity relationship for growing microtubules, *Science* **278**, 856–60.
Gilmore, A.P. and Burridge, K. (1996) Molecular mechanisms for focal adhesion assembly through regulation of protein-protein interactions, *Structure* **4**, 647–51.
Groß, U. (1989) *Ceramic Coating of Metals*. Report to the German Ministry of Research and Technology.
Gunshin, H., Mackenzie, B., Berger, U.V., Gunshin, Y., Boron, W.F., Nussberger, S., Gollan, J.L. and Hediger, M.A. (1997) Cloning and characterization of a mammalian proton-coupled metal-ion transporter, *Nature* **388**, 482–8.
Hernandez, M. and Macia, M. (1996) Free peripheral sulfhydryl-groups CD11/CD18 intergrins, and Ca are required in the cadmium and nickel enhancement of human polymorphonuclear leukocyte adherence, *Arch. Environ. Contam. Toxicol.* **30**, 437–43.
IARC (1990) Monograph on the evaluation of carcinigenic risk to humans in *Chromium, Nickel, Welding*, Vol. 49, International Agency for Research on Cancer, Lyon, France.
Jones, D.B., Doty, S.B. and van den Bos, R.C. (1994) Biomechanics and the foreign body response, in *Failure of Joint Replacement, a Biological, Mechanical or Surgical Problem?* (eds S. Downes and M. Dabestani), Royal National Orthopaedic Hospital.
Kowalec, J.S., Brown, S.A., Payer, J.H. and Merritt, K. (1995) Mixed metal fretting corrosion of Ti6Al4V and wrought cobalt alloy, *J. Biomed. Mater. Res.* **29**, 867–73.
Lacy, S.A., Merritt, K., Brown, S.A. and Puryear, A. (1996) Distribution of nickel and cobalt following dermal and systemic administration with *in vitro* and *in vivo* studies, *J. Biomed. Mater. Res.* **32**, 279–83.
Lyman, S., Gilmore, A., Burridge, K., Gidwitz, S. and White, G.C. (1997) Integrin-mediated activation of focal adhesion kinase is independent of focal adhesion formation or integrin activation – studies with activated and inhibitory β(3) cytoplasmic domain mutants, *J. Biol. Chem.* **272**, 36.
Markovac, J. and Goldstein G.W. (1988) Picomolar concentrations of lead stimulate brain protein kinase C, *Nature* **334**, 71–3.

Merritt, K. and Brown, S.A. (1995) Release of hexavalent chromium from corrosion of stainless-steel and cobalt-chromium alloys, *J. Biomed. Mater. Res.* **29**, 627–33.

Merritt, K. and Brown, S.A. (1996) Distribution of cobalt-chromium wera and corrosion products and biologic reactions, *Clin. Orthop. Rel. Res.* **329**, 233–43.

Meyer, U., Szulczweski, D., Moeller, K., Heide, H. and Jones, D.B. (1993) Attachment kinetics and differentiation of osteoblast on different biomaterials, *Cells and Mater.* **3**, 129–40.

Meyer, U., Szulczewski, D., Barckhaus, R., Atkinson, M. and Jones, D.B. (1994) Biological evaluation of an ionomeric bone cement by osteoblast cell culture methods. *Biomaterials* **14**, 917–24.

Meyer, U., Meyer, T. and Jones, D.B. (1997) No mechanical role for vinculin in strain transduction in primary bovine osteoblasts, *Biochem. Cell Biol.* **75**, 81–7.

Möller, K., Meyer, U., Szulczewski, D., Heide, H., Priessnitz, B. and Jones, D.B. (1994) The influence of zeta potential and interfacial tension on osteoblast-like cells, *Cells and Mater.* **4**, 263–74.

Powis, D.A., Clark, C.L. and O´Brien, K.J. (1994) Lanthanum can be transported by the sodium–calcium exchange pathway and directly triggers catecholamine release from bovine chromaffin cells, *Cell calcium* **16**, 377–90.

Pufahl, R.A., Singer, C.P., Periso, K.L., Lin, S.-J., Schmidt, P.J., Fahmi, C.J., Ciweski-Culotta, V., Peenner-Hahn, J.E. and O'Halloran, T.V. (1997) Metal ion chaperone function of the soluble Cu(I) receptor Atxl., *Science* **278**,.853–5.

Rengel, W. (1994) Metal interactions with voltage-activated and receptor-activated ion channels, *J. Plant Physiol.* **143**, 47–51.

Slikkerveer, A. and de Wolff, F.A. (1996) Toxicity of Bismuth and its compounds, in *Toxicology of Metals* (ed. L.W. Chang), CRC Press, Boca Raton, FL, pp. 439–54

Smith, J.B., Smith, L., Pijuan, V., Zhuang, Y.X. and Chen, Y.C. (1994) Transmembrane signals and proto-oncogene induction evoked by carcinogenic metals, *Environ. Hlth Perspect.* **102**, 181–9.

Sun, Z.L., Wataha, J.L. and Hanks, C.T. (1997) Effects of metal ions on osteoblastlike cell metabolism and differentiation, *J. Biomed. Mater. Res.* **34**.

Takeda, K., Fujita, H. and Shibahara, S. (1994) Differential control of the metal-mediated activation of the human heme oxygenase-1 and metallothionein IIa genes, *Biochem. Biophys. Res. Commun.* **207**, 160–7.

Usami, S., Chen, H.H., Zhao, Y., Chien, S. and Skalak, R. (1993) Design and construction of a linear shear stress flow chamber, *Ann. Biomed. Eng.* **21**, 7–83.

Van Kooten, T.G., Van der Mei, H.C., Schakenraad, J.M. and Busscher, H.J. (1992) Cellular responses to endothelial stimuli, influence of fluid shear and substrate hydrophobicity on adhesion of human fibroblasts, *Biofouling* **5**, 2239–456.

Vijverberg, H.P.M., Leinderszufall, T. and Vankleef, R.G.D.M. (1994) Differential effects of heavy metal ions on Ca^{2+}-dependent K^+ channels, *Cell. Molec. Neurobiol.* **14**, 841–57.

Vroman, L. and Adams, A.L. (1987) Why plasma-proteins interact at interfaces, *ACS Symposium series* **343**, 154–64.

Vroman, L. (1987) The importance of surfaces in contact phase reactions, *Semin. Thromb. Hemost.* **13**, 79–85.

Werrlein, R.J. and Clines, A.D. (1974) Oxygen microenvironment and respiratory oscillations in cultured mammalian cells, *Nature* **251**, 317–19.

Zatta, P., Zamnendetti, P., Bruna, V. and Filippi, B. (1994) Activation of acetyl-cholinesterase by Al(III), *Neuroreport* **5**, 1777–80.

FURTHER READING

BOOKS

ASM Handbooks no. 1 (1990) to no. 19 (1996) (all aspects of metals and ceramics), ASM International, Metals Park, OH, 1995.
ASTM Annual Book of ASTM Standards.
MRS Proceedings of their Annual Fall Meeting.
Handbook of Corrosion (1995) ASM International, Metals Park, OH.
Boyer, R., Welsch, G. and Collings, E.W. (1994) *Materials Properties Handbook: Titanium Alloys*, ASM International, Metals Park, OH.
Guide to Materials Engineering Data and Information (1986) ASM International, Metals Park, OH.
Pollock, D.D. (1993) *Physical Properties for Engineers*, CRC Blackwell Library Services, Oxford.

SOFTWARE

TAPP version 3.0 (1996) A materials database of over 30 000 compound phases, solutions and phase diagrams, ESM Software, USA, Hamilton.

COMPUTERISED MATERIAL DATABASES

Cuthill, J.R., Gokcan, N.A. and Morral J.E. (1988) The Metallurgical Society, Worchdale, USA.
The Materials Property Data Network (1995) STN International, CAS, Columbus, OH.
International Metallic Materials Cross-reference Database Software (1996) Genium Publishing Corporation, Schenectady, NY.
ASTM Stahlschlüssel with CD-ROM (1996) ASTM and Technical Standard Services, Hitchin, Herts.

MATERIALS SELECTION BOOKS

Cornish, E.H. (1985) *Materials Selections and Design*, UK Information Sources, Chameleon Press Ltd.
Waterman, N.A. and Ashby, M.F. (1996) *Elsevier Materials Selector*, Elsevier Applied Science, London.
Ashby, M.F. (1994) Materials Selection Wallchart, Chapman & Hall, London.

MATERIALS SELECTION SOFTWARE

CMS 2.0 Software (1995) Granta Design Limited, Cambridge, UK, Cambridge Materials Selector.

12
X-ray photoelectron spectroscopy

J.J PIREAUX AND J. RIGA
Universtiy of Namur, Namur, Belgium

12.1 INTRODUCTION

X-ray photoelectron spectroscopy (XPS) is applied to the study of any type of material ranging from gases or liquids to the solid state. In the last quarter of a century, studies of surfaces, interfaces and thin films have benefited most from this spectroscopy, which indeed reveals itself as a most powerful, non-destructive method. As a consequence of this, it is present in almost every industrial and university surface laboratory.

Bulk and surface properties of metallic biomaterials are approached by the use of many complementary techniques, such as Auger electron spectroscopy, secondary ion-mass spectroscopy, electron imaging microscopies, Rutherford backscattering spectroscopy and so on.

This chapter aims to present non-specialists with the principles, advantages and limitations of XPS using examples selected from the field of metallic biomaterials. But this should not be considered as a limitation of the method. Examples from other research fields could have been chosen: the XPS technique is also extremely valuable to the study of surfaces and interfaces involving, for example polymers, semiconductors, ceramics, catalysts and glasses. *A priori*, any solid-state material surface can be studied by XPS.

For the purposes of this investigation only practical questions relevant to the study of metallic surfaces will be addressed. Some aspects such as charging effect and binding energy referencing, radiation damage, and theoretical development will not be emphasised here. Therefore, this chapter should not be considered as an exhaustive review; on the contrary, very few references are cited; mostly examples from the authors' laboratory will be used as illustrations. The further reading section will list suggestions on the subject including reference (tutorial) books, handbooks, conference proceedings and reviews on biomaterials.

12.2 PRINCIPLES

The photoelectric effect discovered by Hertz (1887) and explained by Einstein (1905) has resulted through the efforts of Siegbahn *et al.* (1967) in high-resolution spectrometers that are capable, in the range of 0–1000 eV electron energy, of detecting well-defined line structures; these core level electron lines are not only characteristic of the elements present in the samples but also suffer shifts in energy depending on the different chemical states of the atoms (e.g. as in a metal, or in an oxide). Technical developments in high- and ultra-high-vacuum technology in the late 1960s were necessary to the development and applications of X-ray induced photoelectron spectroscopy used in the study of solid-state materials because of extreme surface sensitivity.

12.2.1 THE PHOTOELECTRIC EFFECT

MgKα (1253.6 eV) or AlKα (1486.6 eV) sources are used (after monochromatisation for the latter) to irradiate the sample surface, kept in ultra-high vacuum. The photon energy ($E = h\nu$) absorbed by one electron in an atom has a given probability to provoke the ejection of this electron (hereafter called 'photoelectron'), with a given kinetic energy E_k. Provided the electron does not suffer any further inelastic collision within the solid, it will conserve its kinetic energy until it is detected by an electrostatic analyser. As a consequence of the Einstein's energy conservation relation, this is shown by

$$E_k = h\nu - E_B - \phi \tag{12.1}$$

where E_B is the electron-binding energy on a given orbital, and ϕ is the spectrometer work function. This electron-binding energy may be regarded as a difference between an initial (bound electron) and different final states of the ionised atom: this possibly gives rise to different satellites (Section 12.4.4). In the photoelectron spectrometer, the number of photoelectrons detected at any given energy level, is stored and displayed versus the electron binding energy. As a result, the photoelectron spectrum shows sharp and intense peaks (core-level lines) and some other bands of lower intensity comprising the already mentioned satellites, as well as showing the distribution of electronic states in the valence band of the solid, close to zero binding energy.

The core-level lines correspond to photoelectrons ejected from a specified atom but with a different E_k, according to the electronic levels they are coming from. As the electronic structure of an atom is a unique fingerprint of this atom, photoelectron spectra allow an elemental analysis of the target (except for the detection of hydrogen). Figure 12.1 shows the relative binding energies for the element titanium (metallic state). By definition, the Fermi level corresponds to zero binding energy. Harder X-rays will allow the investigator to probe deeper electronic levels; softer X-

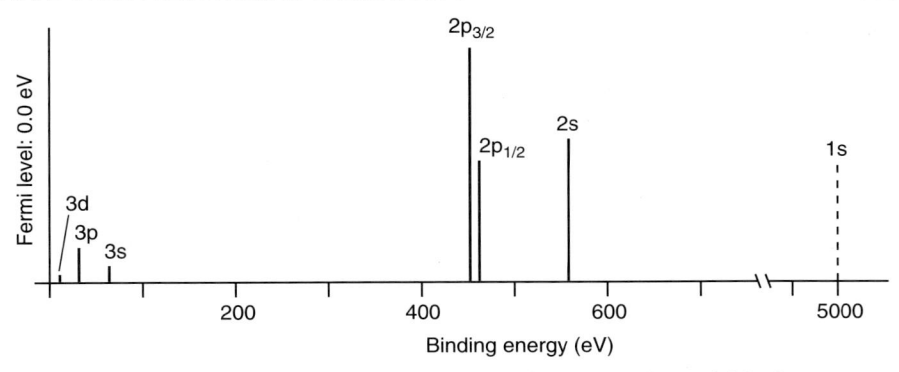

Figure 12.1 Electronic structure of titanium. On the horizontal binding energy scale (relative to the Fermi level), the lines show the positions of the titanium core levels; the line length is proportional to its photoionisation cross-section. See Figure 12.4 for an XPS spectrum of a Ti surface.

rays will only reveal the outer electrons of the atoms; when UV photons are used to probe valence band levels, the technique is called ultraviolet photoelectron spectroscopy (UPS) instead of XPS.

12.2.2 THE EXPERIMENTAL PRINCIPLE

In the study of metals and alloys, a schematic diagram of the XPS apparatus would resemble Figure 12.2; it contains the X-ray source, the electron analyser and optics ensemble, the photoelectron detection and the sample accessories; these are all located in one vacuum chamber. The Mg and Al anode sources cited above are the most frequently used as they allow a sufficient number of core level(s) of any atom to be reached, and as their small natural line width allows the recording of well-resolved photoelectron spectra; for the aluminium source, a monochromator based on X-ray diffraction by quartz crystal(s) is available, to remove spurious excitation channels (see Section 12.4.4). The photoelectron analyser is based on two concentric electrostatic hemispherical sectors, equipped with electrostatic (sometimes magnetic) lenses to collect, retard or accelerate, or to focus, the photoelectron beam. A multiple channeltrons ensemble or a channelplate detector is used to amplify the photoelectric current that is captured versus the electron energy and this results in the XPS spectrum stored on a computer. Common accessories to study metals and alloys are sample temperature control (heating and cooling), ion gun for surface cleaning and depth profiling (see Section 12.4.6), precise sample manipulation for transferring and positioning during angular resolved studies (see Section 12.4.6), and sometimes surface mapping (see Section 12.4.7). Abrasion, fracturing or scraping tools are also sometimes necessary to prepare a clean, fresh surface of the metal.

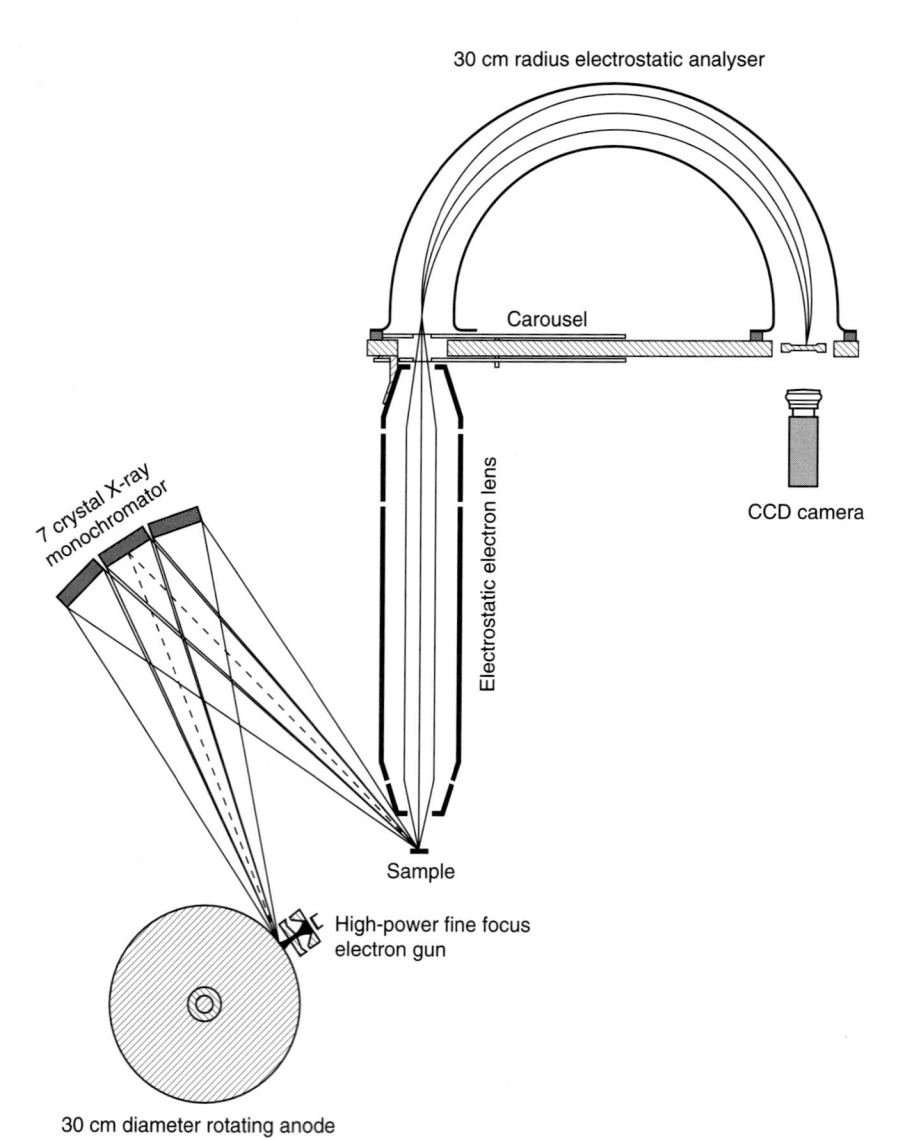

Figure 12.2 Schematic diagram of the ESCA Scienta 300 spectrometer: it shows the rotating anode X-ray source, the monochromator, the electrostatic lens, the hemispherical electron energy analyser and the detector.

12.2.3 PHOTOIONISATION CROSS-SECTION

The XPS sensitivity to detect a specified atom in a sample is first dependent on the probability (σ) for the chosen X-ray to provoke one ionisation in a core level of this atom. This interaction is well described by relativistic quantum chemical (e.g. Hartree–Fock–Slater) calculations, and σ values are readily obtained in published tables. As σ varies for all the electronic levels of a given element and as the natural line width of core levels varies too, the investigator sometimes has to find the best compromise to identify the core level line that will give the most intense signal, for a given set of specified accumulation time, signal to background ratio and memory channels. For example, although σ for the Pt$_{4d}$ level is larger, the Pt$_{4f}$ line is more easily detected because of its smaller inherent width. For an homogeneous sample, the XPS detection limit is about 0.1% for metallic samples; if, for some reason, surface enrichment occurs (inhomogeneous sample), this limit is expressed in terms of 0.1% of monolayer, i.e. 10^{12}–10^{13} atoms cm^{-2} (or 10^{-10}–10^{-9} g cm^{-2}). This extreme surface sensitivity makes XPS an excellent technique to study surface induced modification, contamination, corrosion and thin films.

12.2.4 ELECTRON MEAN-FREE-PATH

Although the X-ray photon penetration depth in solid materials is of a few micrometres, and thus relatively large, the analysed photoelectron spectrum fingerprints only the superficial layers. Indeed, photoelectrons emitted from deeper layers follow the fate of charged particles in a solid, that is they are scattered and disappear from the true photoelectron lines and contribute to the spectrum background (see Section 12.4.4). The photoelectric signal at sample depth d below the surface I_o, is thus attenuated according to a Beer–Lambert law: $I = I_o \, e^{-d/\lambda}$ where λ is the electron mean-free-path. According to empirical laws, it can be described as $\lambda \simeq E_k^{0.75}$, this means that λ varies between 0.5 and 2 nm in the usual photoelectron kinetic energy range. As suggested by Figure 12.3 for an homogeneous solid studied in the 45°/45° geometry, about 99% of a photoelectron core-line intensity originates from a depth of 3λ, i.e. a value of about 6 nm (depending on the electron E_k). Therefore, the XPS method is only sensitive to the extreme surface of the solid materials. This great advantage contains its own limitation: the technique is extremely sensitive to surface contamination. Because of this, it is absolutely essential to handle the samples very carefully in order to avoid contamination; furthermore, the sample has to be analysed in a very good vacuum to preserve its initial surface composition. Ultra-high-vacuum (UHV, defined as pressure below 10^{-9} torr) is mandatory for XPS analysis of reactive surfaces as it is the limit to allow a set of photoelectron spectra to be recorded from a surface free of any external contaminant from the spectrometer vessel.

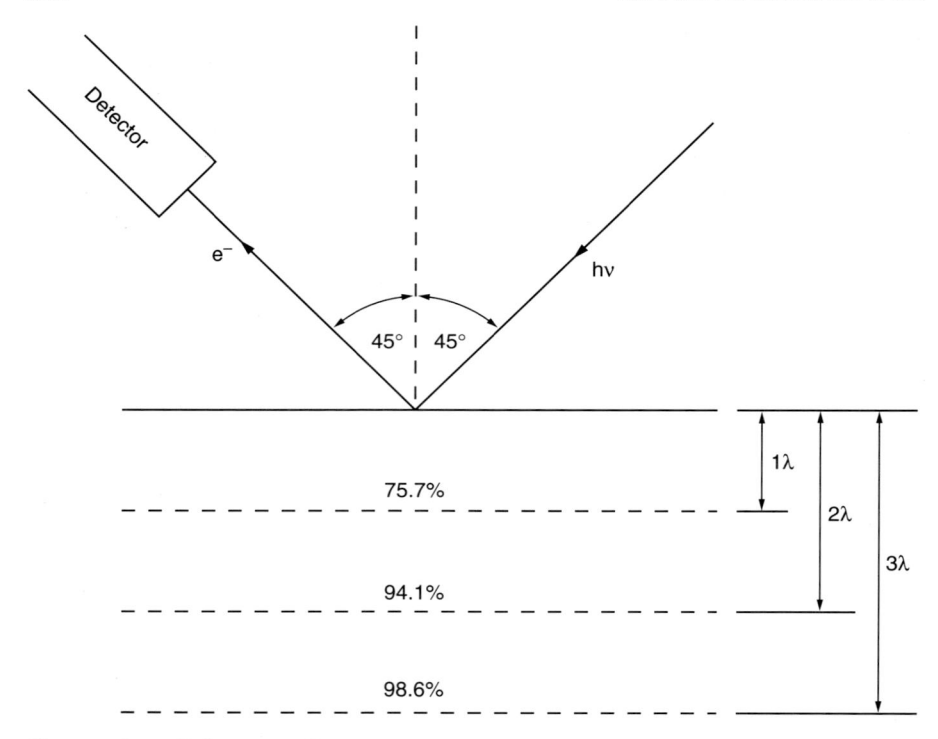

Figure 12.3 Schematic diagram suggesting that the total photoelectron intensity recorded from a homogeneous solid originates from a total depth equal to ±3λ.

12.3 INSTRUMENTAL ASPECTS

The potential buyer/user of an XPS spectrometer can rely now on a few commercial companies offering up-to-date and reliable equipment. The objective parameters that should be taken into account when choosing any instrument for the study of metallic biomaterials are:

- the eventual need to combine XPS with other surface analysis techniques
- the need of specialised accessories to 'manipulate' the samples that might further require a special preparation chamber
- the desire to perform spatially resolved experiments.

Besides the experimental principles already cited (see Section 12.2), the study of metallic biomaterials (i.e. transition or noble metals, such as Cr, Ag, Au, Ti or alloys such as stainless steel or Ti6Al4V) does not require either very specific accessories or highly-skilled personnel. Sample temperature control, ion gun for sample cleaning/ depth profiling should be available accessories; as for abrasion/fracturing/scraping accessories, their use is dependent on the material and the type of research. As current instruments offer measurement times that are often shorter than the time needed for computer-aided data analysis, it seems to make sense not to limit the throughput of the photoelectron spectrometer by the computational facilities: powerful hardware with efficient and easy-to-use interactive software is a must.

In the majority of the XPS analyses, the sample preparation is not critical, provided any external contamination is prevented or removed. The researcher should be aware that any sample preparation might modify the surface composition. However, when studying metals and alloys it is quite safe to recommend a preliminary surface cleaning with an appropriate solvent and also a finish with a rinse in alcohol (isopropyl alcohol is usually the best). All samples should be manipulated with clean gloves and/or tweezers.

12.4 DATA INTERPRETATION

An XPS spectrum contains a wealth of information, useful data can be retrieved at different levels and for different purposes. The most common applications are explained in the following sections.

12.4.1 QUANTIFICATION

The first type of information that one can retrieve from an XPS investigation is the relative concentrations of the various constituents at the surface of the studied materials. This quantification utilises either a survey scan (see Figure 12.4) or more detailed core-level spectra, and rests on measurements of peak areas and on elemental sensitivity factors. Figure 12.4 shows the XPS survey spectrum recorded from one titanium surface: intense doublet at $\cong 450$ eV corresponds to the photoelectrons emitted from the 2p electronic shell of the titanium atoms; the peak at $\cong 530$ eV is assigned to O_{1s} electrons, testifying to some superficial oxidation, whereas a small structure at $\cong 280$ eV fingerprints a superficial carbon contamination. Provided the sample is 'homogeneous', the relative number of photoelectrons emitted from different elements is dictated by the relative number of atoms (for example, N_A and N_B) in the studied volume, the photoionisation cross-sections (σ) of the studied electronic levels, the relative mean-free-paths (λ) of the studied photoelectrons and a correction factor taking into account the characteristics of the spectrometer transmission function (T)

$$\frac{I_A}{I_B} = \frac{N_A}{N_B} \frac{\sigma_A}{\sigma_B} \frac{\lambda_A}{\lambda_A} \frac{T_A}{T_B}. \tag{12.2}$$

Computer tabulated functions usually reassemble the last three terms into one global and/or empirical determined factor F, so that the measurement of relative intensities immediately allows the determination of the N_A/N_B atomic ratios for an unknown sample with an accuracy of the order of 5%

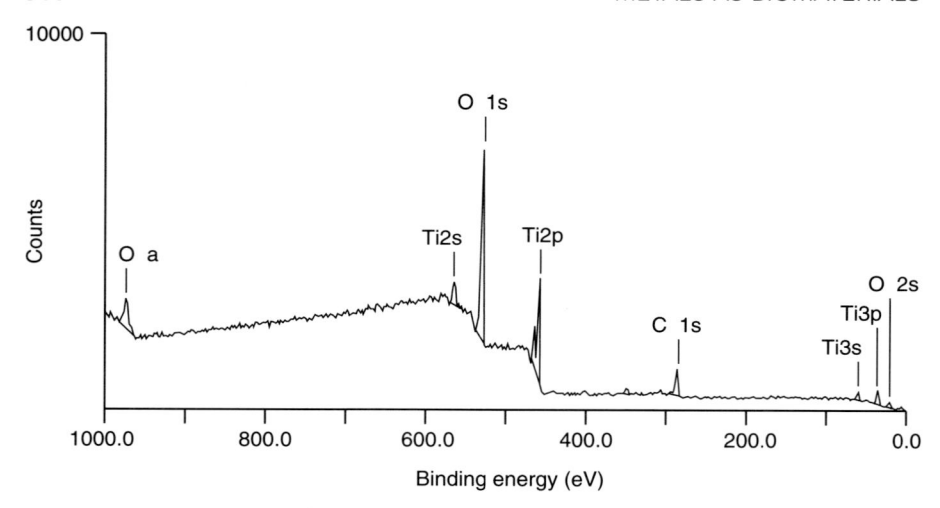

Figure 12.4 XPS photoelectron spectrum of a Ti surface excited with monochromatised AlKα radiation: intensity in accumulated counts versus binding energy in eV. The O_{1s} line testifies of the partial oxidation of the surface; the C_{1s} peak is characteristic of normal contamination. The Ti_{2p} core line is also shown with more detail in Figure 12.5.

$$\frac{N_A}{N_B} = \frac{I_A}{I_B}\frac{F_B}{F_A}, \qquad (12.3)$$

an expression that is indeed valuable for all homogeneous samples provided the F factors are matrix-independent. Applied on Figure 12.4 to the peak heights of the Ti_{2p}, O_{1s} and C_{1S} signals, this last formula allows us to determine that the studied Ti foil contained ≅55 at.% oxygen and 25 at.% carbon; we know that this is not an homogeneous material and that the majority of oxygen and carbon is at the surface. More accurate atomic ratio measurements are obtained from core-level spectra provided one includes in the area measurement any satellite (e.g. shake-up satellites that are particularly intense for transition metal) (see Section 12.4.4).

12.4.2 CHEMICAL SHIFT

XPS, apart from its capability to detect elements in a material, also allows the investigator to determine, with a degree of quantification, the chemical state of the studied element. Variations of core-level binding energies of the same element in different compounds reflect different chemical environments (initial-state effect) and different electronic relaxations in the ionised atom (final-state effect). Figure 12.5 shows Ti_{2p} core-level spectra recorded during depth profiling (see Section 12.4.6) from an oxidised surface to a pure metal. The shift of the Ti_{2p} doublet to a lower

X-RAY PHOTOELECTRON SPECTROSCOPY

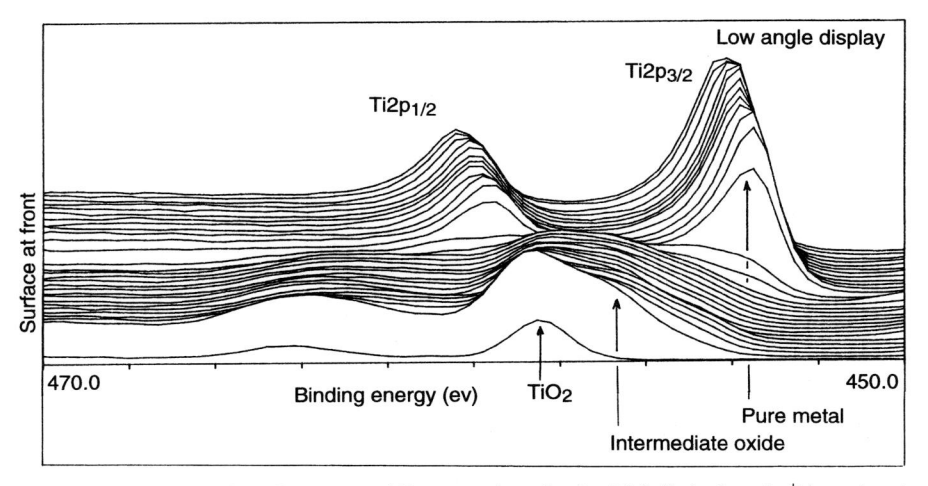

Figure 12.5 Set of XPS spectra (Ti_{2p} core level) of a Ti foil during Ar^+ ion depth profile. The transition from an 'oxidised' surface to a 'pure metallic' material is a clear example of chemical shifts corresponding to different Ti oxidation states.

binding energy is due to different oxidation states of the Ti atoms; typical reference values are shown on the spectra, higher binding energies in general correspond to higher (formal) oxidation states. Between Ti and TiO_2, a chemical shift of +5.5 eV is observed on the Ti_{2p} level. These chemical shifts are already known for most of the compounds and have bean compiled in various textbooks. These can be used provided the photoelectron spectrometer used to record the data has had its binding-energy scale precisely calibrated which is not too difficult, as no spurious surface charging is expected to distort the data used in the study of metallic biomaterials. Table 12.1 reports the values of presently recommended calibration lines, the obtained absolute binding energies are reported against the energy of the Fermi level at 0.0 eV.

However, the researcher should remember that for some elements, final-state effect may completely blur out and supersede the concept of chemical shifts. Table 12.2 shows some values of core-level binding energies for Fe and Ag compounds, the first ones present 'normal' chemical shifts, the second ones testify to the preponderance of relaxation effects.

Table 12.1 Recommended reference binding energies (eV) for calibration of the Al-Kα XPS binding energy scale. Clean metals should be used

Cu_{3p}	$Au_{4f_{7/2}}$	$Ag_{3d_{5/2}}$	CuL_2MM	$Cu_{2p_{3/2}}$
75.14	83.98	368.26	567.96	932.67

Table 12.2 XPS shifts recorded for Fe and Ag compounds showing, respectively, the chemical shift and relaxation effects

Fe compound	$Fe_{2p3/2}$ binding energy (eV)	Chemical shift (eV)	Ag compound	Ag_{3d} binding energy (eV)
Fe	706.8	0	Ag	368 2
FeO	709.8	3.0	Ag_2O	367.8
Fe_2O_3	711.2	4.4	AgO	367.4
FeF_3	714.0	7.2	AgF_2	367.5

12.4.3 THE AUGER EFFECT AND THE AUGER PARAMETER

The photoemission process produces ionised atoms in an excited state. Relaxation may occur rapidly (10^{-14} s) after the photoelectron ejection by emission of either X-ray photon or of Auger electron. The so-called Auger process involves an outer electron relaxing to an inner orbital giving this excess energy to a second electron – the Auger electron – that accompanies the photoelectron emission, thus leaving a doubly ionised atom. However, it should be noted that the Auger electron energy is independent of the mode of the initial photoionisation. Thus, XPS spectra contain both photoelectron and Auger peaks. The Auger peaks are grouped into a series, the most intense of which are catalogued in the literature.

Also, Auger lines present chemical shifts but – although they are often larger – they are more difficult to interpret. In combination with photoelectron chemical shifts they can also be useful to confirm chemical states by using tabulated values. At a more quantitative level, another tool can then be used, the modified Auger parameter α'.

The Auger parameter is defined as the sum of the photoelectron binding energy and of the corresponding Auger electron kinetic energy. It has been shown that α' is very sensitive to final-state effect relaxation phenomena, as this one is significantly larger for a doubly ionised atom. As an example, Table 12.3 shows the measured chemical shifts and Auger parameters for some zinc compounds.

12.4.4 SATELLITES

In XPS, there exist many side-effects generating satellite lines, i.e. non-pure photoelectron or Auger peaks. They are reviewed in the following sections more or less in order of their decreasing importance for quantitative analytical purposes.

Table 12.3 Illustration of the use of the Auger parameter to differentiate some Zn oxidation states when the sole XPS chemical shifts are small

	Zn_{2p} chemical shift (eV)	Auger parameter
Zn	0	0
ZnO	0.3	4.4
ZnS	0.8	5.9

X-RAY PHOTOELECTRON SPECTROSCOPY

Table 12.4 X-ray satellites (relative energies and relative intensities) for the two most common sources: MgK$\alpha_{1,2}$ at 1253.6 eV and AlK$\alpha_{1,2}$ at 1486.6 eV

	α_3	α_4	α_5	α_6	β
Mg: position (eV)	8.4	10.1	17.6	20.6	48.7
intensity (%)	8.0	4.1	0.6	0.5	0.5
Al: position (eV)	9.8	11.8	20.1	23.4	69.7
intensity (%)	6.4	3.2	0.4	0.3	0.6

12.4.4.1 X-ray Satellites

When a non-monochromatised X-ray source is used to produce photoelectrons, the investigator should be aware that some minor intensity peaks – located at lower binding energies – will appear. The relative intensities and positions of those satellite components are known, see Table 12.4 for the most common AlKα and MgKα sources. These satellite peaks should not be assimilated to the true photoelectron peaks and accounted for in order to quantify the elemental composition and chemical shifts. In fact, some computer programs subtract these X-ray satellites peaks before proceeding to any quantitative analysis of the XPS data.

12.4.4.2 Shake-up Satellites

As already mentioned in the description of the Auger process, photoemission leads to some reorganisation of the ensemble of electronic levels of the studied materials. The energy released during this relaxation in or screening of the final state may be partially used to excite a valence electron to an empty electronic level; as a result, the corresponding photoelectron will leave the material with a smaller kinetic energy, thus appearing on the spectrum at a higher binding energy. These shake-up satellite peaks should then be considered as 'disguised' true photoelectron peaks and their intensities must be included in any quantitative data analysis, especially as these satellite intensities may be as large as that of the main line; this is particularly true of transition metals. For those compounds, a rule of thumb is that:

- a metal with all complete d shell (d^{10}) will not present any satellite
- a metal with empty or uncompleted shells will often show shake-up peaks.

It has been shown that the shake-up satellite intensities and positions depend on the nature of the ligand, offering another way, other than the chemical shift, to study the metal-oxidation state. A textbook example (Figure 12.6) is the Cu_{2p} fingerprint spectrum of cuprous and cupric oxides: the Cu^+ ion with a d^{10} electronic configuration does not show any satellite, on the contrary, divalent (d^9) Cu^{2+} ion presents highly characteristic extra peaks to be attributed to the named relaxation process.

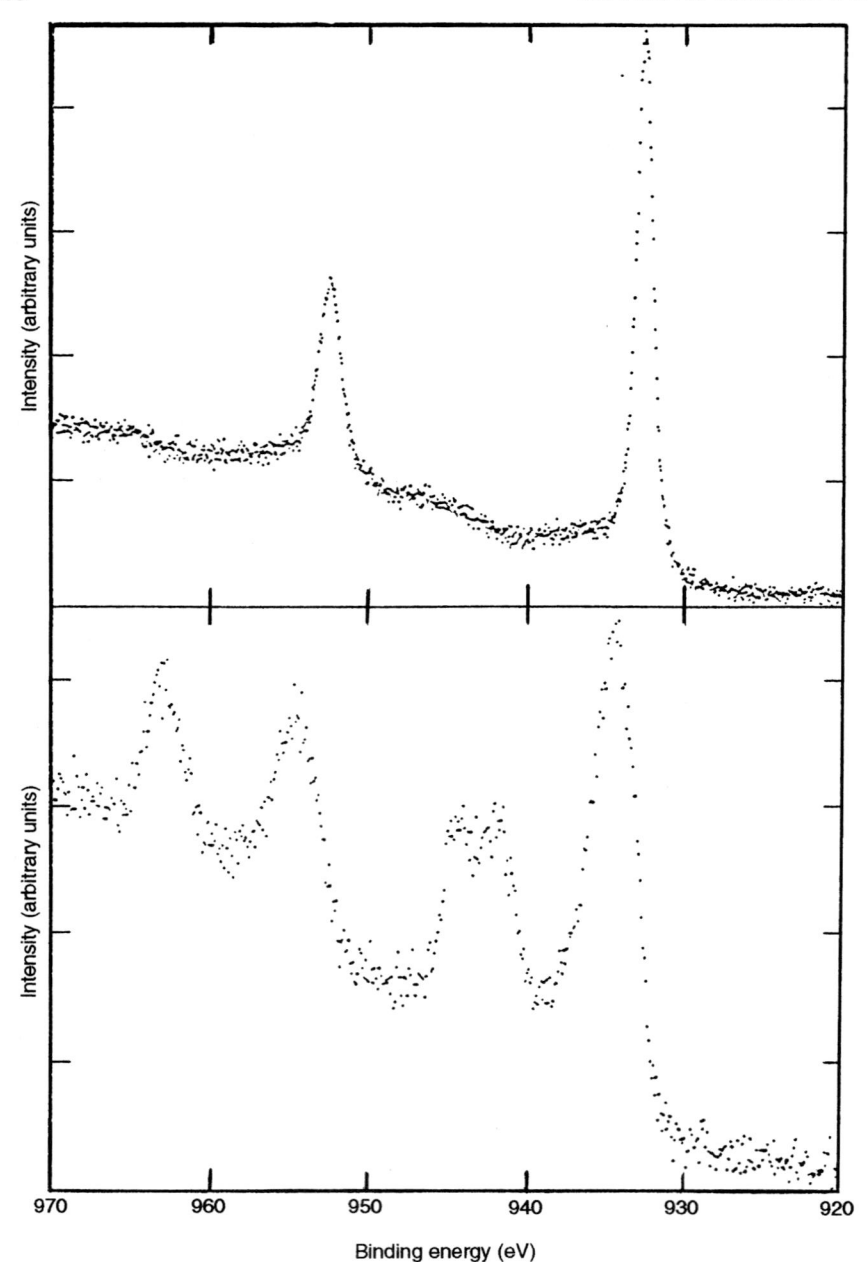

Figure 12.6 XPS spectra of the Cu_{2p} peaks region of the two Cu_2O and CuO oxides. Besides the 2p doublet, the latter compound shows well-defined and very intense shake-up satellites that can be used to corroborate precisely the metal oxidation state.

X-RAY PHOTOELECTRON SPECTROSCOPY

12.4.4.3 Plasmon Satellites

When studying metals the scattering of the photoelectrons on their way out of the sample by electrons of the material can result in the excitation of multiple well-defined energy quanta characteristic of the metals, called (surface and bulk) plasmons. These are collective excitations of the metal free-electrons with quantised energy (between 2 and 20 eV) presenting particularly sharp peaks for the alkali, the alkali earth and group III metals. The successive appearance at regular energy intervals from the original photoelectron (or Auger) line with a progressively reduced intensity constitutes an unmistakable fingerprinting pattern.

12.4.4.4 Energy-loss Line

Similarly, the photo- and Auger-electrons escaping from the material under study might interact with other electrons of the solid and be inelastically scattered. These energy-loss phenomena produce a staircase-like bump on the high binding energy side of the parent line; this bump extends over a few hundred electron-volts energy range and, depending on the metal being studied, may present some fine structure. These energy-loss parts of the XPS spectrum are difficult to use quantitatively; an experienced user might at a glimpse get some insight into the structure (e.g. whether it is homogeneous, inhomogeneous) and element distribution within the material. A more thorough study, producing more quantitative information of the electron-loss spectrum, requires elaborate calculations, computer algorithms are available for this purpose (Tougaard, 1996).

12.4.4.5 Core-level Peak Asymmetry

For some conducting samples the recorded core-level peaks might present a pronounced asymmetry, the half-width at half-maximum to the left (high binding energy) of the peak is significantly larger than the one to the right; the ratio between these two values is around 1.5 for the $3d_{5/2}$ peak of clean Pd. This is attributed to the excitation by the outgoing photoelectrons of very low energy electron-hole pairs. This effect is particularly large when the metal has a high density of electronic states at the Fermi level; it might be analytically used to check whether for example, two metals are, or are not, alloyed.

12.4.4.6 Multiplet Splitting

As electrons have a spin, the photoemission process leaves an uncoupled electron on a core level, whose intrinsic angular momentum may couple in different ways with the spin of unpaired valence electrons, if any. This clearly results in different final states (Figure 12.7), different electronic configurations with different energies, which we have learned will produce multiple peaks. This effect is named multiplet splitting; it is relatively simple for the ionisation of s electrons as in Figure 12.7, but more complex and subtle in its effect when electrons from p orbitals are removed. It

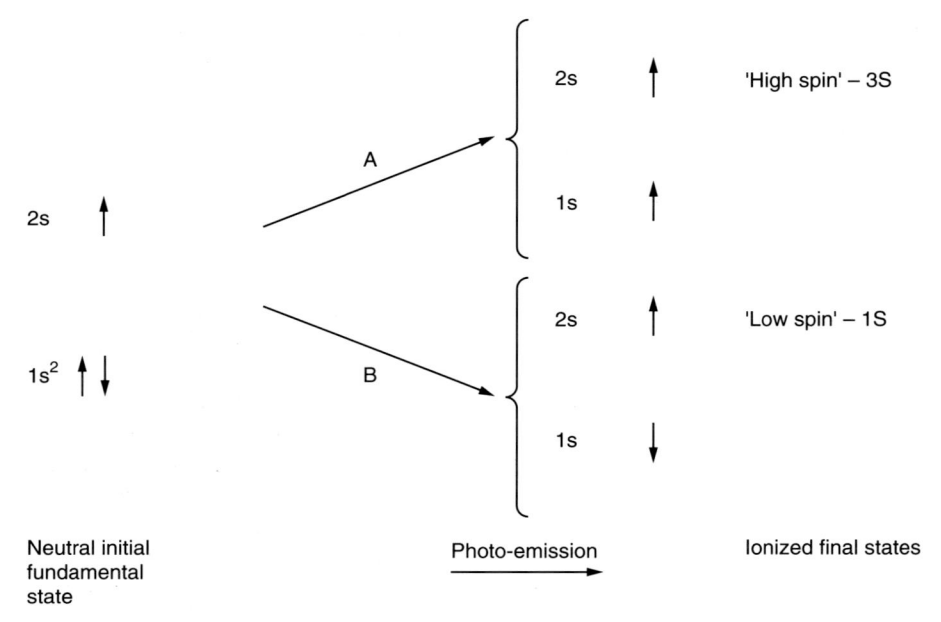

Figure 12.7 Schematic representation of the photoionisation of a 1s electron of a lithium atom (electronic structure: Li $1s^2 2s$). The spin of the remaining 1s electron couples either parallely (high 3S spin-state) or antiparallely (low 1S spin state) to the unpaired 'valence' electron, in this case a 2s electron. This results in a multiplet splitting structure with two energetically different final states, i.e. two photoelectron peaks.

can indeed manifest itself only in a modification of a spin-orbit doublet splitting value and/or peak-shape and -width. The study of multiplet structures is very useful for transition metals with unpaired d electrons as in Table 12.5:

- for an element with a same formal oxidation state but in different compounds, a larger multiplet splitting correlates with a larger electronegativity of the ligand

Table 12.5 Multiplet splitting effect measured on a 3s core level of different (chromium and iron) compounds

Compound	Splitting (eV)	Electronic structure of the metal atom
CrF_3	4.2	d^3
$CrCl_3$	3.8	d^3
$CrBr_3$	3.1	d^3
FeF_3	6.8	d^5
FeF_2	6.0	d^4

- the multiplet splitting amplitude increases with the number of unpaired d electrons in the metal atoms. This is a fourth method (with the chemical shift effect, the Auger lines or Auger parameter, and the shake-up satellites) to ascertain the oxidation state of a metal.

12.4.5 VALENCE BANDS

In the low binding energy region (0–30 eV) of the photoelectron spectrum (Figure 12.4), lines of very low intensity are produced by photoemission from valence bands. These energy bands close to the Fermi level (defined at $E = 0.0$ eV) are characteristic of the solid-state properties of the material as they fingerprint the electronic distribution within the bondings between the atoms in the solid. The low photoelectric cross-section of these electronic states necessitates quite long accumulation time (by comparison to core-level spectra) and any interpretation beyond the fingerprinting level requires sophisticated calculations. Therefore, the recording and use of the valence-band spectra of metals and alloys is usually reserved to basic studies of, for example, density of states at the Fermi level, band-width or band evolution during anneal. Figure 12.8 is a simple example of valence-band fingerprints, sometimes used to complement core level analyses; it shows the valence-band change between two oxides, in this case TiO_2 and RuO_2. The valence bands I and II are identified as the signature of the s and p molecular orbitals, resulting from the combination of the O_{2p} and metal d electrons; structure III is attributed to the metal free d electron band (Riga et al., 1977). TiO_2 is insulating, RuO_2 is conducting – this is indeed clearly indicated on the XPS spectra by band III at the Fermi level, with a binding energy of 0 eV for the latter compound.

12.4.6 DEPTH PROFILE AND ANGULAR ANALYSIS

Intrinsically, the XPS technique is surface sensitive; as mentioned earlier, the element distribution within a depth of about 50 Å below the surface contributes to the photoelectron spectrum. Often there is a need to determine more precisely an element location within this analysed depth or to obtain similar information beyond this depth. In addition to the elemental and chemical information, four different methods can be used to distinguish the depth dimension.

12.4.6.1 Different Core-level Lines

As the photoelectron peak intensity depends on the electron escape depth and thus of its kinetic energy (see Section 12.2), the recording and intensity analysis of different core-level lines from the same element are prone to deliver information on any vertical inhomogeneity in the distribution of this element in the solid. Photoelectron core peaks at low/high binding energies are recorded from electrons with large/small kinetic energies, thus from electrons originating from a deeper/

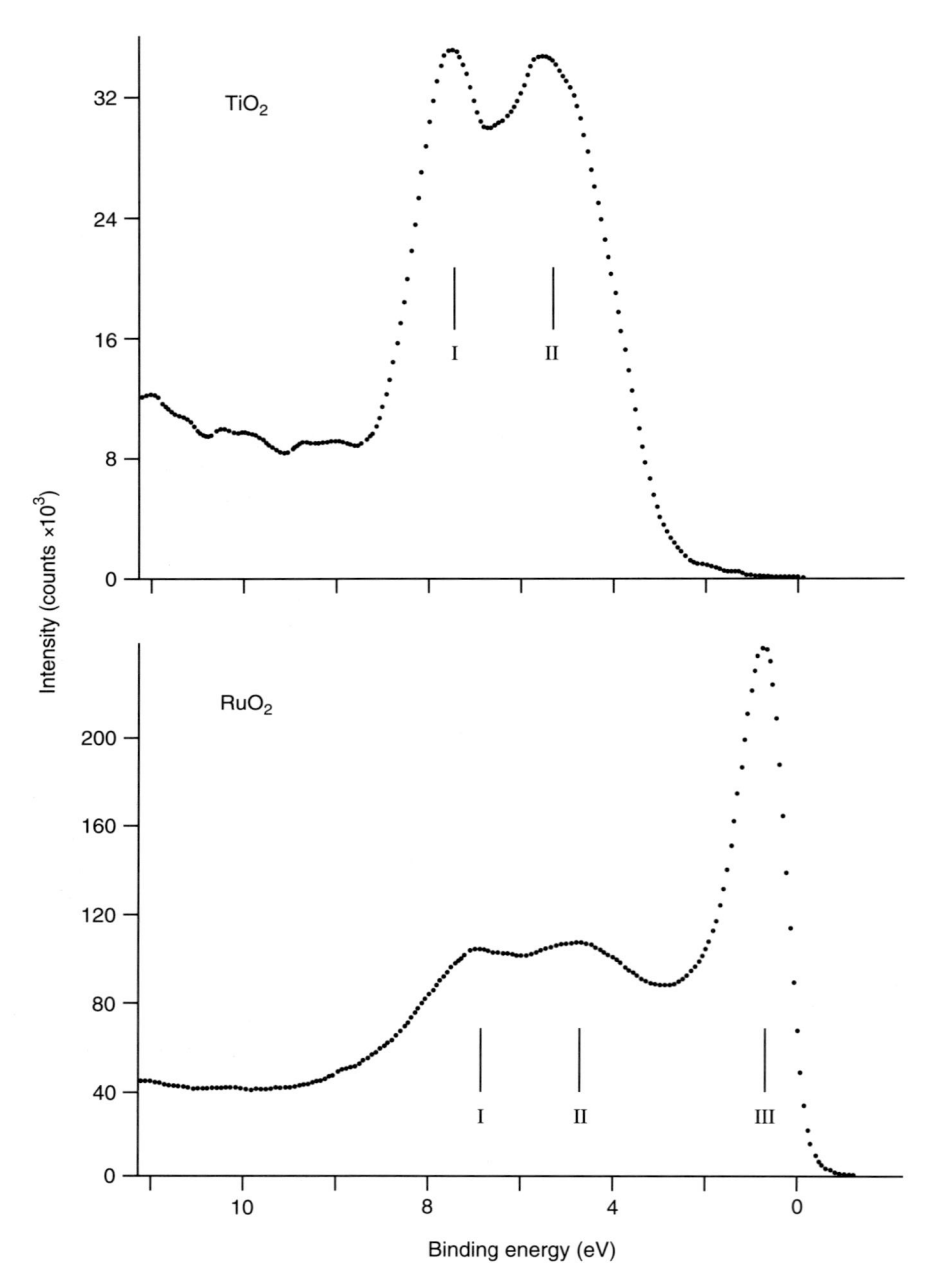

Figure 12.8 XPS valence band spectra of Ti and Ru dioxides. The first one is insulating, the second one is conducting. Indeed, an occupied electronic band (III) is recorded for the latter at the Fermi level (binding energy of 0 eV).

X-RAY PHOTOELECTRON SPECTROSCOPY

shallower section of the solid, their intensity ratios compared to those of a reference homogeneous material allow one to retrieve some kind of 'in depth' distribution.

12.4.6.2 Different X-ray Sources

When the XPS spectrometer is equipped with two or more X-ray sources, they might be used sequentially to record the spectra of the same core-level peaks. Those peaks appearing at the same binding energies correspond, however, to electrons with different kinetic energies and thus originate from different depths in the material.

12.4.6.3 Angular Analysis

When the photoelectron spectrometer is tuned to selectively collect electrons emitted normally to the sample surface, the measured spectrum contains information on the composition of a slice under the material surface, the thickness of which is about 3λ (see Figure 12.3 and Section 12.2). However, if the sample is tilted so that the analysed electrons originate from an almost grazing ejection angle ϑ relative to the surface, than the effective electron escape depth is reduced by a sine function, the smaller this angle ϑ, the higher the surface sensitivity. In this way XPS – which is already surface sensitive – can even highlight more detail by focusing on information gained from extreme surface ($\vartheta \to 0°$) or averaged over the whole electron mean-free-path ($\vartheta \to 90°$). With the recording of spectra at intermediate ϑ values, computer algorithms can be used to 'reconstruct' the in-depth distribution of an element.

12.4.6.4 Ion Profiling

When more detailed depth analysis is required, a frequently used technique is the controlled erosion of the surface by Ar^+ ion sputtering. This is a vacuum technique compatible with XPS; sequential ion erosion and XPS analysis can be programmed to reach depths in the micrometre range. However, this classical way to perform depth analysis is *per se* destructive. Despite this, the technique preserves the advantages of the XPS spectroscopy, keeping available both elemental and chemical information at any step of the process, as is already shown in Figure 12.5. An example of XPS depth profile through a TiO_2 overlayer on a Ti metal is shown in Figure 12.9. This sample is in fact a Ti dental implant. Unfortunately, this method does have some disadvantages as well, such as possible preferential erosion, different sputtering rates not only for different elements but also for the same element involved into various chemical environments and can cause changes in chemical states, so that during a depth profile an exact quantification is difficult to obtain.

12.4.7 SURFACE MAPPING OR MICROANALYSIS

Until recently XPS spectroscopy could not give useful data for studying small areas of a sample or for obtaining a chemical mapping of the elemental distribution on a

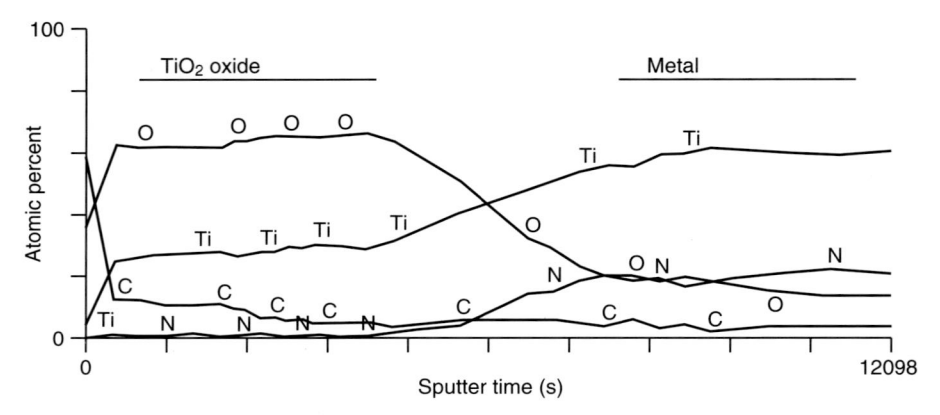

Figure 12.9 XPS 'depth profile' of the varying composition of a Ti dental implant as studied directly after removal of its sterile package. The vertical scale expresses the measured elemental composition in atomic per cent plotted versus sputter time (proportional to depth).

surface. In more recent times, based on different techniques, manufacturers propose instruments whose spatial resolution can reach 5 µm. The technical details are quite complex and are beyond the scope of this chapter. Theoretical and experimental work are very intense in this type of instrumental development and therefore, at present, do differentiate the manufacturers. It should be noted that when the spatial resolution is improved, the X-ray dose has to be increased and this can cause radiation damage in the sample.

12.5 SUMMARY OF XPS FEATURES

The most useful message of this short presentation of the XPS technique is that the spectroscopy, from the surface (0 to about 10 mm below the surface), of a metallic biomaterial or device can be used to:

- detect, non-destructively, any element (except hydrogen), with a sensitivity of about 0.1 monolayer ($\pm 10^{13}$ atoms cm^{-2})
- analyse the chemical environment of the elements
- quantify this elemental and chemical information quite easily, to a few per cent accuracy
- perform depth profile analysis
- produce spatially resolved chemical images with a resolution in the range of 5 µm.

The relatively easy to use XPS technique should not prevent the operator from regularly checking the instrument used. As frequently as possible, the instrument transmission function should be recorded, the binding-energy scale recalibrated and the intensity scale monitored. Keeping these records up-to-date makes it easier to detect any instrument malfunction which would reduce the quality of XPS quantification.

12.6 METALLIC BIOMATERIALS

Using the data of this study, it would appear that the most frequent use of the XPS spectroscopy for studying metallic biomaterials is:

- to determine surface elemental and chemical composition
- to detect contamination, either external (through sample handling) or internal (through segregation of elements from the bulk); this might be very relevant to study the effect of sample manipulation, its toxicity or any sterilisation effect
- to monitor metal passivation and corrosion resistance
- to measure any wear effect
- to gather data on ceramic–metal or polymer–metal interfaces.

As an example, let us briefly consider pure titanium metal. One of the key factors for a favourable osseointegration of Ti implants is the chemical quality and physical structure of the titanium dioxide superficial layer, besides the cleanliness of the implant surface that requires sterilisation (Baier, 1984), although the validity of a rigorous protocol in the handling of the material is questioned (Ameen, 1993). Titanium being a very reactive material, its surface is in any case covered by a native passivating oxide layer about 2–5 nm thick; therefore, it is titanium dioxide which is indeed the real material in contact with body fluids and tissues. In some cases, the otherwise protective oxide layer is not stable; should part of the TiO_2 layer be removed, titanium ion release might be detected (Estassabi *et al.*, 1996; Liu and Burstein, 1996). Most of the time, the implant undergoes dedicated proprietary surface treatments to tailor the oxide thickness, crystallographic structure and roughness (Callen *et al.*, 1995; Pan *et al.*, 1996).

ACKNOWLEDGEMENTS

The research work at the LISE Laboratory is supported by the Belgian National Fund for Scientific Research, the Belgian Ministry for Scientific Research, the Belgian National Program of Interuniversity Research, and the Region Wallonne. Our colleagues are very gratefully acknowledged for their input and many discussions.

NOMENCLATURE

d depth
eV   electron-volt (1 eV: 1.6×10^{-19} joule)

E_k photoelectron kinetic energy
E_B photoelectron binding energy
h Planck's universal constant
I intensity
N_A number of atoms A
T spectrometer transmission function
UPS   ultraviolet photoelectron spectroscopy
XPS   X-ray photoelectron spectroscopy
λ photoelectron mean free path
ν light frequency
ϕ (spectrometer or material) work function
σ photoionisation cross-section

REFERENCES

Ameen, A.P., Short, R.D., Johns, R. and Schwach, G. (1993) The surface analysis of a titanium dental implant material, *Clin. Oral. Impl. Res.* **4**, 144.

Baier, R.E., Mayer, A.E., Natiella, J.R. and Carter, J.M. (1984) Surface properties determine bioadhesion outcomes: methods and results, *J. Biomed. Mater. Res.* **18**, 337–45.

Callen, B.W., Lowenberg, B.F., Lugowski, S., Soothi, R.N.S. and Davies, J.E. (1995) Nitric-acid passivation of Ti6Al4V reduces thickness of surface oxide layer and increases trace-element release, *J. Biomed. Mater. Res.* **29**, 279–90.

Estessabi, A.M., Otsuka, T., Tsuboi, Y., Yekoyama, K., Albrektsson, T., Sennerby, L. and Johansson, C. (1996) Quantitative measurement of metal ion release from orthopedic and dental implants, in *Proceedings of the Fifth World Biomaterials Congress*, 31 May–2 June, Toronto, Canada (abstract), Vol. 2, p. 450.

Liu, C. and Burstein, G.T. (1996) Insights into passive dissolution of titanium *in vitro*, in *Proceedings of the Fifth World Biomaterials Congress*, 31 May–2 June, Toronto, Canada (abstract), ,Vol. 1, p. 555.

Pan, J., Thierry, D. and Leygraf, C. (1996) Hydrogen-peroxide toward enhanced oxide-growth on Titanium in PbS solution. Blue coloration and clinical relevance, *J. Biomed. Mater. Res.* **30**, 393–402.

Riga, J., Tenret-Noel, C., Pireaux, J.J., Caudano, R. and Verbist, J.J. (1977) Electronic structure of Rutile Oxides TiO_2, RuO_2 and IrO_2 studied by XPS, *Phys. Scripta* **16**, 351–4.

Siegbahn, K., Nordling, C., Fahlman, A., Nordberg, R., Hamrin, K., Hedman, J., Johansson, G., Bergmark, T., Karlsson, S.E., Lindgren, J. and Lindberg, B. (1967) *ESCA, Atomic, Molecular and Solid State Structure Studied by Means of Electron Spectroscopy*, Almqvist and Wiksells, Uppsala.

Tougaard, S. (1996) Surface nanostructure determination by XPS peakshape analysis, *J. Vac. Sci. Technol.* **A14**, 1415–23.

FURTHER READING

REFERENCE BOOKS

Briggs, D. and Seah, M.P. (eds) (1990) *Practical Surface Analysis by Auger and X-ray Photoelectron Spectroscopy*, 2nd edition, John Wiley, Chichester.

Brundle, C.R. and Baker, A.D. (eds) *Electron Spectroscopy: Theory, Techniques and Applications*, Vol. 1 (1977); Vol. 2 (1978); Vol. 3 (1979); Vol. 4 (1981); Vol. 5 (1984), Academic Press, London.
Carlson, T.A. (1975) *Photoelectron and Auger Spectroscopy*, Plenum Press, New York.
Hufner, S. (1995) *Photoelectron Spectroscopy*, Springer, Berlin.
Ley, L. and Cardona, M. (eds) (1979) *Photoemission in Solids. Topics in Applied Physics*, Vols 26 and 27, Springer, Berlin.

HANDBOOKS

Beamson, G. and Briggs, D. (1992) *High Resolution XPS of Organic Polymers – the Scienta ESCA 300 Database*, John Wiley, Chichester.
Chastain, J. (ed.) (1992) *Handbook of X-Ray Photoelectron Spectroscopy*, Perkin-Elmer Corp, Eden Prairie, Minnesota.
Handbook of X-Ray Photoelectron Spectroscopy (1991) Jeol.

CONFERENCE PROCEEDINGS

Dekeyser, W., Fiermans, L., Vanderkelen, G. and Vennick, J. (eds) (1973) *Electron Emission Spectroscopy*, Reidel, Dordrecht.
Shirley, D.A. (ed.) (1972) *Electron Spectroscopy*, North-Holland, Amsterdam.
Proceedings of the *International Conference on Electron Spectroscopy* (ICES) series are published in *Journal of Electron Spectroscopy and Related Phenomena*. ICES 2–7 papers appeared in Vols 5, 15, 51–52, 68, 76 and 88–91, respectively.

REVIEWS AND RECENT PAPERS ON BIOMATERIALS

Callen, B.W., Soothi, R.N.S. and Griffiths, K. (1995) Examination of clinical surface preparations on titanium and Ti6AI4V by X-ray photoelectron spectroscopy and nuclear reaction analysis, *Progr. Surf. Sci.* **50**, 269–79.
Kasemo, B. and Lausmaa, J. (1986) Surface science aspects on inorganic biomaterials, *CRC Crit. Rev. Biocompat.* **2**, 335–80.
Lausmaa, J. and Kasemo, B. (1990) Surface spectroscopic characterisation of Ti implants materials, *Appl. Surf. Sci.* **44**, 133–46.
Lewis, G. (1993) X-ray photoelectron study of surface layers on orthopedic alloys, *J. Vac. Sci. Technol.* **A11**, 325–35.
Pan, J, Thierry, D. and Leygraf, C. (1994) Electrochemical and XPS studies of titanium for biomaterial applications with respect to the effect of hydrogen peroxide, *J. Biomed. Mater. Res.* **28**, 113–22.
Ratner, B.D. (ed.) (1988) *Surface Characterization of Biomaterials*, Elsevier, New York.
West, R. and Batts, G. (eds) (1994) *Surface Properties of Biomaterials*, Butterworth-Heinemann, Oxford.

13
Atomic force microscopy

U. HARTMANN
University of the Saarland, Saarbrücken, Germany

13.1 INTRODUCTION

It is not necessary to emphasise the enormous importance of microscopic imaging in the natural sciences, in medicine and in various engineering disciplines. In the past few decades this importance has been recognised repeatedly by the awarding of Nobel prizes to the inventors of a number of new and improved approaches in the field of microscopy. Today, a strong driving force for further developments results from the increasing demand related to key technologies. One of the key technologies is certainly microelectronics where, as a consequence of the decreasing scale of many devices, high-resolution characterisation methods have become fundamentally important for further development in this area. Another discipline where progress is related directly to the availability of powerful microscopy methods is the development of new and functional materials. The latter strongly relies on the characterisation of materials at various and increasing levels of resolution. Structure, microstructure and defect geometry, as well as chemical composition and spatial distribution, are important parameters determining the behaviour of materials and practical applications.

In order to qualify a certain approach as *microscopy*, the method should give spatially localised information on the microstructure and have the potential to provide a magnified real-space image of the sample (Amelincks *et al.*, 1997). Today's materials scientist, for example, has a large number of such methods at his or her disposal. This is necessary because complete characterisation of the given material requires the application of different and complementary characterisation methods, yielding in combination the numerous relevant parameters.

In 1980–1 Binnig, Rohrer and co-workers from the IBM Zürich Research Laboratories invented a new type of microscope (Binnig *et al.*, 1982a, b) which they called the scanning tunnelling microscope (STM). The instrument, which proved capable of imaging solid surfaces with atomic resolution, has revolutionised microscopy and surface analysis in an unprecedented manner. Looking back, it is evident that the outstanding success of STM is not merely due to the ultra-high resolution that can be achieved by this technique. Equally important, if not more

Metals as Biomaterials ISBN 0 471 96935 4 Edited by J.A. Helsen and H.J. Breme. © 1998 John Wiley & Sons Ltd

so, is that STM stimulated the development of a whole family of scanning probe microscopy (SPM) methods, which are all based on instrumental principles very similar to that of the STM. The most popular offspring are atomic force microscopy (AFM) (Binnig et al., 1986) and scanning near-field optical microscopy (SNOM) (Pohl et al., 1984). STM, AFM and SNOM today represent a set of microscopies that can be applied in many different and highly dedicated modes of operation, so that a variety of physical and chemical properties of a material becomes accessible. This versatility of SPM in general is, apart from the inherent high resolution, a major strength. Today's materials scientist can master no more than a few of the microscopy methods based on static electric and magnetic fields, particle beams, electromagnetic radiation, acoustic waves, etc., and presumably would not have access to the instrumentation necessary to apply them in any great number. However, the operational principle of SPM is uniform and a variety of physical properties can often be obtained even by employing only one general-purpose set-up.

The literature in the field is vast. Among others comprehensive introductions have been given by Bonnell (1992), Wiesendanger and Güntherodt (1992/93), Chen (1993), Marti and Amrein (1993), Wiesendanger (1994), Maganov and Whangbo (1996) and Bai (1995). More specific information is found in the various proceedings of the international conferences on STM and related methods. The scope of this contribution is to give a brief introduction to SPM in general and to AFM and its applications in materials science in particular.

13.2 SCANNING PROBE TECHNOLOGY: BASIC FUNDAMENTALS

Two important aspects are essential to all scanning probe methods: scanning and operating the scanned probe in near-field. While scanning has been well established in microscopy for quite some time, e.g. in electron microscopy, consequent near-field operation is a relatively novel approach in microscopy. It implies that the scanned probe has to be operated sufficiently close to the imaged sample surface.

Furthermore, it is conceptually important to consider SPM not simply as a method where a local probe precisely maps the topography or morphology of a surface with high resolution, but as a method where the probe is used to carry out a local experiment at any position met during raster-scanning the sample surface. The results of all successively performed experiments are collected and imaged as a function of the probe's lateral position, respectively. This then yields an image of the scanned surface area from the viewpoint of the particularly chosen experimental parameters. Consequently, different operational parameters will generally result in completely different information on the scanned sample surface.

If a sharp probe, e.g. the tip terminating an extended solid probe, is in very close proximity to a sample surface, a variety of interactions can result. If the probe is at a distance of a few nanometres, van der Waals forces between the probe and the sample will occur. If, in addition, an electrical potential difference is externally applied, electrostatic interactions occur. If the probe and the sample are ferromagnetic, magnetostatic forces will result. If the probe–sample distance is decreased to less than about 1 nm, the application of a small potential difference will lead to a local tunnelling current between the probe and the sample, if both of them are either conducting or semiconducting. This is utilised in STM. If the proximal probe is capable of emitting or collecting light at a sub-wavelength scale, the sample surface can be imaged below the diffraction limit. This is utilised in SNOM. Suitable probes can also be operated in direct mechanical contact with the sample surface, thus providing information on the surface topography, tribological properties, and elastic and/or inelastic response of the sample. Further probe–sample interactions involve near-field acoustics, and thermal and ionic transfer. Apart from the detailed configuration of the probe and the sample and the applied external parameters, the respective probe–sample interaction is also influenced by environmental conditions which can involve liquids as well as gases.

Near-field operation is the prerequisite for obtaining high spatial resolution by breaking diffraction limits. However, in order to utilise experimentally the potential for high resolution the probe has to be permanently kept in the near-field regime with respect to its vertical position, and lateral positioning has to be sufficiently precise. Atomic and even subatomic accuracy in positioning is obtained if piezoelectric actuators are employed. Utilising the inverse piezoelectric effect, a driving voltage applied to the electrodes of the actuator can be converted directly into elongations and contractions. With a suitable arrangement of piezoelectric bars forming a tripod, fully three-dimensional positioning can be achieved (Binnig and Rohrer, 1982). Along each axis the resulting length change upon applying a voltage V is

$$\Delta l = d_{31} \frac{l}{h} V, \qquad (13.1)$$

where d_{31} is the piezoelectric coefficient, and l and h are the length and the thickness of the bar, respectively. An even more efficient conversion of driving voltage into deflection is obtained with piezoelectric bimorphs clamped at both ends (Pohl, 1986). The bimorph consists of a sandwich structure of two piezos with an inner electrode at the interface. For such a device the deflection at the centre between the clamped ends is

$$\Delta h = \frac{3}{8} d_{31} \left(\frac{l}{h}\right)^2 V. \qquad (13.2)$$

A very elegant way to achieve three-dimensional positioning is realised by using a piezoelectric tube of length l, wall thickness h and inner diameter d (Binnig and Smith, 1986). The outer electrode is divided into four segments. If a voltage is applied between the inner and all outer electrodes, the length change of the tube is given by

$$\Delta l = d_{31} \frac{l}{h} V, \qquad (13.3)$$

which corresponds exactly to the result in Equation (13.1). However, since the wall thickness of the tube is usually much smaller than the thickness of the piezoelectric bar, the tube is much more sensitive. Upon applying two voltages of equal magnitude but opposite sign to two opposite pairs of the outer electrodes with respect to the inner electrode, deflections of the tube orientated perpendicular to its axis of symmetry can be obtained (Chen, 1992):

$$\Delta(x, y) = 2\sqrt{2} d_{31} \frac{l^2}{\pi d h} V_{x,y}. \qquad (13.4)$$

The ability to position a probe precisely does not yet allow the stable operation of a near-field microscope. As already emphasised, it is essential that the probe is always kept in the near-field regime of the respective interaction between the probe and the sample (Figure 13.1). In STM the interaction manifests itself in a tunnelling current which depends so sensitively on the probe–sample distance that a change of distance of one atomic diameter results in a current change of one order of magnitude. It is thus essential in any near-field approach to control the probe–sample spacing by a feedback mechanism which ensures that the resulting interaction always corresponds to a preset value. A suitable mode of operation is then given by scanning the probe along the x and y directions upon continuously varying the vertical coordinate (z direction) so that the interaction is kept constant. This is called the *constant-interaction mode* of operation. Displaying the z driving voltage of the piezoelectric actuator as a function of the (x, y) coordinates yields a map of the local interaction all over the scanned area. The feedback-loop system usually has a proportional integral characteristic and is realised by analogue or digital set-ups. The whole system is controlled by a computer which creates the ramp signals for scanning and serves for the acquisition, analysis, processing and visualisation of data. The computer is linked to the microscope and the peripheral electronics by digital-to-analog and analog-to-digital converters. The peripheral electronics contain, apart from the feedback loop, suitable devices to

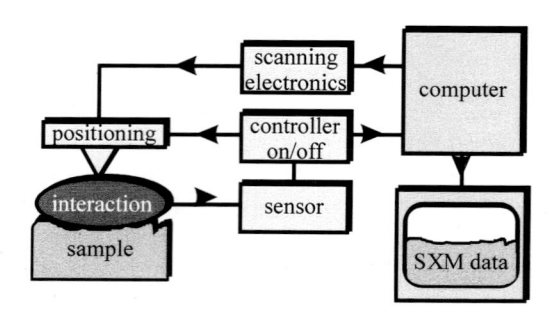

Figure 13.1 Components of a scanning probe instrument.

measure the probe–sample interaction as well as the high-voltage amplifiers for driving the piezoelectric actuators.

In advanced systems the computer control also makes it possible to employ numerous operational modes which deviate from constant-interaction scanning. These modes involve scanning at a constant average probe–sample distance, local spectroscopy, the performance of local surface modifications by increasing the probe–sample interaction and a variety of other features which will be partly discussed below in the context of AFM.

Frequently, the task to be performed by SPM consists of scanning an arbitrary area of the sample upon detecting a particular probe–sample interaction. However, in many applications it is important to analyse a precisely given particular area of a sample, i.e. individual objects on an extended sample surface. The maximum scan range in SPM is usually between 10 and 100 µm. The vertical positioning of the probe achieved by the scanner is typically a few micrometres. It is thus evident that a full three-dimensional positioning of the probe with respect to the sample at a millimetre length scale is convenient. The minimum requirement is, however, that the probe–sample approach has to be performed over a few millimetres in the vertical direction after inserting the sample into the microscope. The steps in forward motion involved in this vertical approach have to be smaller than the total range of the z piezodrive to avoid accidental contact between the probe and the sample during the approach. Furthermore, it is convenient that the two-dimensional positioning of the probe with respect to the sample within the surface plane equally involves steps below the maximum scan range in order to address a particular position on the sample surface. Numerous different coarse positioning devices have been developed over the past 15 years. These involve mechanical constructions on the basis of micrometre screws and reduction levers (Demuth *et al.*, 1986a, b; Coombs and Pethica, 1986; Kaiser and Jaklevic, 1988), spring systems (Smith and Binnig, 1986; Fein *et al.*, 1987; Wiesendanger *et al.*, 1990a), piezoelectric walkers (Binnig and Rohrer, 1982; Mamin *et al.*, 1985; Uozumi *et al.*, 1988; Takata *et al.*, 1989), magnetic walkers (Smith and Elrod, 1985; Corb *et al.*, 1985; Ringger *et al.*, 1986; Wiesendanger *et al.*, 1990a, b), inertial sliders (Pohl, 1987; Anders *et al.*, 1987; Niedermann *et al.*, 1988; Lyding *et al.*, 1988; Frohn *et al.*, 1989) and standard electromagnetic stepper motors which are applied in many commercial instruments today.

The design of the microscope head has to account for numerous sources of imperfections. An instrument which should yield atomic precision is sensitive to external vibrations. This sensitivity can be largely overcome by ensuring high resonant frequencies of the whole device. A sufficiently high resonant frequency and a sufficiently fast feedback system allow a high scan speed. In state-of-the-art instruments, video scan rates can be realised, which is useful for studying dynamic processes. Furthermore, thermal drifts should be as low as possible. Thermal drifts result from differences in the thermal expansion coefficients of different materials and from mechanical constructions of low symmetry. They can be greatly reduced if materials with similar thermal expansion coefficients are used in conjunction with highly symmetrical designs. Non-linearities, hysteresis and creep of the piezoelectric actuators can be eliminated by real-time feedback scan correction or postimaging software corrections. In any case the piezoelectric elements have to be carefully calibrated. Cross-talk between adjacent piezoelectrodes and between the driving voltage and measured signals has to be avoided as far as possible.

A large variety of different home-built instruments has been presented by numerous groups. Additionally, a few commercial instruments are available for STM, AFM and SNOM, involving variants that can be operated in liquids, in ultra-high vacuum (UHV), at low and elevated temperatures, and in high magnetic fields. Of all SPM methods, AFM is certainly the most versatile, which will become evident from the following discussion.

13.3 SCANNING FORCE MICROSCOPY

The most fundamental interaction between the probe and the sample in SPM results in forces. Forces are ever-present between two solids in close proximity and their manifestation does not require any external manipulation. In order to measure forces at a certain spatial resolution the scanning probe instrument has to be equipped with a suitable force sensor. This then leads to an instrument that has even proven capable of imaging atomic structures. It was originally called the AFM (Binnig *et al.*, 1986) and this denotation is still widely used. However, subsequently it turned out that a force microscope can be used to analyse a variety of forces involving short- as well as long-range interactions. Since the resulting applications are much broader than only the analysis of interatomic forces (Sarid, 1991; Güntherodt *et al.*, 1995), it is more appropriate to denote those near-field microscopies that are based on the detection of forces by SFM.

13.3.1 FORCE SENSORS

The general set-up in SFM is absolutely according to what has been discussed in Section 13.2. In order to detect local forces or closely related physical quantities, the sharp probe scanning the sample surface at some distance has to be linked to some sort of force sensor. A convenient way to measure forces precisely is to convert them into deflections of a spring according to Hooke's law

$$\Delta z = \frac{\Delta F}{c}, \qquad (13.5)$$

where the deflection Δz is determined by the acting force ΔF and the spring constant c.

In SFM the force-sensing spring consists of a miniaturised cantilever beam clamped at one end and equipped with the probing tip at the other end. While initially tiny pieces of thin metal foils were equipped with glued diamond tips (Binnig *et al.*, 1986), electrochemically etched metal wires (Figure 13.2) were subsequently found to be easier to handle (Lemke *et al.*, 1990). The increasing demand for cantilevers with integrated sharp tips, tailored reproducibly and for their availability in large numbers soon led to the development of microfabrication techniques based

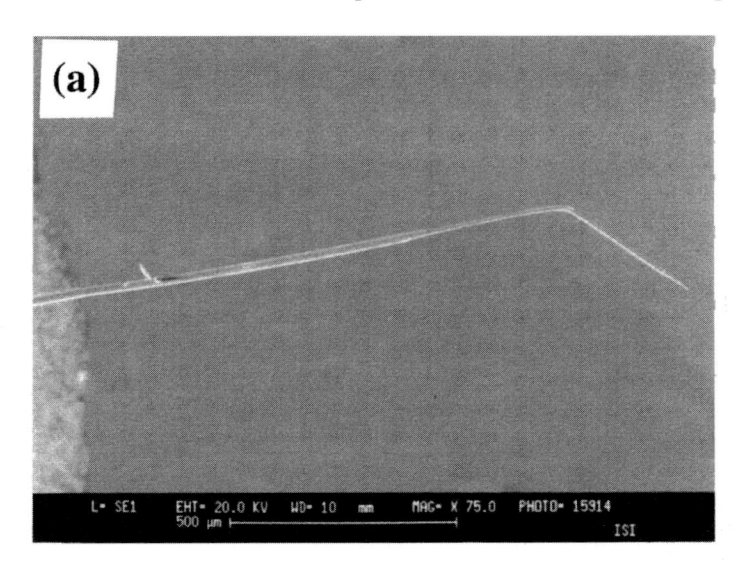

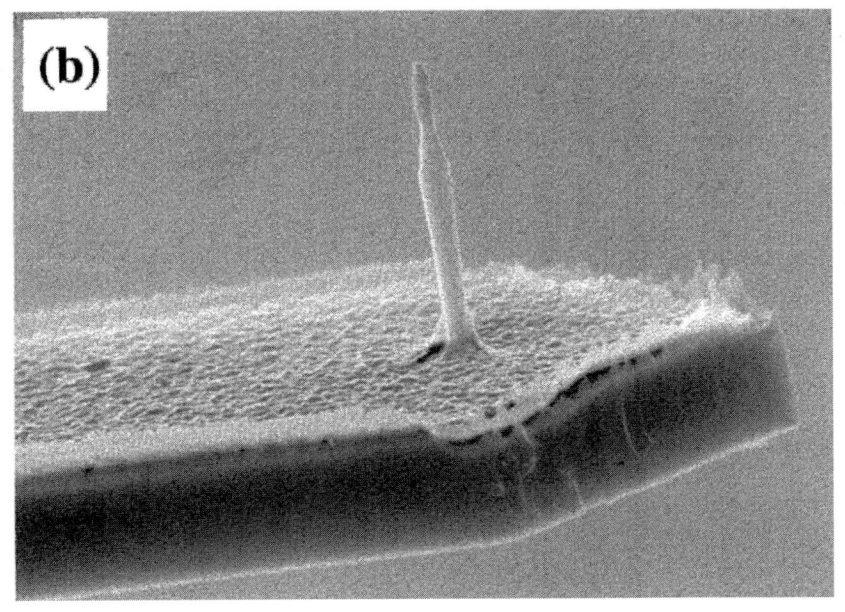

Figure 13.2 (a) Wire cantilever, fabricated by electrochemical etching and bending. (b) Microfabricated silicon cantilever with integrated tip.

on the machining of silicon-related materials (Albrecht *et al.*, 1990b) (Figure 13.2). A variety of cantilevers with different geometries (mainly bar- and V-shaped) and with pyramidal as well as conical tips is now commercially available.

The resonant frequency of a spring with a spring constant c and a lumped effective mass m is given by

$$\omega_0 = \sqrt{\frac{c}{m}}. \tag{13.6}$$

According to Equation (13.5) it is desirable to have a low spring constant in order to achieve maximum force sensitivity. This is, however, contradicted by three aspects. First, according to Section 13.2 the spring constant should be a maximum in order to achieve, via Equation (13.6), a maximum resonant frequency, and thus a minimum vibrational sensitivity and a maximum scan rate. Secondly, the ultimate sensitivity of the force measurement is restricted by the thermal excitation of the cantilever. This latter quantity can be determined from the equipatition theorem (Heer, 1972):

$$(\Delta z)_{rms} = \sqrt{\frac{kT}{c}}, \tag{13.7}$$

where $(\Delta z)_{rms}$ is the rms displacement amplitude of the end of the cantilever due to thermal excitation. Third, if the cantilever is subject to a long-range attractive force, and this will almost always be the case in the probe–sample approach (see Section 13.3.3), its position becomes unstable if the magnitude of the force gradient equals the cantilever's spring constant (Landman *et al.*, 1990). Thus, a certain minimum spring constant is needed in order to approach the sample sufficiently closely without a jump to contact.

In order to estimate the order of magnitude that the spring constant of the cantilever could have, it is straightforward to match c to the respective constant of interatomic coupling in solids (Rugar and Hansma, 1990). Taking in Equation (13.6) $m = 10^{-25}$ kg and $\omega_0 = 10^{13}$ Hz for atomic masses and vibrational frequencies, one arrives at $c = 10$ N m^{-1}. Even smaller spring constants can be easily obtained by minimising the cantilever's mass. Commercial cantilevers have a typical spring constant in the range of $10^{-2} \leq c \leq 10^2$ N m^{-1}, typical resonant frequencies in the range of $10 \leq \omega_0 \leq 500$ kHz and a radius of curvature of the probing tip as small as 10 nm, and are usually fabricated of silicon, SiO_2, or Si_3N_4.

If one again takes the above estimate for the interatomic coupling ($c = 10$ N m^{-1}) for a rough estimate of the resulting deflection of a cantilever which is subject to an interatomic interaction, then according to Equation (13.5), a force of 1 nN causes a deflection of 1 Å, while thermal rms noise according to Equation (13.7) amounts to about 20% of this value. Thus, the task is to measure precisely cantilever deflections smaller than 1 Å.

In the first AFM approaches this was achieved by operating a complete STM on top of the cantilever (Binnig *et al.*, 1986). Since this was not very reliable, numerous schemes based on optical interferometry involving homodyne (McClelland et al., 1987; Erlandsson et al., 1988b; den Boef, 1989) and heterodyne (Martin et al., 1987) detection methods and differential techniques were presented between 1987 and 1989. The most successful interferometric scheme is the fibre-optic approach (Rugar et al., 1988, 1989; Mulhern et al., 1991) shown in Figure 13.3. The interference takes place between the cleaved end of a single-mode optical fibre and the cantilever. By employing a bidirectional fibre coupler the measured interference signal can be related to a reference signal, thus minimising the sensitivity to external noise sources or intensity and mode fluctuations of the diode laser.

A set-up which is even easier to handle is the beam-deflection scheme (Meyer and Amer, 1988; Alexander et al., 1989; Ducker et al., 1990) shown in Figure 13.4. The cantilever deflection is measured by detecting the related displacement of a laser beam reflected off the back of the cantilever. Spatial variations in the reflected laser beam are detected by a position-sensitive photodetector, segmented into four quadrants. If the light beam moves between the upper and lower pairs of segments the deflection of the cantilever can be deduced from a proper treatment of all individual photocurrents

$$\Delta I_{\text{vertical}} = (I_{\text{upper left}} + I_{\text{upper right}}) - (I_{\text{lower left}} + I_{\text{lower right}}). \quad (13.8)$$

$\Delta I_{\text{vertical}}$ is related to the deflection of the laser beam, which is given by

$$\Delta y = \frac{d}{l} \Delta z, \quad (13.9)$$

where l is the length of the cantilever and d that of the light path subsequent to reflection. Usually, the laser beam has a Gaussian intensity profile with a characteristic spot diameter increasing proportionally to the distance d between the cantilever and photodetector. The photocurrent generated in the detector is proportional

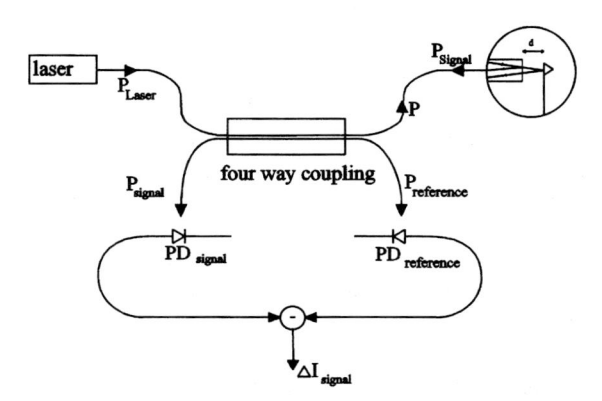

Figure 13.3 Set-up of the fibre-interferometric force microscope.

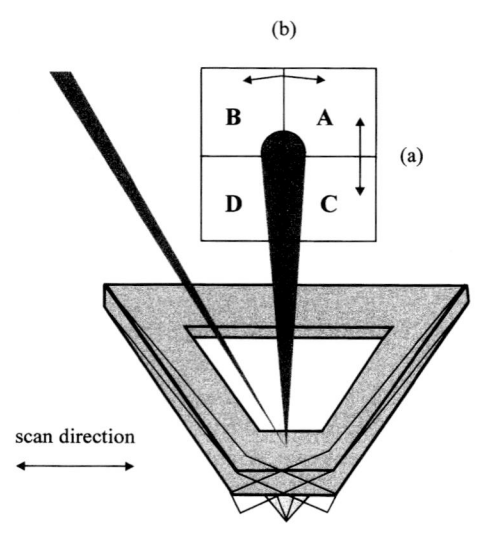

Figure 13.4 Beam-deflection set-up for the simultaneous detection of lateral and vertical force components.

to the flux density j of the photons hitting the photodiode

$$\Delta I_{\text{vertical}} \propto \Delta y d j. \tag{13.10}$$

Since $j \propto 1/d^2$, insertion of Equation (13.9) into Equation (13.10) shows that $\Delta I_{\text{vertical}}$ is independent of the separation d between the cantilever and the detector. This is, however, valid only as long as the deflection Δy is small compared with the spot diameter of the laser beam. For larger deflections non-linearities in $\Delta I_{\text{vertical}}$ (Δy) result. The independence of the force sensor's sensitivity of the separation of the photodetector and the cantilever allows the realisation of very compact beam-deflection schemes.

If a cantilever as shown in Figure 13.4 is scanned in mechanical contact across a sample surface, the surface corrugation causes not only vertical deflections but also a tiny twisting of the cantilever (Mate *et al.*, 1987). This twisting obviously results in a horizontal deflection of the laser spot on the surface of the photodetector

$$\Delta I_{\text{horizontal}} = (I_{\text{upper left}} + I_{\text{lower left}}) - (I_{\text{upper right}} + I_{\text{lower right}}). \tag{13.11}$$

In standard topographical imaging the occurrence of lateral forces acting on the probing tip is often unwanted because the forces affect the images, usually in a complex way (den Boef, 1991). Triangular cantilevers, which are commercially available as standard products, were originally intended to minimise the torsion effects. However, from careful analysis of a huge amount of experimental data, it has been realised that the analysis of lateral forces opens a new avenue in force microscopy.

Lateral force microscopy (LFM) allows the probing of friction forces between the probe and the sample on the nanometer or even at the atomic scale. Since many open questions relate to friction phenomena and their microscopic origin, LFM has gained much importance over the past few years. Unfortunately, it is not easy to calculate the actual lateral force acting on the probing tip from the current difference in Equation (13.11) (Baumeister and Marks, 1967). Thus, absolute values from a sample surface are usually obtained only by first calibrating experimentally the force sensor on suitable reference systems.

In order to make the beam-deflection set-up insensitive to external perturbations or fluctuations of the laser diode, the ratios $\Delta I_{vertical}/\Delta I$ and $\Delta I_{horizontal}/\Delta I$, with ΔI being the sum of all individual photocurrents, are taken for data aquisition. An optimised beam-deflection set-up is then practically almost as sensitive as the interferometer scheme shown in Figure 13.3. Beam deflection offers the advantage of being capable of detecting simultaneously lateral and vertical forces. The mechanical set-up can be kept relatively simple. The fibre interferometer is by far more versatile. It can be implemented under UHV or, for example, under low-temperature conditions. A disadvantage is, however, the more complex mechanical set-up, which allows relative positioning of cantilever and fibre and the restriction to vertical forces.

In comparison with beam deflection and fibre interferometry, the above-mentioned alternative optical deflection sensors, as well as capacitance sensors (Göddenhenrich *et al.*, 1990a; Neubauer *et al.*, 1990) or SQUID-based magnetic detection (Dworak *et al.*, 1997), can be considered to be more or less exotic, or at least not as widely used. These approaches, however, often represent the absolute state of the art with respect to the obtainable sensitivity.

Apart from beam deflection and fibre interferometry, there is one more very elegant and commercially applied approach (Tortonese *et al.*, 1991). Piezoresistive cantilevers change their electrical conductivity owing to tiny deflections. Force measurements can thus be simply performed by probing the actual resistance of the cantilever, preferentially in a bridge set-up. A particularly high sensitivity is obtained if the force microscope is operated in the dynamic mode (see Section 13.3.6). The wide employment of piezoresistive cantilevers is presently restricted by their limited commercial availability. In future, piezoelectric cantilevers (Itoh and Suga, 1993) may also gain some importance and several groups are presently working on their optimisation.

Apart from additional schemes under development to detect sensitively cantilever deflections, some progress has also been made in the further improvement of the monolithically integrated tip of the cantilever. In many applications the sharpness of this tip determines the obtained lateral resolution. Possibilities for increasing the sharpness involve ion etching and local electron-beam-induced deposition of material. Using the latter approach, ultrasharp contamination tips consisting of carbon and carbon compounds can be grown in a scanning electron microscope (SEM) on top

370 METALS AS BIOMATERIALS

of the monolithical tip of the cantilever (Figure 13.5). The tip diameter and aspect ratio can be controlled satisfactorily. A disadvantage of all presently employed tip-refinement methods is, however, that they rule out batch fabrication.

13.3.2 STATE-OF-THE-ART SET-UPS

A maximum versatility of a force microscope is given if the instrument can be operated under the various environmental conditions frequently met in standard experiments in solid-state or soft-matter research. Such a set-up is shown in Figure 13.6 (Euler *et al.*, 1997).

The force microscope is based on the fibre-interferometric scheme shown in Figure 13.3. It can be operated under standard ambient conditions, in a gas atmosphere,

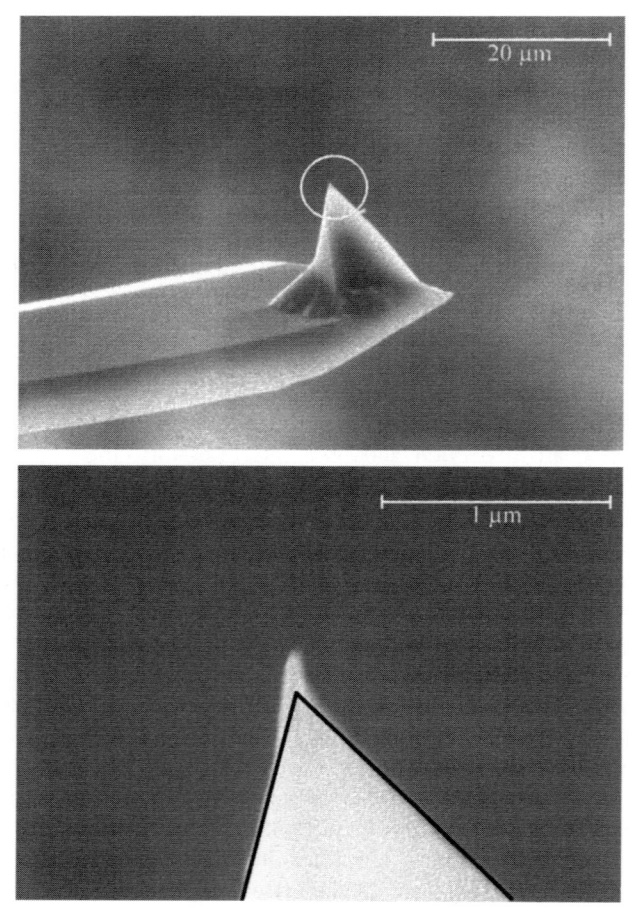

Figure 13.5 Electron-beam deposited supertip on top of an ordinary silicon probe.

ATOMIC FORCE MICROSCOPY

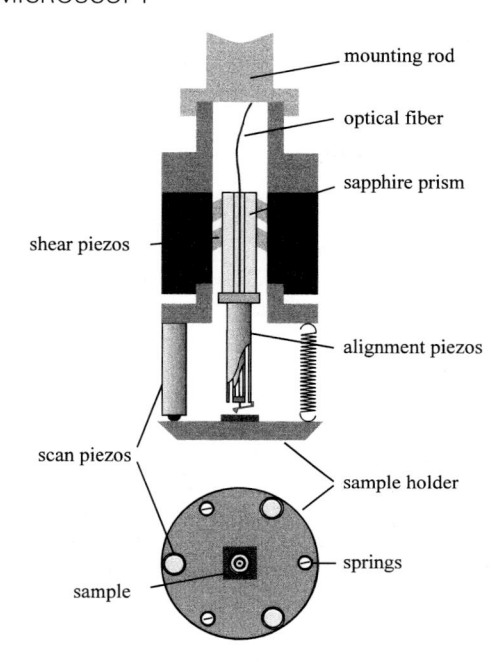

Figure 13.6 Schematics of the set-up of a versatile fibre-interferometric force microscope (Euler *et al.*, 1997).

in UHV, with the sample immersed in a liquid, or upon being inserted in a cryostat containing cold helium exchange gas, or even liquid helium. Such a manifold applicability requires the remote control of all movable parts and a highly sophisticated design largely avoiding the residual thermal drift of mechanical components.

According to the basic considerations in Section 13.2, adjustment of the microscope requires in this case coarse and fine approaches of the fibre end and cantilever, on the one hand, and of the cantilever and sample, on the other. This task is solved by a combination of different piezoelectric actuators involving two concentric piezo tubes for fibre and cantilever positioning, a motor driven by shear piezos for positioning the probe with respect to the sample, and an arrangement of three piezo tubes for scanning (Besocke, 1987). Since the set-up does not contain any element that could be adjusted only manually, fine tuning of the interferometer or the probe–sample separation within a cryostat or a UHV chamber is uncomplicated. The piezoelectric walker can move stepwise over a few millimetres, exhibiting a single-step precision of 100 nm or less. Since the whole microscope head is made from non-magnetic components, it can be operated under the influence of high magnetic fields.

If SFM is to be performed on liquid–solid interfaces, the sample holder in Figure 13.6 is substituted by an electrochemical cell (Siebel *et al.*, 1997). This device contains reference electrodes and is chemically largely inert. The sample, the cantilever

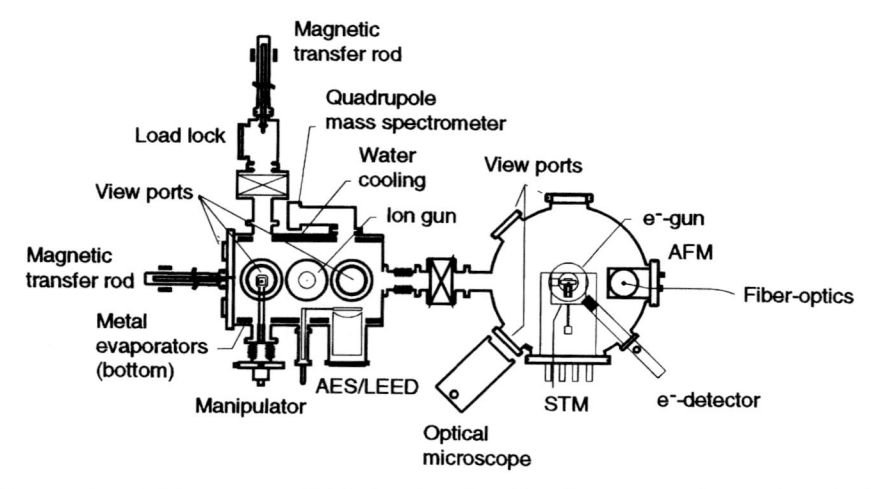

Figure 13.7 Multipurpose UHV chamber for thin film preparation and analysis. The set-up involves an optical microscope, a scanning electron microscope, a STM and an AFM attached to the analysis chamber. The preparation chamber contains standard components for global surface analysis (Memmert *et al.*, 1996).

and the fibre end are all immersed in the liquid environment. A considerable advantage of the fibre interferometer is that no interference between light reflected off the cantilever and at the liquid–gas (or liquid–air) interface affects the measurement. Such interference is often a problem in beam-deflection set-ups.

In UHV operation it is necessary that probes and samples can be exchanged *in situ*. This task is solved by suitable mechanical manipulators which are standard equipment in UHV technology. A complex multichamber UHV system with facilities for sample preparation and general-purpose analysis, and with the capability of performing SEM, STM and AFM investigations, is shown in Figure 13.7 (Memmert *et al.*, 1996).

Even more complex are set-ups that allow additionally a variable sample temperature involving low and elevated values. Some research groups are presently developing such set-ups. The most sophisticated approaches offer the additional option of the application of high magnetic fields. Often, one microscope head can be employed to perform either STM or AFM operation. Commercial solutions will certainly be available in the near future.

13.3.3 PROBE–SAMPLE INTERACTIONS

If two solids are in close proximity to each other many interactions can result, manifesting themselves in forces. The sensitivity of present force microscopes is sufficient for detecting surface forces on a nanometre scale and even intermolecular interactions (Israelachvili, 1985). Figure 13.8 shows the typical variation in the

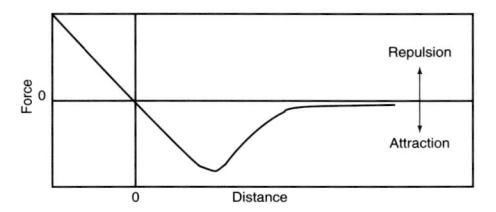

Figure 13.8 Typical variation of the force between the probe and the sample with their relative distance.

interaction potential between the probe and the sample if their separation is successively decreased.

At relatively large separations, typically of the order of 1 nm or more, van der Waals interactions lead to a negative interaction potential and thus to attractive forces (Hartmann, 1990/91a, b). These forces are always present in any environmental situation. Their origins are zero-point quantum fluctuations that depend sensitively on the local probe–sample geometry, on the materials involved and on the medium intervening between the probe and the sample. The van der Waals forces usually increase in magnitude if the probe approaches the sample surface. Often the resulting force–distance curve can be characterised by a simple reciprocal power law (Hartmann, 1994). If the outermost atom of the probe starts to penetrate the sample surface, i.e. if the electronic wave functions of the probe and the sample start to overlap, short-range repulsive forces are introduced. Since the valence- and conduction-band electrons are typically 1–10 Å away from the outermost atomic nuclei of the sample, while the extent of the inner bound electrons is 10–30 pm, the resulting repulsion is indeed very short range. Upon closer approach of the probe to the sample more and more interatomic interactions lead to a continuously increasing repulsion, while the overall long-range probe–sample interaction is still attractive. Thus, the net interaction potential exhibits first a point of inflection, then an absolute minimum, followed by a situation where the repulsive short-range interactions just balance the attractive long-range interactions, and finally a regime where ultimately the repulsive interactions dominate the attractive ones. In this regime the probe seriously penetrates the sample, leading first to elastic and finally to inelastic deformations.

The above scenario occurs for any given experiment since it represents the general behaviour of two solids brought into sufficiently close proximity. However, additional interactions can result if suitable environmental conditions are chosen or if external manipulations are undertaken in a suitable way. If, for example, an electrical potential is applied between the probe and the sample, Coulomb interactions provide an additional long-range attractive contribution. Charges of equal sign on probe and sample would, in contrast, lead to repulsive forces. If the probe and the sample consist of ferromagnetic materials, the resulting long-range magnetostatic interactions can be either repulsive or attractive. In any case the situation is still relatively simple since all long-range interactions mentioned, i.e. van der Waals,

Coulomb and magnetic dipole forces, can be treated in terms of a linear superposition.

Linear physics breaks down if the sample surface is a solid–liquid interface. This situation is not uncommon because sample surfaces are frequently covered by thin adsorbed water or other quasi-liquid contamination layers when subject to ambient conditions. The same situation holds for the cantilever probes. The presence of liquid thin films or even only of a sufficiently high humidity manifests itself in the formation of a liquid capillary between the probe and the sample. The meniscus causes huge attractive interactions which usually dominate all interactions of interest mentioned above (Hartmann, 1994). The problem is not only that capillaries cause large background forces. A more serious consequence is that the overall loading force exerted by the probe on the sample is greatly increased. This limits the lateral resolution obtained in contact-mode SFM and sometimes even leads to the destruction of the sample surface (Section 13.3.4). In addition, liquid menisci are sources of pronounced hysteresis effects in force curves (Section 13.3.8).

There are two possible ways of avoiding capillary formation. The straightforward one is to perform the AFM experiment under UHV conditions. This reduces the adsorption of contaminants to a minimum and allows in many cases the analysis of locally absolutely clean surfaces over a period of time. The second possibility, which excludes liquid meniscus formation between the probing the tip and the sample, is to immerse the cantilever and the sample completely in a suitable liquid. This approach offers a broad avenue of new applications of SPM (Gewirth and Siegenthaler, 1995). The main reason for this is that the surfaces of the sample and the cantilever become solid–liquid interfaces.

A solid–liquid interface represents characteristic properties of both the solid and the adjacent liquid. It generally also involves, however, special physical and chemical phenomena that result only if the selected solid is in contact with the selected liquid. In any case, the presence of the liquid immersion especially changes the aforementioned long-range interactions, with the exception of the magnetostatic forces. Both Coulomb and van der Waals forces depend sensitively on the dielectric properties of the liquid in the intervening gap between the probe and the sample. For the electrostatic force F this dependence is given by $F \propto 1/\varepsilon$. In the case of van der Waals forces the relationship is much more complicated because the interaction depends on the actual static and dynamic dielectric properties of the probe, the sample, and the immersion liquid (Hartmann, 1994). The most striking consequence of the complex relation between van der Waals interactions and electrodynamic properties, especially in the ultraviolet part of the spectrum, is that a repulsive interaction can occur, while van der Waals forces in vacuum or air are always attractive. Thus, an immersion liquid can be used to avoid capillary formation and to lower the magnitude of van der Waals forces. One should be aware of the possibility that the behaviour of the liquid–solid interface can deviate considerably from that of the free sample surface.

One such deviation results from solvation forces that manifest themselves if liquid molecules are squeezed between the probe and the sample when in very close

ATOMIC FORCE MICROSCOPY

proximity to each other (Hartmann, 1994). Other liquid-induced phenomena involve the relevance of hydrophilicity or hydrophobic effects. The most important point, however, is that an immersion liquid can contain a well-defined concentration of positive and/or negative ions, possibly under electrical potential control. In this case an electrochemical environment exists. It is well known that double-layer forces, i.e. ionic Coulomb forces, play an important role in such an environment. The range of these repulsive forces depends on the valence and concentration of the ion species but also on the electrical surface potential. Utilising an electrochemical environment, the forces upon imaging a sample can be successfully controlled and electrochemical investigations can be performed on the nanometre scale.

It was mentioned above that linear approaches to the characterisation of probe–sample interactions often break down if a liquid-immersion medium is present. The reason for this now becomes obvious: van der Waals forces, double-layer forces and solvation forces cannot simply be superimposed in a linear way, nor can they be treated exhaustively in a simple continuous theory. Strong local variations in the ionic or molecular concentrations which are present if double-layer and solvation forces exist result in the local dielectric behaviour of the immersion liquid, which strongly deviates from its bulk behaviour. The local dielectric behaviour, in turn, determines the van der Waals forces acting between the probe and the sample.

It seems worthwhile to emphasise that the presence of liquids as well as that of electrostatic or magnetostatic forces usually modifies significantly the simplest of the probe–sample interaction potential shown in Figure 13.8. This complicates data analysis, in particular if various intermolecular and surface forces are present at the same time. However, the many interactions that can be externally stimulated offers a large number of special applications for SFM, such as electrochemical, magnetic or electric force microscopy.

13.3.4 CONTACT-MODE OPERATION

According to Hooke's law [Equation (13.5)] the cantilever which is raster-scanned across the sample surface exhibits a locally varying deflection that directly represents the corrugation of the sample surface. Since the force microscope is equipped with a feedback loop (Section 13.2), it is convenient to keep the actual cantilever deflection constant by suitably adapting the probe–sample separation continuously during scanning. Thus, the working distance is increased if the local force exerted on the cantilever becomes temporarily relatively high, and it is decreased if the force falls below a prechosen setpoint. The resulting *constant-force mode* is one of the most important modes in which a force microscope can be operated. The very first AFM observations were all performed in this mode (Binnig et al., 1986). Since a proper feedback action which ensures constant forces between the cantilever and the sample is ultimately limited by the response time of the feedback circuit, the scan speed in the constant-force mode is evidently limited. In many cases, especially where only the nanoscale topography of the sample is of interest, an alternative mode of operation is to raster-scan the probe across the sample surface at a constant average height, where the cantilever deflection and thus the force can change during scanning. The *variable-deflection mode* is achieved by limiting the feedback response to relatively low frequencies and by recording higher frequency deflections as a function of the probe position. Compared with the constant-force mode, significantly higher scan rates can be achieved in the variable-deflection mode. Since, however, the recorded maps do not represent exact equiforce surfaces, the recorded data are generally more difficult to interpret. It is thus convenient, if not necessary, to ensure that relative variations in the force do not exceed a few per cent for the whole recorded image.

It is important to note that the term *contact mode* is, at first sight, not very well defined. For example, STM is usually considered as a non-contacting, non-destructive imaging method, where a local wave-function overlap between one atom of the tip with one atom of the sample surface is utilised to obtain local information. In contrast, one would intuitively think of a mechanical contact if the outermost atom of a cantilever tip started to overlap with a sample atom resulting in repulsive forces between the two interacting atoms. Thus, a more precise definition is needed of *contact-mode force microscopy*. Basically, this mode is very similar to the working principle of Edison's gramophone or a classical stylus profilometer (Williamson, 1967/68). While, however, for the latter instrument even in the most advanced set-ups the force exerted by the stylus tip on the sample is in the order of 10^{-4} N, typical values in force microscopy are much smaller. It is most instructive to discuss image formation in the contact mode with the help of Figure 13.8. The feedback setpoint for an operation in the constant-force or variable-deflection mode is chosen within the regime of overall repulsive interaction. This means that the probe exerts a certain loading force on the sample surface. In order to keep this loading force either locally absolutely constant or constant on average during scanning, the probe has to follow the atomic or nanoscale corrugation of the sample surface. In this way it is possible to obtain images like those shown in Figures 13.9 and 13.10. It has been demonstrated that atomic-scale periodicities can be well resolved by AFM in the contact mode on layered materials, ionic crystals and metals. Typical loading forces are of the order of 10^{-8}–10^{-7} N. A cantilever deflection, which can be converted according to Equation (13.5) into a net force, is experimentally accessible. It is important to re-emphasise that this experimentally determined force is composed of a long-range attractive interaction between the probe and the sample and a short-range repulsive interaction between the outermost probe atoms and the sample surface. Consequently, if the force setpoint in contact-mode AFM is given by a certain value, e.g. 10^{-8} N, which represents a net repulsive interaction, the corresponding repulsive force exerted by atoms at the probe apex on the sample is much higher than the setpoint value. Since typical atomic binding forces exhibit a magnitude in the order of 10^{-9} N (Section 13.3.1), it is evident that a loading force in the order of at least 10^{-8} N leads to local deformations or even destruction of the sample surface and eventually of the probe apex. Such deformations lead to an increase in the contact radius, which leads in turn to a reduction in the force acting per atom between the probe and the sample. The increasing extent of the contact

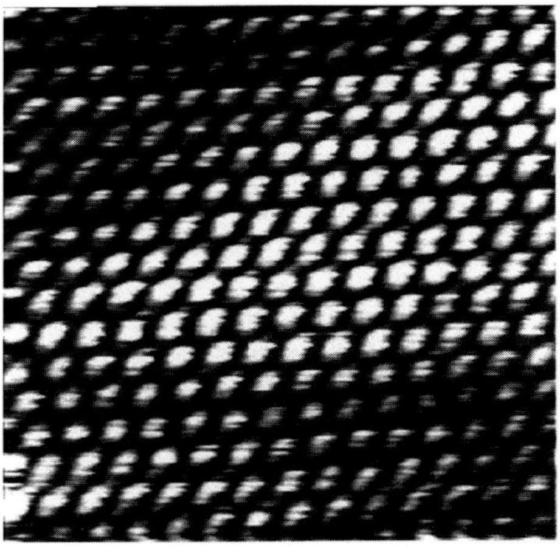

ATOMIC FORCE MICROSCOPY

Figure 13.9 Atomic-scale resolution on Au(111) in the constant-force contact mode. The scanned area is 4×4 nm^2. (Courtesy of P. Güthner, Omicron Vakuumphysik.)

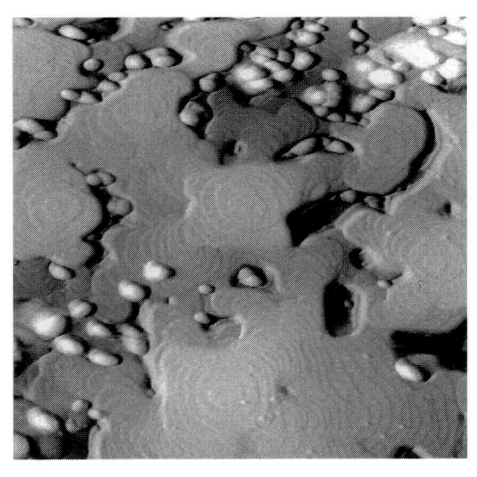

Figure 13.10 Contact-mode image taken at a temperature of 7.8 K. The sample is YBa$_2$Cu$_3$O$_{7-\delta}$ sputter-deposited on a SrTiO$_3$ substrate. The image clearly shows that the superconducting film is composed of screw dislocations. The imaged area is 800×800 nm^2.

radius is the mechanism by which irreversible perturbations of the sample and the probe in the imaging process are largely avoided.

On the one hand, the force per atom for a relatively large contact radius is small enough not to cause surface damage but, on the other hand, a large contact radius exists only if the probing tip is a multi-atom rather than a single-atom tip. This latter conclusion raises the serious question of how an obviously atomic resolution like that shown in Figure 13.9 could be obtained if many atoms of the probe and the sample interact. An important indication for an answer to this question is that almost all of the experimental data acquired in the high-resolution contact mode of operation exhibit only an atomic periodicity rather than a true atomic resolution. This means that generally only the periodic arrangements of unit cells, but neither the inner atomic configuration of this unit cell nor individual atomic lattice defects, are detected. Both features are, however, generally observed in STM images. Two mechanisms are responsible for the majority of pseudoatomic-resolution observations. Moiré interference patterns of atomic periodicity result if the probe's atomic lattice glides across the sample's atomic lattice. In addition, for layered materials such as graphite or mica, the probing tip often carries a piece of sample material picked up during scanning (Abraham and Batra, 1989; Gould *et al.*, 1989). In contrast, on ionic crystals such as LiF, NaCl and AgBr a preferential imaging of the larger negatively charged ions would explain why an atomic periodicity but never an individual atomic lattice defect is visible (Meyer and Amer, 1990; Meyer *et al.*, 1991). The multi-atom imaging mechanisms emphasise once more that true atomic resolution in contact-mode AFM requires ultrasmall loading forces as a prerequisite for a single-atom probe. These can generally not be achieved under ambient conditions (Binnig, 1992).

It is important to consider what theory tells us about the contact-mode imaging mechanism. The key for modelling the occurring forces is the electrostatic Hellman–Feynman theorem (Deb, 1973). According to this theorem the probe–sample interactions can be ultimately obtained from classical electrostatics once the electronic wave functions of the probe and the sample surface have been determined by an accurate quantum-mechanical calculation. The latter is, however, the major problem. Numerical approaches (Ciraci *et al.*, 1990) indicate that there are two relevant contributions to the interatomic forces. A very short-range repulsive interaction with a strong distance dependence results from the Coulomb force between the atomic nuclei of the probe and the sample. Thus, contact-mode AFM can be assumed to probe predominantly the position of atomic nuclei at the sample surface, in contrast to STM which probes the local density of electronic states close to the Fermi level. The second contribution to the total interatomic interaction results from an attractive Coulomb force between the electron clouds of the probe and the atomic nuclei of the sample, and vice versa. This contribution is of longer range than the aforementioned ones and does not decay as rapidly with increasing probe–sample distance. If AFM could be performed within that tiny probe–sample distance region, where the attractive interatomic interaction dominates the repulsive interactions, it would probe primarily the total electronic density of states at the sample surface. This is then more closely related to what is probed by STM. The difference is, however, that the latter technique is restricted to near-Fermi-level electronic states.

13.3.5 LATERAL FORCES

Friction is a well-known phenomenon occurring whenever two bodies in contact are in relative motion with respect to each other. The basic fundamentals of this phenomenon are not very well known and the theory of friction is largely phenomenological. A macroscopic friction force F_f is ultimately related to the microscopic structure of the contact area between the two bodies in direct mechanical contact. Since all surfaces are rough, at least a microscopic scale, the actual contact area is given by relatively few exposed sites establishing a mechanical contact between the two bodies in terms of dominating repulsive forces (Section 13.3.3). The total frictional force is then proportional to the actual contact area A composed by summing up all microscopic contact sites

$$F_f \propto A. \tag{13.12}$$

It has already been discussed (Section 13.3.4) that an increasing loading force F_l leads to an increasing number of microcontacts and thus to a proportionally increasing total contact area

$$A \propto F_l. \tag{13.13}$$

The combination of Equations (13.12) and (13.13) yields Amontons' well-known law

$$F_f = \mu F_l, \tag{13.14}$$

which relates the frictional force to the loading force by the friction coefficient μ and implies that F_f is independent of the interface area between the two contacting bodies. μ is a phenomenological quantity which is characteristic of the involved materials.

It is obvious that AFM is a very well-suited method for analysing friction on an atomic or a nanometre scale because the loading force can be varied over a large range, thus permitting variation in the probe–sample contact radius in the range of one atom up to more than 100 nm (McClelland, 1989; McClelland and Cohen, 1990). LFM as a special application of contact-mode AFM is thus extremely interesting for both the analysis of the microscopic foundations of friction and the imaging of surfaces that exhibit only minor topographic variations but pronounced variations in the chemical composition of the surface. Lateral forces are measured in detecting the cantilever torsion (Figure 13.4). The typical hysteresis obtained by recording this torsion upon scanning the cantilever forwards and backwards across the sample is shown in Figure 13.11. The hysteresis loop is caused mainly by the static friction becoming effective if the scan direction changes. If the loading force is decreased, static friction also decreases, leading to a decreasing loop size.

Even atomic-scale friction can be observed successfully (Mate et al., 1987). The sliding of the probe was found to be non-uniform, exhibiting a pronounced stick–slip

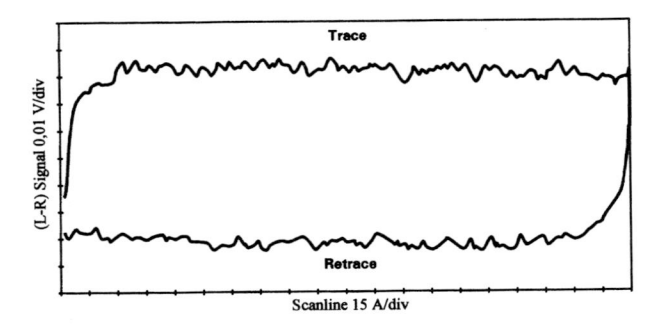

Figure 13.11 Lateral force variations along opposite scans on a glass substrate.

motion. Slips take place instantaneously, while in between the probe and the sample temporarily stick together. A resulting periodicity coincides with the lattice periodicity of the sample surface. This means that the atomic arrangement of probe and sample surfaces determines in a measurable way the frictional properties of the probe–sample interface. The atomic-scale variation of friction can be used for high-resolution imaging (Figure 13.12).

LFM has been performed on a large variety of samples and has proven capable of providing important information, especially on local variation in chemical composition. Studies with the aim of exploiting the microscopic origin of friction were concentrated mainly on layered materials such as graphite or mica. For the latter material the frictional force varies with the periodicity of the hexagonal layer of SiO_4 units (Erlandsson *et al.*, 1988a). The atomic-scale stick–slip behaviour was

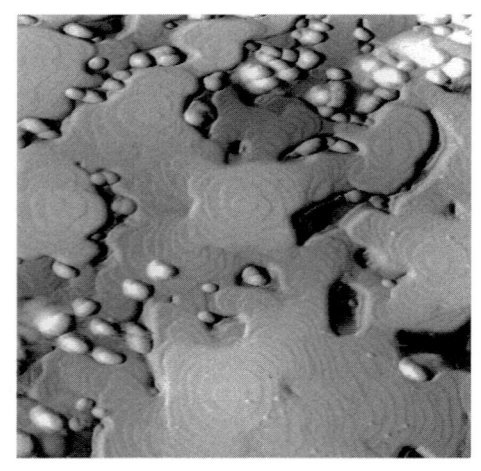

Figure 13.12 Atomic-scale friction on the $23 \times \sqrt{3}$ reconstruction of Au(111). The imaged area is 24×24 nm^2. (Courtesy of P. Güthner, Omicron Vacuumphysik.)

ATOMIC FORCE MICROSCOPY

also found in molecular dynamics simulations concerning a reactive probe–substrate ensemble, where scanning was assumed to be performed under constant loading-force conditions (Landman et al., 1989a, b).

A question of fundamental interest is whether the coefficient of friction μ in Equation (13.14) as determined in the conventional way is the same as that which can be estimated from LFM experiments. A glance at Figure 13.11, however, shows that the frictional force obtained at a certain constant loading force varies along the surface scan. These variations are related to the nanoscale or atomic surface structure. Consequently, μ has to be defined as an average value. Numerous measurements on a large variety of materials have shown that, in general, this average value is not in accordance with the macroscopically determined coefficient. A frequent observation is a more or less pronounced dependence of the microscopic value for μ on the loading force or, in other words, a non-linear relationship between F_f and F_l. This behaviour, which is in contradiction to Equation (13.14), is supported by first-principle theories of atomic-scale friction (Zhong and Tománek, 1990).

LFM is a special variant of contact-mode AFM. Thus, the above considerations concerning true atomic resolution and non-destructiveness also hold for frictional force imaging. In addition, it is difficult to determine absolute forces from the measurements owing to the relatively complex response of the cantilever to torsion. It can, however, be estimated from a large number of experiments that the typical magnitude of lateral forces is in the range of 10^{-10}–10^{-8} N for loading forces that do not cause remanent perturbations of the sample surface.

13.3.6 NON-CONTACT-MODE OPERATION

It is evident that when the probe is lifted by at least 1 nm from the sample surface only long-range interactions will remain. According to the discussion in Section 13.3.3 the relevant forces result in general from van der Waals interactions, electrostatic and magnetostatic interactions and, under ambient conditions, often from the formation of liquid capillaries. Information on the atomic or nanoscale surface structure is completely lost. While van der Waals forces are relatively small and capillary forces can be avoided either by choosing a sufficiently large working distance or by working on clean surfaces, electrostatic and magnetostatic interactions can yield relatively strong forces. This provides important information about the electrical or magnetic charge distribution in the near-surface region of the sample. Since these charge distributions can be manifold, the lateral variation and the range of the resulting interactions are very different on different samples. Near-field operation means in this context that only those charges in the probe and the sample within a certain volume around the probe apex contribute to contrast formation. In other words, if the static interaction is modelled in terms of a multipole expansion of the charge distribution, monopole, dipole and higher contributions are usually found, all of which have to be taken into account to a certain degree. Thus, for the magnetostatic interaction it is very frequently found that the resulting forces are not simply dipole forces but that the monopole term dominates contrast formation (Hartmann, 1994).

In particular, if the microscope is operated in the non-contact mode it is not very reasonable to denote this by AFM and the acronym SFM should clearly be preferred. One of the most important variants of non-contact SFM is magnetic force microscopy (MFM), especially for applied research purposes (Hartmann *et al.*, 1991). In order to image magnetic domains or even interdomain boundaries, a microfabricated cantilever (Figure 13.2) is coated with a magnetic thin film. When it is subjected to the surface stray field of a sample the resulting magnetostatic interactions provide information about the surface magnetisation of the sample. It should be remembered that stray field and magnetisation are generally related in a complex way; however, stray-field mapping sometimes provides clear information on the magnetic domain structure (Figure 13.13). A spatial resolution far below 100 nm can be reached routinely (Hartmann, 1994).

MFM was initially used mainly to investigate components of magnetic recording technology (Martin and Wickramasinghe, 1987; Senz *et al.*, 1987). A large amount of work (Rugar *et al.*, 1990) has strikingly confirmed the usefulness of the technique in applied research. The first image of an interdomain boundary (Göddenhenrich *et al.*, 1988) was a further breakthrough and also made MFM highly interesting for basic research. The main strength of MFM over other magnetic imaging methods is that the investigations can be performed under ambient conditions with little or no surface preparation. MFM has been applied successfully not only to ferromagnetic materials but also to the imaging of vortices in superconductors (Moser *et al.*, 1995). A further important field of application is the analysis of magnetic stray fields caused by electrical currents (Göddenhenrich *et al.*, 1990b; Hartmann, 1994). Since other well-established techniques probe only local variations in the electrical potential, the application of MFM in semiconductor chip analysis will be of growing importance.

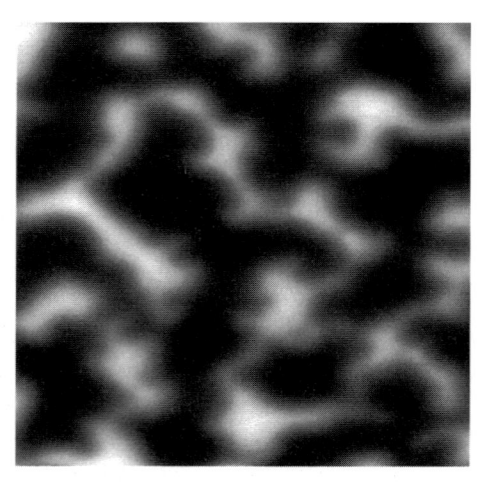

Figure 13.13 MFM image of a $Tb_{30}Fe_{62}Co_8$ thin film showing the bimagnetised-state domain configuration in the material. The scanned area is 5×5 μm^2.

ATOMIC FORCE MICROSCOPY

In Section 13.3.4 it was pointed out that contact-mode force microscopy involves the danger of destructiveness, if the loading force becomes too high. In spite of the relatively large probe–sample separation MFM also involves the potential for sample perturbation. If the stray field produced by the probing tip is too high, the magnetisation of the sample can be affected during scanning (Hartmann, 1988). This phenomenon was found in a number of measurements on soft magnetic samples and successfully modelled in micromagnetic simulations (Scheinfein *et al.*, 1990). The problem can be circumvented in two ways. First, it is possible to deposit a small magnetic particle right at the apex of the probe in such a way that it looks like the tip shown in Figure 13.5 (Leinenbach *et al.*, 1997). Secondly, it is possible to utilise eddy-currents excited in a non-ferromagnetic probe for completely non-destructive magnetic imaging (Hoffmann *et al.*, 1997).

Electrical charges can either be present in the probe and the sample permanently or be introduced by applying an electrical potential between the probe and the sample. Coulomb forces have been measured on a variety of samples (Martin *et al.*, 1988; Stern *et al.*, 1988; Terris *et al.*, 1989/90a, b). One of the most striking demonstrations of the sensitivity obtainable in electric force microscopy is the monitoring of the incremental decay of a charge generated by a voltage pulse in Si_3N_4 (Schönenberger and Alvarado, 1990a). Other experiments concentrated on the study of contact electrification or triboelectrification, where in the latter case charges were produced by bringing the probe into contact with the sample without an externally applied bias voltage (Terris *et al.*, 1989/90a, b). A further important field of application of charge microscopy is the analysis of ferroelectric materials, where even individual domain walls have been imaged (Saurenbach and Terris, 1990).

If a potential difference V is externally applied between the probe and the sample, the resulting Coulomb force is given by

$$F_C = \varphi(d)V^2. \qquad (13.15)$$

φ depends on the geometry of the probe, the local geometrical configuration of the sample surface, the dielectric environment and, explicitly, the probe–sample spacing d. If the probe–sample arrangement is modelled to a first order by a simple parallel-plate capacitor with an electrode area A involving a dielectric medium of relative constant ε_r, one would find $\varphi(d) = \varepsilon_0 \varepsilon_r A/(2d^2)$. F_C exhibits a square dependence in the local electrical potential which opens the possibility of measuring potential variations across sample surfaces. This is particularly interesting for semiconductor devices (Martin *et al.*, 1988; Abraham *et al.*, 1991) and surface-conductance measurements in general (Morita *et al.*, 1989). Furthermore, because of the dependence of φ on ε_r it is also possible to measure dielectric properties of a sample surface, leading to a large variety of applications. Finally, it has been demonstrated that it is also very useful to apply a potential difference for non-electrical measurements in order to separate topographical influences from the long-range interactions of interest (Schönenberger and Alvarado, 1990b).

Up to this point, the impression may have been given that non-contact-mode operation consists simply of lifting the probe of the force microscope to a certain probe–sample distance to measure the long-range interaction in terms of a static force. This is, however, the absolute exception. In discussing the mechanical properties of cantilevers (Section 13.3.1) static characteristics were mainly addressed. It turns out, however, that a broad avenue of new possibilities is opened up if the dynamic properties of the probes are utilised in appropriate approaches (Binnig et al., 1986). As a first characteristic quantity describing these dynamic properties, the resonant frequency was derived in Equation (13.6).

At present, non-contact force microscopy usually involves a sinosoidal excitation of the cantilever with a frequency close to its main resonant frequency, as calculated in Equation (13.6). In order to excite the vibration of the probe, the cantilever can be attached, for example to a bimorph piezoelectric plate. Apart from the cantilever, the sample can also be excited by a suitable piezoelectric actuator. In some applications it is convenient to modulate externally the long-range probe–sample interaction, which also excites a cantilever oscillation. The latter is a particular possibility if electric or magnetic interactions are involved. The non-contact mode of operation involving an oscillating cantilever is also frequently called the dynamic or ac mode.

In contrast to the detection of a quasi-static force, the response of the cantilever in the dynamic mode is, in any case, more complex and deserves more detailed discussion. If the cantilever is excited sinosoidally at its clamped end with a frequency ω and an amplitude δ_0 the probing tip likewise oscillates sinosoidally with a certain amplitude δ exhibiting a certain phase shift α with respect to the driving signal applied to the piezoelectric actuator. The deflection sensor monitors the motion of the probing tip, provided the bandwidth is large enough. The latter requirement clearly favours the optical deflection sensors discussed in Section 13.3.1. The equation of motion, the solution of which is monitored by the deflection sensor, is given by

$$\frac{\partial^2 d}{\partial t^2} + \frac{\omega_0}{Q}\frac{\partial d}{\partial t} + \omega_0^2(d - d_0) = \delta_0 \omega_0 \cos(\omega t), \qquad (13.16)$$

where d_0 is the probe–sample distance at zero oscillation amplitude and $d(t)$ the momentum probe–sample separation. Q is, apart from the intrinsic properties of the cantilever which are the lumped effective mass and the resonant frequency, determined by the damping factor γ

$$Q = \frac{m\omega_0}{2\gamma}, \qquad (13.17)$$

with ω_0 from Equation (13.6). γ introduces the influence of the environmental medium, which could be ambient air, a liquid or UHV. Q thus ranges from values below 100 for liquids, air or other gases at an appropriate pressure, to more than 100 000, which is sometimes obtained in UHV. After the usual building-up, Equation (13.16) leads to the steady-state solution

$$d(t) = d_0 + \delta\cos(\omega t + \alpha) \quad (13.18)$$

for the forced oscillator. The amplitude of the probe's oscillation is given by

$$\delta = \frac{\delta_0 \omega_0^2}{\sqrt{(\omega^2 - \omega_0^2)^2 + 4\gamma^2 \omega^2}}. \quad (13.19)$$

The phase shift between this oscillation and the excitation signal amounts to

$$\alpha = \arctan\frac{2\gamma\omega}{\omega^2 - \omega_0^2}. \quad (13.20)$$

The above simplified formalism is based on the assumption that the oscillation amplitude δ is sufficiently small in comparison with the length of the cantilever. The results derived so far describe only free cantilever oscillations, e.g. oscillations in the absence of any probe–sample interaction. This means that d_0 is still so large that no influence of the sample on the oscillation of the probe can be detected. If d_0 is now so far decreased that a force F affects the motion of the cantilever, a term F/m has to be added to the left-hand side of Equation (13.16). In order to consider almost all interactions that could be interesting in force microscopy one has to assume that

$$F = F\left(d, \frac{\partial d}{\partial t}\right) \quad (13.21)$$

which accounts, apart from static interactions, also for dynamic forces. An example of the latter is hydrodynamic effects or eddy-currents (Hoffmann et al., 1997). Since F describes in the various applications of dynamic-mode force microscopy interactions of various types, for example, of very different dependence on the probe–sample spacing, the $d(t)$ curves monitored by the deflection sensor and found according to Equation (13.16) usually represent enharmonic oscillations. If, however, $F(d)$ can be substituted by a first-order Taylor approximation for $\delta_0 \ll d_0$, the force microscope detects the compliance or vertical component of the force gradient $\partial F/\partial z$. On the basis of this approximation the cantilever behaves under the influence of the probe–sample interaction as if it had the modified spring constant

$$c_F = c - \frac{\partial F}{\partial z}, \quad (13.22)$$

where c is the intrinsic spring constant entering Equation (13.5). An attractive probe–sample interaction with $\partial F/\partial z > 0$ will effectively soften the cantilever spring, to Equation (13.6) the change in the apparent spring constant will modify the cantilever's resonant frequency to

$$\omega = \omega_0 \sqrt{1 - \frac{1}{c}\frac{\partial F}{\partial z}}. \qquad (13.23)$$

Provided that $\partial F/\partial z \ll c$, the shift in resonant frequency is given by

$$\Delta\omega \approx -\frac{1}{2c}\frac{\partial F}{\partial z}. \qquad (13.24)$$

According to Equations (13.19) and (13.20) a modification in the resonant frequency will result in a change of the probe's oscillation amplitude δ and of the phase shift α between the probe oscillation and the driving signal. $\Delta\omega$, δ and α are experimentally accessible quantities that can be used to map the lateral variation in $\partial F/\partial z$. Phase and amplitude also contain information about the damping coefficient γ. Thus, a local variation in this quantity can be separated from the local variation in the compliance by measuring the frequency shift and the change in amplitude or the phase shift. The simple harmonic solution in Equation (13.18) shows that the dynamic mode of operation can conveniently be based on the use of lock-in methods. The additional use of certain feedback mechanisms opens different variants of operation.

The most commonly used detection method, generally referred to as slope detection, involves driving the cantilever at a fixed frequency ω, slightly off resonance. According to Equation (13.23) a change in $\partial F/\partial z$ gives rise to a shift in the resonant frequency $\Delta\omega$ and, according to Equation (13.19), to a corresponding shift $\Delta\delta$ in the amplitude of the cantilever vibration. $\Delta\delta$ is obviously a maximum at that point of the amplitude–frequency curve where the slope is a maximum. As discussed in Section 13.3.1, the sensitivity is ultimately determined by thermal noise. A careful analysis (Dürig et al., 1986; McClelland et al., 1987; Martin et al., 1987) shows that the minimum detectable compliance is given by

$$\left(\frac{\partial F}{\partial z}\right)_{min} = \frac{1}{\delta_{rms}}\sqrt{\frac{2kT\beta}{\omega_0 Q}}, \qquad (13.25)$$

where δ_{rms} is the rms amplitude of the driven cantilever vibration and β is the measurement bandwidth. High Q values can be obtained by the reduction of air damping in vacuum ($<10^{-3}$ mbar). It might thus appear advantageous to maximise sensitivity by obtaining the highest possible Q. With slope detection, however, increasing Q restricts the bandwidth of the system. If $\partial F/\partial z$ changes during scanning, the vibration amplitude settles on a new steady-state value after a sufficient length of time given by

$$\tau = \frac{2Q}{\omega_0}. \qquad (13.26)$$

Thus, for a high-Q cantilever in a vacuum ($Q = 50\,000$) and a typical resonant frequency of 50 kHz the maximum available bandwidth would be only 0.5 Hz, which is unusable for most applications. The dynamic range of the system would be similarly restricted. Because of these restrictions it is not useful to try to increase the sensitivity by raising the Q to such high values. Moreover, if the experiments have to be performed in a vacuum, for example to prevent sample contamination, it may not be possible to obtain a Q low enough for an acceptable bandwidth and dynamic range. Therefore, slope detection is unsuitable for most vacuum applications.

An alternative to slope detection is frequency modulation (FM). In the FM detection system a high-Q cantilever vibrating on resonance serves as the frequency-determining component of an oscillator. Changes in $\partial F/\partial z$ cause instantaneous changes in the oscillator frequency which are detected by a FM demodulator. The cantilever is kept oscillating at its resonant frequency by positive feedback. The vibration amplitude is likewise maintained at a constant level. A variety of methods, including digital frequency counters and phase-locked loops, can be used to measure the oscillator frequency with a very high precision.

In the case of FM detection, a careful analysis (Albrecht et al., 1990c) shows that the minimum detectable force gradient is given by that of Equation (13.25) multiplied by $\sqrt{2}$. However, in contrast to slope detection, Q and β are absolutely independent in FM detection. Q depends only on the damping of the cantilever and β is determined only by the characteristics of the FM demodulator. Therefore the FM detection method allows the sensitivity to be greatly increased by using a very high Q without sacrificing bandwidth or dynamic range.

Contact-mode force microscopy, as discussed so far, relies on the existence of long-range interactions between the probe and the sample. If no static magnetic and electric fields are involved, the only common long-range interactions are, in any case, van der Waals forces and, in the presence of liquids, capillary forces. Van der Waals forces are weak and provide only limited information on the surface structure. Thus, non-contact-mode force microscopy is largely non-destructive but yields only a lateral resolution in the order of the probe–sample spacing. In contrast, contact-mode force microscopy has the potential for high spatial resolution, but it also involves the potential for surface perturbation. The positive aspects of both modes of operation can be combined if the probe is oscillated in such a way that there is only an intermittent contact between the probe and the sample during each oscillation period. This can be realised if the average probe position, i.e. d_0 in Equation (13.16), is sufficiently far from the sample surface. At the same time a sufficiently large driving amplitude δ_0 is chosen to establish the intermittent contact. As a consequence, the small-amplitude approximation in Equation (13.22) is no longer valid and the tip experiences the full variation of the probe–sample interaction potential shown in Figure 13.8. The intermittent-contact mode, which is generally considered as a special variant of the dynamic modes, thus does not probe a simple force gradient. However, the repulsive forces during intermittent contact lower the rms oscillation amplitude, which yields a highly surface-sensitive signal that can be used for feedback support.

The important point is that the energy transferred from the oscillating probe to the sample surface is very much lower in the intermittent-contact mode than that in the standard contact mode of operation. This makes the technique especially interesting for the analysis of delicate, soft-matter samples (Figure 13.14). The intensity of the intermittent contact can be controlled by appropriately setting the free-vibration amplitude as well as the drop in the amplitude, which is kept constant during scanning. Under ambient conditions, amplitudes as large as 10–100 nm are frequently used for cantilevers with resonant frequencies of 100 kHz or more. Under liquid immersion the amplitude and its drop can be set to much smaller values.

Since in all dynamic modes of operation the dynamic properties of the probes are essential, it might be important to search for alternatives with respect to the standard cantilevers as shown in Figure 13.2. High resonant frequencies and high quality factors are of special interest. One such alternative is quartz oscillators. A well-known oscillator type is the tuning fork, commonly used, for example, in watches. With the use of such an element, it is possible to image the surface topography of both conducting and non-conducting samples (Güthner et al., 1989, 1990). The oscillator is driven at its resonant frequency upon approaching the sample surface. Both frequency and amplitude significantly change for typical probe–sample separations below 100 μm. The damping strongly depends on the environmental gas pressure, which leads to the conclusion that mainly hydrodynamic forces are relevant.

The non-contacting force microscope utilising quartz oscillators can be considered as a near-field acoustic microscope. For a 32 kHz oscillator the wavelength in ambient air is about 1 cm. Since the probe–sample spacing is much smaller, the interaction with the sample takes place in the acoustic near-field region. The spatial resolution obtained is thus clearly not limited by the acoustic wavelength and the

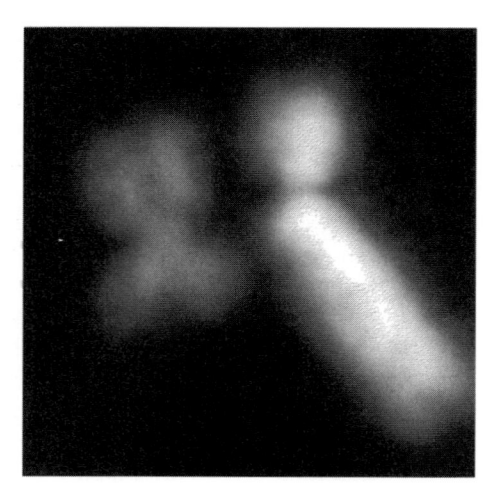

Figure 13.14 Human chromosomes deposited on a glass substrate and imaged by intermittent-contact force microscopy. The image is 3×3 μm^2.

ATOMIC FORCE MICROSCOPY

microscope fulfils the requirements for high-resolution, near-field microscopy discussed in Section 13.2. Recently, the use of quartz rods with high resonant frequency and quality factor has drawn attention to the possibility of performing scanning near-field acoustic microscopy (SNAM) at very high, if not atomic, resolution. This requires a minimum probe–sample spacing obtained by the intermittent-contact operation or in a real contact mode (see also Section 13.3.8).

A considerable technical advantage in using quartz oscillators is that no relative positioning of the oscillator and the deflection sensor is needed. The oscillator provides direct information about the local probe–sample interaction in terms of electrical signals. It is thus of increasing importance to employ such oscillators under UHV and low-temperature conditions where the implementation of conventional deflection sensors is often difficult. The usefulness of quartz or piezoelectric oscillators as elements permitting a precise distance control in various scanning probe applications should be emphasised.

One of the hottest topics in the field of microscopy at present is the achievement of atomic-scale lateral resolution by non-contact force microscopy. High-resolution information can only be obtained if the probe–sample spacing is decreased to a tunnelling distance. If it is possible to stabilise the cantilever oscillation with a relatively small amplitude, with the result that there is only intermittently a sufficient approach between the probe and the sample. The oscillation signal monitored by the deflection sensor will contain some information about this intermittent contact. The long-range interactions, however, still govern the whole oscillation. The FM approach described above is an appropriate way to perform the experiments, which generally have to take place in UHV. If the cantilever is somehow electrically conducting, the intermittent-contact measurements can be combined with intermittent-tunnelling microscopy, thus providing simultaneous information on forces and electronic surface properties. Feedback operation can then be supported by the force measurement, the tunnelling current, or a combination of both. A number of striking experiments (Giessibl, 1995; Shin-ichi and Iwatsuki, 1995; Güthner, 1996; Lüthi *et al.*, 1996) has confirmed that the 7×7 surface reconstruction of the Si(111) surface can be imaged with true atomic resolution (Figure 13.15). Other approaches have shown (Ueyama *et al.*, 1995) that non-contact-mode AFM also has the potential to image III–V compound semiconductors with atomic resolution. Additional experiments performed very recently involve ionic crystals and even metals. It does not have to be emphasised that the capability of investigating a large variety of sample surfaces with atomic resolution independent of the conductivity of the sample or in combination with tunnelling microscopy is an important breakthrough in surface analysis.

13.3.7 SHEAR-FORCE MICROSCOPY

The appearance of shear forces requires that two surfaces be moved laterally with respect to each other. The utilisation of shear interactions opens a new possibility in non-contact force microscopy. If a tip with a suitable resonant frequency and quality

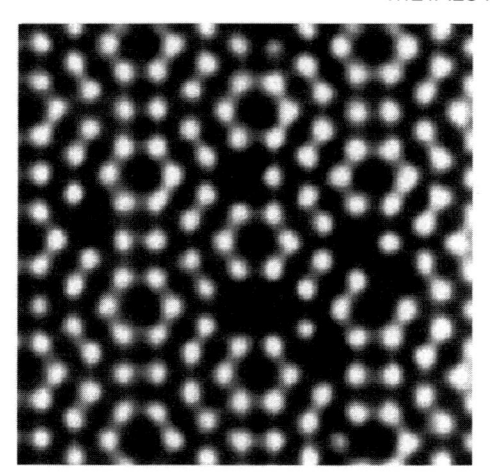

Figure 13.15 Atomic resolution on Si(111) 7 × 7 in non-contact-mode AFM. The grey-scale corresponds to variations of the cantilever's oscillation frequency. (Courtesy of P. Güthner, Omicron Vakuumphysik.)

factor is oscillated, not vertically but largely parallel to the sample surface, a decrease in the oscillation amplitude can be observed upon probe–sample approach. Originally, shear-force detection was introduced as a mechanism to control and keep constant the probe–sample separation in near-field optical microscopy (Betzig *et al.*, 1992; Toledo-Crow *et al.*, 1992; Grober *et al.*, 1994). In this application the probing tip is the end of a glass fibre which is resonantly dithered using a piezo actuator. The detection of the shear force as a function of lateral position provides, apart from feedback purposes, a surprisingly accurate image of the sample surface with nanometre resolution. The glass fibre can be substituted by any other suitable probe. Figure 13.16 shows a comparison between a standard contact-mode AFM image taken on an ordinary CD and a non-contact shear-force image obtained on the same sample. The spatial variation of the shear force clearly represents the surface topography.

The lateral oscillation of the probe and its dependence on probe–sample interactions are fully characterised by the mathematical framework discussed in Section 13.3.6 for a vertical probe oscillation. The axis along which the oscillation takes place has simply to be rotated by 90°. This means, in particular, that F from Equation (13.21) acts along the sample surface and not perpendicular to it. Assuming a permanent or an intermittent probe–sample contact, a decrease in the probe's oscillation amplitude would result from partial sticking or friction in combination with a certain bending of the probe. This mode of operation could be compared with friction-force microscopy, or intermittent-contact force microscopy, as described above. A mechanical contact of small radius between the probe and the sample can even account for the pronounced dependence of the shear force on the probe–sample spacing that has been observed in a vacuum and in liquid helium (Gregor *et al.*, 1996). In changing the probe–sample distance the loading force is changed, which has a direct influence on the measured oscillation amplitude.

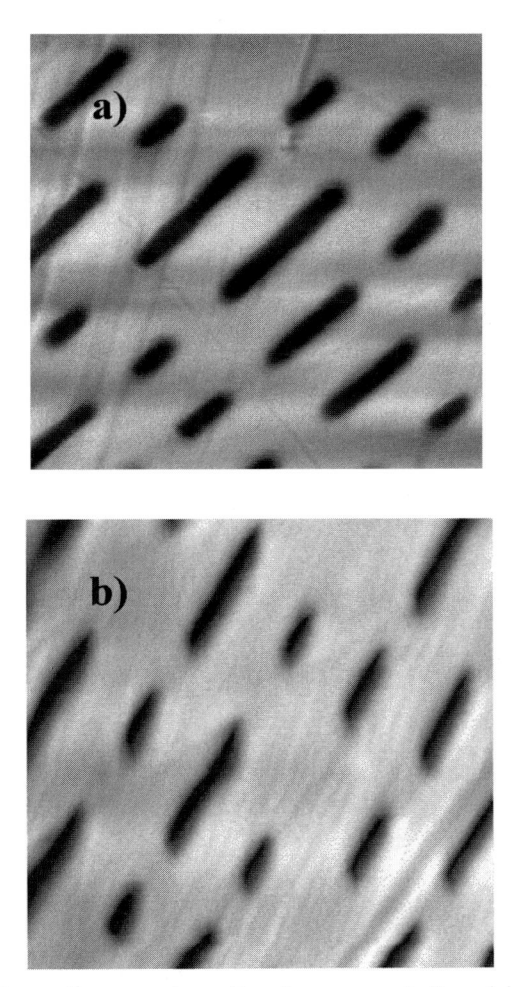

Figure 13.16 Information-carrying pits of a compact disc: (a) was taken in the standard contact mode of operation while (b) represents a shear-force image. The scanned area is 10 × 10 µm².

It is very likely that, apart from direct probe–sample contact, additional phenomena lead to measurable shear forces. Especially under ambient conditions, interactions may be due to viscous drag across the sample between the probe and the sample surface contaminant (Moyer and Paesler, 1993). With this in mind, the force in Equation (13.21) definitely becomes dependent on the probe velocity. More precisely, it becomes proportional to the velocity, since small velocities have negligible higher order dependencies. Furthermore, since the forces are frictional, the decrease in oscillation amplitude is due to an increase in the damping term in Equation (13.19) rather than due to a variation in the resonant frequency. The measured forces are then essentially dissipative but they depend on conservative probe–sample interactions.

The investigations performed so far show that shear-force detection is a convenient method by which to control the working distance in SPM. Shear-force microscopy yields information about the surface topography from the nanometre to the micrometre range, which is qualitatively comparable with the result of standard contact- or non-contact-mode data. However, the actual nature of the shear force is still the subject of considerable controversy. Apart from the mechanisms discussed, further sources of probe–sample interaction dealt with in Section 13.3.3 may also contribute to the interaction. In any case, shear-force data involve the potential for misinterpretation (Durkan and Shvets, 1996) as does any other mode of operation.

13.3.8 FORCE CURVES AND SPECTROSCOPY

Force microscopy is not only capable of providing information about the lateral variation of probe–sample interactions across a sample surface. One can also systematically determine the dependence of the interaction on the probe–sample distance, i.e. the range of the interaction at a given location with respect to the sample surface. Such an investigation is essential in the analysis of the very nature of an unknown interaction. Often the variation in the force appears as shown in the schematical diagram in Figure 13.8. It can, however, also look quite different, as discussed in Section 13.3.3. The basic question now, is the cantilever's response to a given variation in force.

In tracing a force curve the vertical position of the probe with respect to the sample surface is varied systematically. According to Equation (13.5) the acting force leads to a bending Δz of the cantilever. The real probe–sample distance is then given by

$$d = \Delta z - z, \qquad (13.27)$$

where bending of the cantilever towards the sample due to an attractive interaction yields a negative Δz value. The probe–sample approach is described by a decreasing magnitude of $z < 0$, and $\Delta z(z)$ plots are experimentally recorded. Since there is no possibility of independently measuring the distance between the outermost atoms of probe and sample, it is difficult to determine the origin of the $F(d)$ diagram in Figure 13.8. According to Equation (13.27) the probe–sample distance vanishes for $\Delta z = z$, which does not, however, imply that $F(d = 0) = 0$. The net force F vanishes if attractive and repulsive forces balance each other. Then, $\Delta z = 0$, which in turn does not generally imply that $d = 0$.

The most important experimental finding is that a force curve like that shown in Figure 13.8 cannot be traced reversibly, as shown in Figure 13.17a. Upon probe–sample approach attractive forces lead to a bending of the cantilever towards the sample. This causes a non-linear $d(z)$ variation in Equation (13.27). If the vertical component of the force gradient, $\partial F/\partial z$, at a sufficiently small probe–sample spacing

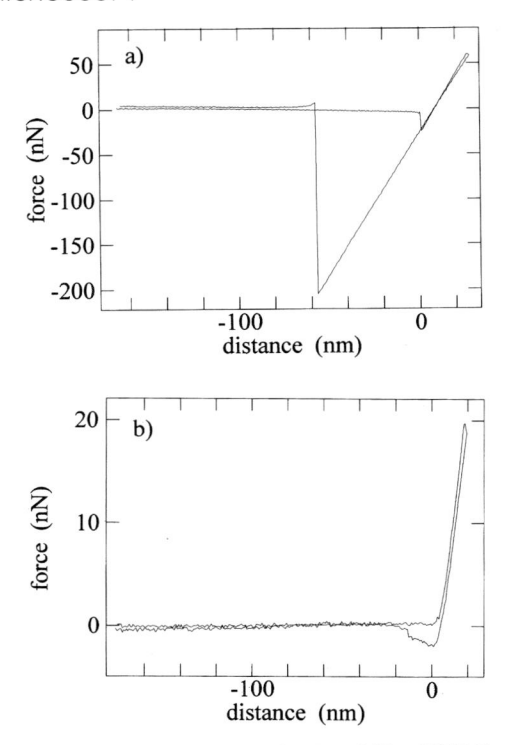

Figure 13.17 Force curves taken on a hydrophilic Si(100) substrate using a silicon cantilever: (a) was taken in ambient air, while (b) was taken under complete immersion of the probe and the sample in water.

d exceeds the cantilever's spring constant c, the instability discussed in Section 13.3.1 causes a jump of the probe to contact. A local minimum in the force curve indicates maximum attraction. A further decrease in the probe–sample spacing increases the loading force and the contact radius. Bending of the cantilever is successively decreased and vanishes when the repulsive forces balance the attractive forces. Further pushing the probe towards the sample causes the cantilever to bend away from the sample. In the absence of elastic deformation of the probe and the sample, $d = 0$ in Equation (13.27) yields a slope of the $\Delta z(z)$ curve equal to unity. The $F(d)$ curve accordingly exhibits an infinite slope because d remains zero independent of the varying z value.

Upon withdrawal of the probe, the motion of the cantilever is reversed. The net loading force continuously decreases. After reversibly reaching the origin of the force curve, which corresponds to the origin of the $\Delta z(z)$ curve, bending of the cantilever again takes place towards the sample surface. In a further attempt to separate the probe and sample, it is found that they adhere to each other. This phenomenon causes an extended motion of the cantilever with $\Delta z = z$. At a certain point of retraction the net force gradient again becomes equal to the cantilever's spring constant and a jump out of contact occurs. From then on, the probe does not experience any interaction with the sample and the cantilever is in its equilibrium position.

Some very important aspects can be concluded from the above comparison between the idealised curve in Figure 13.8 and the experimental curve in Figure 13.17a. Most important is the fact that the full $F(d)$ curve is generally not experimentally accessible (Meyer et al., 1988). For $\partial F/\partial d = c$, with d determined by Equation (13.23), a cantilever instability occurs. Upon probe–sample approach this instability suddenly decreases d by the instantaneous jump of Δz for a certain z value. The actual Δz value now yields the maximum attractive force F_{att}, which is obtained for $z = \Delta z < 0$. From now on, a regime can be reversibly traced with $z = \Delta z$ and $d = 0$ up to repulsive forces, where notable elastic deformation sets in. If there were no adhesion between the probe and the sample at all, the probe would jump out of contact if Δz again becomes smaller than F_{att}/c. In any case a certain regime of the $F(d)$ curve which is determined by the distance interval over which the jump takes place is experimentally not accessible. The questionable interval can be decreased by using sufficiently stiff cantilevers.

Another important aspect is that elastic surface deformations change the slope in the linear regime of $\Delta z(z)$. Since in this case $z > 0$, $d < 0$ is obtained and information about the involved elasticity is additionally provided by the $F(d)$ curve. For negative values of d the probe penetrates the sample surface and the slope of the $F(d)$ curve changes to a finite value. Inelastic surface deformation leads to irreversibilities and eventually to characteristic jumps in the $\Delta z(z)$ curve (Landman et al., 1990). Under such circumstances the force microscope can be operated as a nanoindentor with some advantages over conventional indentation hardness testers (Pethica et al., 1983).

Even if no inelastic surface deformation is involved, force curves generally exhibit considerable hysteresis (Figure 13.17a). This hysteresis is due to an adhesive force between the probe and the sample. For clean probe and sample surfaces adhesion can result from covalent or metallic binding between the probe and the sample atoms (Landman et al., 1990). The pronounced hysteresis, however, which is usually observed under ambient conditions, is due to capillary forces (Hartmann, 1994). These often already initiate the jump to contact upon the approach of the probe to the sample. If the probe is then retracted the liquid meniscus deforms, with increasing substrate–probe separation. Sometimes it can be elongated to a length of more than 100 nm. Upon reaching the maximum adhesive force, F_{adh}, the capillary breaks and the cantilever jumps back to its equilibrium position. Usually, the magnitude of F_{adh} is much larger than that of F_{att}, which causes a huge hysteresis. In contrast, F_{adh} should be reduced to the real substrate–probe adhesion if the force curve is taken in a liquid (Weisenhorn et al., 1989). Indeed, the hysteresis is greatly reduced under liquid immersion (Figure 13.17b).

As an alternative to the $F(d)$ curve, the $\partial F/\partial z(d)$ curve can also be taken. The probe is then operated in the dynamic mode as described in Section 13.3.6. The quantity

ATOMIC FORCE MICROSCOPY

derived from the cantilever oscillation is, however, only equal to the numerically calculated derivative of the $F(d)$ curve if no hydrodynamic or other dissipative interactions are involved. In tracing the range of the probe–sample interaction, the interaction is systematically varied with respect to magnitude and sign. This is often called force spectroscopy. As in other spectroscopies, however, it is not always important to vary the energy over the whole accessible range. Sometimes it is more interesting to map local variations of a given characteristic feature within the whole spectrum. With respect to the force curves discussed above, characteristic quantities are F_{att}, F_{adh} and the surface elasticity, c_s.

Spatial adhesion maps represent the lateral variation of F_{adh} due to material inhomogeneities and the surface topography (Mizes et al., 1991). If F_{adh} is dominated by capillary interactions, the nanoscale behaviour of liquid thin films, in particular that of polymers, can be studied in detail (Mate et al., 1989). This provides qualitatively new information on the surface forces of molecular film arrangements (Burnham et al., 1990; Blackman et al., 1990). F_{att} can also be mapped, in the same way as F_{adh}.

The surface elasticity is roughly characterised by an effective spring constant, c_s. If a sample exhibits a finite c_s, a sufficient loading force makes the probe penetrate the sample. This process is described by Equation (13.27) for a negative probe–sample spacing d. For a given loading force F the cantilever deflection Δz then depends on the local value of c_s and, of course, on the probe's spring constant c

$$\Delta z = \frac{c_s}{c} d. \tag{13.28}$$

With Equation (13.27) one obtains

$$c_s = \frac{\Delta z}{z - \Delta z} c \tag{13.29}$$

in terms of the experimentally accessible quantities. This result tells us in particular that the cantilever's spring constant has to be chosen appropriately. Experimentally, elasticity maps are obtained in a dynamic-contact or intermittent-contact mode by modulating z (Maivald et al., 1991). This causes a corresponding oscillation of Δz from which the surface elasticity c_s can be derived according to Equation (13.29).

13.4 NANOMETRE-SCALE MODIFICATION OF SURFACES

An image acquired by SFM is a collection of data representing the result of the particular experiment performed at any addressed location of the raster-scanned area.

This point of view that applies to any SPM investigation was discussed in detail in Section 13.2. In the ideal case the probe–sample interactions involved in any kind

396 METALS AS BIOMATERIALS

of microscopy are weak enough not to permanently modify either the probe or the sample. However, any interaction involves forces. If these forces do not permanently or temporarily affect the sample, there must be a restoring force that allows the sample to recover after the probe is taken away, or even allows the sample to balance the interaction in the presence of the probe. A great advantage of SFM is that the probe–sample interaction, e.g. the loading force exerted by the probe on the sample, can be varied over a considerable range. This range generally includes a regime in which the chosen strength of interaction exceeds a critical value leading to more or less durable sample modifications. In the present context such a modification is considered as a generated nanostructure if it is at least stable enough to survive after removing the probe from the respective location. Usually, the modification should be at least stable enough to be imaged by the same probe with which it was generated. *A priori*, surface manipulations thus involve metastable as well thermodynamic equilibrium configurations of the sample. Nanomodifications at sample surfaces can be produced by utilising several of the interactions discussed in Section 13.3.3. Sufficiently strong interactions between the probe and the sample can be generated in the contact-mode as well as in the non-contact-mode operation.

Nanotechnology deals with individual objects, the lateral dimensions of which are in the range of 0.1–100 nm. For such small objects the physical properties are strongly influenced by size and surface effects because the geometrical dimensions approach characteristic lengths associated with elementary processes. Examples of such lengths are the electron mean path, the de Broglie wavelength, the coherence lengths in a superconductor and the ferromagnetic exchange length. Nanotechnology is considered to be a key technology with a strong influence on future technical develop-

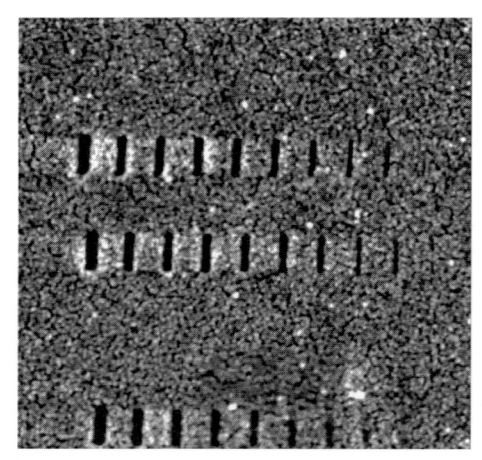

Figure 13.18 Nanomodifications in a gold thin film, performed by AFM in an intermittent-contact mode. The structures were imaged with the same probe with which they were produced. The scanned area is 3.2 × 3.2 μm^2. The smallest structures are about 100 nm in width.

ATOMIC FORCE MICROSCOPY

ments, in particular in the field of information technology. The well-defined production of nanometre-scale structures involves basic research on nanopositioning and nanocontrol approaches, nanoprecision machining, the possibilities of utilising self-assemblence and autoreproduction phenomena, and the possibilities of linking nanostructures to conventional microstructures. Most important, however, is a profound understanding of all relevant physical properties of matter on the nanometre scale and the resulting properties of nanodevices. For this task, SFM, and SPM in general, are very valuable tools for the fabrication and the analysis of nanoscale structures.

A straightforward method for modifying the surface of a sample is to operate the force microscope in the contact or intermittent-contact mode with sufficiently high loading forces (Figure 13.18). Modifications can be performed on conducting,

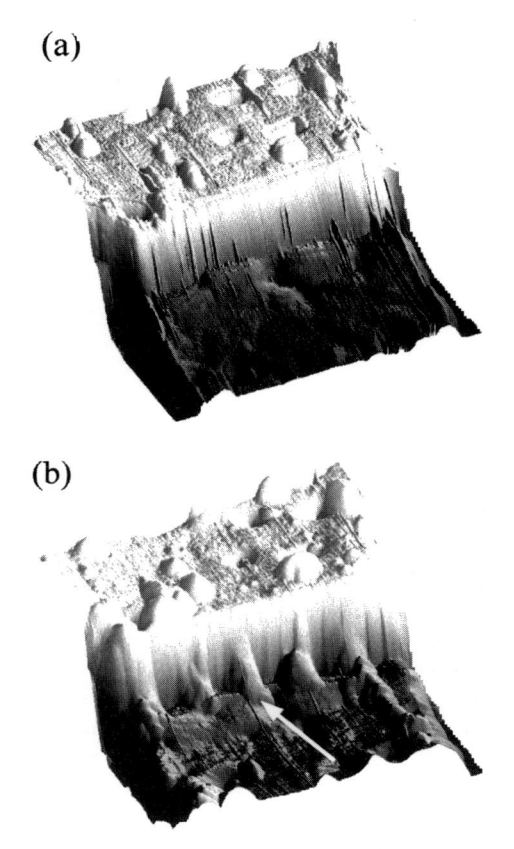

Figure 13.19 Step-etch Josephson junction in a high-T_c superconducting thin film. (a) Original junction; (b) junction after mechanical modification by AFM. The arrow indicates one out of five clearly visible nanobridges which have been deposited at the step. The procedure can be used to tune and optimise the junctions of a SQUID. The scan range is 5×5 μm^2 (Drechsler et al., 1997).

semiconducting and insulating samples. On appropriate substrates and through careful choice of the operational parameters, structures with dimensions below 10 nm can be generated reproducibly (Albrecht, 1989; Jung *et al.*, 1992). AFM-induced mechanical surface manipulations with sufficient stability can be used either to produce complete thin film devices or, in a proper combination with microfabrication techniques, to optimise particular components of a given microstructure (Figure 13.19). As well as direct surface structuring, the usefulness of nanostructured masks in combination with conventional etching techniques has been demonstrated. In the non-contact mode of operation sufficiently strong probe–sample interactions are obtained by using long-range electromagnetic, electrostatic and magnetostatic fields. This offers a variety of possibilities for modifying and functionalising surfaces with high resolution. It has, for example, been shown that a considerable amplification of the electromagnetic field can result locally if a probing tip is illuminated by a laser beam (Jersch and Dickmann, 1996). Using this phenomenon, the sample surface can be modified by local thermal treatment. It has further been demonstrated that by applying voltage pulses to the tip, patterns of trapped charge can be written into insulating thin films with a very high resolution (Barrett and Quate, 1991). By using ferromagnetic probes with a sufficiently high magnetic stray field, the magnetisation of a ferromagnetic sample can be locally reversed (Figure 13.20). Thus, it is even possible to write well-defined magnetic patterns into quite hard magnetic materials (Moreland and Rice, 1990; Göddenhenrich *et al.*, 1992).

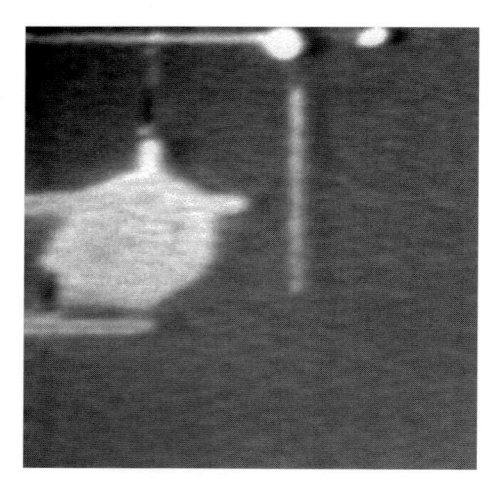

Figure 13.20 Magnetic domains in a 10 nm thick iron film. The domains were generated by approaching a ferromagnetic probe to the thin film. In thermodynamic equilibrium the easy axis of magnetisation lies in the sample surface. The stray field of the magnetic probe locally produces a metastable state where the magnetisation is directed along the surface normal in either direction (black and white domains). After lifting the probe to a certain minimum probe–sample separation, the magnetic configuration can be imaged without any destructive influence. The imaged area is 18×18 μm^2.

ATOMIC FORCE MICROSCOPY

At present, the various approaches towards manipulating surfaces on a nanometre scale can be considered as basic research yielding the basis for future directions in nanotechnology. SPM makes nanolithography accessible to almost everyone because large and expensive facilities, as known from electron-beam or X-ray lithographies, are no longer necessarily required to produce small structures for basic investigations. The industrial production of nanoscale devices, however, requires batch fabrication approaches, i.e. the parallel processing of large areas. The latter task cannot yet be solved by AFM-based approaches. This may, however, change in the future. The first steps towards the microfabrication of multiple sensor tips and whole SPM instruments have already been presented (Busta *et al.*, 1989; Akamine *et al.*, 1989; Albrecht, 1989; Albrecht *et al.*, 1990a; Tsukamoto *et al.*, 1991).

13.5 CONCLUSIONS AND OUTLOOK

AFM is presently the most widely used variant in the field of SPM. Within 10 years the technique has become an extremely powerful tool in surface analysis. It has been discussed in detail that possible investigations are not restricted to contact-mode surface profilometry but that intermittent-contact and non-contact modes of operation open up the possibilities for measuring manifold interactions between a local probe and the sample surface. It is thus more appropriate to denote the whole family of possible variants by the abbreviation SFM, emphasising that various scanning force methods are being used. One of these methods is AFM, which is capable of achieving atomic resolution. Contact-mode operation also involves LFM, which maps frictional forces on an atomic or nanometre scale. A link between contact-mode operation and real non-contact-mode operation is intermittent-contact force microscopy. This variant is particularly useful in imaging delicate, soft-matter samples at very high resolution. Non-contact force microscopy opens the possibility for detecting long-range interactions such as van der Waals forces, electrostatic forces and magnetostatic forces. Detailed information about the nature and range of an unknown interaction can be obtained from force–distance curves. With suitable operation these curves also provide information about surface elasticity and adhesion forces.

Force microscopes can be operated in static as well as in dynamic modes, utilising all the relevant mechanical properties offered by the microfabricated probes. In state-of-the-art instruments the sensitivity is limited only by the thermal excitation noise of the probes. It is thus interesting to operate force microscopes under low-temperature conditions and considerable effort is presently being devoted to the development of respective instruments. In addition, force microscopes can be operated in a gas atmosphere, in UHV or under liquid immersion.

Apart from largely non-destructive probing, force microscopes can also be employed as instruments that are suitable for modifying and functionalising sample surfaces on a nanometre scale. For this application a large advantage is that nanomanipulation and subsequent imaging can be performed with the same instrument merely by changing appropriate parameters of operation. Nanolithography thus becomes accessible to everyone who employs force microscopy. This aspect provides an optimum basis for developing new approaches in nanotechnology in many laboratories.

Future efforts in force microscopy will be concentrated on both further improving the instrument and employing the technique for more and more applications in basic as well as applied research. Further technical developments will predominantly involve the application of force microscopy in UHV, under high magnetic fields and at a variable sample temperature. These developments are strongly related to the development of improved cantilever-deflection sensors avoiding complicated mechanical adjustments. Microfabrication and the batch production of arrays of force probes are essential to further advance some approaches being considered as very promising in nanotechnology. Applications already established in basic research will become equally well established in industrial production processes, e.g. for purposes of quality control. New applications will again first be introduced in basic research. These will involve the use of particular probe–sample interactions that have yet not been used for high-resolution imaging. An example of the latter is spin resonance force microscopy (Rugar *et al.*, 1992). Force microscopes will gain considerable importance, especially in soft-matter science. The analysis of individual intermolecular interactions will open up completely new possibilities in biology and biochemistry. In this field it will be of predominant importance to functionalise systematically probes with specific molecular structures and to operate the force microscope at the highest sensitivity in physiological environments.

ACKNOWLEDGEMENTS

The author would like to thank all members of his research group who provided high-quality viewgraphs. In particular, U. Memmert and R. Houbertz made a large contribution by collecting experimental data. Mrs S. Neumann exhibited a great deal of patience in carefully processing the typescript.

REFERENCES

Abraham, D.W., Williams, C.C., Shinkman, J. and Wickramasinghe, H.K. (1991) *J. Vac. Sci. Technol. B* **9**, 703.
Abraham, F.F. and Batra, I.P. (1989) *Surf. Sci.* **209**, L125.
Akamine, S., Albrecht, T.R., Zdeblick, M.J. and Quate, C.F. (1989) *IEEE Electron Device Lett.* **10**, 490.
Albrecht, T.R. (1989) Ph.D. Thesis, Stanford University.
Albrecht, T.R., Akamine, S., Carver, T.E. and Quate, C.F. (1990a) *J. Vac. Sci. Technol. A* **8**, 3386.
Albrecht, T.R., Akamine, S., Zdeblick, M.J. and Quate, C.F. (1990b) *J. Vac. Sci. Technol. A* **8**, 317.
Albrecht, T.R., Grütter, P., Horne, D. and Rugar, D. (1990c) *IBM Research Report* RJ 7681.
Alexander, S., Hellemans, L., Marti, O., Schneir, J., Elings, V., Hansma, P.K., Longmire, M. and Gurley, J. (1989) *Appl. Phys. Lett.* **65**, 164.

Amelincks, S., van Dyck, D., van Landuyt, J. and van Tendeloo, G., eds (1997) *Handbook of Microscopy General Introduction*, VCH, Weinheim.
Anders, M., Thaer, M. and Heiden, C. (1987) *Surf. Sci.* **181**, 176.
Bai, Ch. (1995) *Scanning Tunneling Microscopy and its Application*, Springer, Berlin.
Barrett, R.C. and Quate, C.F. (1991) *J. Appl. Phys.* **70**, 2725.
Baumeister, T. and Marks, L.S. (1967) *Standard Handbook for Mechanical Engineers*, McGraw-Hill, New York.
Besocke, K. (1987) *Surf. Sci.* **181**, 139.
Betzig, E., Finn, P.L. and Weiner, J.S. (1992) *Appl. Phys. Lett.* **60**, 2484.
Binnig, G. (1992) *Ultramicroscopy* **42–44**, 7.
Binnig, G. and Rohrer, H. (1982) *Helv. Phys. Acta* **55**, 726.
Binnig, G. and Smith, D.P.E. (1986) *Rev. Sci. Instrum.* **57**, 1988.
Binnig, G., Quate, C.F. and Gerber, Ch. (1986) *Phys. Rev. Lett.* **56**, 930.
Binnig, G., Rohrer, H., Gerber, Ch. and Weibel, E. (1982a) *Phys. Rev. Lett.* **49**, 57.
Binnig, G., Rohrer, H., Gerber, Ch. and Weibel, E. (1982b) *Appl. Phys. Lett.* **40**, 178.
Binnig, G., Rohrer, H., Gerber, Ch. and Weibel, E. (1982c) *Physica B* **109/110**, 2075.
Blackman, G.S., Mate, C.M. and Philpott, M.R. (1990) *Phys. Rev. Lett.* **65**, 2270.
Bonnell, D.A., ed. (1992) *Scanning Tunneling Microscopy: Theory, Techniques and Applications*, VCH Press, New York.
Burnham, N.A., Dominguez, D.D., Mowery, R.L. and Colton, R.J. (1990) *Phys. Rev. Lett.* **64**, 1931.
Busta, H.H., Shadduck, R.R. and Orvis, W.J. (1989) *IEEE Trans. Electron Devices* **36**, 2679.
Chen, C.J. (1992) *Appl. Phys. Lett.* **60**, 132.
Chen, C.J. (1993) *Introduction to Scanning Tunneling Microscopy*, Oxford University Press, New York.
Ciraci, S., Baratoff, A. and Batra, I.P. (1990) *Phys. Rev. B* **41**, 2763.
Coombs, J.H. and Pethica, J.B. (1986) *IBM J. Res. Dev.* **30**, 443.
Corb, B.W., Ringger, M. and Güntherodt, H.-J. (1985) *J. Appl. Phys.* **58**, 3947.
Deb, B.M. (1973) *Rev. Mod. Phys.* **45**, 22.
Demuth, J.E., Hamers, R.J., Tromp, R.M. and Welland, M.E. (1986a) *J. Vac. Sci. Technol. A* **4**, 1320.
Demuth, J.E., Hamers, R.J., Tromp, R.M. and Welland, M.E. (1986b) *IBM J. Res. Dev.* **30**, 396.
den Boef, A.J. (1989) *Appl. Phys. Lett.* **55**, 439.
den Boef, A.J. (1991) *Rev. Sci. Instrum.* **62**, 88.
Drechsler, A., Pitzius, P. and Hartmann, U. (1997) unpublished result.
Ducker, W.A., Cook, R.F. and Clarke, D.R. (1990) *J. Appl. Phys.* **67**, 4045.
Dürig, U., Gimzewski, J.K., Pohl, D.W. and Schlitter, R. (1986) *IBM Research Report* RZ 1513.
Durkan, C. and Shvets, I. (1996) *J. Appl. Phys.* **79**,1219.
Dworak, V., Pitzius, P. and Hartmann, U. (1997) unpublished result.
Erlandsson, R., Hadziioannou, G., Mate, C.M., McClelland, G.M. and Chiang, S. (1988a) *J. Chem. Phys.* **89**, 5190.
Erlandsson, R., McClelland, G.M., Mate, C.M. and Chiang, S. (1988b) *J. Vac. Sci. Technol. A* **6**, 266.
Euler, R., Memmert, U. and Hartmann, U. (1997) *Rev. Sci. Instrum.* **68**, 1776.
Fein, A.P., Kirtley, J.R. and Feenstra, R.M. (1987) *Rev. Sci. Instrum.* **58**, 1806.
Frohn, J., Wolf, J.E., Besocke, K. and Teske, M. (1989) *Rev. Sci. Instrum.* **60**, 1200.
Gewirth, A.A. and Siegenthaler, H., eds (1995) *Nanoscale Properties of the Solid/Liquid Interface*, Nato ASI Series E, Vol. 288, Kluwer, Dordrecht.
Giessibl, F.J. (1995) *Science* **267**, 68.
Göddenhenrich, Th., Hartmann, U. and Heiden, C. (1988) *J. Microsc.* **152**, 527.
Göddenhenrich, Th., Hartmann, U. and Heiden, C. (1992) *Ultramicroscopy* **42–44**, 256.

Göddenhenrich, Th., Lemke, H., Hartmann, U. and Heiden, C. (1990a) *J. Vac. Sci. Technol. A* **8**, 383.
Göddenhenrich, Th., Lemke, H., Mück, M., Hartmann, U. and Heiden, C. (1990b) *Appl. Phys. Lett.* **57**, 2612.
Gould, S.A.C., Burke, K. and Hansma, P.K. (1989) *Phys. Rev. B* **40**, 5363.
Gregor, U.J., Blome, P.G., Schöfer, J. and Ulbrich, R.G. (1996) *Appl. Phys. Lett.* **63**, 307.
Grober, R.D., Harris, T.D., Trautman, J.K., Betzig, E., Wegscheider, W., Pfeiffer, L. and West, K. (1994) *Appl. Phys. Lett.* **64**, 1421.
Güntherodt, H.-J., Anselmetti, D. and Meyer, E., eds (1995) *Forces in Scanning Probe Methods*, Nato ASI Series E, Vol. 286, Kluwer, Dordrecht.
Güthner, P. (1996) *J. Vac. Sci. Technol. B* **14**, 2428.
Güthner, P., Fischer, U. and Dransfeld, K. (1989) *Appl. Phys. B* **48**, 89.
Güthner, P., Schreck, E., Dransfeld, K. and Fischer, U. (1990) in *Scanning Tunneling Microscopy* (eds R.J. Behm, N. Garcia, and H. Rohrer), Kluwer, Dordrecht, p. 507.
Hartmann, U. (1988) *J. Appl. Phys.* **64**, 1561.
Hartmann, U. (1990/91a), *Phys. Rev. B* **42**, 1541.
Hartmann, U. (1990/91b) *Phys. Rev. B* **43**, 2404.
Hartmann, U. (1994) *Adv. Electron. Electron Phys.* **87**, 49.
Hartmann, U., Göddenhenrich, T. and Heiden, C. (1991) *J. Magn. Magn. Mat.* **101**, 263.
Heer, C.V. (1972) *Statistical Mechanics, Kinetic, Theory, and Stochastic Processes*, Academic Press, New York.
Hoffmann, B., Houbertz, R. and Hartmann, U. (1997) *European Workshop on Microtechnology and Scanning Probe Microscopy*, Mainz, Germany, Extended Abstract.
Israelachvili, J.N. (1985) *Intermolecular and Surface Forces*, Academic Press, London.
Itoh, T. and Suga, T. (1993) *Technnical Digest International Conference on Solid State Sensors and Actuators*, Transducer's 93, Yokohama, p. 610.
Jersch, J. and Dickmann, K. (1996) *Appl. Phys. Lett.* **68**, 868.
Jung, T.A., Moser, A., Hug, H.J., Brodbeck, D., Hofer, R., Hidler, H.R. and Schwarz, U.D. (1992) *Ultramicroscopy* **42–44**, 1446.
Kaiser, W.J. and Jaklevic, R.C. (1988) *Rev. Sci. Instrum.* **59**, 537.
Landman, U., Luedtke, W.D., Burnham, N.A. and Colton, R.J. (1990) *Science* **248**, 454.
Landman, U., Luedtke, W.D. and Nitzan, A. (1989a) *Surf. Sci.* **210**, L177.
Landman, U., Luedtke, W.D. and Ribarsky, M.W. (1989b) *J. Vac. Sci. Technol. A* **7**, 2829.
Leinenbach, P., Memmert, U., Schelten, J. and Hartmann, U. (1997) *European Workshop on Microtechnology and Scanning Probe Microscopy*, Mainz, Germany, Extended Abstract.
Lemke, H., Göddenhenrich, Th., Bochem, H.-P., Hartmann, U. and Heiden, C. (1990) *Rev. Sci. Instrum.* **61**, 2538.
Lüthi, R., Meyer, E., Bammerlin, M., Baratoff, A., Lehmann, T., Howald, L., Gerber, Ch. and Güntherodt, H.-J. (1996) *Z. Phys. B Condensed Matter* **100**, 165.
Lyding, J.W., Skala, S., Hubacek, J.S., Brockenbrough, R. and Gammie, G. (1988) *Rev. Sci. Instrum.* **59**, 1897.
Maganov, S.N. and Whangbo, M.H. (1996) *Surface Analysis with STM and AFM*, VCH, Weinheim.
Maivald, P., Butt, H.J., Gould, S.A.C., Prater, C.B., Drake, B., Gurley, J.A., Elings, V.B. and Hansma, P.K. (1991) *Nanotechnology* **2**, 103.
Mamin, H.J., Abraham, D.W., Ganz, E. and Clarke, J. (1985) *Rev. Sci. Instrum.* **56**, 2168.
Marti, O. and Amrein, M., eds (1993) *STM and SFM in Biology*, Academic Press, San Diego.
Martin, Y., Abraham, D.W. and Wickramasinghe, H.K. (1988) *Appl. Phys. Lett.* **52**, 1103.
Martin, Y. and Wickramasinghe, H.K. (1987) Appl. Phys. Lett. **50**, 1455.
Martin, Y., Williams, C.C. and Wickramasinghe, H.K. (1987) *J. Appl. Phys.* **61**, 4723.
Mate, C.M., Lorenz, M.R. and Novotny, U.J. (1989) *J. Chem. Phys.* **90**, 7550.
Mate, C.M., McClelland, G.M., Erlandsson, R. and Chiang, S. (1987) *Phys. Rev. Lett.* **59**, 1942.

McClelland, G.M. (1989) in *Adhesion and Friction* (eds M. Grunze and H.J. Kreuzer), Springer, Berlin, p. 1.
McClelland, G.M. and Cohen, S.R. (1990) in *Chemistry and Physics of Solid Surfaces VIII*, (eds R. Vanselow and R. Howe), Springer, Berlin, p. 419.
McClelland, G.M., Erlandsson, R. and Chiang, S. (1987) in *Review of Progress in Quantitative Non-destructive Evaluation*, Vol. 6 (eds D.O. Thompson and D.E. Chimenti), Plenum, New York, p. 307.
Memmert, U., Hodel, U. and Hartmann, U. (1996) *Rev. Sci. Instrum.* **67**, 2269.
Meyer, E., Heinzelmann, H., Brodbeck, D., Overnay, G., Overnay, R., Howald, L., Hug, H., Jung, T., Hidber, H.-R. and Güntherodt, H.-J. (1991) *J. Vac. Sci. Technol. B* **9**, 1329.
Meyer, E., Heinzelmann, H., Grütter, P., Jung, Th., Weisskopf, Th., Hidler, H.-R., Lapka, R., Rudin, H. and Güntherodt, H.-J. (1988) *J. Microsc.* **152**, 269.
Meyer, G. and Amer, N.M. (1988) *Appl. Phys. Lett.* **53**, 1045.
Meyer, G. and Amer, N.M. (1990) *Appl. Phys. Lett.* **56**, 2100.
Mizes, H.A., Loh, K.G., Miller, R.J.D., Ahuja, S.K. and Grabowski, E. (1991) *Appl. Phys. Lett.* **59**, 2901.
Moreland, J. and Rice, P. (1990) *Appl. Phys. Lett.* **57**, 310.
Morita, S., Ishizaka, T., Sugawara, Y., Okada, T., Mashima, S., Imai, S. and Mikoshiba, N. (1989) *Jpn. J. Appl. Phys.* **28**, L1634.
Moser, A., Hug, H.J., Parashikov, I., Stiefel, B., Fritz, O., Thomas, H., Baratoff, A. and Güntherodt, H.-J. (1995) *Phys. Rev. Lett.* **74**, 1847.
Moyer, P.J. and Paesler, A. (1993) *SPIE Conf. Proc.* **1855**, 58.
Mulhern, P.J., Hubbert, T., Arnold, C.S., Blackford, B.L. and Jericho, M.H. (1991) *Rev. Sci. Instrum.* **62**, 1280.
Neubauer, G., Cohen, S.R., McClelland, G.M., Horne, D. and Mate, C.M. (1990) *Rev. Sci. Instrum.* **61**, 2296.
Niedermann, Ph., Emch, R. and Descouts, P. (1988) *Rev. Sci. Instrum.* **59**, 368.
Pethica, J.B., Hutchings, R. and Oliver, W.C. (1983) *Phil. Mag. A* **48**, 293.
Pohl, D.W. (1986) *IBM J. Res. Dev.* **30**, 417.
Pohl, D.W. (1987) *Rev. Sci. Instrum.* **58**, 54.
Pohl, D.W., Denk, W. and Lanz, M. (1984) *Appl. Phys. Lett.* **44**, 651.
Ringger, M., Corb, B.W., Hidber, H.-R., Schlögl, R., Wiesendanger, R., Stemmer, A., Rosenthaler, L., Brunner, A.J., Oelhafen, P.C. and Güntherodt, H.-J. (1986) *IBM J. Res. Dev.* **30**, 500.
Rugar, D. and Hansma, P. (1990) *Physics Today*, October, p. 23.
Rugar, D., Mamin, H.J. and Guethner, P. (1989) *Appl. Phys. Lett.* **55**, 2588.
Rugar, D., Mamin, H.J., Erlandsson, R., Stern, J.E. and Terris, B.D. (1988) *Rev. Sci. Instrum.* **59**, 2337.
Rugar, D., Mamin, H.J., Güthner, P., Lambert, S.E., Stern, J.E., McFadyen, I. and Yogi, T. (1990) *J. Appl. Phys.* **68**, 1169.
Rugar, D., Yannoni, C.S. and Sidles, J.A. (1992) *Nature* **360**, 563.
Sáenz, J.H., Garcia, N., Grütter, P., Meyer, E., Heinzelmann, H., Wiesendanger, R., Rosenthaler, L., Hidber, H.R. and Güntherodt, H.-J. (1987) *J. Appl. Phys.* **62**, 4293.
Sarid, D. (1991) *Scanning Force Microscopy with Applications to Electric, Magnetic, and Atomic Forces*, Oxford University Press, New York.
Saurenbach, F. and Terris, B.D. (1990) *Appl. Phys. Lett.* **56**, 1703.
Scheinfein, M.R., Unguris, J., Pierce, D.T., Celotta, R.J. (1990) *J. Appl. Phys.* **67**, 5932.
Schönenberger, C. and Alvarado, S.F. (1990a) *Phys. Rev. Lett.* **65**, 3162.
Schönenberger, C. and Alvarado, S.F. (1990b) *Z. Phys. B* **80**, 373.
Shin-ichi, K. and Iwatsuki, M. (1995) *Jpn. J. Appl. Phys.* **34**, L145.
Siebel, E., Memmert, U., Vogel, R. and Hartmann, U. (1998) *Appl. Phys.* A**66**, 83.
Smith, D.P.E. and Binnig, G. (1986) *Rev. Sci. Instrum.* **57**, 2630.
Smith, D.P.E. and Elrod, S.A. (1985) *Rev. Sci. Instrum.* **56**, 1970.

Stern, J.E., Terris, B.D., Mamin, H.J. and Rugar, D. (1988) *Appl. Phys. Lett.* **53**, 2717.
Takata, U., Hosoki, S., Hosaka, S. and Tajima, T. (1989) *Rev. Sci. Instrum.* **60**, 789.
Terris, B.D., Stern, J.E., Rugar, D. and Mamin, H.J. (1989/90a) *Phys. Rev. Lett.* **63**, 2669.
Terris, B.D., Stern, J.E., Rugar, D. and Mamin, H.J. (1989/90b) *J. Vac. Sci. Technol. A* **8**, 374.
Toledo-Crow, R., Yang, P.C., Chen, Y. and Vaez-Iravani, M. (1992) *Appl. Phys. Lett.* **60**, 2957.
Tortonese, M., Yamada, H., Barret, R.C. and Quate, C.F. (1991) *Technical Digest International Conference on Solid State Sensors and Actuators*, Transducers '91, San Francisco, p. 448.
Tsukamoto, S., Lin, B. and Nakagiri, N. (1991) *Rev. Sci. Instrum.* **62**, 1761.
Ueyama, H., Ohta, M., Sugawara, Y. and Morita, S. (1995) *Jpn. J. Appl. Phys.* **34**, L1068.
Uozumi, K., Nakamoto, K. and Fujioka, K. (1988) *Jpn. J. Appl. Phys.* **27**, L123.
Weisenhorn, A.L., Hansma, P.K., Albrecht, T.R. and Quate, C.F. (1989) *Appl. Phys. Lett*, **54**, 2651.
Wiesendanger, R. (1994) *Scanning Probe Microscopy and Spectroscopy*, Cambridge University Press, Cambridge.
Wiesendanger, R., Anselmetti, D. and Güntherodt, H.-J. (1990a) *Europhys. News* **21**, 72.
Wiesendanger, R., Bürgler, D., Tarrach, G., Anselmetti, D., Hidber, H.R. and Güntherodt, H.-J. (1990b) *J. Vac. Sci. Technol. A* **8**, 339.
Wiesendanger, R. and Güntherodt, H.-J., eds (1992/93) *Scanning Tunneling Microscopy I–III*, Springer, Berlin.
Williamson, J.B.P. (1967/68) *Proc. Inst. Mech. Engng. London* **182** (3K), 21.
Zhong, W. and Tománek, D. (1990) *Phys. Rev. Lett.* **64**, 3054.

14
Electrochemical impedance spectroscopy as a surface analytical technique for biomaterials

J. HUBRECHT
Catholic University of Leuven, Leuven, Belgium

14.1 INTRODUCTION

Electrochemical impedance spectroscopy (EIS) is an ideal tool for studying and monitoring the status and behaviour of interfaces between conducting phases. The application area of the technique is very wide, as is supported by the abundant literature on the subject. A biometal facing, directly or indirectly, a real or simulated biological environment forms such an interface system. EIS can image the way in which the transfer of charges between the different phases is conducted or impeded under the influence of a corrosion process, a passive film or coating, or other interface phenomena (Gabrielli, 1980, 1990; Macdonald, 1993; Mansfeld, 1993; Scully, 1993; Vereecken, 1996).

When applying the technique and making the connections to the measurement devices, the biometal forms one electrode, called the working electrode (WE). In order to impose an electrical signal and measure the system response, a three-electrode circuit is usually set up, where the other two electrodes are the reference electrode (RE) and the auxiliary or counter electrode (CE). In most cases the electrical signal applied is a voltage and the system response is a current, which means that the measurement is potentiostatically controlled, while a galvanostatically controlled measurement works the other way round. Considering the former case, the voltage signal may be a sine wave of single frequency and small amplitude, say 10–20 mV, coming from a function generator. The controlling device, the potentiostat, receives this ac signal and applies it between the WE and the RE, and it further measures the ac current response in the circuit between the WE and the CE. From the experimental point of view it may be necessary to superimpose the ac voltage on a dc voltage,

Metals as Biomaterials ISBN 0 471 96935 4 Edited by J.A. Helsen and H.J. Breme. © 1998 John Wiley & Sons Ltd

which is different from the individual open-circuit potential of the system itself, and the response is then ac current superimposed on dc current. The reason for the small amplitude is that the system investigated, which in principle is not linear, may then be treated as being approximately linear and that the ac response is of the same single frequency as the applied signal; moreover, a small signal has the advantage of not disturbing or modifying the system during the measurement.

The ac current response, characterised by an amplitude and a phase shift with respect to the applied ac voltage, depends on the actual load between the WE and the RE, and thus on all processes occurring between them. The ratio of the amplitudes of the applied and the response signal on the one hand and the phase shift between both signals on the other determine the impedance, which may be represented by a complex number. When the frequency of the applied ac signal is varied within a certain range, e.g. from 100 kHz to 1 mHz, then for each frequency another value of the impedance, Z, is measured, which in the complex plane (the Nyquist representation) leads to an impedance spectrum. It is common practice to plot the negative value of the imaginary impedance part, Z'', on the upward ordinate axis against the real impedance part, Z', on the abscissa. The scales on both axes should be the same. Another popular way of representing the results graphically is the Bode plot, which is a separate representation of the logarithm of the impedance modulus, $|Z|$, and the phase, φ, vs the logarithm of the frequency [see Chapter 4, Equations (4.19) and (4.20)]. Whereas the Nyquist plot has the advantage of giving an overall view of the impedance spectrum, which is convenient for acquiring promptly an insight into the model, the Bode plot offers a complete and detailed view of the frequency dependence of the impedance, which links specific parts in the spectrum to characteristic frequency ranges and avoids hidden responses in the spectrum. The spectrum is characteristic of the situation occurring between the WE and the RE at the moment of the measurement. A situation that is changing in time or under the influence of changing experimental parameters is translated into a changing spectrum.

The actual ac voltage applied between the WE and the RE, and the ac current response of the system, are passed to another device, which may be a frequency response analyser (FRA) or a lock-in amplifier (LIA), in order to measure the signal characteristics and calculate the impedance value for each frequency. Often the measurement set-up is controlled by a personal computer (PC), which receives the measurement data, presents them in real time on the screen and stores them in memory. The PC may even take over some of the functions of the other devices mentioned, thus entailing the evolution from formerly voluminous to presently more compact and cheaper measurement equipment.

Some variations are possible on this general technical outline. For instance, the sequential series of single frequencies of the applied ac voltage may be replaced by one multisine, a combined signal consisting of many simultaneous sine waves of different frequency. When the small amplitude condition is respected, the current response comprises the same frequencies as the signal applied and may be deconvoluted into the separate frequencies using a Fourier transformation.

ELECTROCHEMICAL IMPEDANCE SPECTROSCOPY

The market presently offers a broad choice of EIS measurement systems, varying in characteristics such as available frequency range, range of measurable impedance magnitudes, quality of noise rejection, software control, monitoring capabilities, compactness, portability and price. It should be pointed out that although the application of the EIS measurement technique is becoming easier and more straightforward, some know-how and experience may be an asset and some technical precautions may be necessary in order to obtain valuable and useful results.

Apart from these technical aspects of EIS the analysis and interpretation of data is another important issue. Many physicochemical phenomena, the impedance of which is measured, show a resistive, capacitive or inductive behaviour or a behaviour that is a combination of these. Then the link with the characteristics of simple electrical elements or circuits is easily seen. An electrical equivalent circuit, consisting of serial and/or parallel combinations of resistors, capacitors and inductors, and assembled on the basis of the electrically familiar shape of a spectrum, may indeed form a reasonable model for the system investigated, translating the impedance spectrum into a physicochemical insight.

When a metal WE is inert with respect to the solution it faces, as is the case for the noble metals or alloys in many solutions, it then behaves purely capacitively, because of the presence of an electrochemical double layer at the interface. Purely capacitive behaviour is also experienced when the WE is a metal or alloy that forms a stable and intact passive or oxide layer at the interface with the given environment. The complex expression for the impedance, Z, of a capacitor is

$$Z = \frac{1}{j\omega C} = -j\frac{1}{\omega C}, \qquad (14.1)$$

where $j = \sqrt{-1}$, the imaginary unit, $\omega = 2\pi f$ is the pulsation or angular frequency, f is the frequency and C is the capacitance. The Nyquist spectrum is then a vertical straight line (A in Figure 14.1). It may not coincide with the vertical axis because of the presence of a resistive layer of electrolyte between the WE and the RE, which shifts the line to the right of the complex plane parallel to itself. This model is represented in Figure 14.2a and its expression is

$$Z = R_e + \frac{1}{j\omega C}, \qquad (14.2)$$

where R_e is the resistance of the electrolyte layer. Depending on the system considered, C is called the capacitance of the electrochemical double layer, the passive layer or the oxide layer. An ideal capacitive spectrum is, however, seldom found. The electrode interface is never completely homogeneous or smooth at all scales of magnification and this heterogeneity or roughness, sometimes called fractality when the structure is repeatedly self-similar, may cause a slope of less than 90° (B in Figure 14.1). In other cases distributed relaxation phenomena at the interfacial region of the WE may have the same consequence. The impedance expression for

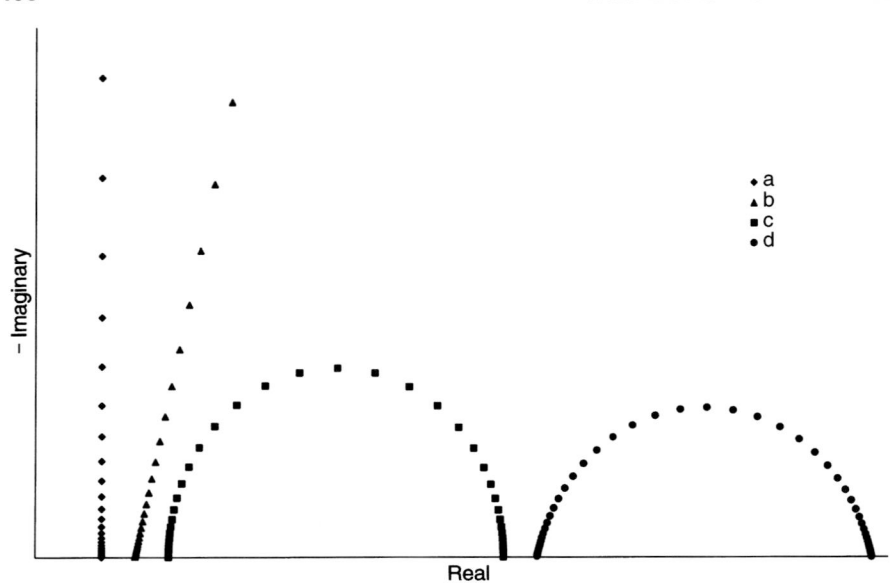

Figure 14.1 Typical Nyquist spectra according to the equivalent circuits of Figure 14.2.

the model capacitor then receives an exponent, α, which is between 0 and 1, and the new model is called a constant phase element (CPE)

$$Z = R_e + \frac{1}{(j\omega Q)^\alpha}, \qquad (14.3)$$

where the magnitude, Q, now replaces the capacitance, C, from the ideal case. This model is represented in Figure 14.2b.

When one or more redox processes are taking place at the WE, charges are passed across the interface between the electrode and the solution. The model then has to be supplemented with a parallel resistor (Figure 14.2c, d), leading to a semicircle (C in Figure 14.1) or depressed semicircle spectrum (D in Figure 14.1) in the complex plane. This happens when charges are exchanged at the WE between electroactive species in the solution or between the active electrode material and the solution, e.g. in the case of corrosion processes or when the passive or oxide layer is being attacked. The impedance expression becomes:

$$Z = R_e + \frac{1}{\frac{1}{R} + j\omega Q} \qquad (14.4)$$

in the ideal case, or

ELECTROCHEMICAL IMPEDANCE SPECTROSCOPY

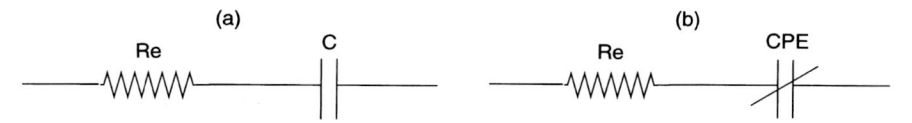

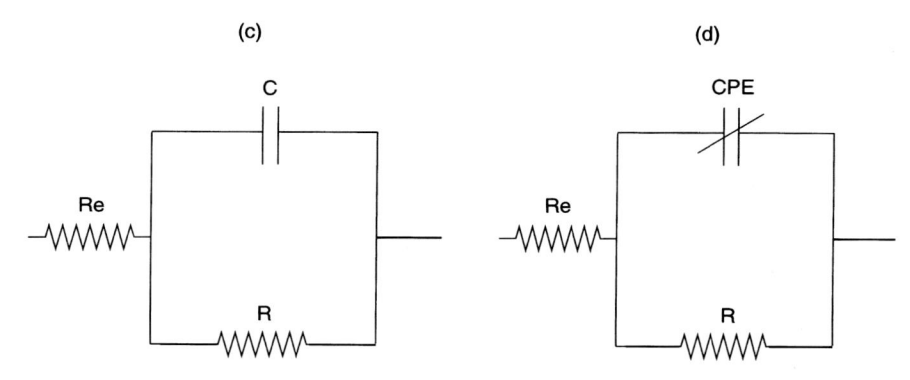

Figure 14.2 Simple equivalent circuits.

$$Z = R_e + \frac{1}{\frac{1}{R} + (j\omega Q)^\alpha} \tag{14.5}$$

in the non-ideal case, where R is the resistance.

Depending on the system considered, R is called the charge transfer resistance, or polarisation resistance or faradaic resistance. The charge transfer resistance is usually related to simple redox processes, whereas the polarisation and faradaic resistance are more general terms usually pointing to combined phenomena such as a corrosion process. The choice of the term depends on the author reporting and sometimes on the technique used to determine it. The resistive value, R, deduced from the diameter of the semicircle, may be inversely proportional to the rate of the electrochemical reaction mentioned.

The above *RC* circuit can be retained as a model for a different phenomenon: when a non-conducting coating is applied to the WE metal or alloy. The coating material acts as the dielectric of a model capacitor; furthermore, in contact with a solution pores in the coating are filled with electrolyte and form conducting paths, which together lead to the parallel model resistor. In this case R and C are called the coating resistance and capacitance, respectively.

Both kinds of *RC* circuits model different processes and normally differ in corresponding time constant; however, they may appear together in one model, for instance when a corrosion process occurs at the basis of the pores in the coating, and the spectrum may contain two distinct semicircles. Many real systems require even more complicated modelling.

The Bode plots for the models shown in Figure 14.2 are given in Figures 14.3 and 14.4 for the impedance modulus and phase, respectively.

When interpreting and comparing impedance data, it is important to distinguish between the impedance values measured as such and the values reduced to the unit surface area of the electrode, and the same holds true for the value of the modelling elements. The reader is warned that throughout this text the same symbol is used for the full and for the unit surface area of the electrode, but the actual meaning of the symbol and the units of the data will be clear in each individual case described.

When, by electrochemical means, a passive film or oxide film is intentionally formed on a metal or alloy, then at a certain potential a certain current or charge is passed across the interface. If the impedance spectrum of such an electrode reveals capacitive behaviour, then the charge or potential dependence of the capacitance may be investigated in addition to the frequency dependence of the impedance.

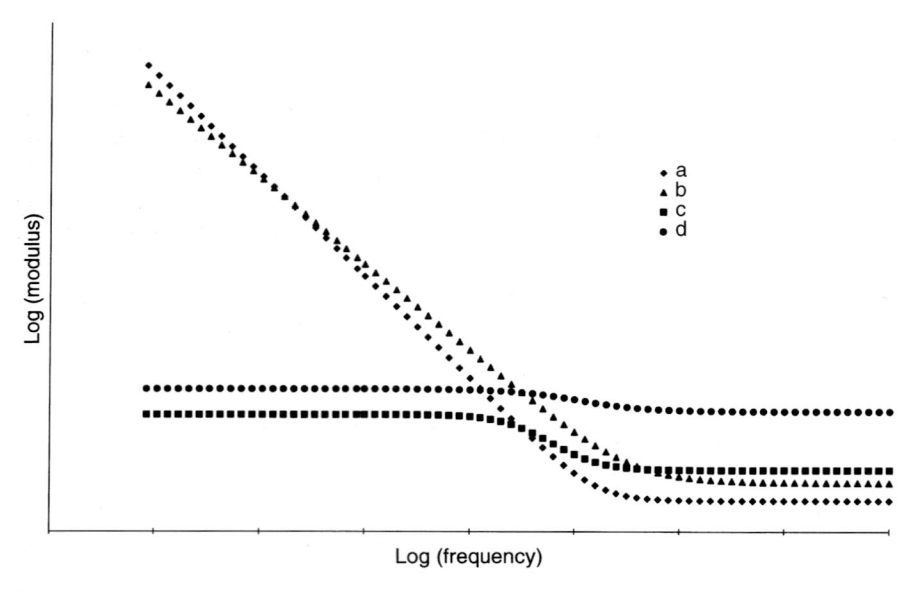

Figure 14.3 Bode plots of the impedance modulus according to the equivalent circuits of Figure 14.2. Each division of the frequency axis corresponds to one decade. The absolute value depends on the variables of the circuit but the shape is constant irrespective of the absolute value. No numerical values are indicated on the modulus axis because these depend on the variables of the measured system.

ELECTROCHEMICAL IMPEDANCE SPECTROSCOPY

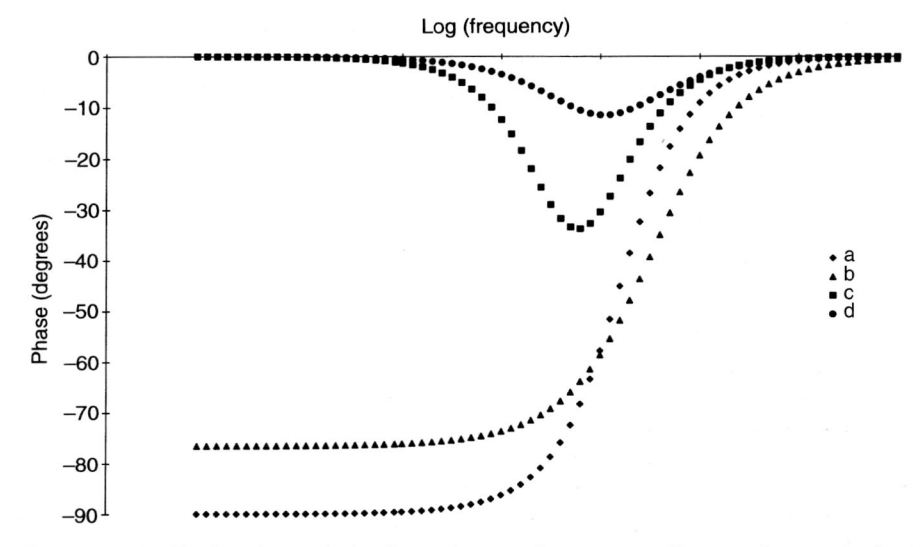

Figure 14.4 Bode plots of the impedance phase according to the equivalent circuits of Figure 14.2. See caption to Figure 14.3 for details of the axes.

The resulting information concerns the dielectric or semiconductive (from the Mott–Schottky plot) properties of the film.

Considering the above modelling possibilities it may seem a delicate job to derive physicochemical data from the carefully measured spectra, although some routine skill is soon acquired. Sometimes data are easily obtained at first sight from the graphical plots themselves, but the latest commercial set-ups usually contain suitable software packages to facilitate the data analysis, fit the spectra with several selected models and estimate the model parameters.

In the following sections some typical EIS case studies are treated in relation to the interfacial behaviour of biometals with respect to their environment.

14.2 PASSIVE AND OXIDE FILMS: DIELECTRIC AND ELECTRONIC PROPERTIES

One of the first attempts to study the nature of the passive layer on surgical implant alloys through the determination of a differential capacitance was made by Solar *et al.* (1979). Although not an impedance measurement in the now classical sense of the term, as the measurement was done via the pulse potentiostatic technique, the work points quite clearly to the perspectives offered by EIS.

The implant materials chosen were commercially pure titanium and ELI grade Ti6Al4V alloy, surface finished to different degrees. These were tested in Ringer's physiological solution at 37°C, in which the amino acid content, oxygen content and pH were varied in order to simulate *in vivo* conditions for the implant material. In the electrical model used by the authors, the electrode, constituted by the implant metal, behaved as a parallel plate condensor, with the passive layer acting as the dielectric.

At increasing anodic potentials the electrode capacitance was measured and found to decrease. This decreasing capacitance, C_f, indicates that the passive film became thicker as the applied potential increased, in accordance with the following equation

$$C_f = \frac{\varepsilon_r \varepsilon_0 A_{\text{eff}}}{d}, \tag{14.6}$$

where ε_r is the relative dielectric constant of the oxide, ε_0 is the permittivity of the vacuum, A_{eff} is the effective electrochemical surface area and d is the total oxide thickness.

It was also observed that when the reciprocal capacitance was plotted against the total charge, a linear relationship was found. The explanation is that the increase in the oxide film thickness, Δd, with increasing applied potential may be related to the charge measured, ΔQ, using Faraday's law

$$\Delta d = \frac{M}{zF\rho} \frac{\Delta Q}{A_{\text{eff}}}, \tag{14.7}$$

where M is the molecular mass of the oxide, z is the number of electrons involved in the charge transfer reaction, F is Faraday's constant and ρ is the oxide material density.

When the individual thickness increments, according to Equation (14.6), produced at each applied potential are summed and combined with Equation (14.7) a linear relationship can indeed be established between the reciprocal capacitance and the cumulative charge, Q

$$\frac{1}{C_f} = \frac{M}{\varepsilon_r \varepsilon_0 zF\rho A_{\text{eff}}^2} Q, \tag{14.8}$$

and the effective electrochemical surface area can be calculated from the slope of the straight line. Figure 14.5 shows such plots and the influence of solution pH. Using the appropriate oxide constants in Equation (14.8), values for A_{eff} are obtained which are smaller than the apparent geometrical surface area. A_{eff} is apparently dependent on the pH and degree of mechanical polishing: it increases as the size of the polishing compound is increased or as the solution pH is decreased. The latter effect is only minor at pH values between 9.0 and 4.4, but in more acid solutions such as pH 1.5 A_{eff} approaches the geometrical surface area of the specimen. A physical model of the natural passive film on titanium and Ti6Al4V is conceived, consisting of a smooth planar oxide layer and oxide needles at surface irregularities, formed through mechanical polishing. During electrochemical measurements the current will preferably flow via the thin planar oxide, resulting in a decreased effective surface area. When the pH is decreased, the oxide needles may dissolve, and

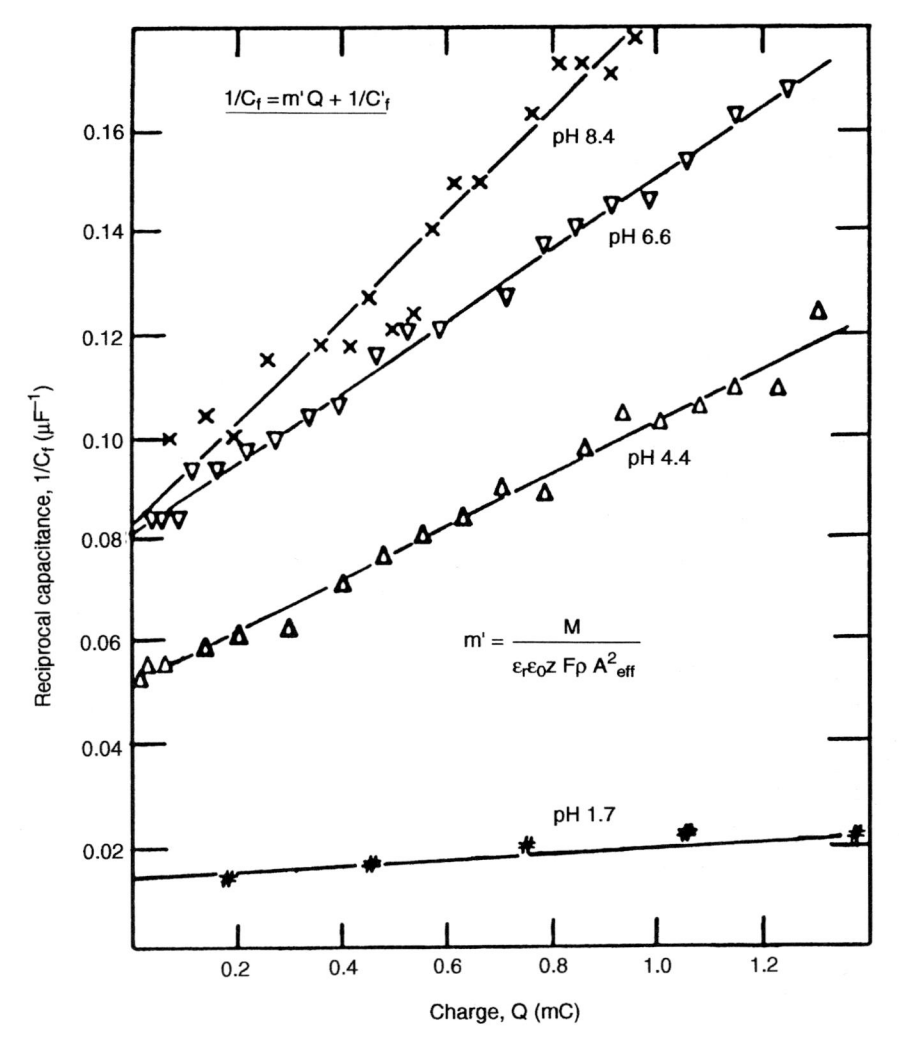

Figure 14.5 Reciprocal capacitance vs charge for commercially pure titanium and Ti6Al4V alloy in Ringer's solution, and effect of pH. (Reprinted with permission, Solar et al., 1979, Copyright ASTM.)

when the size of the polishing compound is increased, the number of surface irregularities, and thus the number of oxide needles, is decreased. From both phenomena a larger effective surface area follows.

Further interest in passive film behaviour on biomaterials is shown in Silva et al. (1990), where in particular the electronic properties of passive films are studied in order to elucidate the corrosion behaviour of biomaterials in physiological media and finally in the human body.

The materials chosen were AISI 316L stainless steel (composition in wt%: Cr 18.0, Ni 12.5, Mo 2.8, Si 1.2, Mn 1.6, C 0.025, Fe balance) and the alloy Ti6Al4V (composition in wt%: Al 6.5, V 4.14, C 0.02, Fe 0.19, Ti balance). Specimens were cylindrical, with a diameter of 10 mm and a thickness of 2 mm. The specimens were heat treated for 1 h in a nitrogen atmosphere at 1050 and 720°C, respectively, then quenched in water at 0°C and cooled in air, respectively. Using epoxy resin each specimen, connected to an electrical conductor, was cemented into a glass tube with an internal diameter equal to that of the specimen, so that a free surface area of 0.785 cm^2 was obtained. The specimens were wet ground onto 500 grit SiC paper 24 h before the test.

The materials were immersed in artificial extracellular fluid, the composition of which is given in Table 14.1. One of these solutions contains lactic acid, which simulates the metabolic products in the body when infection occurs. The solutions were kept at 37 ± 0.5°C and deaerated with nitrogen.

The cell was equipped with a WE, which was the specimen, a saturated calomel RE (SCE) and a platinum wire CE.

Passive films were formed at open-circuit potentials and at applied potentials in the anodic region, where passivity was checked with polarisation tests and where no localised corrosion occurred, and this forming process was conducted over various periods.

The EIS measurements were controlled at a constant potential using an EG&G M273 potentiostat. Frequencies were scanned between 5 mHz and 100 kHz. The measurement set-up was supplemented with an EG&G M5208 LIA, which measured the impedance data in the high-frequency range using sequential single sine perturbations. In the low-frequency region a multisine of equal amplitude signals was applied and the impedance data were then calculated with the aid of a Fourier transformation of the cell response.

An example of an EIS spectrum is given in Figure 14.6 for the unit surface area of the Ti6Al4V alloy in solution 2 at an open-circuit (or corrosion) potential of −0.57 V vs SCE. From the almost vertical straight line the impedance spectrum is interpreted as being dominated by the film capacitance.

Table 14.1 Solution composition (mM) (Silva et al., 1990)

Species	Solution 1	Solution 2
Na^+	137.0	137.0
K^+	4.0	4.0
Ca^{2+}	6.6	6.6
Mg^{2+}	50.0	5.0
Cl^-	1100.0	110.0
Acetate	36.8	–
Lactate	–	53.2
pH	6.7	4.0

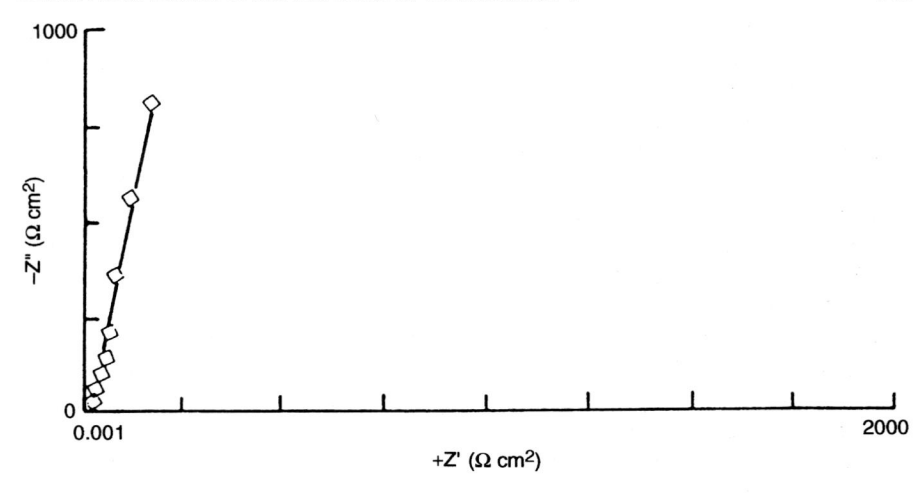

Figure 14.6 Complex plane plot of Ti6Al4V alloy in solution 2 at the corrosion potential ($E_{corr} = -0.57$ V/SCE) (Silva et al., 1990).

More tests were performed at a constant frequency of 1 kHz and a varying applied potential. For the film capacitance, assuming it is determined directly from the impedance measured, the Mott–Schottky equation for n-type semiconductors is valid

$$\frac{1}{C_f^2} = \frac{2}{\varepsilon_r \varepsilon_0 e N_D} \left(E - E_{fb} - \frac{kT}{e} \right), \qquad (14.9)$$

where C_f is the capacitance of the semiconductor per unit surface area, e is the electron charge, N_D is the density of charge carriers, E is the electrochemical potential, E_{fb} is the flat band potential, k is Boltzmann's constant and T is the absolute temperature.

The graphical representation of the square of the reciprocal semiconductor capacitance vs the potential leads to the Mott–Schottky plot, an example of which is shown in Figure 14.7 for Ti6Al4V in solution 2 and in Figure 14.8 for 316L stainless steel in solution 1, both 1 h after immersion at open circuit. E_{fb} can be determined from extrapolation of the linear part of the curve towards the zero on the ordinate axis, and N_D can be calculated from the slope of the straight line. Moreover, there is a simple relation between the capacitance of the semiconductor and the thickness of the space charge layer, W, similar to that of Equation (14.6):

$$W = \frac{\varepsilon_r \varepsilon_0}{C_f}. \qquad (14.10)$$

Considering Equation (14.9) it follows that W is also a function of the applied potential

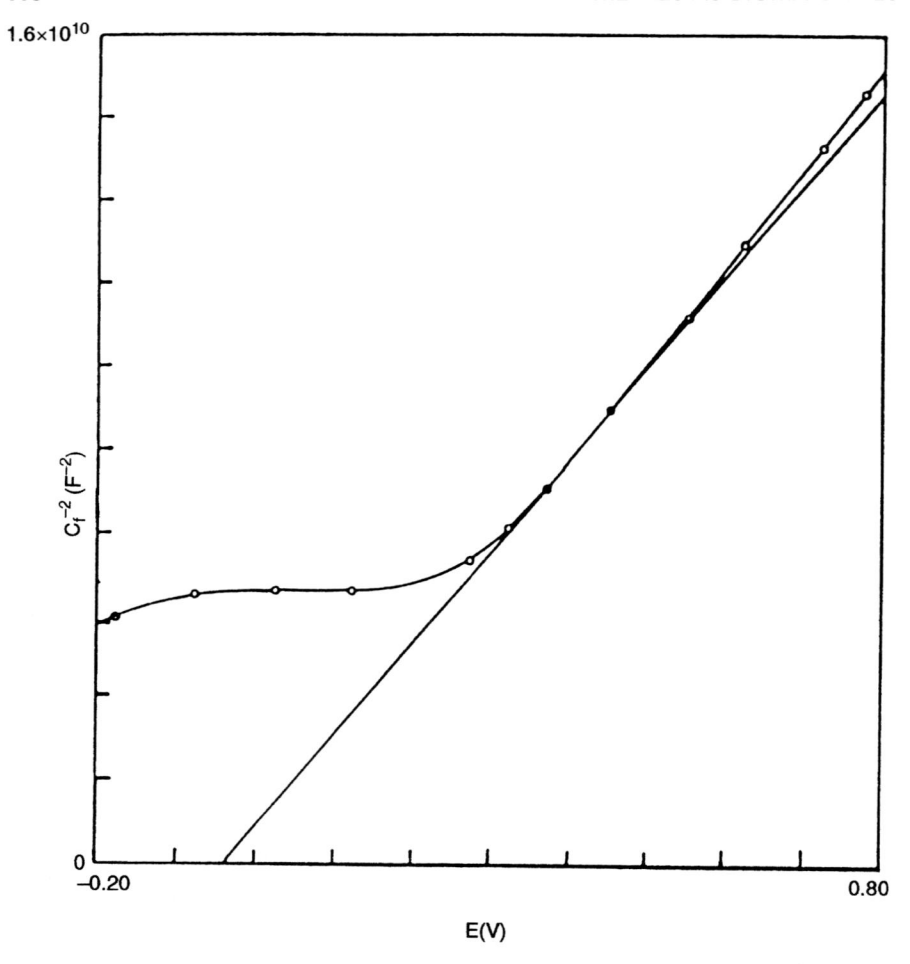

Figure 14.7 Mott–Schottky plot for Ti6Al4V alloy in solution 2 (Silva et al., 1990).

$$W = \sqrt{\frac{2\varepsilon_r \varepsilon_0}{eN_D}\left(E - E_{fb} - \frac{kT}{e}\right)}. \quad (14.11)$$

In this study a maximum thickness of the space charge layer is estimated. Table 14.2 collects some of the data. In the calculations ε_r is given a value of 12 for the film on 316L stainless steel and a value of 170 for the film on the Ti6Al4V alloy. Concerning the 316L stainless steel, the general form of the Mott–Schottky plot is a bell shape, where the capacitance first decreases with increasing E, then reaches a minimum at about 0.200–0.300 V and finally increases again. The explanation is that the first part is due to a decreasing number of charge carriers, N_D, the minimum to a constant N_D,

ELECTROCHEMICAL IMPEDANCE SPECTROSCOPY

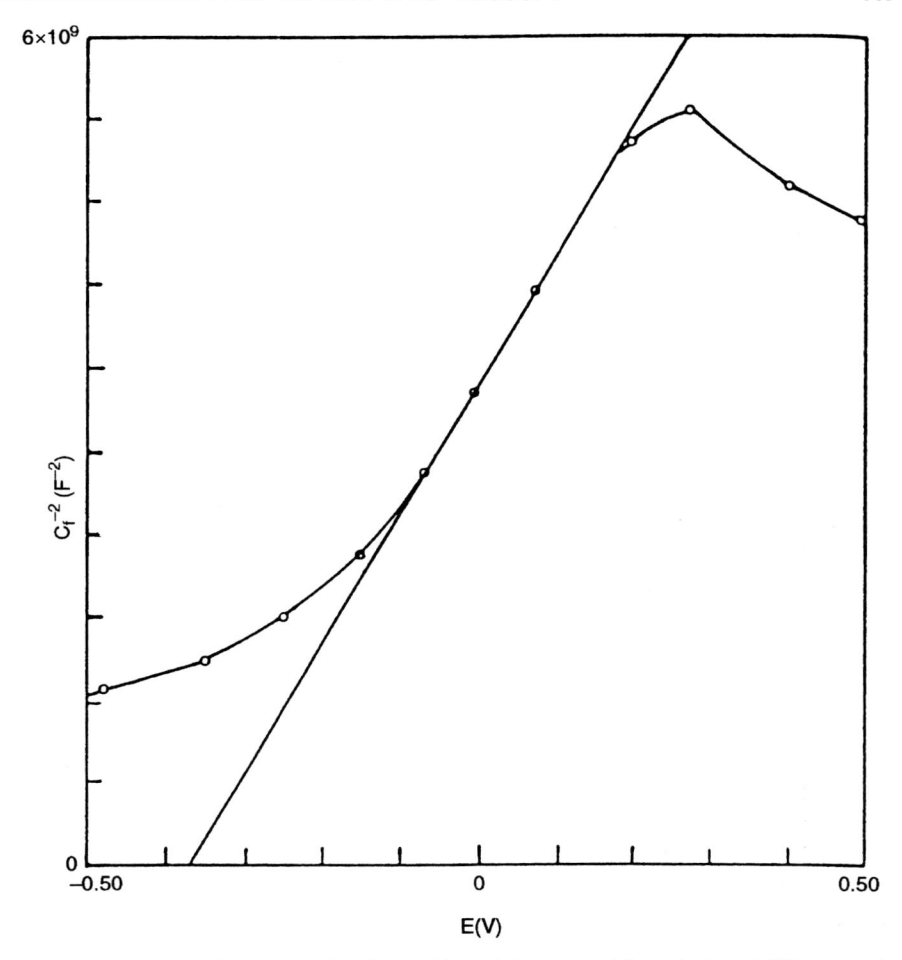

Figure 14.8 Mott–Schottky plot for 316L stainless steel in solution 1 (Silva *et al.*, 1990).

the oxide being exhausted of donors, and the third part to the participation of the valence band. Table 14.2 shows that for this material in solution 1, without lactic acid, E_{fb} decreases during the first 22 h of the open-circuit test and is constant afterwards, because of a rearrangement within the film with an increasing crystallinity. In solution 2, with lactic acid, E_{fb} rises during the first 22 h of the open-circuit test. For the same material after 1 h of immersion, E_{fb} is seen to increase with decreasing pH at a rate of 60 mV per pH unit, which is called Nernstian behaviour. For longer periods such behaviour is no longer observed, probably because of structural changes at the interface, where the contribution of the oxides Fe_2O_3 and Cr_2O_3 varies depending on their relative thickness. The Mott–Schottky plot of

Table 14.2 Data from Mott–Schottky impedance tests for 316L stainless steel and Ti6Al4V alloy in solutions 1 and 2 (Silva et al., 1990)

Solution[a]	Immersion time[b] (h)	E_{fb} (V/SCE)	C_{sc} (µF cm^{-2})	W (nm)	N_D (atoms cm^{-3})
316L					
1	1	−0.365	21.3	0.62	2.1×10^{21}
	22	−0.533	21.6	0.42	3.8×10^{21}
	72	−0.531	21.5	0.51	3.2×10^{21}
	24[c]	−0.340	0.89	0.51	1.5×10^{21}
	7[d]	−0.280	–	–	1.3×10^{21}
2	1	−0.213	21.1	0.51	2.3×10^{21}
	22	−0.145	28.1	0.62	1.9×10^{21}
Ti6Al4V					
1	1	−1.48	14.2	0.16	4.5×10^{19}
	22	−1.53	11.9	0.16	5.5×10^{19}
2	1	−0.037	11.9	0.15	7.6×10^{19}
	22	0.019	11.9	0.16	6.0×10^{19}

[a]Solution 1, pH 6.7; solution 2, pH 4.0.
[b]Under open-circuit conditions unless otherwise indicated.
[c]Controlled at 0.25 V/SCE.
[d]Controlled at 0.40 V/SCE.

Figure 14.9 shows the influence of different applied potentials and immersion times for 316L in solution 1. The values for N_D derived from experiments at an applied potential are lower than those at open circuit, and the values for E_{fb} are higher. This phenomenon could be due to a reduction in the number of structural and electronic defects acting as electron donors in the passive film as the film grows thicker. The maximum thickness of the space charge layer is found to be about 0.6 nm for 316L.

Concerning the Ti6Al4V alloy, the general form of the Mott–Schottky plot first indicates a small variation with increasing potential, but above 0.300 V the curve becomes steeper and finally turns into a linear part. The pH affects the slope of this linear part, which in turn has a considerable effect on the E_{fb} value derived and a smaller effect on the N_D value. The density of charge carriers is about one order of magnitude lower for this material than for 316L, resulting in a less conductive passive film consequence as well as a higher corrosion resistance of the Ti6Al4V alloy in physiological media. The maximum thickness of the space charge layer for Ti6Al4V is estimated at about 0.16 nm.

In much the same way as in Solar et al. (1979) and Silva et al. (1990), the work of Pan et al. (1994) is concentrated around the determination of dielectric and electronic properties of the oxide film on a biomaterial in order to obtain better knowledge of its corrosion behaviour and the release of products into the surrounding tissue, and also to warrant better control.

Here the material was a commercially pure titanium rod, wet ground with 2400 grit paper and rinsed with deionised water, ethanol and acetone. The medium was a

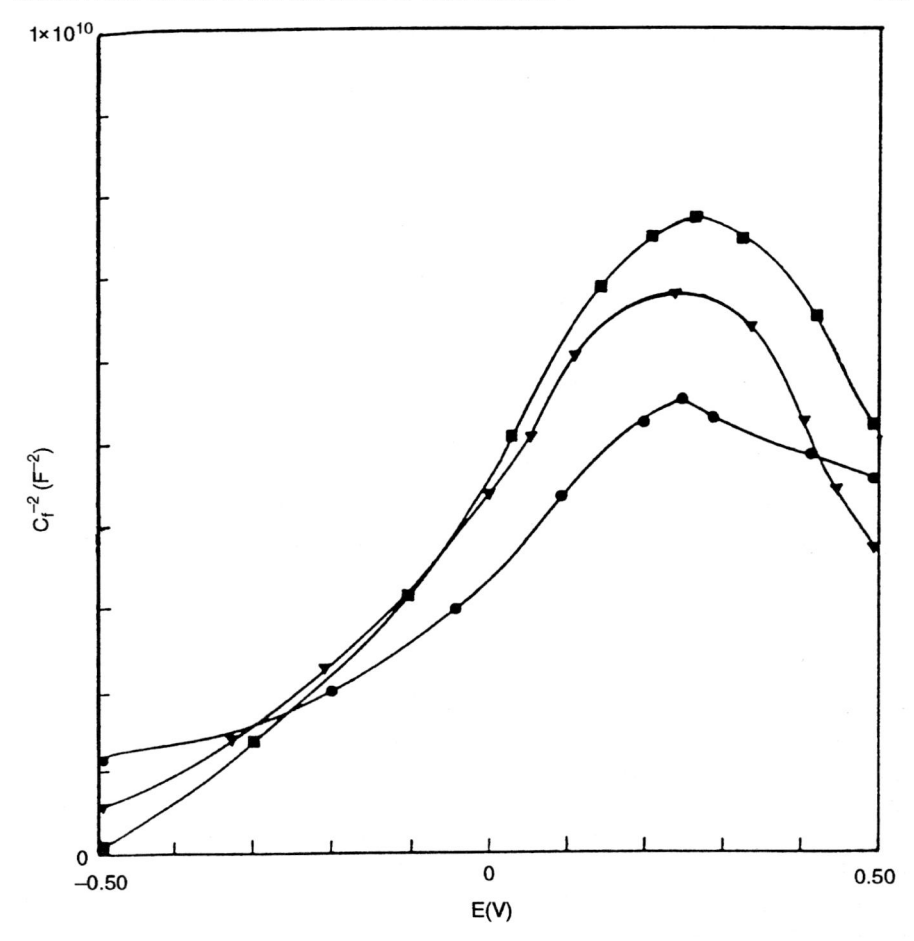

Figure 14.9 Mott–Schottky plots for 316L stainless steel for different applied potentials and immersion exposures in solution 1: ●, 1 h after immersion under open-circuit conditions; ▼, prepolarised for 24 h at 0.25 V/SCE; ■, prepolarised for 7 h at 0.40 V/SCE (Silva et al., 1990).

Table 14.3 Composition (g l^{-1}) and pH of the PBS solution. (From *Journal of Biomedical Materials Research*, Vol. 28, Pan *et al.*, Electrochemical and XPS studies of titanium for biomaterial applications with respect to the effect of hydrogen peroxide, pp. 113–22, 1994. Reprinted by permission of John Wiley & Sons, Ltd)

NaCl	$Na_2HPO_4 \cdot 12H_2O$	KH_2PO_4	pH
8.77	3.58	1.36	7.2–7.4

phosphate-buffered saline (PBS) solution, composed as in Table 14.3, with chemicals of analytical grade. The pH was adjusted with NaOH and the effect of addition of H_2O_2 was studied in the concentration range from 1 to 100 mM, as the presence of H_2O_2 in living tissues is linked to inflammation processes and may play a part in the implant performance. The solutions were deaerated with nitrogen and kept at 25°C. The three-electrode cell was further provided with a platinum wire, as a CE, and a SCE, which was the reference for all potential measurements, except for the flat band potential, which is expressed vs the standard hydrogen electrode (SHE). The measurements were performed using an EG&G, Parc, Model 273A potentiostat/galvanostat and a Solartron 1254 FRA.

For the measurement of the dielectric constant, the titanium electrode was first cathodically reduced at a potential 0.2 V lower than the open-circuit potential for 5 min to clean the surface, then the specimen was potentiostatically polarised and the charge measured during anodic formation of the passive layer. The electrode impedance was simultaneously determined with an ac signal of 10 mV amplitude, and the capacitance of the oxide film was calculated from the impedance recorded at a constant higher frequency of 1 kHz, to exclude the effect of the capacitance of the

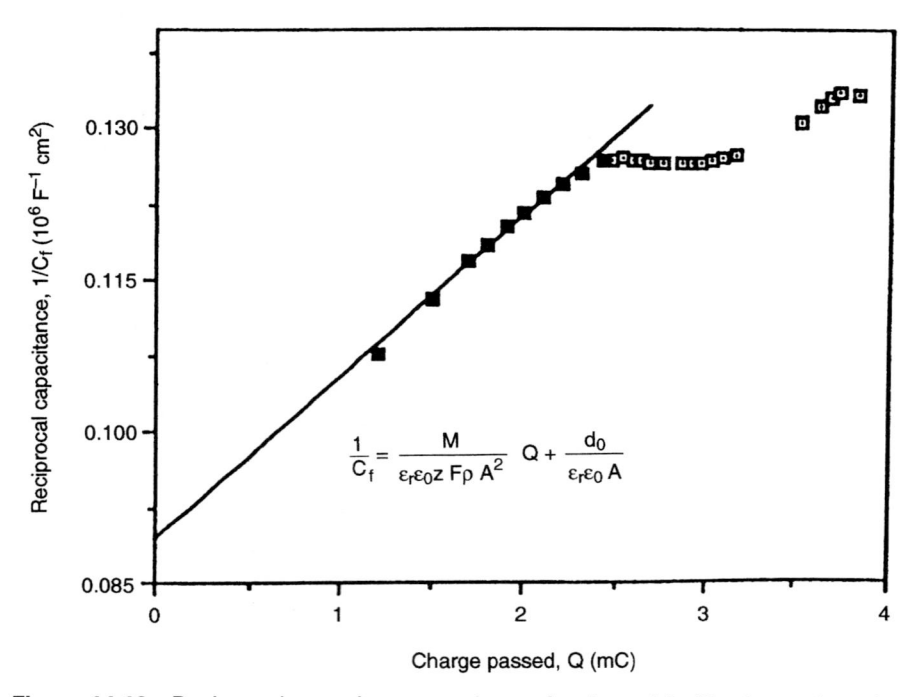

Figure 14.10 Reciprocal capacitance vs charge for the oxide film formed on titanium in the PBS solution at 0.4 V/SCE. (From *Journal of Biomedical Materials Research*, Vol. 28, Pan *et al.*, Electrochemical and XPS studies of titanium for biomaterial applications with respect to the effect of hydrogen peroxide, pp. 113–22, 1994. Reprinted by permission of John Wiley & Sons, Ltd.)

electrochemical double layer. In Figure 14.10 the reciprocal value of the film capacitance per unit surface area is plotted against the charge measured during formation of the anodic oxide film on a titanium specimen in a PBS solution at a potential of 0.4 V. The linear part of the curve at the beginning of the anodic polarisation, according to the growing phase of the film, is observed immediately and its slope does not appear to be affected significantly by the applied potential in the range under study. After the linear part the curve comes to a stationary phase, pointing to a limiting thickness of the passive film. The charge necessary to reach this limit increases slightly with the applied potential, which is apparently typical of the anodic oxide film on titanium, acting as a dielectric. On the basis of the assumption that all of the charge measured stems from the growth of the oxide film, its dielectric constant and/or its thickness may be calculated from the slope of the linear part of the curve. An equation similar to Equation (14.8) for the reciprocal value of the film capacitance is used, except for a term representing the contribution of the original film thickness

$$\frac{1}{C_f} = \frac{M}{\varepsilon_r \varepsilon_0 z F \rho A^2} Q + \frac{d_0}{\varepsilon_r \varepsilon_0 A}, \qquad (14.12)$$

where A is the geometrical exposed surface area of the electrode and d_0 is the original film thickness.

Table 14.4 summarises some calculated values, which are averages of five parallel measurements, of the apparent dielectric constant, determined from the geometrical surface area of the electrode, and of the original thickness of the oxide film grown on titanium in a deaerated PBS solution at 0.4 V in the presence of various concentrations of H_2O_2. ρ is assumed to have the value for rutile, TiO_2, of 4.26 g cm^{-3}. Here the electrochemical effective surface area is assumed to be equal to the geometrical exposed area, i.e. the roughness factor is 1. If the real surface roughness were taken into account, the dielectric constant would be smaller, as the anodising process as well as the addition of H_2O_2 are known to roughen the surface. The addition of H_2O_2 raises the slope of the linear part of the curve and consequently diminishes ε_r. This probably occurs because the charge measured no longer results from the oxide formation process alone, but also from oxygen evolution and enhanced film dissolution in the presence of H_2O_2. The original film thickness decreases as well, which can be

Table 14.4 Apparent dielectric constant and original film thickness of the oxide layer on titanium measured at 0.4 V/SCE in the PBS solution. (From *Journal of Biomedical Materials Research*, Vol. 28, Pan et al., Electrochemical and XPS studies of titanium for biomaterial applications with respect to the effect of hydrogen peroxide, pp. 113–22, 1994. Reprinted by permission of John Wiley & Sons, Ltd)

	No H_2O_2	10 mM H_2O_2	100 mM H_2O_2
ε_r	65	43	48
d_0 (Å)	54	39	48

explained by the dissolution of the passive film on addition of H_2O_2. A second increase in the reciprocal value of the capacitance with the charge is observed, leading to a higher dielectric constant. This may be due to the formation of another layer with a higher dielectric constant or the rearrangement of the structure of the surface oxide film, e.g. the formation of a porous outer layer or slow hydration processes.

For the Mott–Schottky plots, the oxide film was first grown through potentiostatic polarisation at 0.4 or 0.8 V or through galvanostatic polarisation at 5 µA cm^{-2} for 2 h. During a downward potential scan the capacitance was then measured to obtain the Mott–Schottky plots for various H_2O_2 concentrations. Such a plot is represented in Figure 14.11 for the oxide film on titanium in deaerated PBS solution with and without the addition of H_2O_2, the films being potentiostatically formed at 0.4 V. These films are considered to behave as n-type semiconductors, so the applicability of the Mott–Schottky equation [Equation (14.9)] is obvious. The space charge capacitance, for which the equation holds, is taken to be equal to the measured film capacitance. The linear part of the curves offers the opportunity to calculate a donor density of 1.2×10^{20} cm^{-3} and 1.5×10^{20} cm^{-3} on the basis of the dielectric constants measured and a flat band potential of −0.65 and −0.70 V vs the SHE for the oxide formed in the

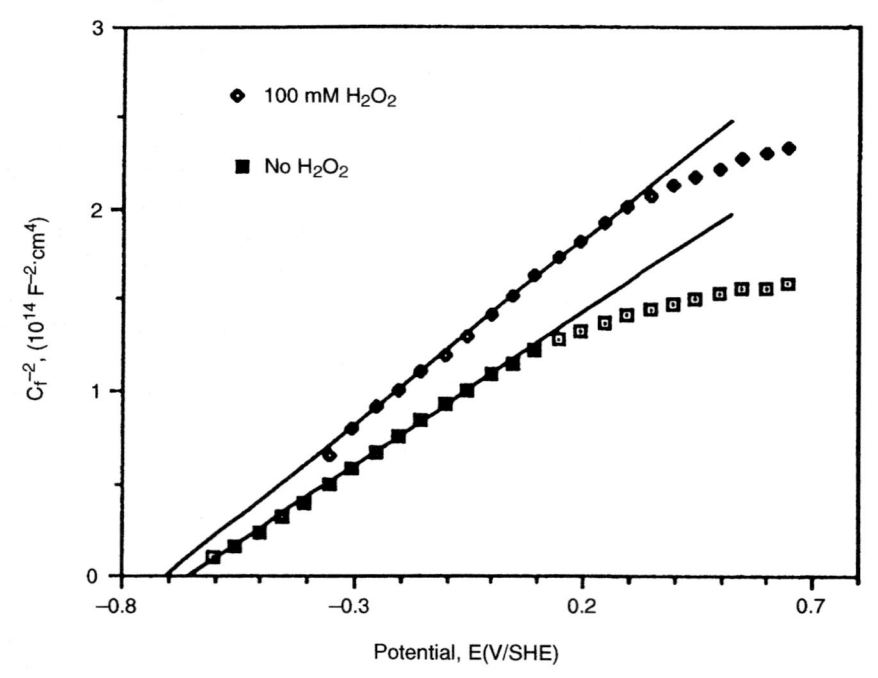

Figure 14.11 Mott–Schottky plots for the oxide films on titanium in the PBS solution with and without H_2O_2; films are formed potentiostatically at 0.4 V/SCE. (From *Journal of Biomedical Materials Research*, Vol. 28, Pan et al., Electrochemical and XPS studies of titanium for biomaterial applications with respect to the effect of hydrogen peroxide, pp. 113–22, 1994. Reprinted by permission of John Wiley & Sons, Ltd.)

ELECTROCHEMICAL IMPEDANCE SPECTROSCOPY

deaerated PBS solution, without the addition of H_2O_2 and with 100 mM H_2O_2, respectively. So, the addition of H_2O_2 raises the donor density slightly and shifts the flat band potential to a more negative value, and the same effect holds for galvanostatically formed films. It follows that the addition of H_2O_2 implies a more defective oxide film, as the donor states in titanium oxides are determined by oxygen vacancies and the flat band potential by the concentration of impurities. The deviation of the plots from the linear behaviour at higher potentials indicates an amorphous or strongly disordered and/or non-stoichiometric passive film.

14.3 PASSIVE AND OXIDE FILMS: CORROSION AND REDOX PROCESSES

Later, the same group conducted a more profound investigation into the system described above (Pan, 1996a, b). One set of titanium specimens was immersed in a PBS solution without H_2O_2, for several weeks, while another set was immersed in the same solution with 100 mM H_2O_2 for 1 or 2 weeks until a blue coloration of the titanium surface ensued. The latter phenomenon, effected owing to interference, was kept under control by shielding the cell from light using an aluminium foil. Each set of experiments was run three times in parallel. The specimens were arranged into a three-electrode cell and an impedance spectrum was recorded once a day at the open-circuit potential after gently shaking the cell in order to remove from the titanium surface any gas bubbles caused by H_2O_2 decomposition. The measurement set-up consisted of a Solartron 1260 impedance/gain-phase analyser and an EG&G Parc Model 273A potentiostat/galvanostat, controlled by a computer. The signals applied had an amplitude of 10 mV and a frequency varying between 1 kHz and 5 mHz (sometimes 1 mHz). The spectra were analysed using computer software and interpretation was based on equivalent circuit modelling and a non-linear least- squares fitting technique. Because of the occurrence of the distributed relaxation phenomenon, the spectra were modelled using the CPE instead of the ideal capacitance; nevertheless, the value supplied by the fitting procedure was taken as a capacitance. The quality of the fit was tested by the χ^2-value and by the plot of error distribution vs frequency, comparing experimental with simulated data.

Figure 14.12 shows Bode plots for the unit surface area of titanium in the medium without H_2O_2 after 1 day and 30 days of immersion. An almost purely capacitive spectrum is observed with a phase angle close to $-90°$ over a wide frequency range, which is typical for a thin passive oxide film on titanium. Moreover, it does not change with time, providing evidence of a stable oxide film. When 100 mM of H_2O_2 was initially added to the medium the spectra evolved as in Figure 14.13, in which the Bode plots after 1, 15 and 30 days are represented. In the early phase a slow variation in the spectrum is observed from Figure 14.13a and b. In a later phase a blue coloration of the titanium surface occurs and the impedance spectrum is highly modified (Figure 14.13c). Consequently, H_2O_2 changes the passive oxide film on titanium, as well as its electrochemical properties.

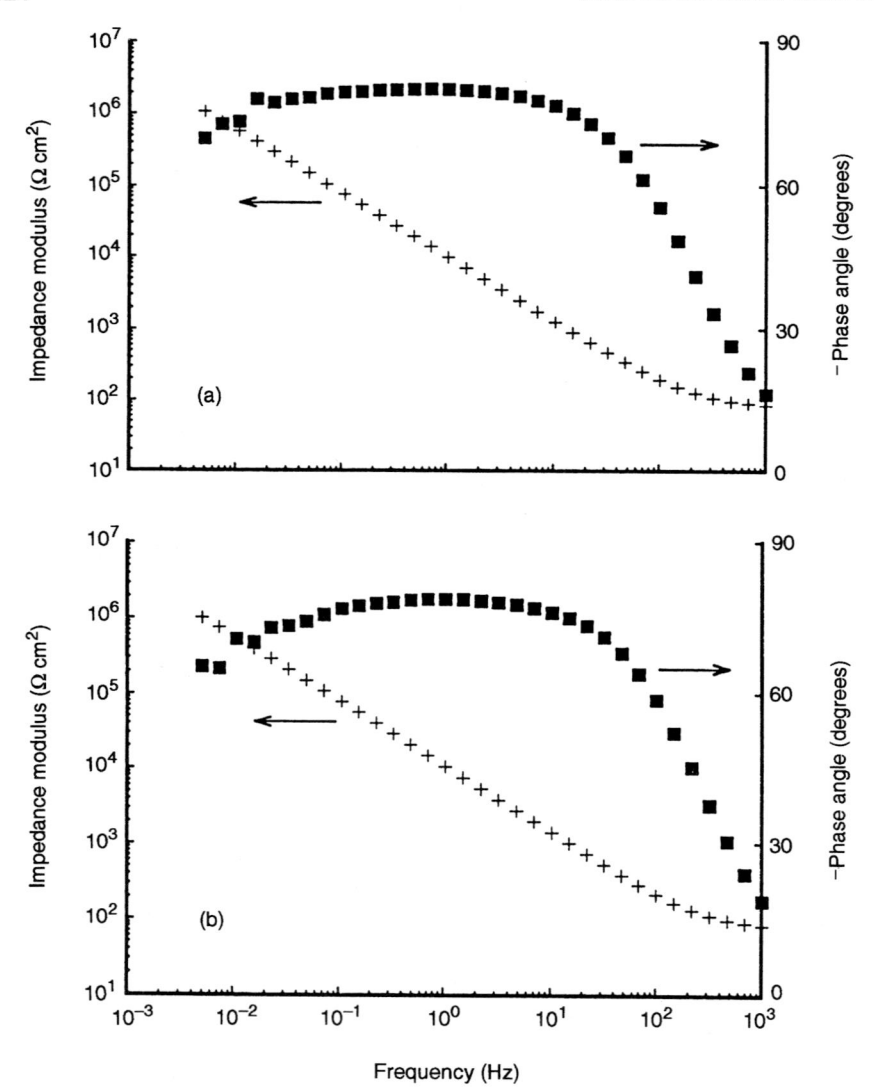

Figure 14.12 Bode plots for titanium exposed in the PBS solution without H_2O_2 addition: (a) 1 day; (b) 30 days of exposure. (From *Electrochimica Acta*, Vol. 41, Pan *et al.*, Electrochemical impedance spectroscopy study of the passive oxide film on titanium for implant application, pp. 1143–53, 1996, with kind permission from Elsevier Science Ltd, UK.)

In order to reach a more quantitative interpretation of the spectra related to the three typical situations cited above, two equivalent circuits are proposed on the basis of the two-layer model of an oxide film (Figure 14.14). This model, which, using other independent techniques, is proved to hold for titanium in many conditions

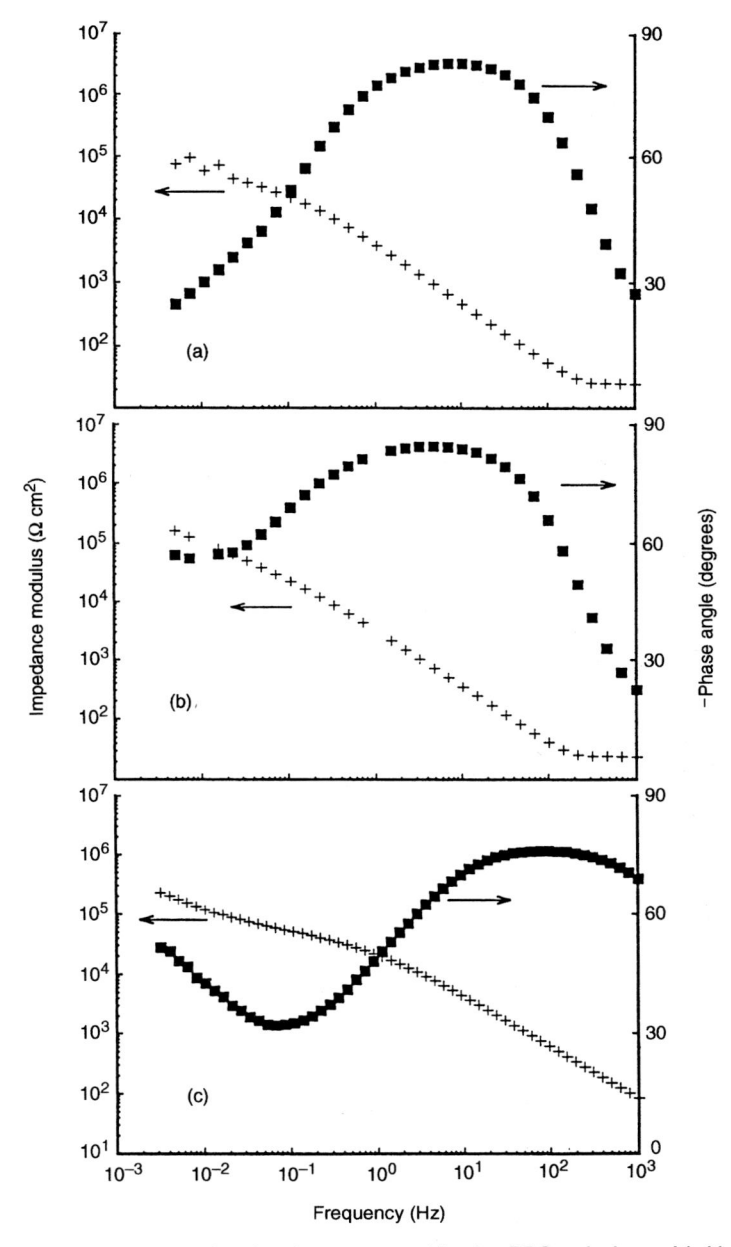

Figure 14.13 Bode plots for titanium exposed in the PBS solution with H_2O_2 addition with an initial concentration of 100 mM: (a) 1 day; (b) 15 days; (c) 30 days of exposure. (From *Electrochimica Acta*, Vol. 41, Pan et al., Electrochemical impedance spectroscopy study of the passive oxide film on titanium for implant application, pp. 1143–53, 1996, with kind permission from Elsevier Science Ltd, UK.)

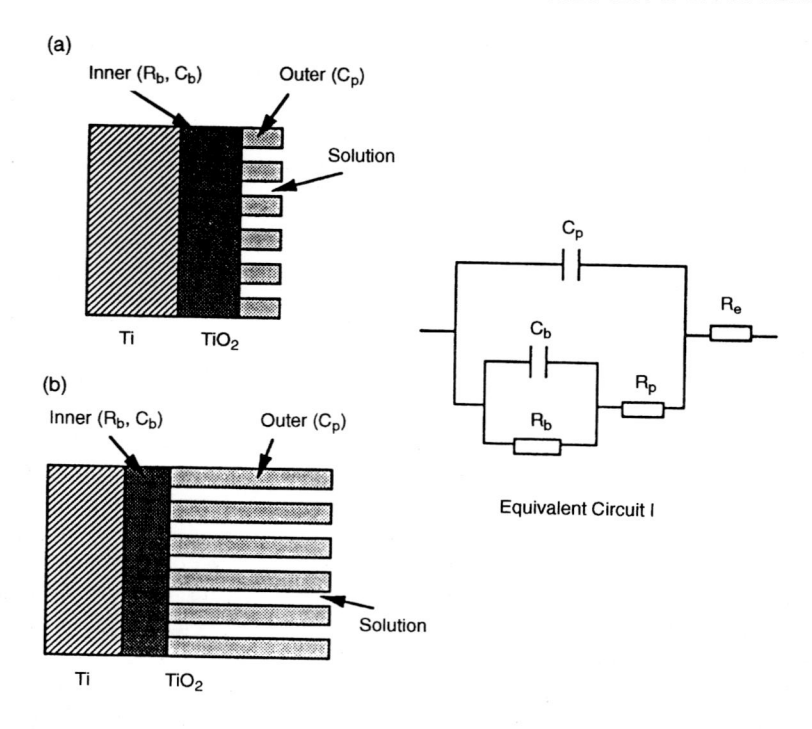

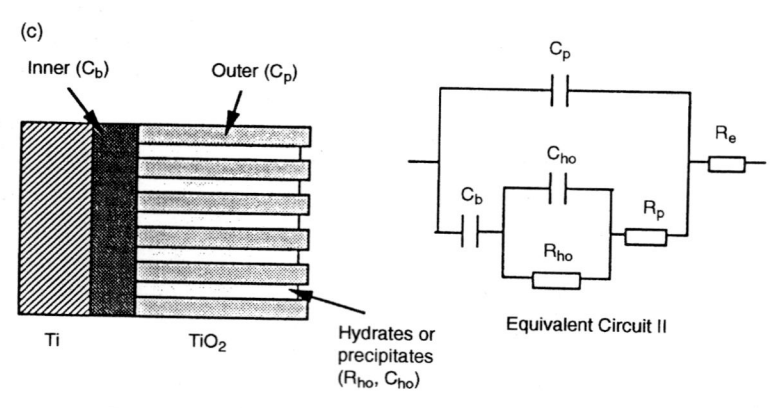

Figure 14.14 Equivalent circuits used for the two-layer oxide film on titanium: (I) porous layer unsealed; (II) porous layer sealed; schematic representation of the oxide film on titanium under different exposure conditions in the PBS solution: (a) without H_2O_2; (b) with H_2O_2, earlier stage; (c) with H_2O_2, later stage, when the titanium surface appears blue. (From *Electrochimica Acta*, Vol. 41, Pan *et al.*, Electrochemical impedance spectroscopy study of the passive oxide film on titanium for implant application, pp. 1143–53, 1996, with kind permission from Elsevier Science Ltd, UK.)

including the present one, considers an inner oxide layer of dense structure, located immediately against the titanium metal. An outer porous oxide layer is situated on top of the dense layer. The pores in the outer oxide layer may or may not be filled with hydrated compounds or precipitates, and in the former case the oxide film is said to be sealed. Situation a in Figure 14.14 represents schematically the case of the oxide film on titanium exposed to the medium without H_2O_2, resulting in a stable film. Situation b is the case of the medium with H_2O_2, in the early phase, and situation c in the later phase, when blue coloration of the titanium surface occurs. The equivalent circuit I in Figure 14.14 is typical for unsealed anodic oxide films, where the pores in the outer layer are simply filled with electrolyte. Circuit I leads to a good fitting of spectra measured in situations a and b. The equivalent circuit II is typical for sealed anodic oxide films, where the pores in the outer layer are filled with hydrated compounds and is a good fit with the spectra measured in situation c. The circuit elements, each time expressed for the unit surface area, are: R_e, the solution resistance; C_b, the inner layer capacitance; R_b, the inner layer resistance; C_p, the outer layer capacitance; R_p, the outer layer resistance or the electrolyte resistance inside the pores; C_{ho}, the capacitance of the hydrates/precipitates inside the pores; and R_{ho}, the resistance of the hydrates/precipitates inside the pores.

Circuit I models the two parallel oxide layers as two nested resistance/capacitance parallel circuits. In circuit II a supplementary resistance/capacitance parallel circuit, accounting for the hydrates in the pores, is built in with respect to circuit I, and the part of the inner layer is simplified into one single capacitance.

At this point the impedance results indicate that the process of adding H_2O_2 to the medium containing the titanium specimen is comparable to the process of sealing an anodic oxide film. As mentioned above, the oxide film on top of the titanium specimens consists of a dense inner layer and a porous outer layer. Moreover, owing to the action of H_2O_2, the porous layer has grown thicker and contains hydrates/precipitates together with ions from the medium.

The fitting of circuit I to the spectra relating to the experiments without H_2O_2 results in a very high resistance of the inner barrier layer, about 5 MΩ cm^2 (see Figure 14.15), which involves a high corrosion resistance and thus a low rate of titanium release and oxide growth. The capacitance of the same layer is relatively small, decreasing slightly with the immersion time to a stationary value of about 10 µF cm^{-2}. This is an indication of a slowly growing titanium oxide film and the long-term stability of the thin passive film. The resistance of the porous layer is low, increasing slightly with time from 100 to 200 Ω cm^2, meaning that the pores are probably only filled with solution, while the capacitance of the porous layer is about 25 µF cm^{-2}. As it appears that the porous layer is rather thin, it follows that the corrosion of titanium must be prevented mainly by the presence of the dense inner layer, which also contributes for the major part to the measured impedance.

When H_2O_2 is added to the medium, circuit I still leads to a good fitting of the impedance data, although only in the early phase of the exposure. During the initial period of the early phase, when the H_2O_2 concentration is high but quickly descends, the dense inner layer has a low resistance and a high capacitance. The limit of the

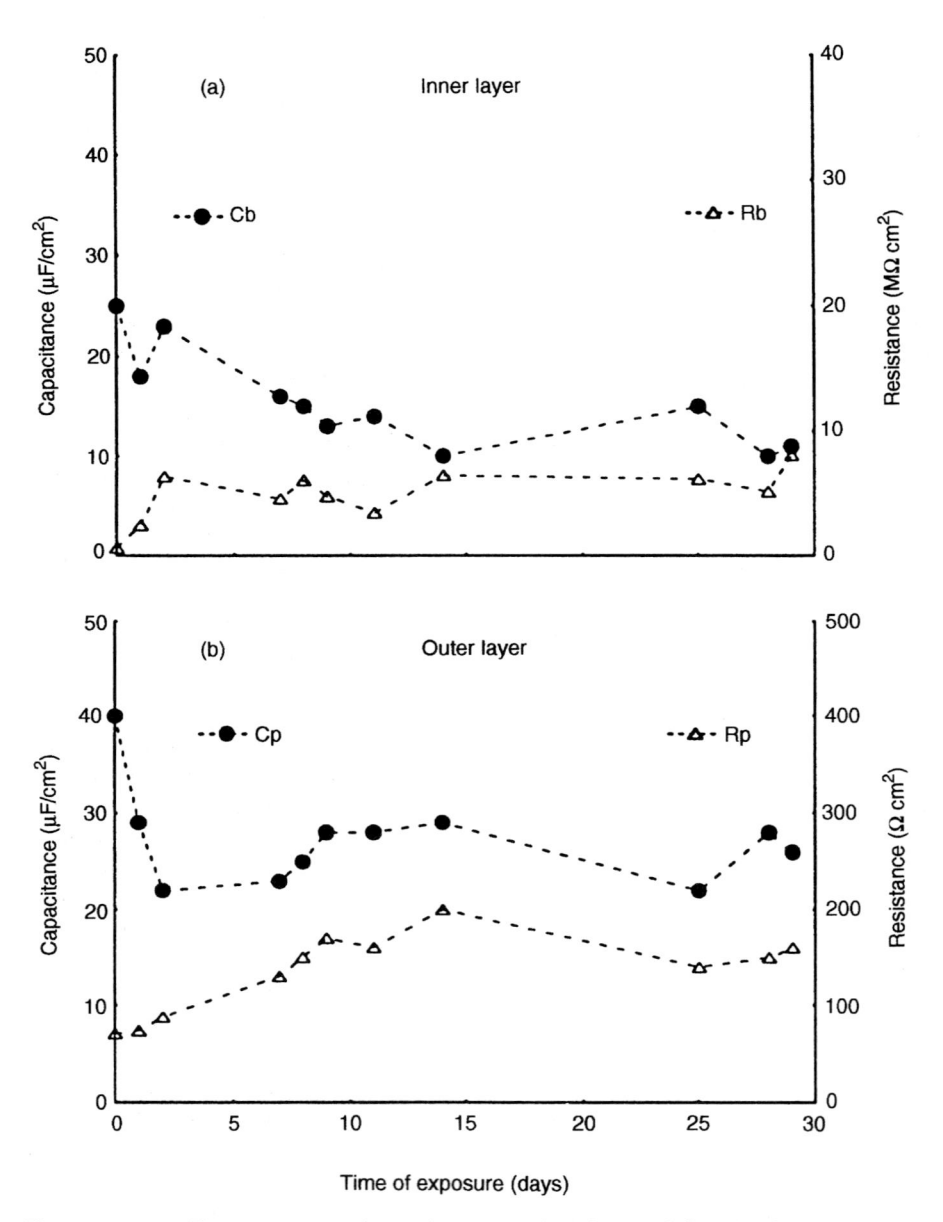

Figure 14.15 Fit parameters (capacitance and resistance) for titanium exposed in the PBS solution without H_2O_2 as a function of exposure time: (a) inner layer; (b) outer layer. (From *Electrochimica Acta*, Vol. 41, Pan *et al.*, Electrochemical impedance spectroscopy study of the passive oxide film on titanium for implant application, pp. 1143–53, 1996, with kind permission from Elsevier Science Ltd, UK.)

impedance modulus at low frequencies is about 100 kΩ cm^2, which means an important decrease with respect to the situation without an addition of H_2O_2. Thus the original dense oxide layer is partly dissolved and becomes more defective through the addition of H_2O_2. The corrosion resistance is relatively low, the rate of dissolution/oxidation of titanium increases and a high amount of titanium may be released into the solution. After the initial period, the H_2O_2 concentration is low and stable. The capacitance of the dense inner layer becomes stable (Figure 14.16). The resistance of this layer increases and reaches a high value in the order of magnitude of MΩ cm^2, almost as in the situation without H_2O_2. The inner layer thus regrows or undergoes a self-healing process and the film again becomes protective. The increased porosity of the outer layer emerges from its capacitance, which at first remains stable at a relatively high value and finally seems to descend. It also appears that hydrates and/or precipitates are generated in the pores, as the resistance of the porous layer is rather high, in the order of magnitude of several tens of kΩ cm^2, and still increasing.

In the later phase, when blue coloration of the titanium surface occurs, circuit II leads to the best fit of the impedance data. The evolution of the circuit element values with the exposure time is recorded in Figure 14.17. The capacitance of the outer layer is stabilised at a low value of about 3 μF cm^{-2}, reflecting a thick outer layer. Concerning the hydrates and/or precipitates in the pores, the corresponding resistance is about 50 kΩ cm^2 and the corresponding capacitance decreases. These magnitudes may give an image of the ongoing process of hydration and/or precipitation. The limit of the impedance modulus at low frequencies has increased and it seems that the film has again reached a high corrosion resistance. R_{ho} appears to increase again up to 400 kΩ cm^2 after drying in air for 1 h and immersion in the same solution, which is proof for the link between this model element and the hydrates/precipitates within the pores including the amount of water bound or absorbed. Pan *et al.* (1996b) translated the various measured capacitances into thicknesses of the corresponding dielectric oxide layers, using an equation similar to Equation (14.6) (see Table 14.5). For the relative dielectric constant a value of 65 was taken, which is that of TiO_2. A surface roughness factor was also considered: 1 for the dense barrier layer and 1–2 for the porous outer layer. In this way, total oxide thicknesses were calculated, varying from about 10 ± 2 nm in the medium without H_2O_2 to about 30 ± 10 nm in the medium with H_2O_2.

The literature, however, contains some warning messages as to what exactly determines biocompatibility. It appears that not only corrosion processes or corrosion products are to be considered, but also electron exchange processes and reaction products of redox processes involving tissue compounds. The warning also concerns the kind of information revealed from electrochemical measurements and impedance measurements in particular (e.g. Kovacs, 1991a). Test specimens were made from 316L stainless steel, CoCrMo alloy and Ti6Al4V alloy, mechanically polished to a mirror finish and immediately immersed. The media were Ringer's solution with lactic acid on the one hand, and Ringer's solution with lactic acid and the redox couple 0.01 M $K_4Fe(CN)_6$/0.01 M $K_3Fe(CN)_6$ on the other, at 37°C. The tests were continued for 20 h. Impedance measurements were executed at various time intervals, in the region from 0.1 to 10 Hz for the intermediate measurements, and from 0.001 Hz to 100 kHz for the

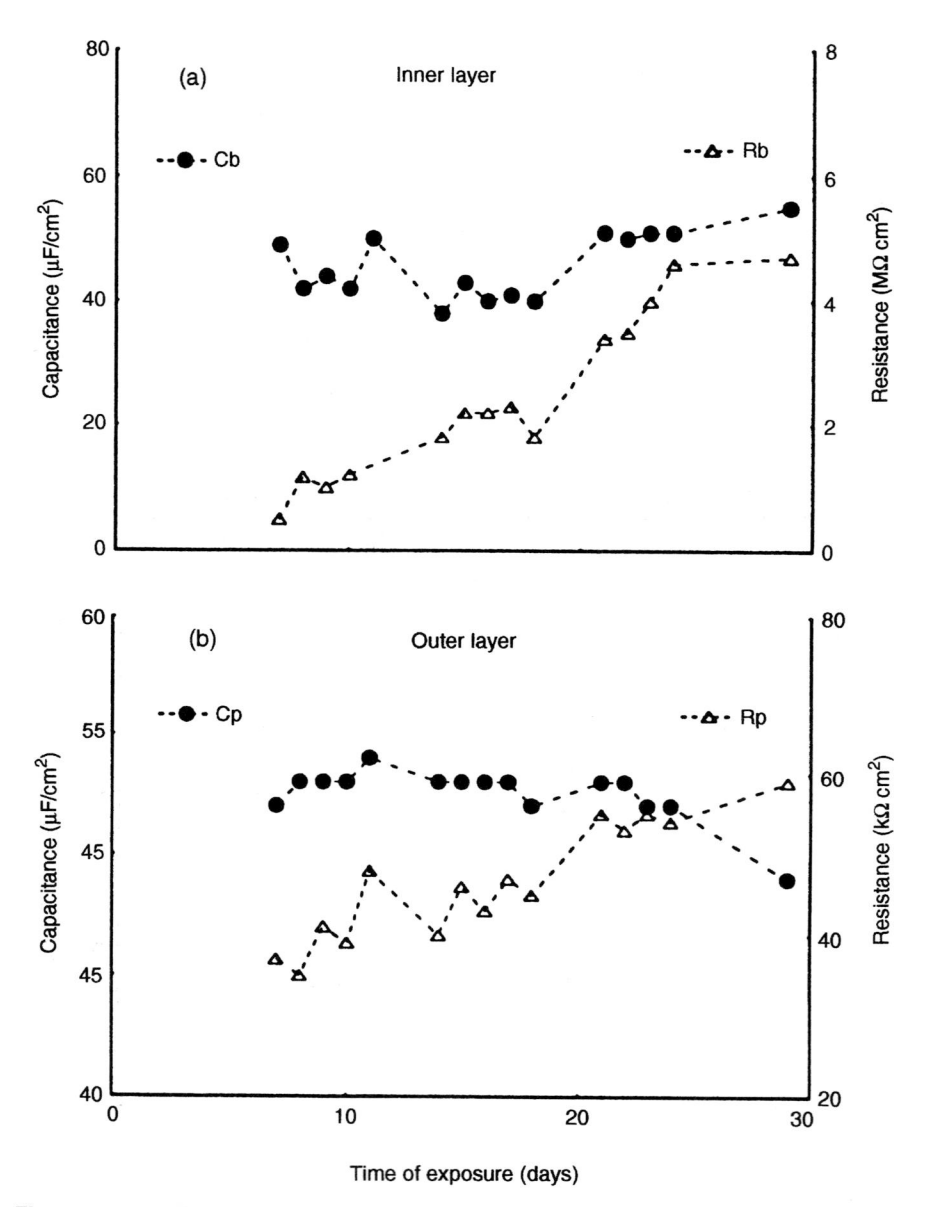

Figure 14.16 Fit parameters (capacitance and resistance) for titanium exposed in the PBS solution with H_2O_2 as a function of exposure time during the earlier stage of exposure: (a) inner layer; (b) outer layer. (From *Electrochimica Acta*, Vol. 41, Pan et al., Electrochemical impedance spectroscopy study of the passive oxide film on titanium for implant application, pp. 1143–53, 1996, with kind permission from Elsevier Science Ltd, UK.)

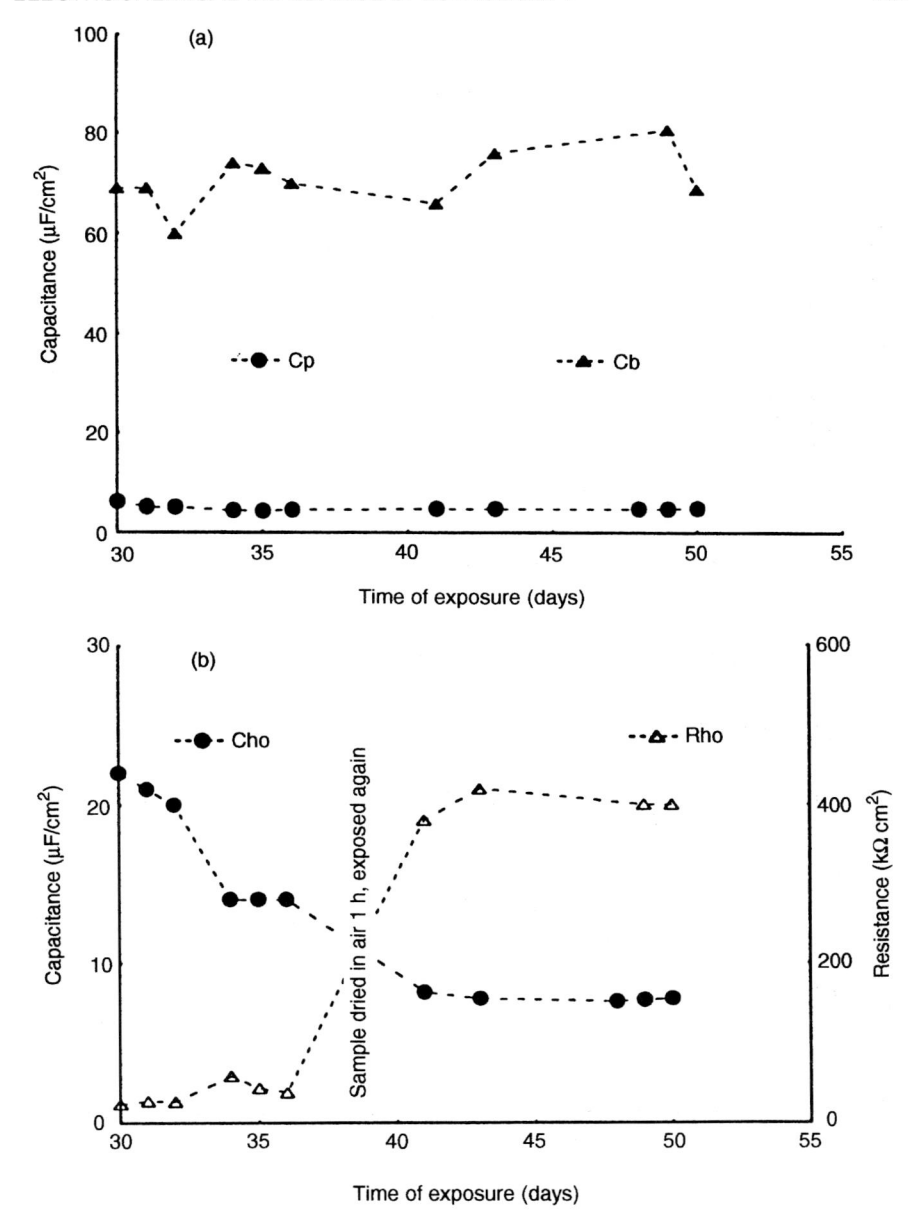

Figure 14.17 Fit parameters for titanium exposed in the PBS solution with H_2O_2 as a function of exposure time during the later stage: (a) capacitance for the inner and outer layers; (b) capacitance and resistance for the hydrates or precipitates inside the pores. (From *Electrochimica Acta*, Vol. 41, Pan *et al.*, Electrochemical impedance spectroscopy study of the passive oxide film on titanium for implant application, pp. 1143–53, 1996, with kind permission from Elsevier Science Ltd, UK.)

Table 14.5 Estimated thickness (nm) of the oxide film on titanium in the PBS solution. (From *Journal of Biomedical Materials Research*, Vol. 30, Pan et al., Hydrogen peroxide toward enhanced oxide growth on titanium in PBS solution: blue coloration and clinical relevance, pp. 393–402, 1996. Reprinted by permission of John Wiley & Sons, Ltd)

Titanium sample	Inner layer	Outer layer	Total thickness
Yellow (PBS without H_2O_2)	6	2.5–5.0	8.5–11.0
Blue (PBS with H_2O_2)	1	20–40	21.0–41.0

Thickness based both on EIS results and on optical measurements.

final measurements. The result deduced from the impedance measurements was the polarisation resistance for the unit surface area, R_p. In Figure 14.18, representing the logarithm of the reciprocal value of the polarisation resistance vs the logarithm of the time, t, for the various implant materials in Ringer's solution with lactic acid, two separate linear parts can be distinguished. The materials were compared with carbon in order to determine the polarisation resistance in the absence of corrosion processes as well as protective passive layers, as carbon shows no pronounced time dependence. The two linear parts indicate that the rate determining process changes during the passivation of the alloys. In the early phase the polarisation resistance is probably determined by the rate of the corrosion process, but after 1 or 2 h the electron exchange process may assume control. This reasoning leads to the following equations:

$$\frac{1}{R_p} = \frac{1}{R_{p,c}} + \frac{1}{R_{p,e}} \tag{14.13}$$

$$\frac{1}{R_{p,c}} = b_c t^{-k_c} \tag{14.14}$$

$$\frac{1}{R_{p,e}} = b_e t^{-k_e}, \tag{14.15}$$

where $R_{p,c}$ is the polarisation resistance for the metal corrosion on the unit surface area, $R_{p,e}$ is the polarisation resistance for the electron exchange on the unit surface area, and b_c, b_e, k_c and k_e are constants.

When $R_{p,e}$ is much larger than $R_{p,c}$, it is inferred from Equations (14.13) and (14.14) that

$$\log\left(\frac{1}{R_p}\right) = \log b_c - k_c \log t. \tag{14.16}$$

When $R_{p,c}$ is much larger than $R_{p,e}$, it follows from Equations (14.13) and (14.15) that

$$\log\left(\frac{1}{R_p}\right) = \log b_e - k_e \log t. \tag{14.17}$$

ELECTROCHEMICAL IMPEDANCE SPECTROSCOPY

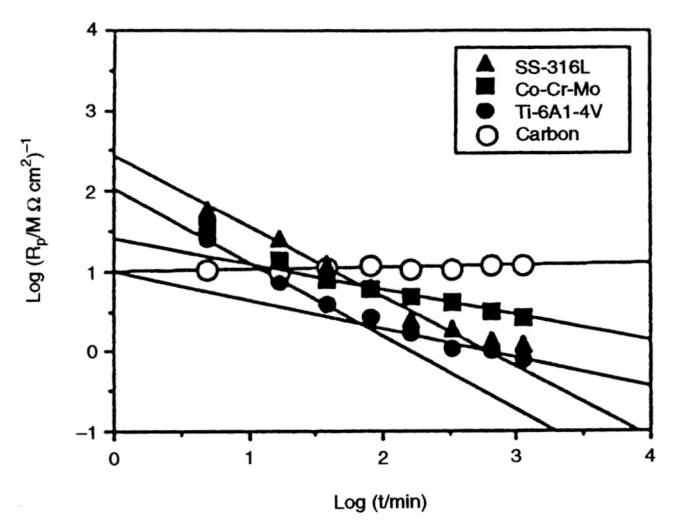

Figure 14.18 Log ($1/R_p$) vs log t plots for orthopaedic implant alloys and carbon in Ringer's solution (Kovacs, 1991a, with permission of The Electrochemical Society, Inc.).

Figure 14.18 consequently illustrates that the implant materials in the medium mentioned undergo an electrochemical process which first, for a short time, is a corrosion process and soon is mainly a process of electron exchange, being slower than the process at the carbon specimen.

When the medium is Ringer's solution with lactic acid and the redox couple, Figure 14.19 is the result, showing that, with the addition of a fast redox system to the electrolyte, the polarisation resistance of the implant materials is one to three orders of magnitude larger with respect to carbon, and that the mutual distinction between the materials is becoming more pronounced: Ti6Al4V > CoCrMo > 316L. The only linear slope for each material seems to refer to the process of electron exchange, which assumes control after less than 5 min of exposure. Thus care should be taken when interpreting polarisation resistances in terms of rates of electrochemical processes, as a polarisation resistance recorded at a passive film may be related as much to the rate of electron exchange as to that of a corrosion process. Although both kinds of potential phenomena seem to affect biocompatibility, a clear distinction should be made, as interpreting all electrochemical interactions at implant materials in any medium in terms of corrosion phenomena could lead to serious overestimations of their real corrosion rates.

In order to investigate the relative contribution of the pure alloying elements in the formation of the protective passive layer on the biomaterial alloy and in its release of soluble corrosion products, the experiments were repeated with the metals iron, chromium, nickel, molybdenum, manganese, cobalt, titanium, aluminium and vanadium in otherwise identical conditions except for the medium, which was only Ringer's solution with lactic acid (Kovacs, 1991b).

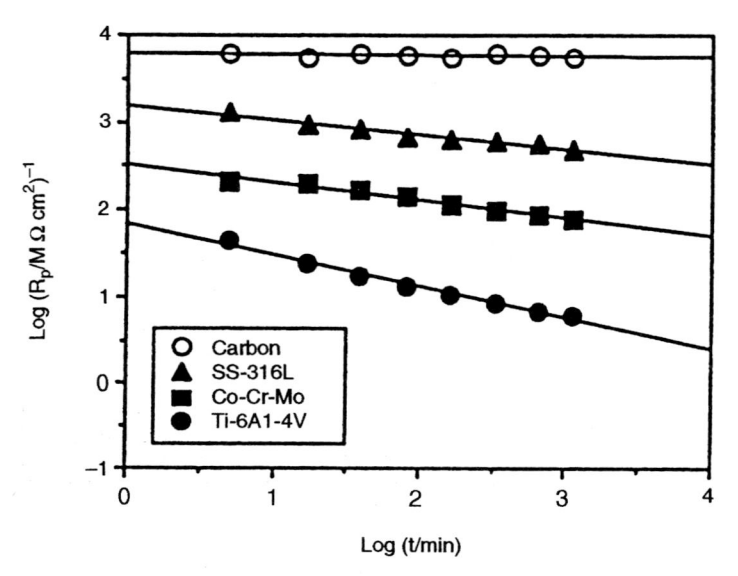

Figure 14.19 Log ($1/R_p$) vs log t plots for orthopaedic implant alloys and carbon in Ringer's solution with 0.01 M $K_4Fe(CN)_6$/0.01 M $K_3Fe(CN)_6$ (Kovacs, 1991a, with permission of The Electrochemical Society, Inc.).

The plot of the logarithm of the reciprocal polarisation resistance for the unit surface area vs the logarithm of time for the metals chromium and titanium is similar to that for the implant alloys themselves. Two separate linear parts are discernible, corresponding to equations similar to (14.14) and (14.15) or:

$$\log\left(\frac{1}{R_{p,c}}\right) = c_c - k_c \log t \tag{14.18}$$

and

$$\log\left(\frac{1}{R_{p,e}}\right) = c_e - k_e \log t, \tag{14.19}$$

where c_c and c_e are constants.

The author ascertains that these plots for the three alloys and for chromium and titanium may be further split up into plots of the logarithm of the reciprocal polarisation resistance vs the open-circuit potential (Figure 14.20) on the one hand, and plots of the open-circuit potential vs the logarithm of time (Figure 14.21) on the other, claiming that:

$$\log\left(\frac{1}{R_{p,c}}\right) = c'_c - \left(\frac{1}{b_{c,c}}\right) E_{oc,c} \tag{14.20}$$

ELECTROCHEMICAL IMPEDANCE SPECTROSCOPY

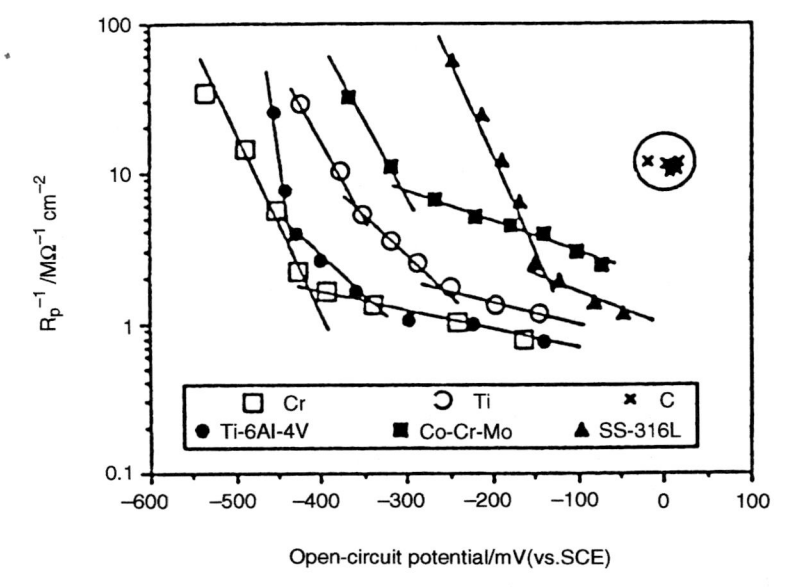

Figure 14.20 Log ($1/R_p$) vs open-circuit potential plots for orthopaedic implant alloys, chromium, titanium and carbon (Kovacs, 1991b, with permission of The Electrochemical Society, Inc.).

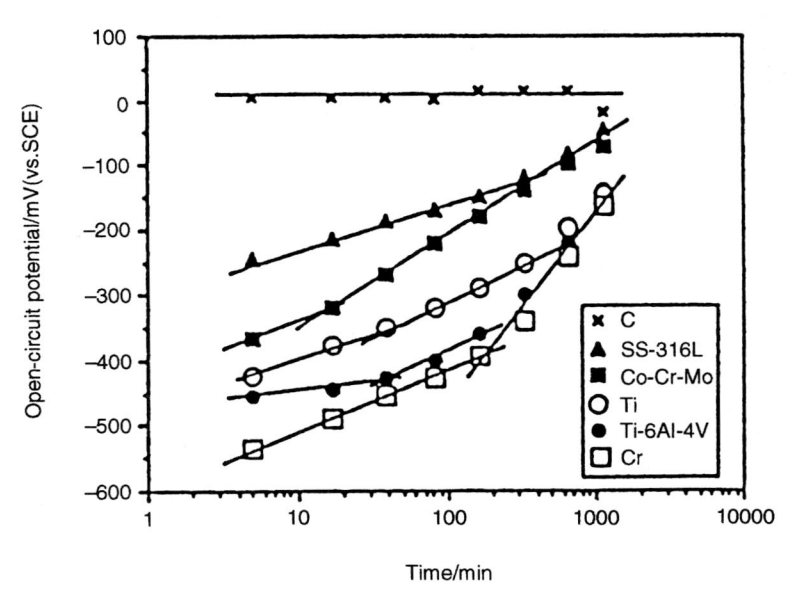

Figure 14.21 Open-circuit potential vs log t plots for orthopaedic implant alloys, chromium, titanium and carbon (Kovacs, 1991b, with permission of The Electrochemical Society, Inc.).

$$\log\left(\frac{1}{R_{p,e}}\right) = c'_e - \left(\frac{1}{b_{c,e}}\right) E_{oc,e} \quad (14.21)$$

$$E_{oc,c} = c''_c + \frac{b_{a,c} b_{c,c}}{b_{a,c} + b_{c,c}} \log t \quad (14.22)$$

$$E_{oc,e} = c''_e + \frac{b_{a,e} b_{c,e}}{b_{a,e} + b_{c,c}} \log t, \quad (14.23)$$

where $E_{oc,c}$ is the open-circuit potential in the region of metal corrosion control, $E_{oc,e}$ is the open-circuit potential in the region of electron exchange control, c'_c, c'_e, c''_c, c''_e are constants, and $b_{a,c}$, $b_{a,e}$, $b_{c,c}$ and $b_{c,e}$ are the anodic and cathodic Tafel constants for the corrosion process and the electron exchange process. The potentials are expressed versus the SCE.

The slopes of the linear parts of the plots corresponding to Equations (14.22) and (14.23) offer a means to determine the factor, containing the Tafel coefficients necessary to calculate the corrosion current density or the exchange current density from the respective polarisation resistance.

Figures 14.22–14.27 show the plots of the logarithm of the reciprocal polarisation resistance for the unit surface area vs the logarithm of time and of the open-circuit potential vs the logarithm of time for the three alloys, each time accompanied by the

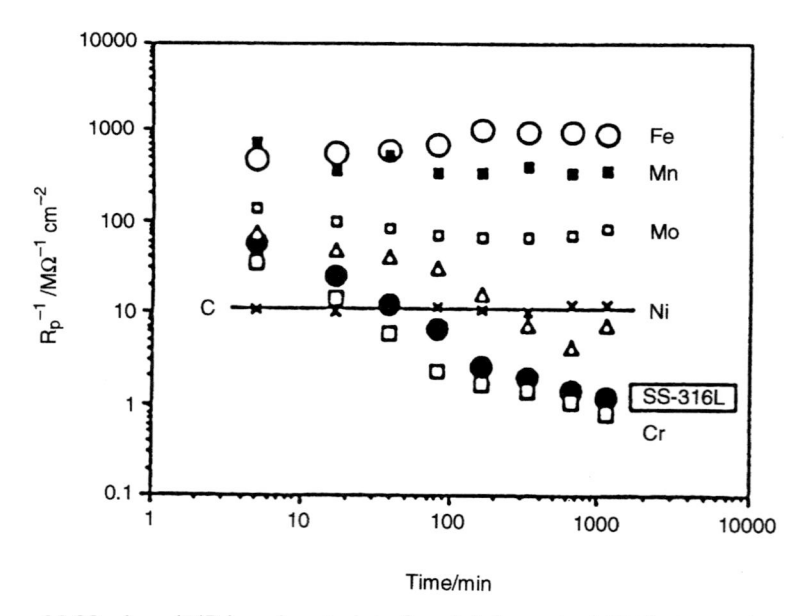

Figure 14.22 Log ($1/R_p$) vs log t plots for stainless steel 316L, iron, chromium, molybdenum, nickel, manganese and carbon (Kovacs, 1991b, with permission of The Electrochemical Society, Inc.).

ELECTROCHEMICAL IMPEDANCE SPECTROSCOPY

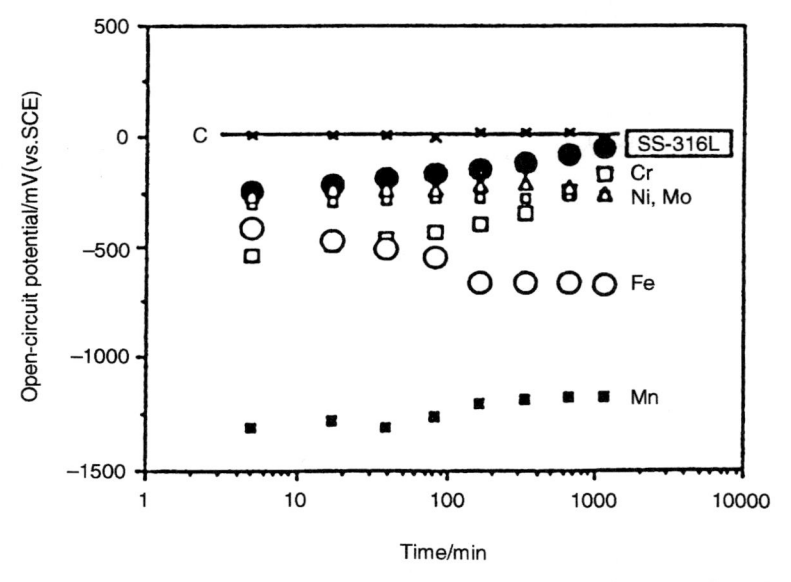

Figure 14.23 Open-circuit potential vs log t plots for stainless steel 316L, iron, chromium, molybdenum, nickel, manganese and carbon (Kovacs, 1991b, with permission of The Electrochemical Society, Inc.).

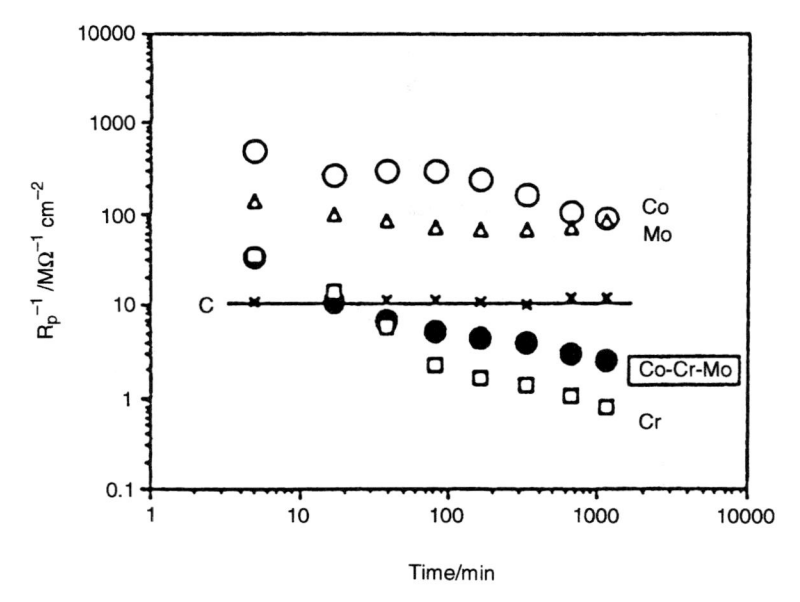

Figure 14.24 Log ($1/R_p$) vs log t plots for CoCrMo alloy, cobalt, chromium, molybdenum and carbon (Kovacs, 1991b, with permission of The Electrochemical Society, Inc.).

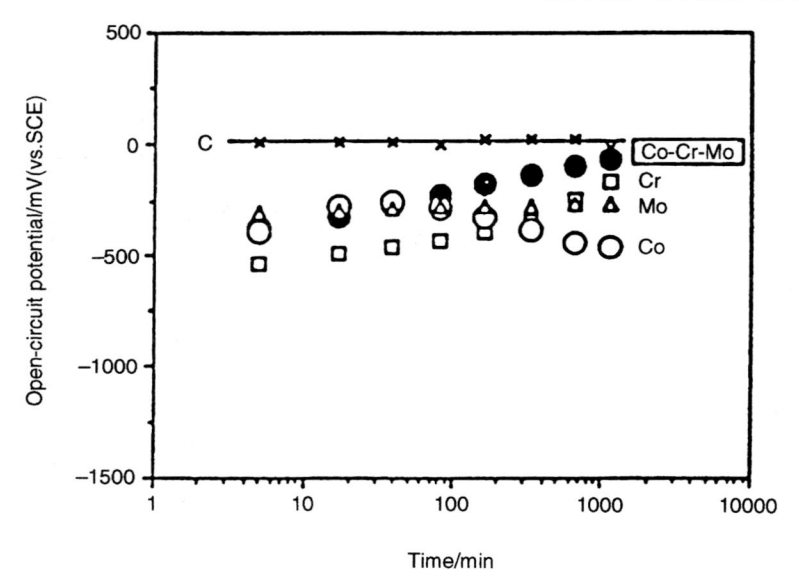

Figure 14.25 Open-circuit potential vs log t plots for CoCrMo alloy, cobalt, chromium, molybdenum and carbon (Kovacs, 1991b, with permission of The Electrochemical Society, Inc.).

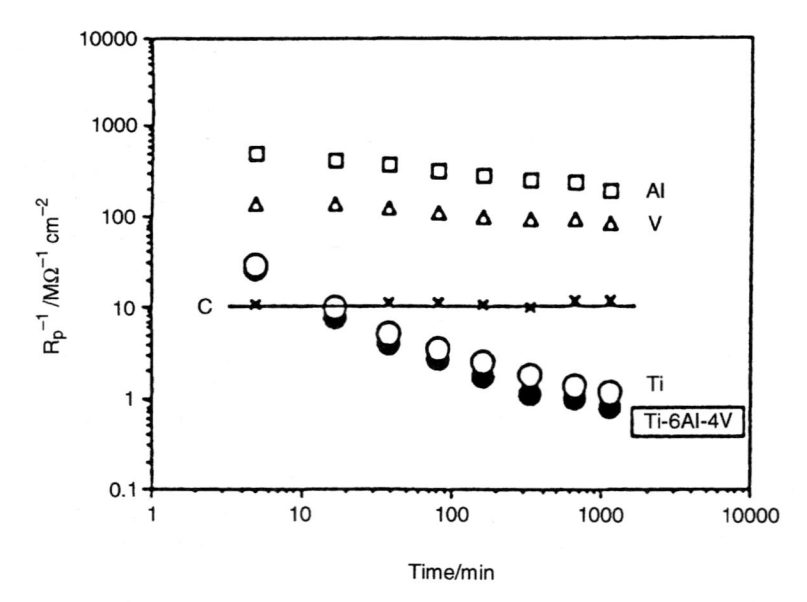

Figure 14.26 Log ($1/R_p$) vs log t plots for Ti6Al4V alloy, titanium, aluminium, vanadium and carbon (Kovacs, 1991b, with permission of The Electrochemical Society, Inc.).

ELECTROCHEMICAL IMPEDANCE SPECTROSCOPY

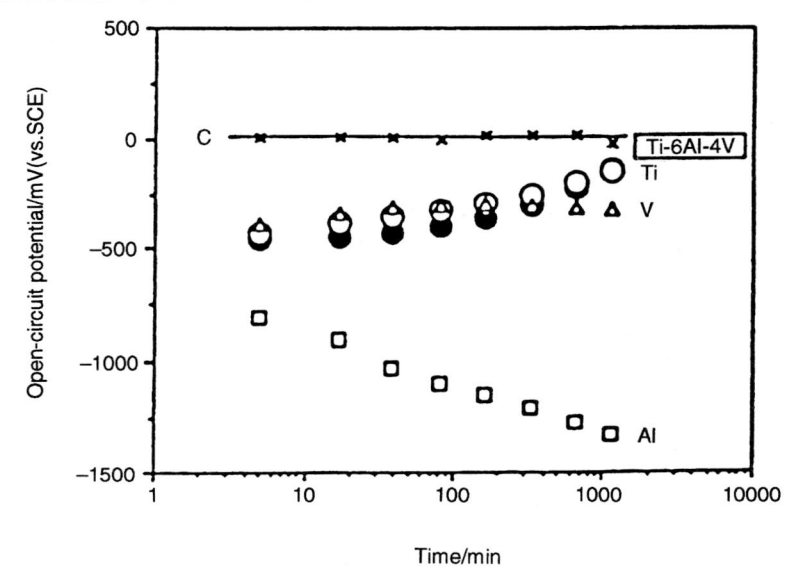

Figure 14.27 Open-circuit potential vs log t plots for Ti6Al4V alloy, titanium, aluminium, vanadium and carbon (Kovacs, 1991b, with permission of The Electrochemical Society, Inc.).

behaviour of the pure alloying metals. They show that the alloys 316L stainless steel and CoCrMo follow a behaviour similar to that of chromium and that the alloy Ti6Al4V behaves in a similar way to titanium. This confirms that the protective passive layer on 316L stainless steel and the CoCrMo alloy is formed by the oxides of chromium, even though it is only an alloying element, and the passive layer on the Ti6Al4V alloy by the oxides of titanium, which is the base metal itself. Both the region where the corrosion process and the region where the electron exchange determine the polarisation resistance, and thus the current density, may be distinguished in the plots for the pure metals as well as for the alloys.

The author further remarks that a clear distinction should be made between two kinds of anodic corrosion processes: the formation of a soluble corrosion product, including non-protective oxides and hydroxides, i.e. the release of a metal ion, on the one hand, and the formation of a protective oxide/hydroxide on the other. Although one process may represent the major part, both may occur at the same time and their current contributions should be summed to obtain the total corrosion current. The corrosion rate of 316L stainless steel and the CoCrMo alloy is determined mainly by the dissolution process and the formation of non-protective oxides or hydroxides of metals other than chromium, which becomes enriched at the surface. The corrosion rate of Ti6Al4V, however, is determined by the formation of a protective oxide layer of titanium, and not by the dissolution process of the elements aluminium or vanadium. When fretting wear mechanically degrades the passivity of an implant alloy, different amounts of ions from the various alloying elements may be released into the biological environment, depending on the occurrence of the processes mentioned above, and this affects biocompatibility. In particular, the present study shows that the alloying elements molybdenum and aluminium will be released as dissolved metal ions into the medium selected rather than form protective layers.

In order to test the behaviour of an implant material in variously conditioned solutions, similar experimental routes may be followed (Kovacs, 1992). Figures 14.28–14.30 represent the open-circuit potential with respect to the SCE vs the logarithm of the reciprocal polarisation resistance for the unit surface area of 316L stainless steel, CoCrMo and Ti6Al4V, respectively, in Ringer's solution with different additives or pH values to simulate different *in vivo* environments. EDTA was added to simulate the complexing action of serum proteins in the biological environment and H_2O_2 was added to simulate inflammatory tissue responses. The pH may vary as a consequence of surgery or may be low in an occluded location. The figures also illustrate the monitoring capabilities of the technique: the arrows show the direction of changes with time. In this respect, the CoCrMo alloy, for example, is seen to be repassivated more efficiently in the presence of the complexing agent, EDTA.

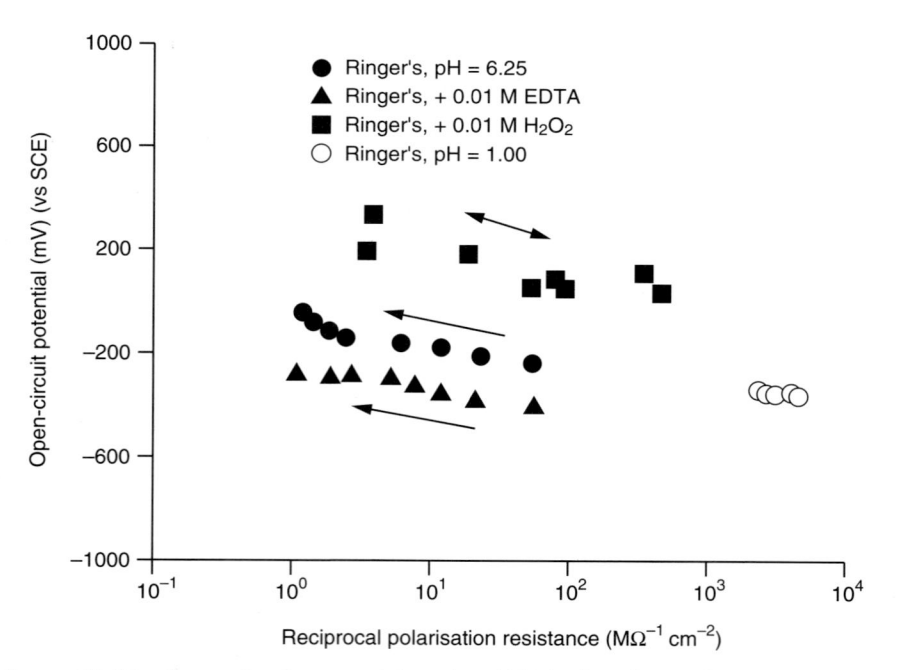

Figure 14.28 Open-circuit potential vs log $(1/R_p)$ plots for stainless steel 316L conditioned in various electrolytes (Kovacs, 1992, with permission of NACE International).

ELECTROCHEMICAL IMPEDANCE SPECTROSCOPY

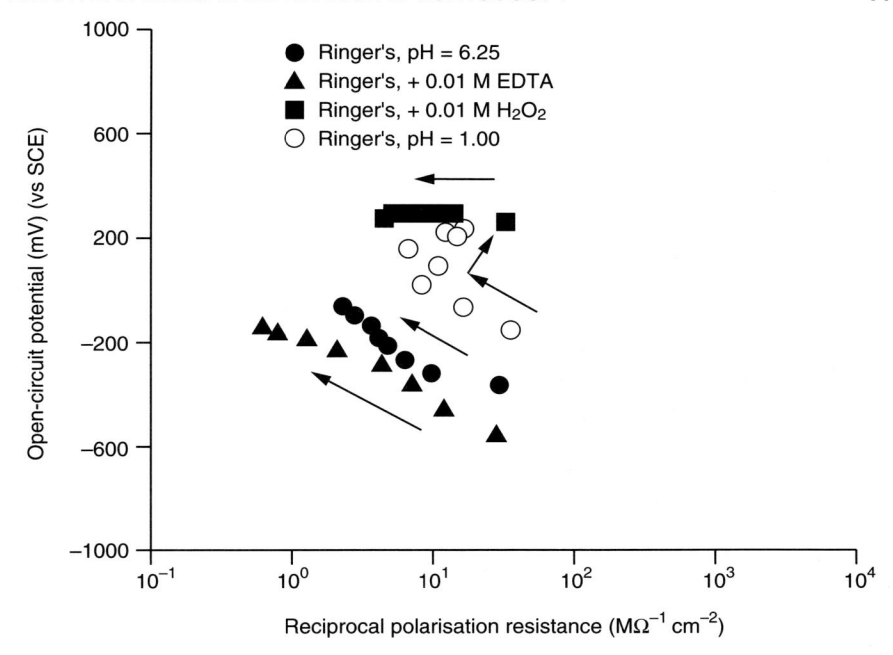

Figure 14.29 Open-circuit potential vs log ($1/R_p$) plots for CoCrMo alloy conditioned in various electrolytes (Kovacs, 1992, with permission of NACE International).

Similar work was performed by Gluszek and Masalaski (1993), who studied the corrosion behaviour of 316L stainless steel in Ringer's solution conditioned at different pH values simulating different tissue environments. The composition of the steel in wt% was: C 0.03, Mn 1.96, Si 0.19, P 0.024, S 0.03, Cr 17.28, Ni 14.8, V 0.35, Mo 2.8, Cu 0.07, Fe balance. The specimens were discs of 15 mm diameter, which were ground with abrasive paper 600, degreased with ethanol and mounted in a special holder designed to avoid crevice corrosion. The composition of Ringer's solution is shown in Table 14.6, the temperature of the solution was 37°C and it was enriched in oxygen before each measurement, and the pH values selected were 7.4, 5.5 and 9.0. A three-electrode cell was installed, which was sealed during the measurements. Potentials were referenced vs the SCE.

The electrochemical impedance data were measured using a Solartron FRA 1255 and a Solartron ECI 1286 controlled by a computer. The frequency was scanned from 0.004 Hz to 10 kHz at an amplitude of 10 mV, and spectra were recorded after 10 min, 1 h, 4 h and 24 h of exposure to the solution. All spectra, when represented in the Nyquist complex plane, formed single, depressed semicircles, so they were modelled with an *RC* circuit containing a CPE. The semicircle best fitting the data was extrapolated to obtain an estimation of the polarisation resistance. It is assumed that the corrosion current, and thus the corrosion rate, is inversely proportional to the polarisation resistance.

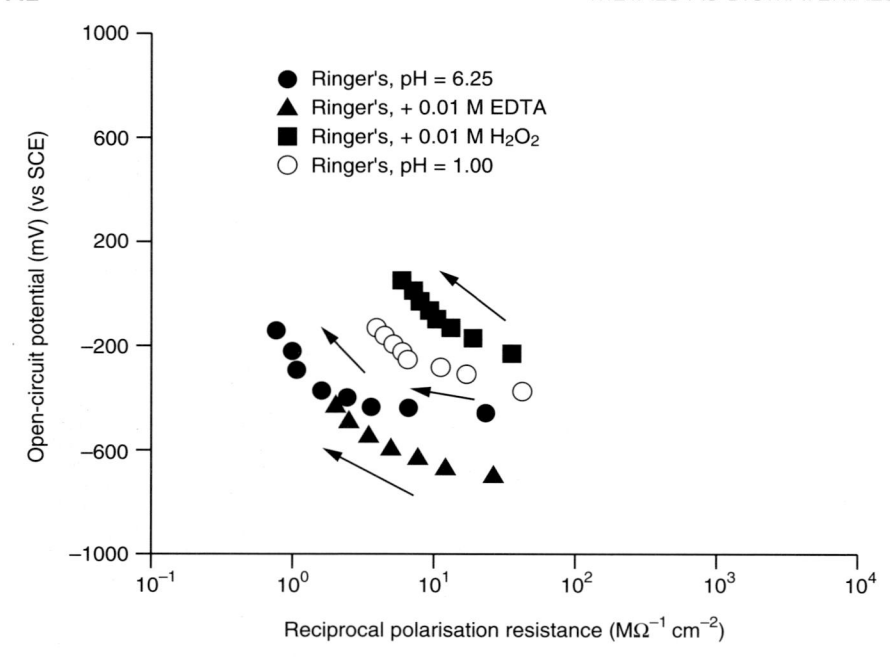

Figure 14.30 Open-circuit potential vs log ($1/R_p$) plots for Ti6Al4V alloy conditioned in various electrolytes (Kovacs, 1992, with permission of NACE International).

The bar chart in Figure 14.31 represents the polarisation resistance for the unit surface area of 316L stainless steel at the three pH values selected and for different exposure times. The corrosion rate does not seem to be affected by the pH value of Ringer's solution, but it is strongly affected by the immersion time, as it decreases considerably. The latter phenomenon should be explained by the growing thickness of the passive layer on top of the steel surface. Figure 14.32 is a similar bar chart for the capacitance per unit surface area. As it decreases with exposure time, the figure confirms the growing tendency of the passive film. In general, the capacitance decreases, and thus the film thickness increases, with increasing pH of Ringer's solution. It is concluded that the best corrosion resistance is maintained in a normal physiological environment of pH 7.4 or in a slightly alkaline medium of pH 9.0, whereas the worst resistance is maintained in a slightly acidic environment of pH 5.5.

Table 14.6 Chemical composition of Ringer's solution (Gluszek and Masalaski, 1993, with permission of The Institute of Materials)

NaCl	8.60 g dm^{-3}	Na$^+$	147.16 mEq dm^{-3}
CaCl$_2$	0.48 g dm^{-3}	Ca^{2+}	4.38 mEq dm^{-3}
KCl	0.30 g dm^{-3}	K$^+$	4.02 mEq dm^{-3}
		Cl$^-$	155.56 mEq dm^{-3}

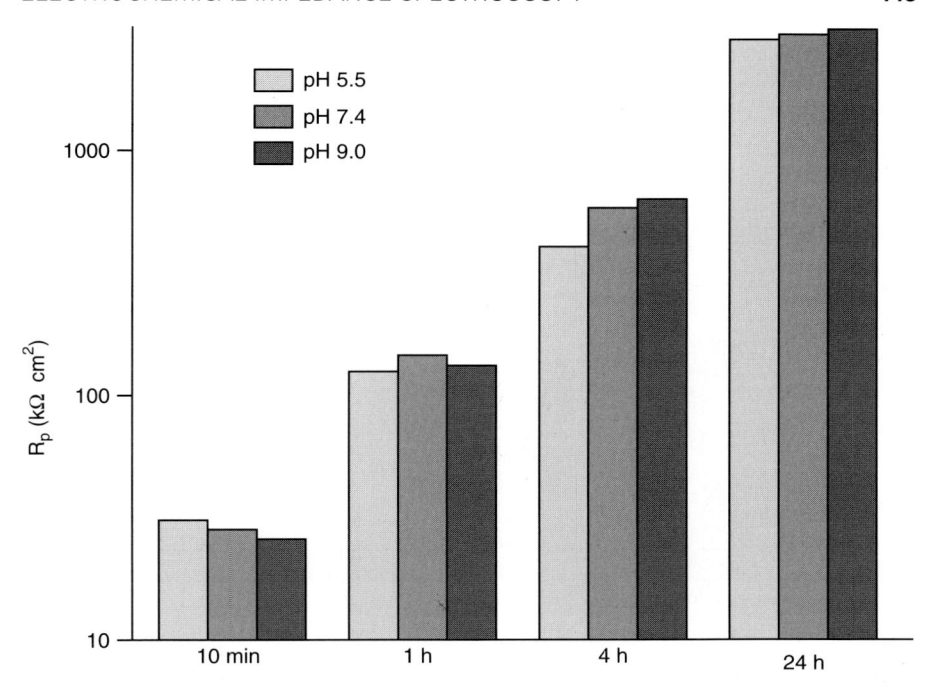

Figure 14.31 Polarisation resistance values of surgical steel 316L after different times of exposure in Ringer's solutions of different pH values (Gluszek and Masalaski, 1993, with permission of The Institute of Materials).

Another team also presented work in the research area of the protective character of passive and oxide layers (Escudero *et al.*, 1995). In this study the material was MA-956, an iron-based superalloy of nominal composition in wt%: Cr 20, Al 4.5, Ti 0.5, Y_2O_3 0.5, Fe balance. It was strengthened by oxide dispersion and processed by mechanical alloying and powder metallurgy. The specimens were in the shape of rods of 30 mm length and 4 mm diameter, and sharp edges on the surface contacting the electrolyte were eliminated by machining the ends of the rods to a round shape. The specimens were further ground with 600 grit SiC paper, degreased and ultrasonically cleaned in alcohol. In the as-received condition the superalloy spontaneously forms a passive film of a few ångströms thickness. Some samples were preoxidised by isothermal treatment at 1100°C in air for a relatively long period of 100 h and after annealing the samples were cooled outside the furnace. This kind of treatment ensures the formation on top of the alloy of a fine and tightly adherent α-alumina layer with an approximate thickness of 5–7 μm. Finally, the corrosion behaviour of these intact samples was also compared to that of defect samples. Two small scratches about 1 mm in length were mechanically punched on to the surface of a preoxidised sample and the intersection of the scratches produced

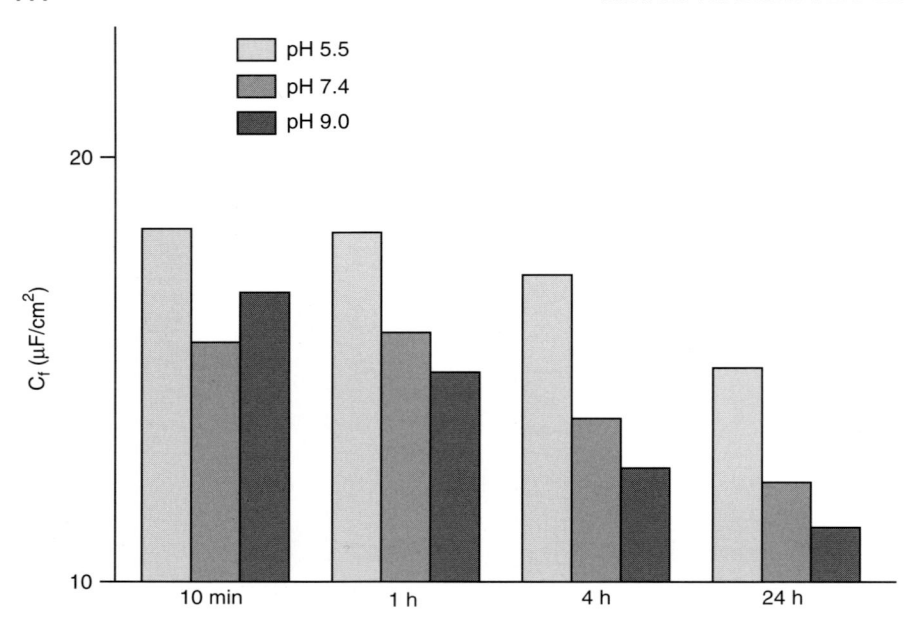

Figure 14.32 Influence of exposure time on the capacitance, C_f, for surgical steel 316L in Ringer's solutions of different pH values (Gluszek and Masalaski, 1993, with permission of The Institute of Materials).

a free metal surface of a few micrometres. The specimens were embedded in epoxy resin to isolate the electrical contact from the test medium, which was Hanks solution, pH 7.4, and the free surface area of the specimen was about 4 cm^2. A three-electrode cell was arranged according to Figure 14.33: the RE is a SCE and the CE is a platinum wire.

The electrochemical impedance measurements were potentiostatically controlled. The applied signal had an amplitude of 10 mV and a frequency varying between 100 kHz and 10 mHz. The specimens were tested in periods from a few hours up to 6 months. The spectra for the samples with the natural passive film and for the pre-oxidised samples were interpreted via an electrical equivalent circuit (Figure 14.34a), where R_e is the ohmic resistance of the electrolyte and, depending on the nature of the specimen, C_f is the capacitance of the passive film and R_f is the resistance of the passive film, or C_{Al} is the capacitance of the alumina layer and R_{Al} is the resistance of the alumina layer. Figure 14.34b shows the corresponding typical Nyquist spectrum and the graphical method of determining the circuit parameters.

Figure 14.35 is the Nyquist and Bode representation of the as-received and preoxidised samples after immersion for 1 day in Hanks solution. The Nyquist plot shows both systems to behave almost purely capacitively within the frequency range selected. From the high-frequency part of the Bode plot of the impedance modulus an ohmic electrolyte resistance is deduced of about 23 Ω for the as-received

ELECTROCHEMICAL IMPEDANCE SPECTROSCOPY

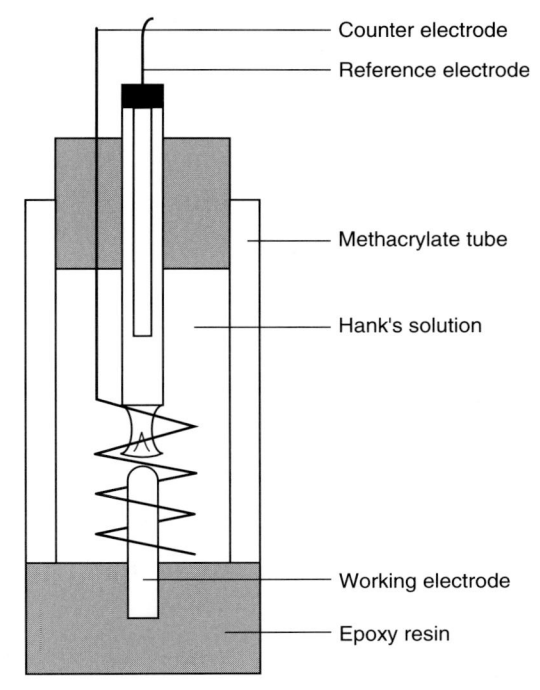

Figure 14.33 Sketch of the cell used in the electrochemical tests in Escudero et al. (1995). (From *Biomaterials*, Vol. 16, Escudero et al., Electrochemical impedance spectroscopy of preoxidized MA956 superalloy during *in vitro* experiments, pp. 735–40, 1995, with kind permission from Elsevier Science Ltd.)

specimen, and the same plot leads to the capacitance values of both kinds of specimens, according to:

$$C_f \text{ or } C_{Al} = \frac{1}{|Z|\omega}, \quad (14.24)$$

where ω is taken to be 1. The authors claim that when Z', the real part of the impedance, is plotted against $-\omega Z''$, the negative imaginary part of the impedance times the angular frequency, the slope of the oblique region is given by $-RC$, which allows the calculation of R_f or R_{Al}, even if only a part of the semicircle is obtained in the Nyquist spectrum. This procedure is illustrated in Figure 14.36 for the as-received and the preoxidised samples, based on the results of Figure 14.35. Table 14.7 groups the circuit parameters for the unit surface area, determined in the way described, of both kinds of samples and for different exposure times. The natural passive film of the as-received samples demonstrates a high resistive value, R_f, and a low capacitive value, C_f, in the order of magnitude $10^5 \ \Omega \ cm^2$ and $10^{-5} \ F \ cm^{-2}$, respectively, for all exposure times, and these values are a sign of good corrosion behaviour. They are, however, superseded by at least two orders of magnitude when the specimens are

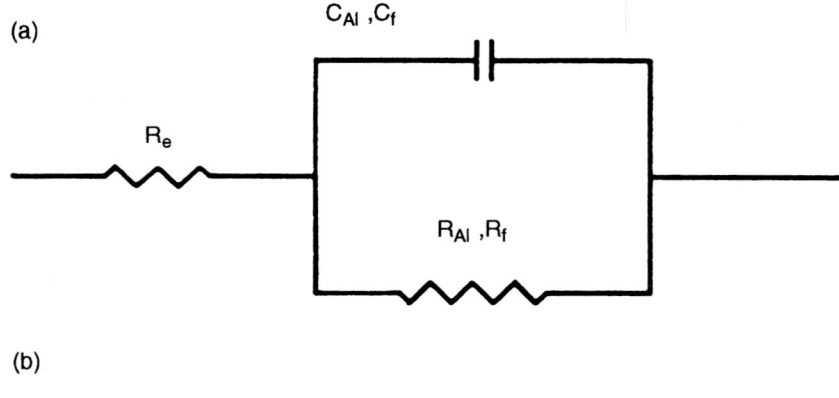

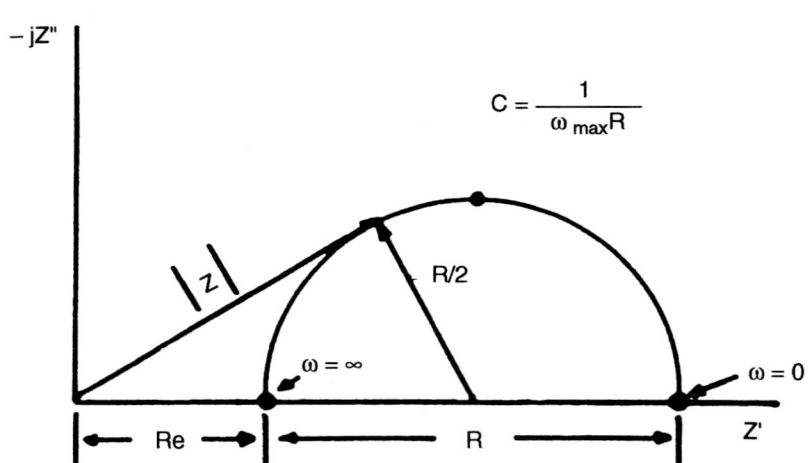

Figure 14.34 (a) Equivalent circuit for MA-956 alloy in the as-received or pre-oxidised condition; (b) typical Nyquist plot for the circuit (Escudero et al., 1995). (From *Biomaterials*, Vol. 16, Escudero et al., Electrochemical impedance spectroscopy of preoxidized MA956 superalloy during *in vitro* experiments, pp. 735–40, 1995, with kind permission from Elsevier Science Ltd.)

preoxidised and tested shortly after immersion: R_{Al} is about $10^8 \ \Omega \ cm^2$ and C_{Al} is about $10^{-8} \ F \ cm^{-2}$. For longer exposure times the corrosion resistance first appears to decrease slightly and then, after some 270 days, almost returns to the original value. This is because the alumina layer contains a discontinuous pattern of microdefects. The high resistance measured in the beginning of the test is related to the rather slow penetration of the electrolyte into the defects. When penetration is complete and the electrolyte has finally reached the metal substrate, then the resistance is at a minimum value, say $10^6 \ \Omega \ cm^2$ after 30 days. Afterwards, when corrosion products form that block the defects, higher resistances are again obtained.

ELECTROCHEMICAL IMPEDANCE SPECTROSCOPY

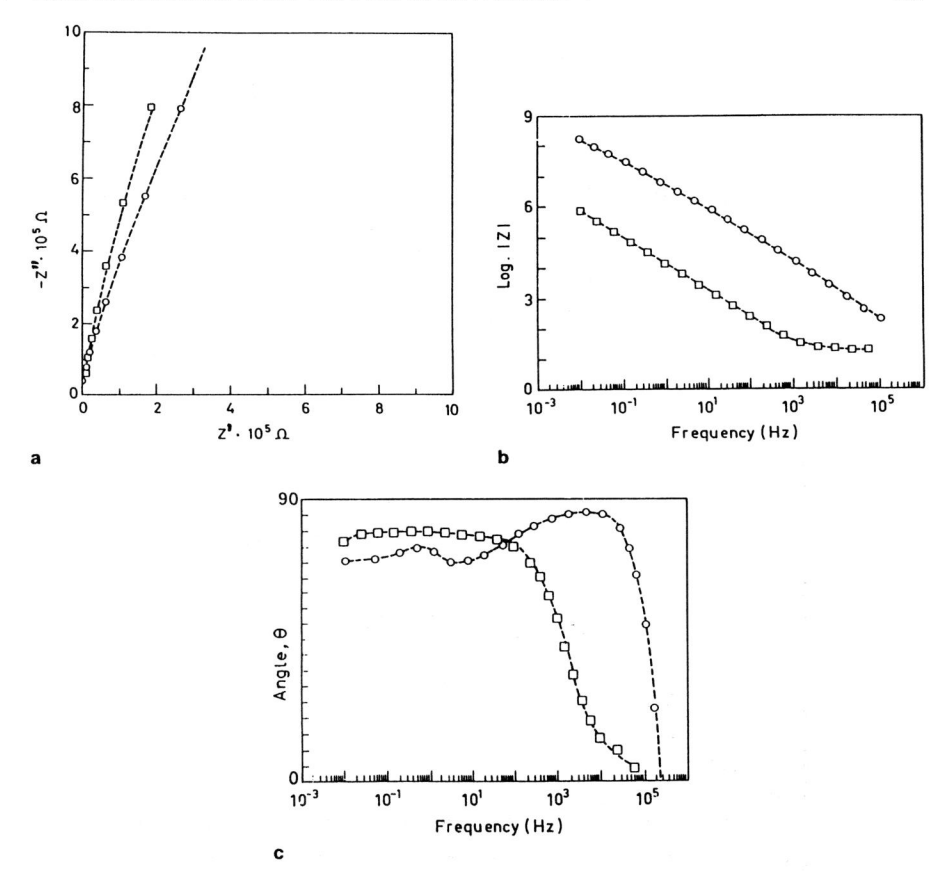

Figure 14.35 (a) Nyquist and (b,c) Bode plots for MA-956 alloy in both the as-received (□) and preoxidised (○) conditions, after 1 day in Hanks' solution (Escudero *et al.*, 1995). (From *Biomaterials*, Vol. 16, Escudero *et al.*, Electrochemical impedance spectroscopy of preoxidized MA956 superalloy during *in vitro* experiments, pp. 735–40, 1995, with kind permission from Elsevier Science Ltd.)

Opposite to these intrinsic microdefects, externally applied defects may affect the protective power of the alumina layer, and therefore scratched samples, as described above, are also tested. As new channels, parallel to the existing microchannels, are thus created in the alumina layer, the circuit model should be completed in that sense (Figure 14.37). The new circuit elements, which represent phenomena at the substrate interface, i.e. at the base of pores or defects, are C_d, the double-layer capacitance, and R_t, the charge transfer resistance, which is inversely proportional to the corrosion rate.

In Figure 14.38 the Nyquist and Bode plots for the defective specimen are shown for different exposure times. After 1 day the shape of the spectrum has not changed

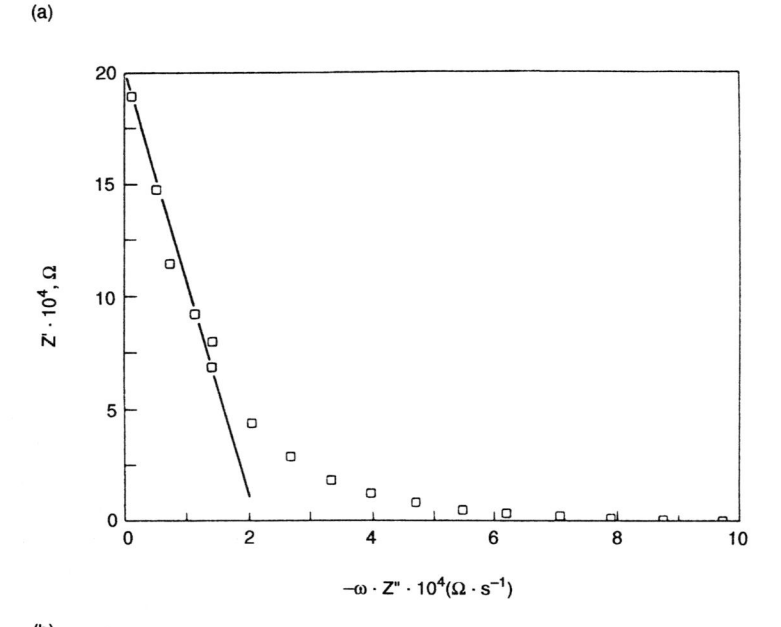

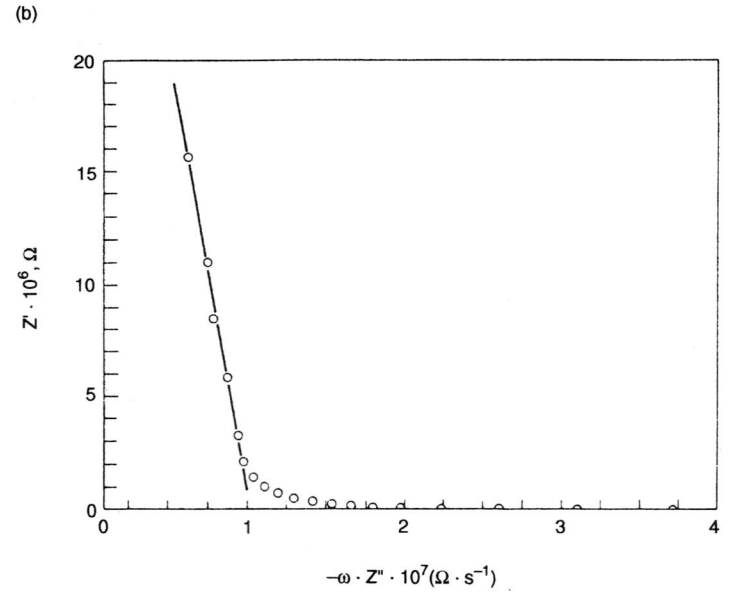

Figure 14.36 Representation of Z' against $\omega Z''$ for MA-956 alloy in (a) as-received and (b) preoxidised conditions, after 1 day in Hanks' solution (Escudero *et al.*, 1995). (From *Biomaterials*, Vol. 16, Escudero *et al.*, Electrochemical impedance spectroscopy of preoxidized MA956 superalloy during *in vitro* experiments, pp. 735–40, 1995, with kind permission from Elsevier Science Ltd.)

ELECTROCHEMICAL IMPEDANCE SPECTROSCOPY

Table 14.7 Evolution with time of the electrochemical parameters for both preoxidised and as-received MA-956 alloy samples (Escudero et al., 1995)

Time (days)	Alumina layer		Passive film	
	C_{Al} (F cm^{-2})	R_{Al} (Ω cm^2)	C_f (F cm^{-2})	R_f (Ω cm^2)
1	2.9×10^{-8}	1.3×10^8	7.1×10^{-5}	2.1×10^5
7	2.3×10^{-8}	9.0×10^{-7}	1.0×10^{-4}	0.7×10^5
30	1.6×10^{-7}	8.3×10^6	5.7×10^{-5}	0.8×10^5
180	4.7×10^{-8}	1.0×10^7	0.9×10^{-5}	0.7×10^5
270	6.5×10^{-8}	1.8×10^8	3.9×10^{-5}	0.8×10^5

very much compared with the intact samples, while after 8 days the curve is a clear semicircle followed by a straight line, which becomes another semicircle after longer exposure times, e.g. 180 days. The second semicircle obtained in the Nyquist plot at lower frequencies is confirmed by the two maxima in the Bode plot of the phase angle of the impedance and provides evidence for corrosion phenomena under charge transfer control. Both semicircles lead to values for the parameters of the circuit represented in Figure 14.37. The parameters obtained at the higher frequencies describe the protective capacity of the alumina layer in the non-defective zones, while those obtained at the lower frequencies reflect the corrosion process at the base of the defect. The parameters are listed in Table 14.8 for different immersion times. Shortly after immersion the corrosion resistance of the defective sample is slightly lower than that of the intact preoxidised sample, but higher than that of the as-received specimen. After 8 days, however, the resistance is decreasing to below that of the as-received one and after very long exposure times, e.g. 180 days, the sample has degenerated.

The corrosion behaviour of this MA-956 superalloy, in the as-received and the preoxidised state, was further compared with more conventional materials, i.e. CoNiCr, TiAlV and stainless steel coated with a γ-alumina layer, the chemical

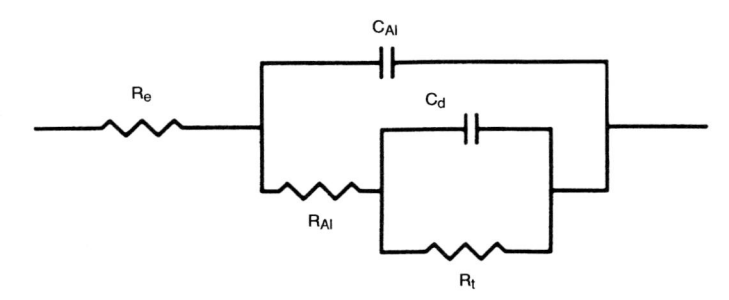

Figure 14.37 Equivalent circuit for preoxidised MA-956 alloy with defects in the alumina layer (Escudero et al., 1995). (From *Biomaterials*, Vol. 16, Escudero et al., Electrochemical impedance spectroscopy of preoxidized MA956 superalloy during *in vitro* experiments, pp. 735–40, 1995, with kind permission from Elsevier Science Ltd.)

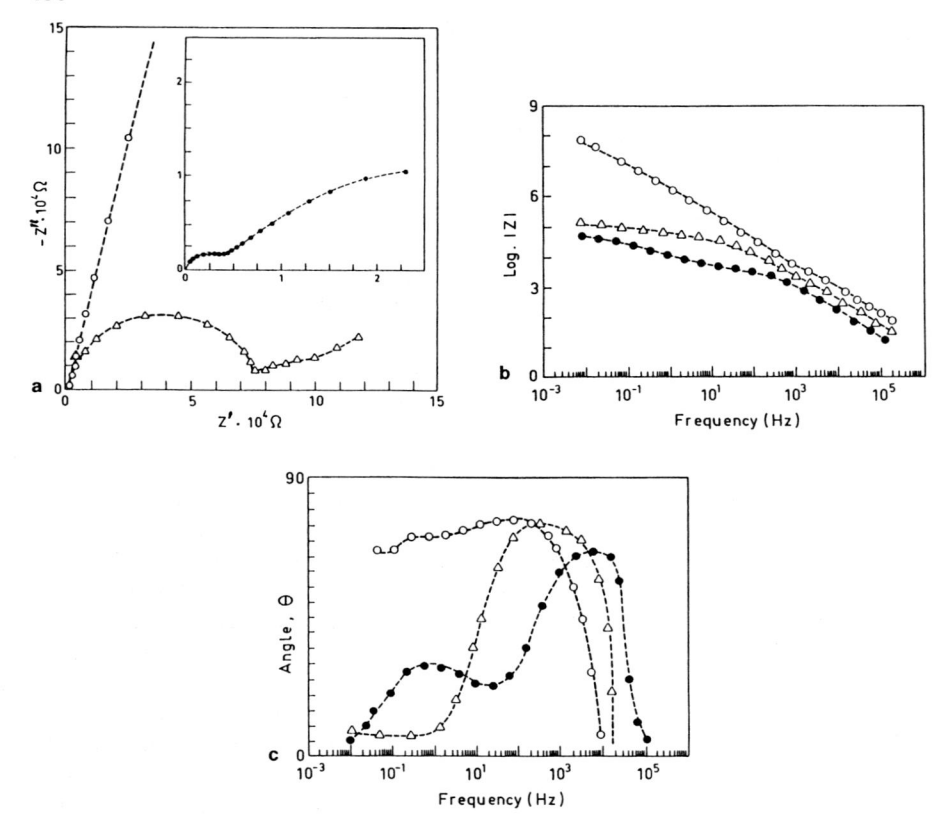

Figure 14.38 (a) Nyquist and (b,c) Bode plots for a preoxidised MA-956 alloy sample with an extrinsic defect in the oxide layer after different immersion times in Hanks' solution: ○, 1 day; △, 8 days; ●, 180 days (Escudero et al., 1995). (From *Biomaterials*, Vol. 16, Escudero et al., Electrochemical impedance spectroscopy of preoxidized MA956 superalloy during *in vitro* experiments, pp. 735–40, 1995, with kind permission from Elsevier Science Ltd.)

Table 14.8 Evolution with time of the electrochemical parameters for preoxidised MA-956 alloy samples in the presence of an extrinsic defect in the alumina layer (Escudero et al., 1995). (From *Biomaterials*, Vol. 16, Escudero et al., Electrochemical impedance spectroscopy of preoxidized MA956 superalloy during *in vitro* experiments, pp. 735–40, 1995, with kind permission from Elsevier Science Ltd)

Time (days)	Capacitance (F)	Resistance (Ω)
1	1.4×10^{-7}	1.3×10^{7}
8	2.4×10^{-7}	8.0×10^{4}
180	First semicircle 2.4×10^{-7}	First semicircle 5.2×10^{3}
	Second semicircle 1.7×10^{-5}	Second semicircle 7.0×10^{4}

Table 14.9 Chemical composition of the different metallic biomaterials investigated in Escudero *et al.* (1996). (From *Journal of Biomedical Materials Research*, Vol. 31, Escudero *et al.*, Comparative study of the corrosion behavior of MA-956 and conventional metallic biomaterials, pp. 313–7, 1996. Reprinted by permission of John Wiley & Sons, Ltd)

Metallic materials	Composition (wt%)
CoNiCr alloy	35Co35Ni20Cr10Mo
TiAlV alloy	6Al4V, Ti balance
MA-956 superalloy	20Cr4.5Al0.5Ti0.5Y_2O_3, Fe balance
Stainless steel	18Cr12Ni2.5Mo, <0.003C, Fe balance

composition of which is listed in Table 14.9 (Escudero *et al.*, 1996). The samples had a cylindrical shape and an exposed surface area between 10 and 15 cm². The MA-956 superalloy samples, both polished and preoxidised, were prepared as described above, and the preoxidised samples thus obtained a typical α-alumina thickness of 4 μm. The TiAlV and CoNiCr alloy samples were first polished with 600 grit SiC paper, then degreased and cleaned ultrasonically in alcohol. The stainless steel sample received its alumina coating via plasma spraying. α-Alumina powder was applied directly on to the stainless steel surface, and after the plasma spraying a face-centred cubic γ-alumina layer was obtained, of approximate thickness 200 μm.

The test medium was again Hanks solution, pH 7.4, at room temperature. The specimens were arranged as WEs into a three-electrode cell, where the RE was a SCE and the CE was a stainless steel wire. Electrochemical impedance measurements were performed using an applied sine wave of amplitude 10 mV between 1 mHz and 64 kHz.

As an example, the Nyquist plots for the polished MA-956 superalloy and the TiAlV alloy after 100 days' exposure to Hanks solution are given in Figure 14.39. For TiAlV a charge transfer resistance may be inferred from the diameter of the semi circle, when it is extrapolated towards the lower frequencies. This procedure is more difficult for the capacitive arc related to the polished MA-956 superalloy, in which an approximate charge transfer resistance is deduced from the impedance value at the lowest frequency. For all the materials investigated such a charge transfer resistance is determined and the next step is the calculation of a maximum threshold of the corrosion current density, i_{corr}. Figure 14.40 is a bar chart comparing these maximum corrosion rates after 100 days in Hanks solution, and the authors state that all materials tested behave in a stationary way during the testing period. Although the difference in performance among the conventional alloys is not very pronounced, the CoNiCr alloy shows the best corrosion resistance, with a maximum corrosion current density level of 3×10^{-2} μA cm^{-2}. The polished MA-956 superalloy performs better than the conventional materials and for the preoxidised MA-956 sample the improvement even amounts to two orders of magnitude. The

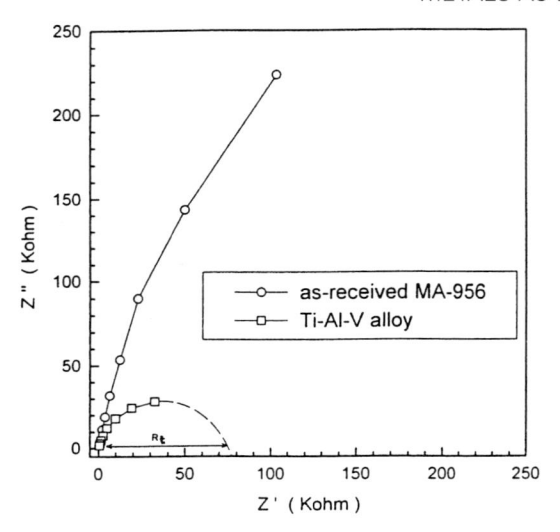

Figure 14.39 Nyquist plot for TiAlV alloy (□) and as-received MA-956 superalloy (○) after 100 days' exposure to Hanks' solution. (From *Journal of Biomedical Materials Research*, Vol. 31, Escudero et al., Comparative study of the corrosion behavior of MA-956 and conventional metallic biomaterials, pp. 313–7, 1996. Reprinted by permission of John Wiley & Sons, Ltd.)

large difference between the two alumina-coated alloys, stainless steel and MA-956 superalloy, relates to the nature of the crystallinity of the respective alumina layers: the plasma sprayed γ-alumina is highly porous, which easily allows contact between the electrolyte and stainless steel substrate, whereas the thermally induced α-alumina is a compact and dense material acting as a perfectly insulating dielectric. The conclusion is that the preoxidised MA-956 superalloy experiences very slow corrosion kinetics with respect to the conventional biomaterials.

14.4 THE EFFECT OF A COATING

In the work referenced in Barbosa (1991) the step was made from the study of passive films towards the study of purposely induced coatings on biomaterials, which are meant to improve the corrosion resistance of those materials *in vivo* and to improve the biocompatibility. With regard to the corrosion behaviour, the question is raised of whether the possibly better material performance may have resulted solely from the barrier effect of the coating or from a chemical interaction between the coating material and the substrate material leading to an interface which inhibited further (corrosion) reactions. In particular, the work relates to the effect of hydroxyapatite coatings on the corrosion resistance of AISI 316L stainless steel and commercially pure titanium, and investigates the degree to which Ca^{2+} and PO_4^{3-} ions, released by the dissolution of such coatings, affect the electrochemical properties of the materials mentioned.

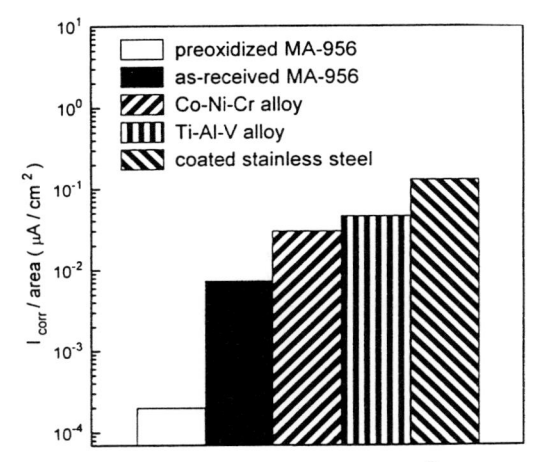

Figure 14.40 Corrosion current density i_{corr} (µA cm^{-2}) for the different studied biomaterials after 100 days' immersion in Hanks' solution. (From *Journal of Biomedical Materials Research*, Vol. 31, Escudero *et al.*, Comparative study of the corrosion behavior of MA-956 and conventional metallic biomaterials, pp. 313–7, 1996. Reprinted by permission of John Wiley & Sons, Ltd.)

The metal specimens had a thickness of 1 mm and an exposed surface area of 0.5×0.8 mm^2. They were wet ground with 600 grit SiC paper and connected to an electrical conductor.

The solutions selected were: 0.154 M NaCl as a control (solution 1), 0.154 M NaCl saturated with hydroxyapatite (solution 2), and 0.154 M NaCl with 1 mM CaCl$_2$ and 2.7 mM Na$_2$HPO$_4$ (solution 3), made on the basis of distilled water, commercially available hydroxyapatite and pro analysis grade chemicals. Under stationary conditions the concentrations in the second solution were 0.38 mM in Ca^{2+} and 0.26 mM in PO$_4^{3-}$, and in the third solution the concentrations of Ca^{2+} and HPO$_4^{2-}$ were such that there was supersaturation with respect to octacalcium phosphate, although precipitation was not observed during the tests. The solutions were not deaerated and were kept at room temperature (20 ± 2°C).

The electrochemical cell consisted of two compartments, each containing 5 cm^3 of solution. One compartment held the SCE and the other the WE, which was the specimen, and the CE, which was a platinum foil with a surface area of 800 mm^2. EIS measurements were performed with a set-up similar to that described by Silva *et al.* (1990) and controlled by a computer and appropriate software. The frequency was varied between 0.05 Hz and 100 kHz. Measurements were made after exposure during well-determined periods under an open circuit in solutions 1 and 2, or after 30 min under potentiostatic control at −100, 0 or +100 mV in solutions 1 and 3.

All EIS spectra were reported to have the typical depressed semicircle form in the Nyquist representation, as is demonstrated in Figure 14.41 for titanium in solution 1 after 12 h at open circuit. The impedance was reduced to the unit surface area of the electrode. Using a computer program, the curves were fitted to a semicircle, the

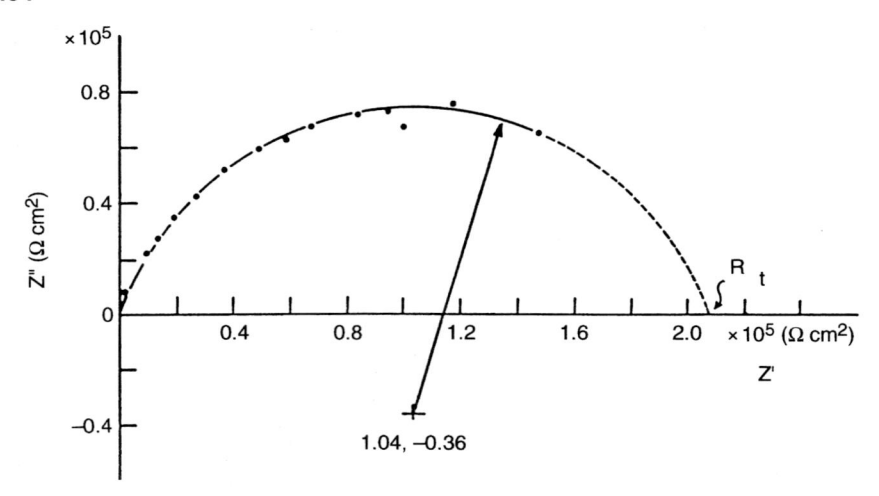

Figure 14.41 Nyquist plot of the impedance spectrum of a titanium electrode immersed in solution 1 for 12 h under open circuit (Barbosa, 1991). (With permission from Butterworth-Heinemann Ltd.)

centre of which lay below the real axis. The square of the correlation coefficient is usually 0.999 or better. One characteristic of the spectra, called the charge transfer resistance for the unit surface area, R_t, is determined from the intersection of the depressed semicircle and the real axis at low frequencies, taking into account the solution resistance. Another characteristic, called in general terms the interface capacitance per unit surface area, C_i, is approached by an equation similar to (14.24):

$$C_i = \frac{1}{|Z|_{\omega=1}} \tag{14.25}$$

where $|Z|_{\omega=1}$ is the modulus of the impedance for the unit surface area measured at an angular frequency of 1 rad s^{-1}.

The differences among the experiments and their spectra is reflected in different sets of the characteristics, R_t and C_i.

In Figure 14.42 the behaviour of titanium in open circuit in solutions 1 and 2 after 3 and 24 h of exposure is plotted in the Bode representation of the logarithm of the impedance modulus for the unit surface area. The impedance modulus is always smaller in solution 2 than in solution 1, and it is inferred that the same holds for the respective charge transfer resistances, which means that the dissolution process becomes easier in the presence of hydroxyapatite.

Table 14.10 gives values of the interface capacitance, C_i, calculated from the impedance spectra of titanium in the same solutions after the same periods. C_i diminishes in time in both solutions, meaning that the thickness of the passive film increases if the contribution of the double layer is neglected and if a relation analogous to that of Equation (14.10) is considered. As the films in solution 2 have

ELECTROCHEMICAL IMPEDANCE SPECTROSCOPY

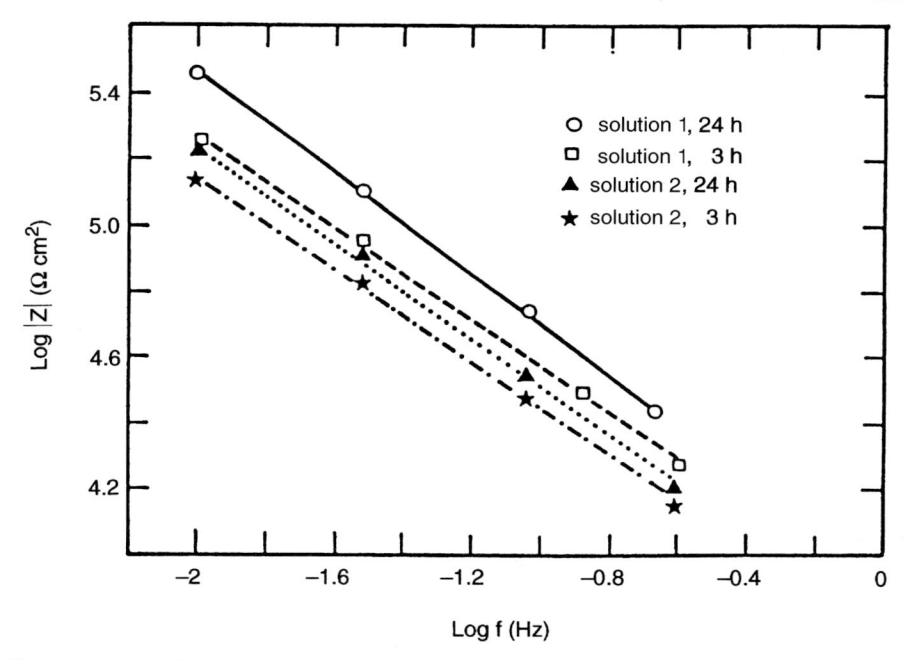

Figure 14.42 Bode magnitude representation of the impedance data obtained for titanium in NaCl and hydroxyapatite (HAP) solutions after 3 and 24 h of immersion (Barbosa, 1991). (With permission from Butterworth-Heinemann Ltd.)

a larger interface capacitance than in solution 1, it follows that the former have a smaller thickness, e.g. if one takes $\varepsilon_r = 100$ for the film, then in solution 1 after 24 h the thickness is 3.2 nm and in solution 2 after 24 h it is 2.1 nm.

In the bar chart of Figure 14.43 the charge transfer resistance for stainless steel is compared in solutions 1 and 3 and at different applied potentials, while in Figure 14.44 the same is done for titanium. The presence of Ca^{2+} and HPO_4^{2-} ions raises the charge transfer resistance of stainless steel at the three applied potentials, whereas that of titanium is reduced. Thus, the film on stainless steel becomes more resistive in the presence of Ca^{2+} and HPO_4^{2-} ions and the film on titanium becomes less

Table 14.10 Interfacial capacitance of titanium in solutions 1 (NaCl) and 2 (NaCl + hydroxyapatite) (Barbosa, 1991). (With permission from Butterworth-Heinemann Ltd)

Solution	Duration of immersion (h)	C_i ($\mu F\ cm^{-2}$)
1	3	35
	24	27
2	3	50
	24	42

resistive. The conclusion is that a lower corrosion rate should result for stainless steel coated with hydroxyapatite and a higher one for titanium. Further, the charge transfer resistance is lower for stainless steel than for titanium, which confirms the lower corrosion rate of titanium.

Table 14.11 lists the values of the interface capacitance calculated from the impedance spectra for stainless steel and titanium in solutions 1 and 3 at three applied potentials. For stainless steel it appears that at 0 and 100 mV the interface capacitance is larger in solution 1 than in solution 3, so the film thickness is smaller, whereas at −100 mV the difference is not significant. Another observation is that the higher the applied potential, the smaller the interface capacitance, and thus the thicker the film.

For titanium the interface capacitance remains almost unchanged in solutions 1 and 3 at all applied potentials.

This work was continued by Sousa and Barbosa (1995), who investigated stainless steel coated with hydroxyapatite of different thicknesses. The substrate material was 350L duplex stainless steel, with a semiquantitative composition, expressed in wt% and determined by energy dispersive spectrum analysis, of: Fe 56.3, Cr 21.3, Ni 13.2, Mn 5.8, Si 0.4, Mo 3.0. The hydroxyapatite coating was applied by plasma spraying in two different nominal thicknesses, 50 and 200 µm. The coated samples were compared with polished passivated surfaces. The samples were cylindrical and their preparation is described in Sousa and Barbosa (1996). They were provided with an electrical contact via a threaded rod and their upper part was covered with a lacquer. The medium selected was Hanks balanced salt solution, kept at 37 ± 1°C.

The 100 ml polymer cell was equipped with the specimen as the WE, a SCE and a square platinum sheet of 800 mm^2 surface area as a CE. The measurement set-up consisted of a potentiostat, a FRA and a computer. The applied ac signals had an amplitude of ± 10 mV and a frequency varying between 10 kHz and 1 Hz. They were superimposed on the corrosion potential, measured after 30 min in open circuit.

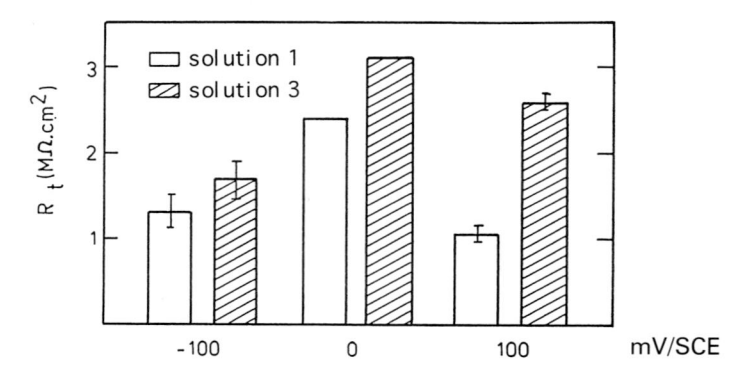

Figure 14.43 Charge transfer resistance of 316L stainless steel in solutions 1 and 3 at −100, 0 and 100 mV/SCE (Barbosa, 1991). (With permission from Butterworth-Heinemann Ltd.)

ELECTROCHEMICAL IMPEDANCE SPECTROSCOPY

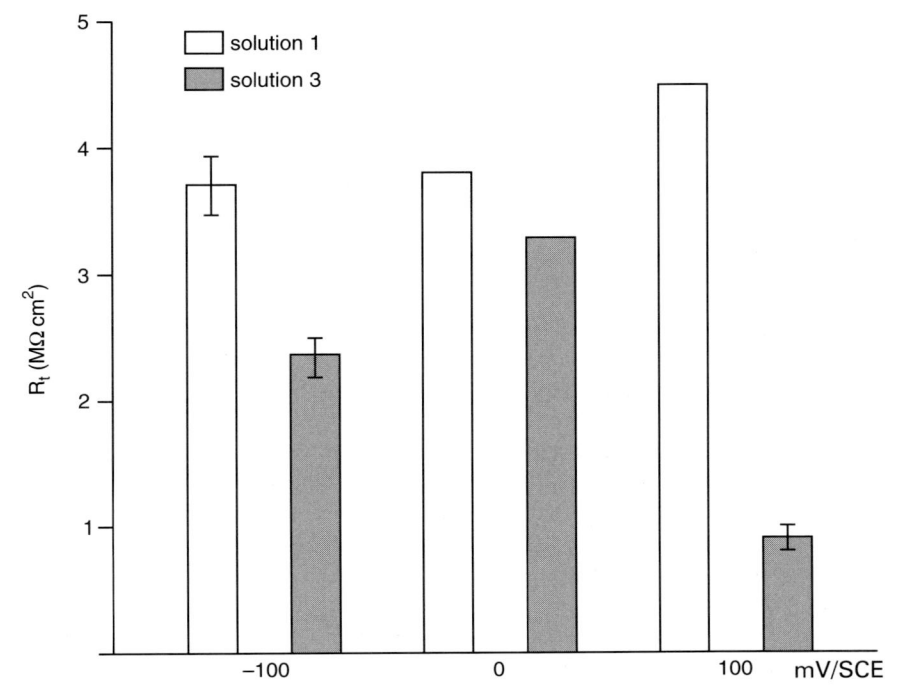

Figure 14.44 Charge transfer resistance of titanium in solutions 1 and 3 at −100, 0 and 100 mV/SCE (Barbosa, 1991). (With permission from Butterworth-Heinemann Ltd.)

Table 14.11 Interfacial capacitance of 316L stainless steel and titanium in solutions 1 and 3 at three applied potentials (Barbosa, 1991). (With permission from Butterworth-Heinemann Ltd)

Material	Solution	Potential (mV)	C_i ($\mu F\ cm^{-2}$)
Stainless steel	1	−100	38
		0	35
		100	33
	3	−100	40
		0	26
		100	24
Titanium	1	−100	20
		0	23
		100	22
	3	−100	26
		0	25
		100	26

As the Nyquist representation of the EIS spectra did not appear to fit to a simple model, the authors listed the impedance moduli for the unit surface area, averaged over three measurements, at a high frequency, 1000 Hz, and a low frequency, 1 Hz (Table 14.12). At low frequencies the impedance is mainly determined by charge transfer and mass transfer processes. A thicker coating raises the impedance values, owing to a reduction in real surface area and/or in the oxidation rate of the substrate, and it therefore offers a higher degree of protection.

The surface roughness of the metal is another important parameter in a discussion of interface phenomena of an implant material, even if it is coated (Sousa and Barbosa, 1996). Cylindrical specimens (Figure 14.45) were made from the Ti6Al4V alloy. The diameter was 8 mm and the height of the exposed part 30 mm. Three surface conditions were considered: polished/passivated, grit-blasted/passivated and grit-blasted/coated with hydroxyapatite. The preparation of the first type was as follows: pickling in a solution of 1% HF and 15% HNO_3 (v/v%) for 4 min at room temperature, wet grinding with SiC paper down to 600 grit, polishing with diamond down to 1 μm and passivating in 30% HNO_3 (v/v%) at 60°C for 10 min. After each step the specimen was rinsed in distilled and deionised water in an ultrasonic bath for 3 min, except for after the last step, when the ultrasonic bath was omitted, and then the specimen was rinsed in alcohol and dried. The second type was grit-blasted with alumina particles and passivated as before. The third type was grit-blasted in the same way and coated using plasma spraying with hydroxyapatite grains of 60 μm approximate diameter in a thickness of 50 and 200 μm. The medium was again Hanks balanced salt solution, the composition of which is shown in Table 14.13, at 37 ± 1°C. Other experimental details are as described above.

In Table 14.14 the impedance moduli are listed for the geometrical unit surface area of the different specimens at two frequencies, 1043 and 1.63 Hz. The numbers are averages of two measurements, with the ratio of that value to the one measured on the polished surface in parentheses. The impedance moduli of the grit-blasted specimens are about one-third of those of the polished ones, a ratio which is believed to correspond to the surface roughness factor obtained through the grit-blasting process. An important result is that deposition of a 50-μm-thick hydroxyapatite coating makes the impedance modulus decrease in spite of the covering of the metal surface, and the suggestion is made that some characteristics of the interface

Table 14.12 Impedance moduli ($\Omega\ cm^2$) at two frequencies for 350L duplex stainless steel coated with hydroxyapatite of different thicknesses (Sousa and Barbosa, 1995). (From *Journal of Materials Science: Materials in Medicine*, Vol. 6, Sousa and Barbosa. The effect of hydroxyapatite thickness on metal ion release from stainless steel substrates, Table 3, pp. 818–23, 1995, with kind permission of Chapman & Hall)

Frequency (Hz)	50 μm	200 μm
1000	23.5	59.6
1.00	1992	2549

ELECTROCHEMICAL IMPEDANCE SPECTROSCOPY

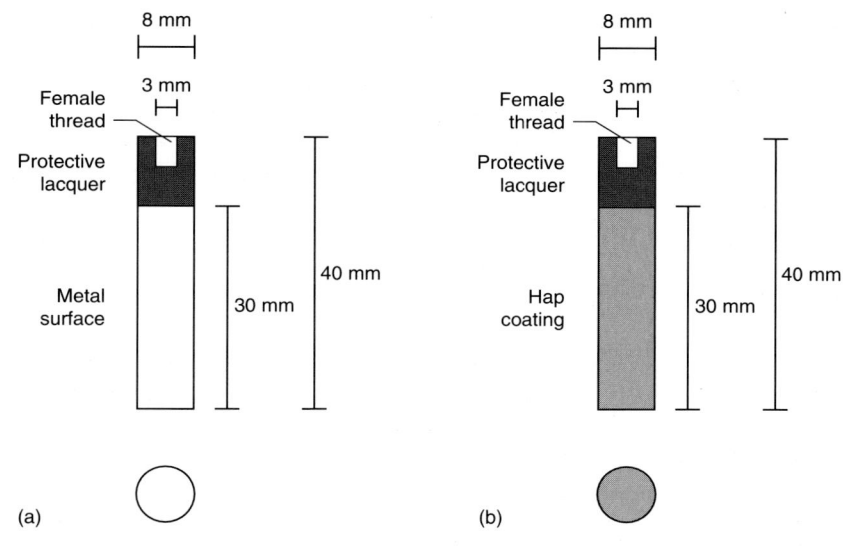

Figure 14.45 Configuration of the cylindrical specimens used in Sousa and Barbosa (1996): (a) uncoated; (b) coated with hydroxyapatite. (From *Biomaterials*, Vol. 17, Sousa and Barbosa, Effect of hydroxyapatite thickness on metal ion release from Ti6A14V substrates, pp. 397–404, 1996, with kind permission from Elsevier Science Ltd.)

between the metal and the solution may have been changed by the application or the presence of the coating. Deposition of a 200-μm-thick coating, however, makes the impedance modulus increase again, as the real exposed surface area of the substrate has probably become smaller with respect to the specimens with the thinner coating.

Table 14.13 Composition of Hank's balanced salt solution used in Sousa and Barbosa (1996). (From *Biomaterials*, Vol. 17, Sousa and Barbosa, Effect of hydroxyapatite thickness on metal ion release from Ti6A14V substrates, pp. 397–404, 1996, with kind permission from Elsevier Science Ltd)

Inorganic salts	Concentration (g l^{-1})
$CaCl_2$, anhydrous	0.14
KCl	0.40
KH_2PO_4	0.06
$MgCl_2 \cdot 6H_2O$	0.10
$MgSO_4 \cdot 7H_2O$	0.10
NaCl	8.00
$NaHCO_3$	0.35
$Na_2HPO_4 \cdot 7H_2O$	0.09
Other components	
D-Glucose	1.00
Phenol Red	0.01

Table 14.14 Impedance moduli (Ω cm^2) at two frequencies for the various surface states of Ti6Al4V in Hank's balanced salt solution (Sousa and Barbosa, 1996). (From *Biomaterials*, Vol. 17, Sousa and Barbosa, Effect of hydroxyapatite thickness on metal ion release from Ti6A14V substrates, pp. 397–404, 1996, with kind permission from Elsevier Science Ltd)

Frequency (Hz)	Polished surface	Grit-blasted surface	50-μm-thick HA coating	200-μm-thick HA coating
1043	47.3 (1.0)	18.5 (0.39)	16.2 (0.34)	40.0 (0.85)
1.63	3676 (1.0)	1220 (0.33)	1062 (0.29)	2242 (0.61)

HA, hydroxyapatite.

As metal ions are released from the surface of the implant material, local acidification through hydrolysis may enhance the dissolution process of the hydroxyapatite coating and its detachment. Because of the enlargement of the real surface area through grit-blasting, this dissolution is even accelerated with respect to the polished specimens, but surface roughness appears to be an important requirement to obtain a strong physical bond between the substrate and the coating; however, the thicker the coating, the slower this degradation process. It is thus important to find a coating thickness that delays the interface degradation until it is no longer critical for the performance of the implant. This work shows that a 200-μm-thick coating on a grit-blasted Ti6Al4V alloy gave a higher degree of protection than a polished/passivated surface which, in turn, performed better than a 50-μm-thick coating.

14.5 THE ROUGHNESS OF IMPLANT ELECTRODES

When implantation of an electrode is to be considered, the performance of the electrode is again dependent on the condition of the interface with the tissue (Bolz *et al.*, 1995). The high-pass filtering capability is important when an electrode serves in the transmission of pacing pulses or the measurement of organ signals. Translating the electrochemical interface behaviour of the electrode into an electrical equivalent circuit, the authors proposed a faradaic resistance in parallel with a double-layer or Helmholtz capacitance, which together form a high-pass filter. As the capacitance value is directly related to the surface area of the electrode, increasing the surface area means increasing the double-layer capacitance and decreasing the cut-off frequency, thus improving the characteristics of the electrode. However, the dimensions and thus the geometrical surface area of the implant electrode are restricted, so the active surface area, the real interface area between the electrode and the environment considering all surface irregularities, roughness or porosity, must be made as large as possible. The present work compares the results of two coating techniques.

One technique is the sintering of spheres with a diameter of about 200 μm, resulting in a porous coating of several layers of spheres on top of the electrode material and an active surface area which is larger than the geometrical surface area. The other technique is called fractally coating, in which the electrode material receives several coatings of hemispheres of decreasing size each time. If each coating doubles the active surface area, then N coatings enlarge the active surface area with a final factor of 2^N. The result is a fractal structure, a self-similar structure independent of the scale. The very large active surface area is directly accessible to the electrolytic charge carriers, whereas the sintered active surface area is only accessible via the pores. The fractal coating is obtained via plasma-enhanced physical vapour deposition (PVD), a sputter technique that can be applied to many elements or even combinations of elements.

Figure 14.46 shows the Bode plot of the impedance modulus for a smooth, a sintered and a fractally coated electrode of the same geometrical surface area of 10 mm^2. The cut-off frequency for the fractally coated electrode is more than three orders of magnitude lower than that for the smooth electrode, which indicates an increase in active surface area with a factor of at least 1000. The spectra show that only the fractally coated electrode was able to ensure a perfect transmission of signals. The present study used fractal coatings of iridium and TiN, and it appears that the quality of the electrode is determined initially not by the nature of the coating, as long as biocompatibility is respected, but by the structure of the coating.

Fröhlich *et al.* (1996) tested another method to decrease the impedance and cut-off frequency. When an electroactive material is applied to the electrode surface, a local reversible redox system is created that allows charge transfer across the interface between the electrode and the environment. The result is that a potential fluctuation is more readily followed by a current, i.e. that the impedance is diminished. As iridium is well known for its biocompatibility and possesses four oxidation states, an electroactive coating was chosen of iridium oxides or hydroxides applied electrolytically on top of either 316L stainless steel or platinum. The coating process was as follows: the

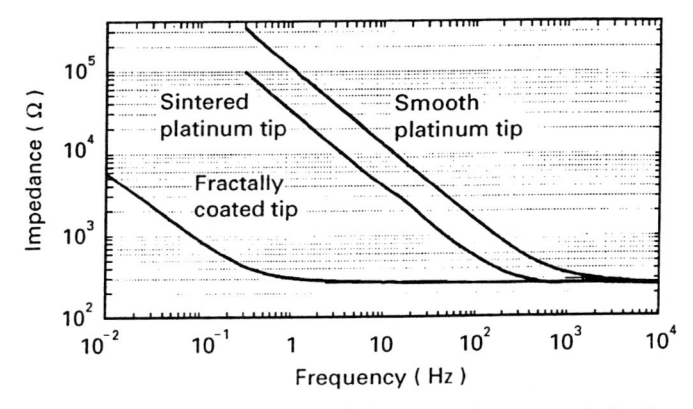

Figure 14.46 Bode plot comparison of the impedance moduli of a smooth, a sintered and a fractally coated electrode with the same geometrical surface area of 10 mm^2 (Bolz *et al.*, 1995). (From *Journal of Materials Science: Materials in Medicine*, Vol. 6, Bolz *et al.*, Effect of smooth, porous and fractal surface structure on the properties of an interface, Figure 5, pp. 844–8, 1995, with kind permission from Chapman & Hall.)

substrate was electrolytically cleaned in a commercial basic solution, Galvarol, at a current density of −20 A dm^{-2}. Oxide layers were dissolved in an acid solution, Solvamet, at the same current density. When 316L stainless steel was used as a substrate it was coated with a thin gold layer using an Auromet solution to obtain a surface with a high and uniform conductivity and a good adhesion to the iridium oxide coating. The final iridium oxide coating was electrolytically applied from an aqueous, conditioned iridium (IV) chloride solution at 25°C using an anodically pulsed current varying from 5 to 0 A dm^{-2}. The current pulses were 0.2 s wide and separated by 3 s. Figure 14.47 shows the Bode spectra of the impedance modulus of a 316L stainless steel electrode with and without an iridium oxide coating immersed in PBS solution. The smaller impedance of the coated with respect to the uncoated electrode in the frequency region below 1 kHz is evident: the cut-off frequency for the former was estimated at 0.4 Hz and that of the latter at 1.5 kHz. Similarly, an interface capacitance could be attributed of 36 mF cm^{-2} and 6.6 µF cm^{-2}, respectively, making a difference of more than three orders of magnitude. In order to test the long-term behaviour of the iridium oxide coatings, anodic and cathodic voltage pulses of amplitude 10 V, width 1 ms and frequency 2 Hz were applied for 4 weeks. Figure 14.48 shows that behaviour under anodic load and it can be seen that only during the first 24 h did a minor modification of the impedance spectrum occur. The authors state that cathodic loads lead to similar behaviour; moreover, the electrochemical properties of the iridium oxide coating were not changed during storage in either physiological saline solution or air.

14.6 CONCLUSIONS

Biometals may have many different functions when implanted into the (human) body. On this basis several selections may be made regarding the nature of the bulk

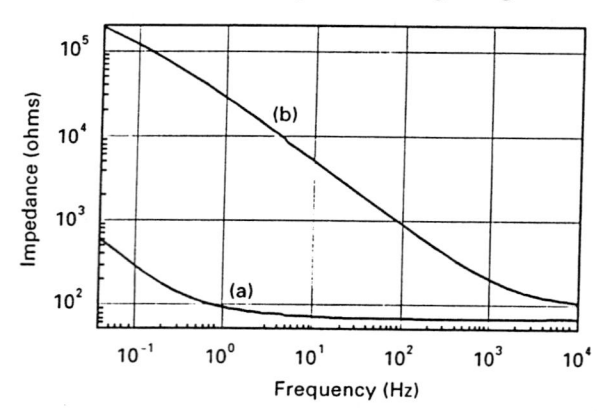

Figure 14.47 Bode plot of the impedance moduli of (a) an iridium oxide-coated and (b) an uncoated electrode made of 316L stainless steel in PBS solution (Fröhlich et al., 1996). (From *Journal of Materials Science: Materials in Medicine*, Vol. 7, Fröhlich et al., Electroactive coating of stimulating electrodes, pp. Figure 4, 393–7, with kind permission from Chapman & Hall.)

ELECTROCHEMICAL IMPEDANCE SPECTROSCOPY

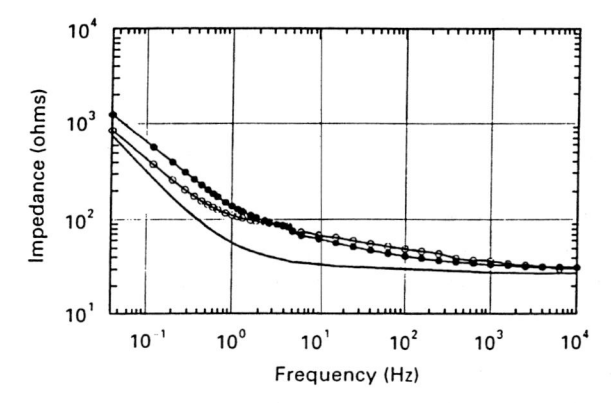

Figure 14.48 Bode plot of the impedance modulus showing the long-term behaviour under anodic loads in PBS solution: —, no load: ○, anodic load, 1 day; ●, anodic load, 32 days (Fröhlich *et al.*, 1996). (From *Journal of Materials Science: Materials in Medicine*, Vol. 7, Fröhlich *et al.*, Electroactive coating of stimulating electrodes, pp. Figure 4, 393–7, with kind permission from Chapman & Hall.)

material, the top metal layer, the physical, mechanical or chemical treatment, the surface roughness, the top non-metal coating, the method of application, etc., although choices may be restricted by, for instance, strength and biocompatibility. In combination with real and relevant simulated bioenvironments this leads to many examples of interfaces that can be studied with EIS, and of which only a few are presented in the works cited here. That is to say, the work is not finished, it has only started. Moreover, when making purchasing decisions for EIS equipment, cost limitations become less and less important.

Concerning the data analysis, progress can certainly be made in undertaking more systematic EIS research of selected systems and refining the models. Care must be taken not to carry one particular model, together with its interpretation, from one case to another.

NOMENCLATURE

A	geometrical exposed surface area of the electrode
A_{eff}	effective electrochemical surface area
$b_{a,c}$	anodic Tafel constant for the corrosion process
$b_{a,e}$	anodic Tafel constant for the electron exchange process
b_c	constant
$b_{c,c}$	cathodic Tafel constant for the corrosion process
$b_{c,e}$	cathodic Tafel constant for the electron exchange process
b_e	constant
c_c	constant
c'_c	constant
c''_c	constant

c_e	constant
c'_e	constant
c''_e	constant
C	capacitance
C_{Al}	capacitance of the alumina layer (per unit surface area)
C_b	inner-layer capacitance per unit surface area
C_d	double-layer capacitance
C_f	capacitance of the passive or oxide or semiconductor film (per unit surface area)
C_{ho}	capacitance of the hydrates/precipitates inside the pores per unit surface area
C_i	interface capacitance per unit surface area
C_p	outer-layer capacitance per unit surface area
d	total oxide thickness
d_0	original film thickness
e	electron charge
E	electrochemical potential
E_{corr}	corrosion potential
E_{fb}	flat band potential
$E_{oc,c}$	open-circuit potential in the region of metal corrosion control
$E_{oc,e}$	open-circuit potential in the region of electron exchange control
f	frequency
F	Faraday's constant
i_{corr}	corrosion current density
j	imaginary unit
k	Boltzmann constant
k_c	constant
k_e	constant
M	molecular mass of the oxide
N	number of coatings
N_D	density of charge carriers
Q	cumulative charge or magnitude replacing the capacitance in the impedance expression for the CPE
R	resistance
R_{Al}	resistance of the alumina layer (for the unit surface area)
R_b	inner-layer resistance for the unit surface area
R_e	ohmic resistance of the electrolyte layer (for the unit surface area)
R_f	resistance of the passive film (for the unit surface area)
R_{ho}	resistance of the hydrates/precipitates inside the pores for the unit surface area
R_p	outer-layer resistance or electrolyte resistance inside the pores for the unit surface area or polarisation resistance for the unit surface area
$R_{p,c}$	polarisation resistance for the metal corrosion on the unit surface area

$R_{p,e}$	polarisation resistance for the electron exchange on the unit surface area
R_t	charge transfer resistance (for the unit surface area)
t	time
T	absolute temperature
W	thickness of the space charge layer
z	number of electrons involved in the charge transfer reaction
Z	complex impedance (for the unit surface area)
Z'	real impedance part (for the unit surface area)
Z''	imaginary impedance part (for the unit surface area)
$|Z|$	impedance modulus (for the unit surface area)
α	CPE exponent
Δd	increase in the oxide film thickness
ΔQ	increase in the charge measured
ε_0	permittivity of the vacuum
ε_r	relative dielectric constant of the oxide
ρ	oxide material density
φ	impedance phase
ω	pulsation or angular frequency

REFERENCES

Barbosa, M.A. (1991) Electrochemical impedance studies on calcium phosphate-metal interfaces, in *Bioceramics*, Vol. 4 (eds W. Bonfield, G.W. Hastings and K.E. Tanner), *Proceedings of the 4th International Symposium on Ceramics in Medecine*, London, September 1991, Butterworth-Heinemann, London, pp. 325–33.

Bolz, A., Fröhlich, R., Schmidt, K. and Schaldach, M. (1995) Effect of smooth, porous and fractal surface structure on the properties of an interface, *J. Mater. Sci. Mater. Med.* **6**, 844–8.

Escudero, M. L., González-Carrasco, J.L., García-Alonso, C. and Ramírez, E. (1995) Electrochemical impedance spectroscopy of preoxidized MA 956 superalloy during *in vitro* experiments, *Biomaterials* **16**, 735–40.

Escudero, M.L., López, M.F., Ruiz, J., García-Alonso, M.C. and Canahua, H. (1996) Comparative study of the corrosion behavior of MA-956 and conventional metallic biomaterials, *J. Biomed. Mater. Res.* **31**, 313–17.

Fröhlich, R., Rzany, A., Riedmüller, J., Bolz, A. and Schaldach, M. (1996) Electroactive coating of stimulating electrodes, *J. Mater. Sci. Mater. Med.* **7**, 393–7.

Gabrielli, C. (1980) *Identification of Electrochemical Processes by Frequency Response Analysis*, Technical Report no. 004/83, Solartron Instruments, Farnborough.

Gabrielli, C. (1990) *Use and Applications of Electrochemical Impedance Techniques*, Technical Report, Schlumberger Instruments, Farnborough.

Gluszek, J. and Masalaski, J. (1993) The influence of variations in pH of Ringer's solution on corrosion behaviour of surgical steel, in *Progress in the Understanding and Prevention of Corrosion*, Vol. 2 (eds J.M. Costa and A.D. Mercer), Institute of Materials, London, pp. 1289–96.

Kovacs, P. (1991a) *In vitro* studies on the electrochemical behavior of orthopaedic implant alloys, in *Extended Abstracts of the Electrochemical Society Meeting*, Washington, DC, 5–10 May 1991, The Electrochemical Society, Pennington, NJ, Vol. 91-1, Abstract no. 61, p. 93.

Kovacs, P. (1991b) *In vitro* studies on the electrochemical behavior of pure metals used in orthopaedic implant alloys, in *Extended Abstracts of the Electrochemical Society Meeting*, Phoenix, AZ, 13–17 October 1991, The Electrochemical Society, Pennington, NJ, Vol. 91-2, Abstract no. 173, pp. 255–6.

Kovacs, P. (1992) Electrochemical techniques for studying the corrosion behavior of metallic implant materials, in *Techniques for Corrosion Measurement, Proceedings of the Corrosion/92 Symposium*, NACE, Houston, TX, pp. 5/1–14.

Macdonald, D.D. ed. (1993) *Second International Symposium on Electrochemical Impedance Spectroscopy, Electrochim. Acta* (Special Issue) **38** (14).

Mansfeld, F. (1993) *Analysis and Interpretation of EIS Data for Metals and Alloys*, Technical Report no. 26, Schlumberger Instruments, Farnborough.

Pan, J., Thierry, D. and Leygraf, C. (1994) Electrochemical and XPS studies of titanium for biomaterial applications with respect to the effect of hydrogen peroxide, *J. Biomed. Mater. Res.* **28**, 113–22.

Pan, J., Thierry, D. and Leygraf, C. (1996a) Electrochemical impedance spectroscopy study of the passive oxide film on titanium for implant application, *Electrochim. Acta* **41** (7/8), 1143–53.

Pan, J., Thierry, D. and Leygraf, C. (1996b) Hydrogen peroxide toward enhanced oxide growth on titanium in PBS solution: blue coloration and clinical relevance, *J. Biomed. Mater. Res.* **30**, 393–402.

Scully, J.R., Silverman, D.C. and Kendig, M.W., eds (1993) *Electrochemical Impedance: Analysis and Interpretation*, ASTM Special Technical Publication no.1188, West Conshohocken, PA.

Silva, R., Barbosa, M.A., Rondot, B. and Cunha Belo, M. (1990) Impedance and photoelectrochemical measurements on passive films formed on metallic biomaterials, *Br. Corros. J.* **25**, 136–40.

Solar, R.J., Pollack, S.R. and Korostoff, E. (1979) Titanium release from implants: a proposed mechanism, in *Corrosion and Degradation of Implant Materials* (eds B.C. Syrett and A. Acharya), ASTM Special Technical Publication no. 684, Proceedings of an ASTM Symposium, Kansas City, MO., 22–3 May 1978, West Conshohocken, PA, pp. 161–72.

Sousa, S.R. and Barbosa, M.A. (1995) The effect of hydroxyapatite thickness on metal ion release from stainless steel substrates, *J. Mater. Sci. Mater. Med.* **6**, 818–23.

Sousa, S.R. and Barbosa, M.A. (1996) Effect of hydroxyapatite thickness on metal ion release from Ti6Al4V substrates, *Biomaterials* **17**, 397–404.

Vereecken, J., ed. (1996) *Third International Symposium on Electrochemical Impedance Spectroscopy, Electrochim. Acta* (Special Issue) **41** (7/8).

15
Retrieval analysis

P. LAFFARGUE,[1] H.J. BREME,[2] J.A. HELSEN[3] AND H.F. HILDEBRAND[4]
[1]Hôpital Roger Salengro, Lille, France
[2]University of the Saarland, Saarbrücken, Germany
[3]Catholic University of Leuven, Leuven, Belgium
[4]University of Lille, Lille, France

15.1 INTRODUCTION

The ultimate test of the biological performance of any implant is the overall health and comfort of the patient, the degree and duration of this comfort, the physiological status of the organ or tissues contacting the implant, the interface and the implant itself, after retrieval during revision or from post-mortem retrieval. The success of an arthroplasty or any other temporary support or permanent substitution of a defective organ is, however, a function of a complex interplay of a burden of factors, one of which is the bulk and surface properties of the materials making up the implant. The statement that 'The stability of a prosthesis in its bony bed determining the subsequent fate, success or failure of surgical reconstructions primarily depends on the surgical technique and design of the implant' (Boss *et al.*, 1994) is too narrow. The design parameters are also dictated by the capabilities of the materials available, although it is true that the violation of sound engineering laws quickens and intensifies failures. For readers especially interested in bone implants the paper of Boss *et al.* (1994) gives an excellent review on the nature of the bone–implant interface and '... the lessons learned from implant retrieval and analysis in man and experimental animals'. Reading is highly recommended for those interested in retrieval analysis.

The common knowledge on the bulk and surface properties of metals and alloys was collated in the preceding chapters. The toxicity and mutagenicity of individual metals and alloys are well documented. Consequently, it may be accepted that modern designers and manufacturers of metal implants select metals and alloys that meet general biomedical safety criteria. Implants still fail, despite the vast body of *in vitro* and *in vivo* experimental evidence, material and design testing. In this chapter a few case studies of failed implants will be presented and it will be shown

---

Metals as Biomaterials ISBN 0 471 96935 4 Edited by J.A. Helsen and H.J. Breme. © 1998 John Wiley & Sons Ltd

how small instances of neglect can be catastrophic. In Section 15.2 failures of metals and alloys collected from the current literature will be mentioned. In the paragraphs thereafter non-published case studies will be discussed.

A valuable tool in the assessment of the success or failure of an implant is the post-mortem retrieval of implants. Specimens obtained in revision surgery may not necessarily reflect the status of the devices in patients who are functioning normally and are asymptomatic (Pidhorz et al., 1993). It should be noted here that retrieved specimens represent a potential biohazard for the transmission of human immunodeficiency and hepatitis viruses, and the safety of all personnel involved in the analysis is of paramount importance. One way of lowering the risk is, according to McCaskie et al. (1995), screening the donor for disease (but this should be done with the consent of the relatives) while another is complete sterilisation (but this may alter the biomechanical properties). A well-documented retrieval procedure should be followed throughout, from storage to chemical and histological analysis. If skeletal implants are involved, care should be taken to sample surrounding soft tissue as well, an often forgotten detail (Pidhorz et al., 1993). Post-mortem retrieval is also one of the many means of helping to reduce the number of animal experiments.

In the following paragraphs a non-exhaustive summary of retrieval studies from the literature and a number of case studies will be discussed.

15.2 SUMMARY OF LITERATURE DATA

Hereafter only experimental evidence for non-ideal behaviour of the materials is discussed. Histology and medical consequences are beyond the scope of this chapter.

15.2.1 POST-MORTEM RETRIEVAL

15.2.1.1 Porous-coated Titanium-alloy Hip Components

Not much interest is shown in the current literature to reactions of the coating itself in retrieved, well-functioning prostheses, despite the intimate tissue contact and the load transfer function. In none of the cases described by Collier et al. (1992a) and Pidhorz et al. (1993) is any reference made to corrosion or other degradation mechanisms of the coating or the metal substrate. From more than 1 month of implantation time all showed ingrowth which increased up to 80% after 4 years. The ingrowth contact was either continuous or in islands. It started with woven bone, gradually transformed into lamellar bone in 2–4 months and subsequently became denser in the course of time. Fibrous encapsulation was present in voids, with loci of large separation between the cortex and implant, and along the smooth part of partially porous stems. Younger and older patients reacted in the same way and bony ingrowth occurred for patients. Metal debris was found at the holes in the acetabular cup but the histolytic response was small and localised and no granulomas or evidence for bone lysis were detected (Pidhorz et al., 1993).

RETRIEVAL ANALYSIS

15.2.1.2 Hydroxyapatite-coated Prostheses

All apatite-coated parts showed good bone contact with bony bridges extending from the endosteum to the implant interface, even after a very short implantation time of 3 weeks (up to 10% of the surface of the coated femoral component and 20% of the acetabular component), with as much as 54% more bone contact than for the non-coated parts. No fibrous tissue was seen around coated parts and no metal degradation in the substrate was reported (Bloebaum *et al.*, 1991; Collier *et al.*, 1992a; Bauer *et al.*, 1993).

15.2.1.3 Cemented Prostheses

Of many reported cases only one was loose but not painful. The cement–bone interface was intact and there was only rare fibrous tissue formation. New bone was intimately apposed. Frequent findings were that the cement interface was separated and circumferential and radial fracture of the cement mantle was frequent. 'Cement' is a misnomer because the material does not adhere to the metal surface but only fills the space. Fracture of the cement is considered to be a frequent initiation of (mechanical) failure. Debonding cement–implant creates voids which may accumulate debris (e.g. polyethelene and metal) (Collier *et al.*, 1992a; Schmalzried *et al.*, 1993).

15.2.2 RETRIEVAL ANALYSIS FROM REVISION

Animal studies are an easy way to document implantation experiments fully from the setting up of the experiment to the analysis of the retrieved devices. As implantation periods in animals are generally restricted to 2 or 3 years, for dogs a period roughly considered to be equivalent to 6–10 years of human implantation, failure by fatigue fracture or corrosion is almost never observed. Moreover, orthopaedic implants for animals are generally overdimensioned compared with real loading in human applications and this contributes to absence of fractures (e.g. DeYoung *et al.*, 1992; Cheng *et al.*, 1995).

Another consequence of overdimensioning is a reduction of wear, fretting and many other direct or indirect causes of corrosion, which is definitely underestimated. As far as the authors are aware, no fractures or corrosion problems have been reported for customised human total hip arthroplasties. This observation might also be attributed to slight mechanical overdimensioning of customised prostheses (due to more complete space filling). Of the 74 total hip replacements (THR) implanted and assessed by Lombardi *et al.* (1995) with a follow-up of 11–46 months, no fractures or fatigue failures were reported. Metal substrate problems specific to phosphate-coated prostheses were not found in the literature within the vast body of references to hydroxyapatite-coated prostheses (e.g. Dhert, 1994; Buma and Gardeniers, 1995).

The relation between stiffness or the Young's modulus E of metals and alloys and bone response does not seem to be clear. A relatively recent paper reports a coherent comparison of bone density measurements of the calcar femorale around 15 CoCr and 15 titanium alloy implants. The proximal parts of the prostheses were porous coated and the prostheses were of similar design and dimensions. The data indicated that the use of a titanium stem, with a two-fold decrease in the modulus of elasticity and a 33% increase in the bending deflection in the mediolateral plane, does not provide any more protection from bone loss for a preponderance of the proximal part of the femur than does the use of a stiffer CoCr stem (Hughes *et al.*, 1995).

The most frequently reported problems are wear and the consequences of wear particles, fatigue and corrosion.

15.2.2.1 Wear

All titanium alloy implants are very susceptible to severe abrasive wear of the articulation surfaces. Abrasive wear is enhanced in the presence of acrylic debris from cement. Metallosis was reported for 22 patients with THR with Ti6Al4V articulating on ultrahigh molecular weight polyethylene (UHMWPE) by Nasser *et al.* (1990). Metallosis is defined as 'aseptic fibrosis, local necrosis or loosening of a device due to metallic corrosion and release of wear debris' (Black *et al.*, 1990). Intracellular deposits were observed by Hildebrand *et al.* (1996) in macrophages, fibroblasts, histiocytes and multinucleated giant cells (MGC) upon retrieval of the implants and tissue from 31 patients with loosening THR. Helsen and coworkers measured the extent of wear of a cemented CoCr hip prosthesis provoked by micromovements between the cement mantle and the stem after 8 years of implantation. These authors estimated the number of particles produced at 1.5×10^9, assuming a particle size of 2 μm (Helsen *et al.*, 1997). Six cases of abnormal wear due to ceramic screws developed in bipolar prostheses. All patients had metallosis to a greater or lesser extent (Matsuda and Yamamuro, 1994). Wear debris was reported in 12 patients after the removal of stainless steel osteosynthesis plates. Metal particles were disseminated, particularly in soft surrounding tissues and (fewer) in bone. This resulted in mild inflammatory changes in an area wider than areas of metal impregnation (Torgersen *et al.*, 1995). It is absolutely clear that wear particles introduce a non-favourable physiological response. To the best of the authors' knowledge, the long-term consequences are not yet known.

15.2.2.2 Fatigue Failure

The incidence of this type of failure was high in the 1970s and early 1980s (as much as 11% has been reported) but this incidence rate certainly decreased with the vanishing use of stainless steel and its gradual replacement by CoCr and titanium alloys. Cook and Thomas (1991) reported two broken porous-coated CoCrMo alloy components out of 137 retrievals and three broken porous-coated Ti6Al4V components from 22 retrievals: (1) fatigue fracture initiated at the medial edge of the posterior condyle of the CoCrMo femoral component near the junction of the coated and uncoated region (male, 69 years old, after 20 months); (2) fracture of the fixation

RETRIEVAL ANALYSIS 471

spikes of a CoCrMo patellar component, initiated at the junction of the pegs and the metal backing (male, 74 years old, after 12 months); (3) fracture of the metal backing of a Ti6Al4V acetabular shell, initiated at the screwhole (female, 52 years old, after 48 months); (4) fracture of the medial part of a Ti6Al4V tibial component, initiated at the medial end of the strut of the central stabilising stem (female, 62 years old, after 28 months); and (5) fracture of the posteromedial part of a Ti6Al4V tibial component, initiated at the medial edge of the device, posterior to the central stabilising strut (male, 46 years old, after 35 months). Metallurgical analysis revealed all of these cases to have microstructures typical of porous-coated substrates, however within the accepted ASTM standards. No metallurgical defects, non-metallic inclusions, voids or porosities were present in the area of failure. The fatigue strength of porous-coated CoCr and titanium alloys is inferior to that of uncoated wrought or forged materials (one-third strength). Stress concentration by the porous coating and non-uniform bone ingrowth caused these implants to break.

15.2.2.3 Corrosion

In 1991 Mathiesen and collaborators reported an analysis of nine uncemented hip prostheses of modular design, which were revised for various reasons, but for four of these tissue discoloration was found, located at the head–neck junction. The tissue showed extensive necrosis associated with metal particles. The head and stem were made of a cast CoCr alloy, the exact composition of which was not determined. These four cases of corrosion were not well documented but the presence of corrosion was beyond doubt. At that time reports on corrosion of CoCr alloys were rare. It was hypothesised to be crevice corrosion, facilitated by structural imperfections and poor mechanical fitting of the tapered head to the stem. None of the nine prostheses was broken (Mathiesen *et al.*, 1991). In the same journal 1 year later, Collier and his colleagues reported on 139 modular femoral components of hip prostheses, revised for a variety of reasons. In 91 specimens the stem and head were made of the same alloy and none of the tapered interfaces showed signs of corrosion. In 25 of the remaining 48 with a stem of a titanium alloy and a head of a CoCr alloy, corroded tapered heads were found. Moreover, the corrosion was time dependent and all those that had been in place for more than 40 months were damaged. The damage was interpreted as a galvanically accelerated crevice corrosion. The implantation time was between 11 and 78 months, and not one was broken (Collier *et al.*, 1992b). Worse cases were two modular hip prostheses retrieved after a fracture in the neck region slightly distal to the taper at 85 and 70 months after implantation. Both had stems of a titanium alloy and heads of a CoCr alloy. Intergranular corrosion initiated a crack which progressed by cyclic fatigue loading. A typical feature of the surface was the presence of pits, formed by egression of surface grains following grain boundary attack. The cracks progressed in the taper interface. The described fractures were the logical result of the processes reported earlier (Gilbert *et al.*, 1994). With the huge number of modular prostheses made with dissimilar alloys and implanted since the early 1980s, more of these fractures can be expected in the future. The results discussed above were not predicted. The behaviour of the couple TiAlV–CoCrMo was predicted to be safe, based on thorough electrochemical *in vitro* testing (Barbosa, 1991).

15.3 ILLUSTRATED CASE STUDIES

15.3.1 FAILURE OF A HIP PROSTHESIS

In Figure 15.1 a hip prosthesis made of a CoCrMo alloy is shown which failed under service conditions. The fracture, which had occurred in the region of the neck, represents a peculiarity. Greenish corrosion products could be observed on the surface of the fracture.

From the metallographic investigations (Figures 15.2 and 15.3), which were performed in the neighbourhood of the failure, it became clear that the prosthesis had been implanted in the cast condition. The unfavourable dendritic microstructure contains many shrinkage voids caused by the solidification. These shrink holes act as notches which lead to increases in the working stresses. In addition, brittle, blocky CoCrMo carbides can be observed on the grain boundaries of the dendrites. An enrichment of chromium occurs in the region of these carbides with a resulting derichment of chromium in the neighbouring matrix. As a consequence of this decrease in chromium the corrosion resistance of the material is diminished. Because of this unfavourable microstructure of the as-cast CoCrMo alloy a great number of prosthesis stems failed in the 1970s and 1980s (Schmid *et al.*, 1980). For this reason an annealing (homogenisation) of the as-cast condition was recommended (Semlitsch and Wintsch, 1972). Owing to this homogenisation the blocky carbides are dissolved in the matrix, which results in an improvement of the corrosion resistance (Süry, 1974). In the case of the failure of the prosthesis neck, the fracture of the as-cast material with the unfavourable microstructure was obviously generated by crevice

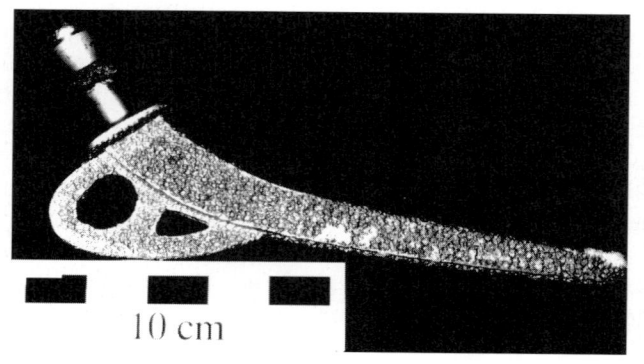

Figure 15.1 Broken hip prosthesis.

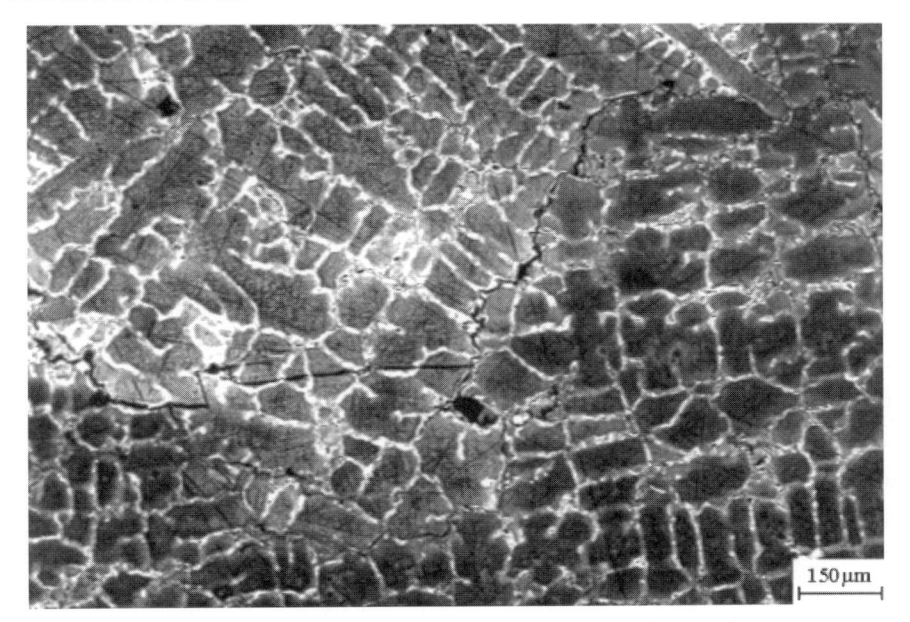

Figure 15.2 Microstructure in the neighbourhood of the fracture.

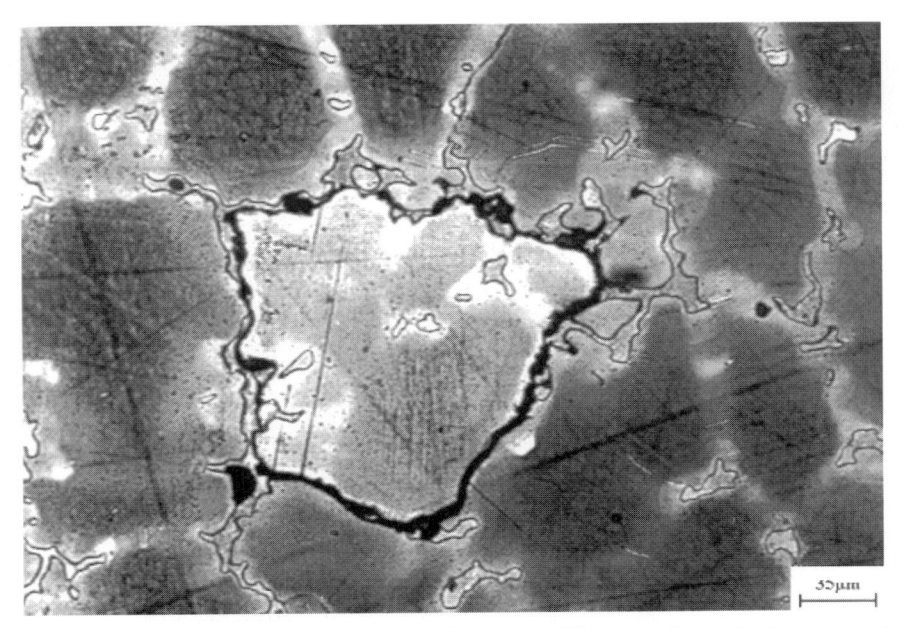

Figure 15.3 Microstructure at a higher magnification than that shown in Figure 15.2.

474 METALS AS BIOMATERIALS

corrosion. In the gap between the head and the neck the oxygen content was consumed, causing a decrease in the pH value of the body fluid and an increase in the corrosion rate, especially in areas with a derichment of chromium.

15.3.2 FAILURE OF A KNEE SLEDGE

Figures 15.4 and 15.5 show, respectively, the X-ray and the macroscopic photographs of a broken knee sledge which was made of the alloy Ti6Al4V in the forged ($\alpha + \beta$) condition.

For improved friction and abrasion behaviour the implant surface was coated with TiN by physical vapour deposition (PVD). In order to enlarge the surface of the underside of the sledge, where the maximum bending stresses occur under service conditions, the sledge was sand blasted with alumina before coating. Because of the high blast energy the material was penetrated by small (<10 μm) Al_2O_3 particles.

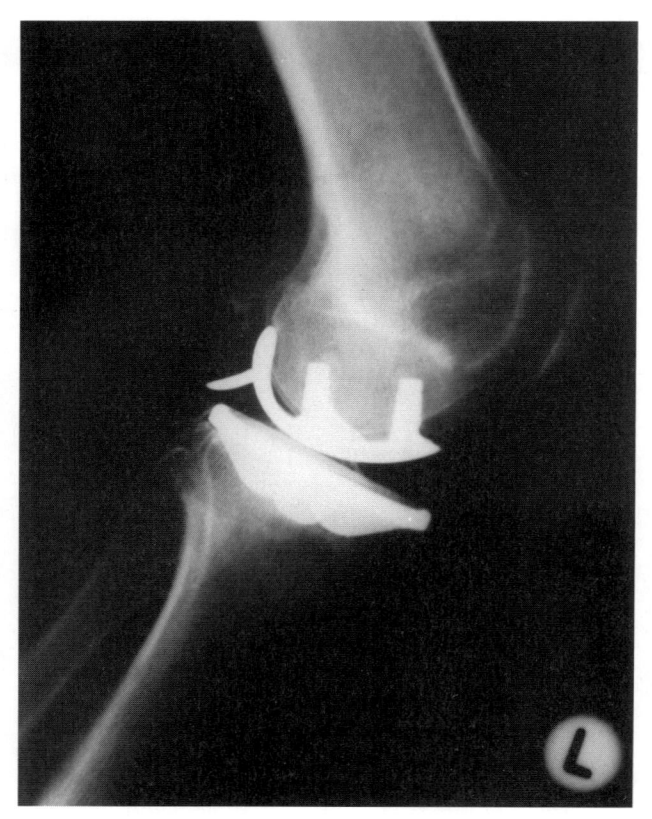

Figure 15.4 X-ray photograph of a broken knee sledge.

RETRIEVAL ANALYSIS

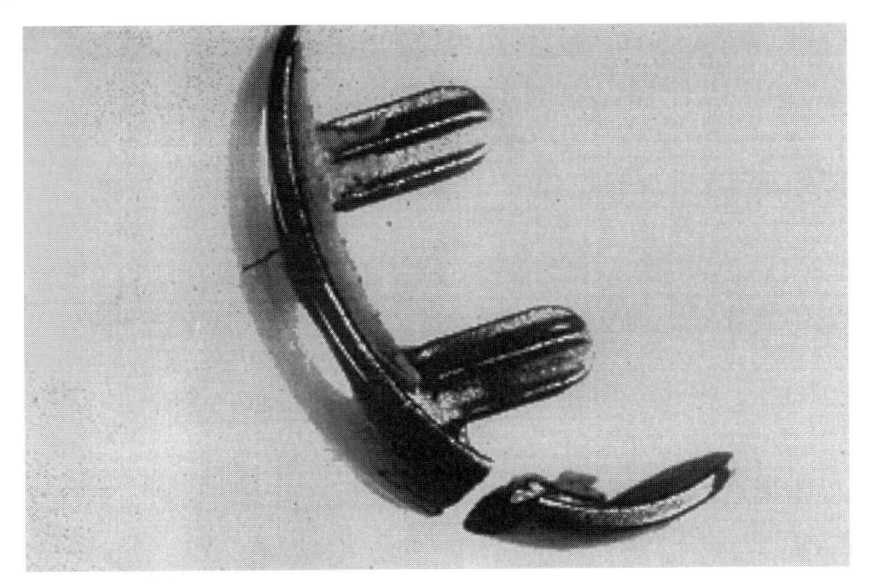

Figure 15.5 Retrieved broken knee sledge.

Al_2O_3 grains sticking to the underside were detected by energy dispersive X-ray spectrometry (EDX) analysis of a scanning electron microscope (SEM) (Figure 15.6). These particles are able to produce a strong notch effect, whereby during loading of the implant the working bending stresses may be drastically increased,

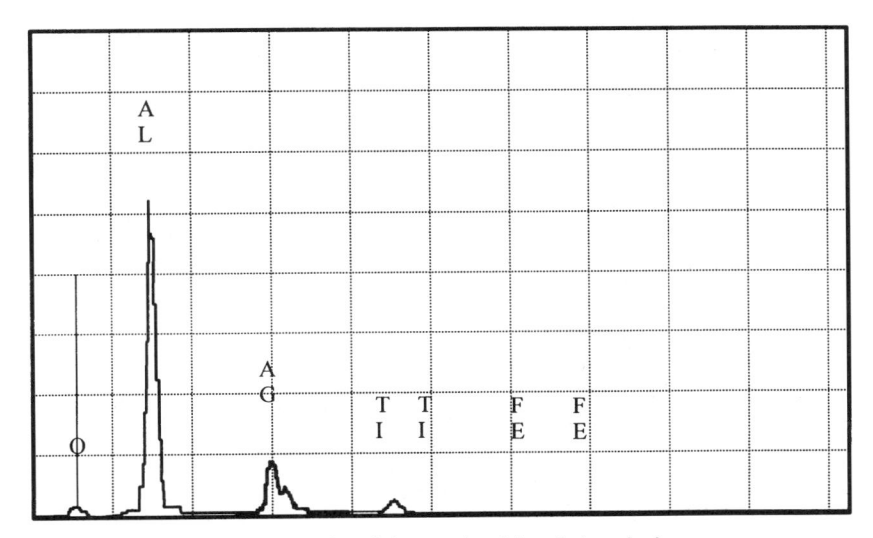

Figure 15.6 SEM EDX analysis of the underside of the sledge.

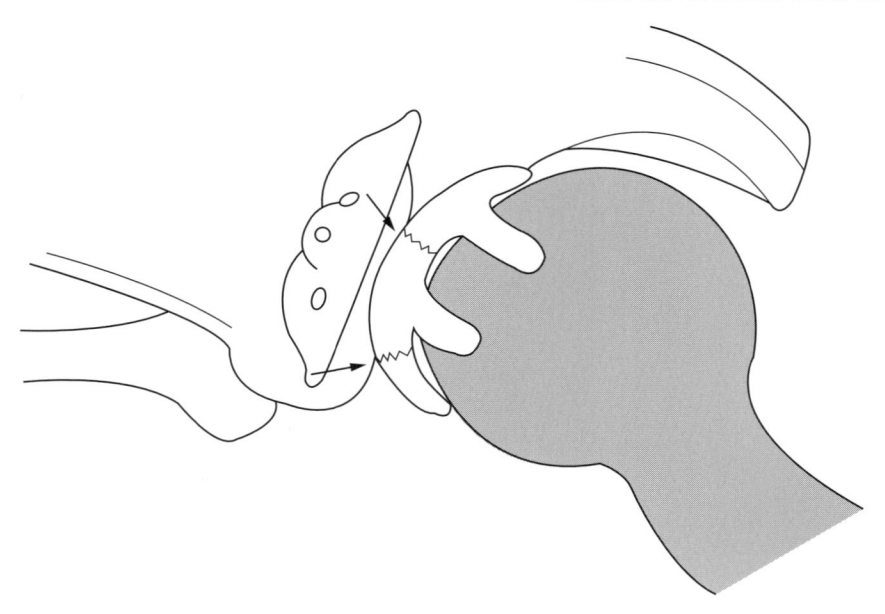

Figure 15.7 Position of the sledge after implantation.

especially if, as in the given case, the implantation technique promotes the formation of bending stresses. By means of the X-ray photographs taken immediately after the operation it could be proved that the landscape of the knee was not precisely adapted to the implant (Figure 15.7). The gap between the sledge and the knee was filled with bone cement, which was also used to fix the implant. Because of the different (especially elastic) properties of the metal and cement under loading a debonding occurred, with high bending stresses acting on the underside of the sledge. These stresses were additionally increased by the notch effect of the Al_2O_3 particles.

15.3.3 LETHAL BLOCKAGE OF AN ARTIFICIAL HEART VALVE

Figure 15.8 shows a broken Bjørk–Shiley heart valve which had caused the death of the patient. Both ends of the strut were broken. From the metallurgical study it became clear that the frame and outlet strut had been joined by fusion welding. For this purpose two holes were drilled in the frame and both strut ends inserted before welding. The broken ends of the strut which, as well as the frame, was made from Haynes 25 (Co20Cr15W10Ni3Fe), showed two totally different structures. While one surface fracture occurred in a brittle manner (Figure 15.9), the other had the typical features of a fatigue fracture with striations and the ductile endurance fracture (Figure 15.10). Several factors were acting at once to initiate the failure of the heart valve. The metallographical investigation of the heat-affected zones showed different grain sizes. Since the microstructure of the end with the brittle

RETRIEVAL ANALYSIS

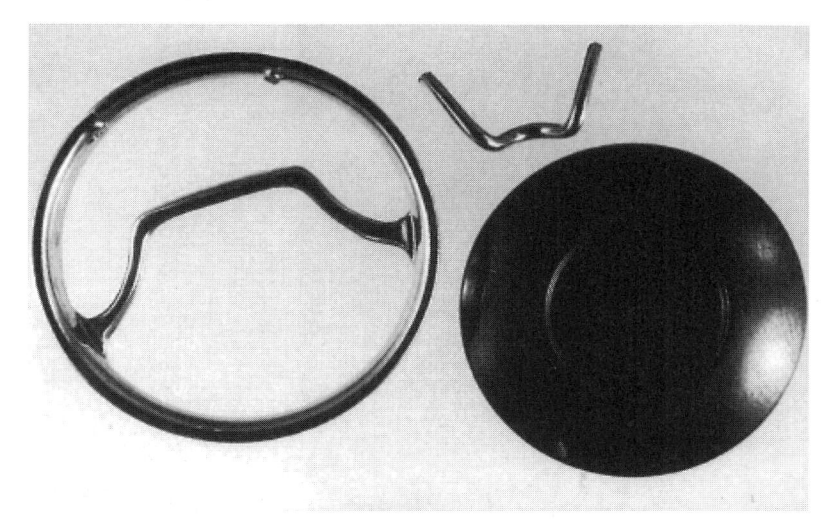

Figure 15.8 Broken heart valve.

fracture was fine grained, it is clear that on this side of the strut less heat had been applied during welding than on the other end, which had a coarse-grained structure. As a result, the strut end welded with less heat was not completely joined to the frame, whereby a fissure with a severe notch effect and a stress concentration, respectively, were present. It is known that in cracks or fissures, the pH value of the

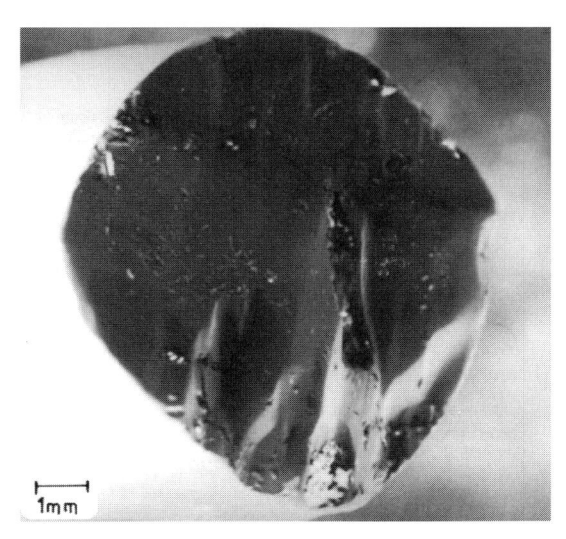

Figure 15.9 Brittle fracture of one end of the strut.

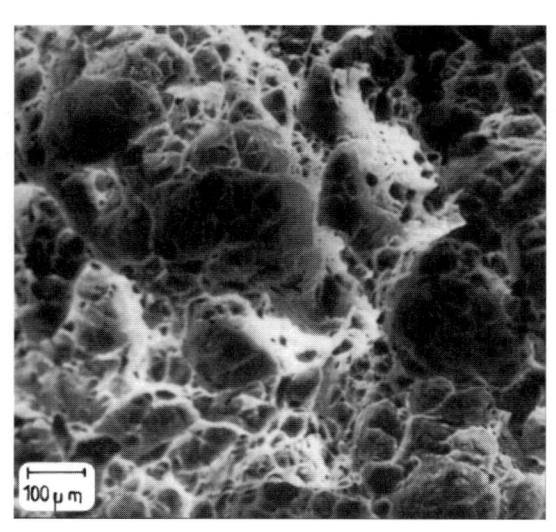

Figure 15.10 Fatigue fracture of the other end of the strut to that shown in Figure 15.9.

fluid is drastically decreased because of oxygen consumption. This causes the corrosion resistance of the material to be diminished, an effect which is enhanced even more because conductive contacts exist between the base metal with its globular structure and the solidified primary crystallization zone of the weld. In the electrolytic body fluids these contacts produce local cells with an increased corrosion rate of the less noble metal. In addition, because the strut ends are welded one after the other, the secondary end is welded under stress, thus producing residual (tension) stresses which can contribute to the brittle failure of the material. Because of the interaction of these various effects the brittle fracture occurred first. The valve was still working for a certain period until fatigue of the other strut end took place (Röckelein et al., 1989).

15.4 METAL DISTRIBUTION IN BODY FLUIDS AND TISSUES

Biological fluids and tissue samples were analysed from 31 patients with THR made of three different alloys. Normal values are given in Table 15.1. The metal content in body fluids was generally very high for the three types of alloy (Table 15.2). Stainless steel THR showed the lowest increase of metals in body fluids, with mostly normal values for chromium.

NiCrMo THR released high amounts of all elements and a more than 45-fold concentration of nickel in the total blood and more than 30-fold concentration in the plasma were recovered. CoCr THR showed significant increases of chromium and about 15-fold concentrations of cobalt in total blood plasma. The highest concentrations were generally correlated to long-term exposure.

RETRIEVAL ANALYSIS

Table 15.1 Normal nickel, cobalt and chromium levels in human biological samples

Biological samples	Ni	Co	Cr	Reference
Total blood (mg l^{-1})	<1.80	<0.11	<3.00	Hildebrand et al. (1988)
Plasma (mg l^{-1})	<0.90	<0.10	<1.40	Hildebrand et al. (1988)
Urine (mg g^{-1} creatinine)	<3.30	<0.36	<3.00	Hildebrand et al. (1988)
Articular capsule (mg g^{-1} dry weight)	0.20	0.05	0.20	Hofmann et al. (1982)
Fascia lata (mg g^{-1} dry weight)	0.50	0.20	0.50	Hofmann et al. (1982)
Connective tissue (mg g^{-1} dry weight)	0.50	0.10	0.50	Michel and Zilkens (1987)

Particular interest was devoted to three patients in whom the ceramic head of the THR had broken and was replaced by a metallic head, without replacement of the polyethylene acetabulum. Remaining ceramic particles then abraded the metallic head and consequently produced a large amount of metallic wear particles. Although these patients had had the THR for only 3 years, the concentrations of chromium and nickel were higher than in patients without the failure of the ceramic head. Moreover, extremely high values of cobalt were noted, with a more than 15-fold increase in urine and a more than 400-fold increase in total blood and plasma compared with upper normal values.

After retrieval of the THR and implantation of a titanium THR, these patients were studied for over 2 years to assess the elimination of the three metals concerned. Only nickel reached normal values after this period, whereas chromium and cobalt were still detected in five- to 10-fold concentrations (Figure 15.11).

In order to estimate the possible storage of corrosion products in implant-surrounding tissue, quantitative analyses were performed of different tissue samples obtained during the removal of the THR. In this tissue a similar metal distribution was found to that in body fluids (Table 15.3).

The tissue around stainless steel THR contained the smallest amounts of metal. NiCrMo THR released a large amount of nickel which was recovered particularly in the bone and the fascia lata. The chromium was predominantly present in granuloma and connective tissue.

Regarding CoCr THR, there was no significant difference between the two groups of patients, and in all tissue samples higher cobalt than chromium levels were obtained, in particular in the bone and fascia lata, where cobalt reached concentrations 1000 and 600 times higher than maximal normal values, respectively.

The metal ion release in patients with THR has aroused growing interest during the last few years. Elevated nickel values were described by Dobbs and Minski (1980) and high cobalt levels were mentioned previously by Coleman et al. (1972, 1973). Since these initial investigations, several authors have confirmed these findings (Sarmiento and Gruen, 1985; Griffith et al., 1987; Black, 1988; Hildebrand et al., 1988; Dorr et al., 1990; McKellop et al., 1990; Nasser et al., 1990; Weissman et al., 1991).

Table 15.2 Distribution of nickel, cobalt and chromium in urine, plasma and blood from patients with THR (from Hildebrand et al., 1996)

Alloy (n)	Exposure time (years)	Urine (µg g^{-1} creatinine)			Total blood (µg l^{-1})			Plasma (µg l^{-1})		
		Ni	Co	Cr	Ni	Co	Cr	Ni	Co	Cr
NiCrMo (5)	2–8	43.2 ± 9.2	5.5 ± 1.2	45.8 ± 10.7	83.3 ± 20.9	1.9 ± 1.1	12.3 ± 7.9	27.4 ± 7.6	1.5 ± 0.8	13.6 ± 11.5
Stainless steel (9)	3–15	5.6 ± 4.8	0.4 ± 0.1	1.1 ± 0.8	10.4 ± 8.8	0.4 ± 0.3	1.2 ± 1.0	6.6 ± 2.5	0.3 ± 0.2	1.6 ± 1.1
CoCr (14)	2–12	6.3 ± 4.7	2.6 ± 1.9	29.8 ± 17.2	5.1 ± 3.8	1.5 ± 1.2	8.4 ± 5.4	2.6 ± 2.2	1.3 ± 1.2	18.9 ± 11.3
CoCr strong wear (3)	2–3	11.2 ± 3.8	62.9 ± 2.9	33.4 ± 8.3	10.8 ± 3.9	41.4 ± 6.0	19.5 ± 4.0	10.9 ± 1.4	44.5 ± 4.1	25.4 ± 9.1
Normal	0	<3.3	<0.4	<3.0	<1.8	<0.1	<3.0	<0.9	<0.1	<1.4

Table 15.3 Typical distribution of nickel, cobalt and chromium in tissue samples from patients with THR loosening ($\mu g\ g^{-1}$ dry weight) (from Hildebrand et al., 1996)

Alloy	Exposure time (years)	Tissue sample	Ni	Co	Cr
Stainless steel	2	Granuloma	4.95	4.35	6.62
		Bone	1.52	1.21	1.43
		Connective tissue	1.12	0.93	0.83
NiCrMo	5	Granuloma	54.73	4.71	49.19
		Connective tissue	33.44	3.55	27.83
		Bone	53.15	2.84	62.64
		Fascia lata	47.52	8.32	67.24
CoCr	12	Connective tissue	0.26	2.00	1.37
		Bone	0.74	59.50	32.50
		Fascia lata	3.34	117.70	83.70

The high concentrations should be considered either as the result of corrosion and consequently the quality of the alloy, or as the consequence of clinical complications such as loosening related to allergic reactions and/or infections.

In conclusion, alloys containing cobalt, chromium and nickel corrode *in vivo* and release metal ions in biological fluids as well as in implants surrounding tissue. The metabolism and clearance of the metal ions varies for different alloys. Nickel and especially chromium are observed in the form of extracellular and intracellular precipitates, whereas cobalt seems to be bound to whole tissue in an unprecipitated form. In contrast to occupational exposure, orthopaedic implants are an internal and quite distinct source of contamination by allergic and toxic elements. Sometimes, alarmingly high concentrations of these elements are recovered in tissue and body fluids, so that more intensive monitoring of patients with such implants is to be strongly recommended.

15.5 FAILED AND VERY SUCCESSFUL IMPLANTS

Since the beginning of the twentieth century the rapid development of orthopaedic surgery has been based on the use of metal for implants, including osteosynthesis materials such as plates, screws, pins, nails and articular prostheses. At present, implants used in orthopaedic surgery are made of three kinds of alloys (Black, 1988):

- stainless steel alloys, containing iron and a high content of chromium
- CoCr alloys containing 25–30% chromium, 5–7% molybdenum and small amounts of other minerals (nickel, manganese, iron, silicon, etc.), or wrong CoCr alloys, containing about 20% chromium, 10% nickel and 15% tungsten
- alloys containing 90% titanium with a low content of aluminium, vanadium and/or iron, or commercially pure titanium.

Four different biological effects are observed, depending on the concentration, the length of contact and the method of administration.

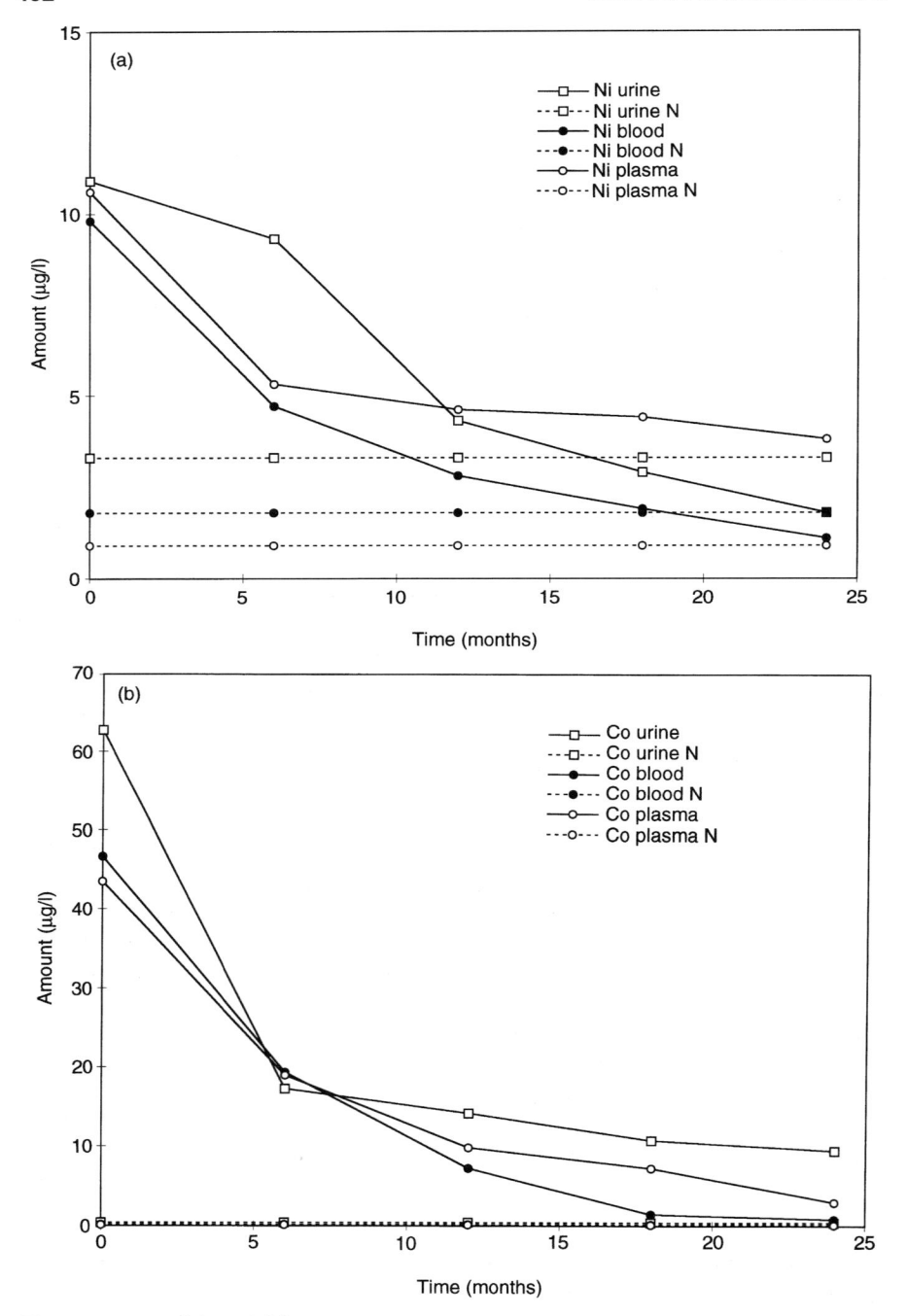

Figure 15.11 (a) and (b).

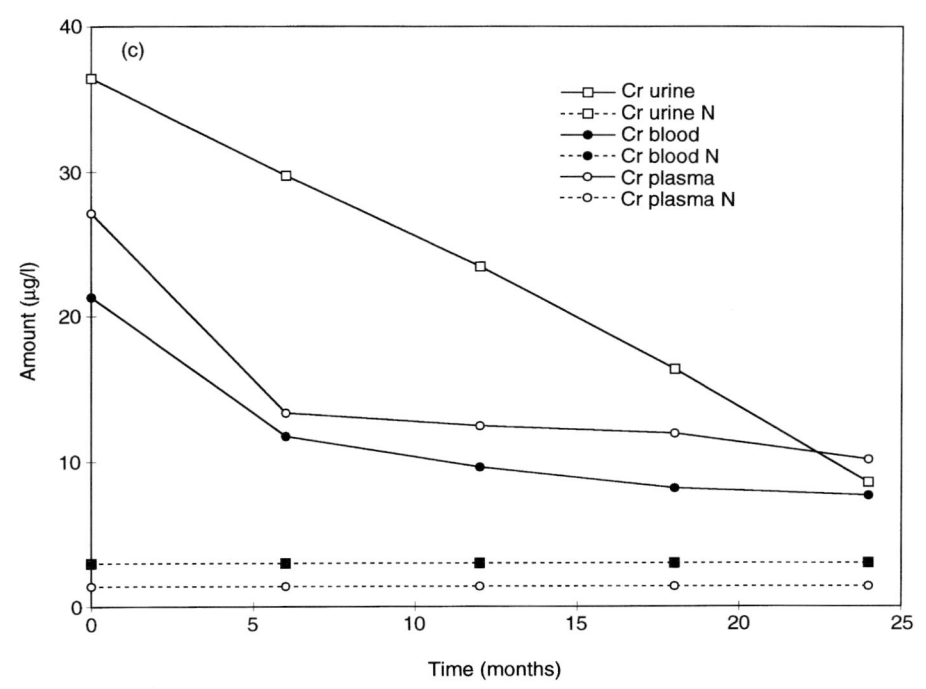

Figure 15.11 Nickel, chromium and cobalt clearing in a patient studied for over 2 years after retrieval of a CoCr THR. Only nickel reached normal upper values after this period. Horizontal dotted lines indicate normal upper values. These are too low for cobalt and thus do not appear in the graph (Hildebrand *et al.*, 1996)

- At very low concentrations, metals such as zinc, copper, nickel and cobalt for instance, are considered to be essential elements (Anke *et al.*, 1980).
- In contrast, high or excessive concentrations of these same substances can produce toxic effects, which are well known for arsenic, cobalt, nickel, lead and others. The cytotoxic effects of metallic ions have also been demonstrated on different cell-culture systems (Frazier and Andrews, 1979).
- Metals also have a high allergenic potency. In particular, nickel ions, chromates and cobalt salts are recognised to be redoubtable sensitising agents (Barrière *et al.*, 1979; Wall and Calcan, 1980).
- Numerous metal compounds are considered to be carcinogenic in animals. At present, the mechanism of this effect is not elucidated (Sunderman, 1989a). However, there is no clinical or statistical evidence of cancer induced by implants or prostheses made of alloys containing chromium, cobalt or nickel (Sunderman, 1989b).

The main reason for unwanted secondary biological and/or clinical effects is the release of ions from orthopaedic and dental alloys. It is induced by aggressive biological milieu such as plasma, serum, lymph or saliva, which may contain numerous oxidising enzymes. In addition, the electrogalvanic phenomena, which appear in the presence of different alloys in the oral cavity cannot be precluded, but may also be due to the use of different materials for orthopaedic implants, e.g. plates and screws, and articular prostheses.

Wear and abrasion particles released from articular prostheses and from mobile or non-stabilised implants are another risk factor. They can provoke directly a foreign-body response and, later on, other tissue reactions by their further dissolution in metallic ions. Other wear particles such as polyethylene and ceramics can also be the consequence of the continuous abrasion existing in the metal–polyethylene or metal–ceramic couples in articular prostheses. This wear debris is able to induce considerable tissular damage, leading to the loosening of the prosthesis, and the consequences may be osteolysis, loss of normal bone architecture, serious macrophagic reactions, granulomas, cysts, inflammation and allergic reactions.

An analysis of the reasons for the failure of implants will be given in the following paragraph, which also deals with articular prostheses and osteosynthesis materials.

15.5.1 ARTICULAR PROSTHESES

15.5.1.1 Total Hip Prostheses

Total hip arthroplasty has undergone a rapid development since the 1960s. The number of hip arthroplasties performed world-wide annually is estimated at 500 000. Numerous models of total hip prostheses have been performed and implanted, and they can be differentiated by:

- design of femoral and acetabular implants
- implant material
- bearing couples: metal–polyethylene, metal–metal, ceramic–polyethylene, ceramic–ceramic
- diameter of the femoral head (22, 28, 32 mm)
- fixation: cemented or uncemented implants, with or without hydroxyapatite coating.

The major problems leading to failure are aseptic loosening and periprosthetic bone resorption.

15.5.1.2 Aseptic Loosening

Loosening of a total hip prosthesis can be defined as a modification of the position of the implant. Harris *et al.* (1982) defined criteria of definite, probable or possible loosening, including all cases (symptomatic or not) of radiolucency at the bone–cement interface or cement–stem interface. Published loosening rates vary from 1.7 to 47%, depending on the surgical intervention, the implant used and the duration of follow-up. Such cases require surgical revision, sometimes with difficult problems of reconstruction.

Many causes for the occurrence of loosening have been cited, including the design of the implant, malposition, cementing technique, ageing of the cement (microfrag-

RETRIEVAL ANALYSIS

mentation by fretting or cement mantle fracture), fracture of the femoral stem and instability of uncemented implants (primary or secondary due to the lack of osteointegration of the porous metal surface). All these factors can generate micromobility of the implant, which becomes progressively worse, leading to osteolysis with mobilisation and sinking of the prosthesis. A case of femoral and acetabular hip prosthesis loosening is shown in Figure 15.12.

These mechanical phenomena can be aggravated or even caused by osteolytic periprosthetic reactions subsequent to the liberation of wear particles. For some few years, the causes of these osteolytic reactions have been considered to be biological rather than due to mechanical loosening factors. In most cases, however, it is difficult to separate clearly these mechanical and biological factors leading to the implant failure.

15.5.1.3 Periprosthetic Osteolysis

Retrieval and autopsy studies on patients with total hip replacements have shown that bone resorption induced by wear debris is one of the most important processes that can generate aseptic loosening and also one of the main reasons for late failures in THR.

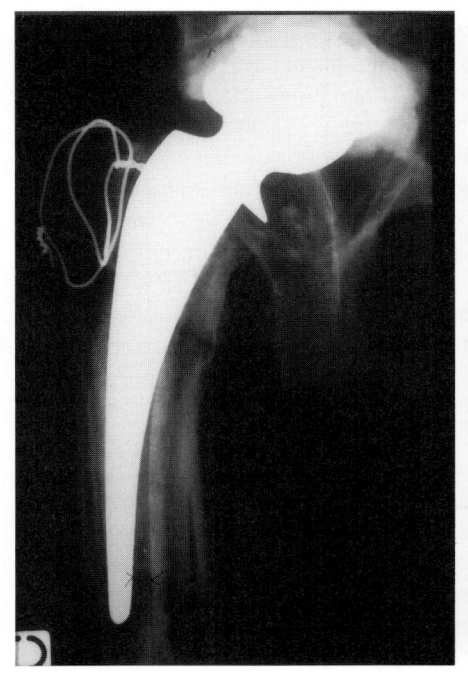

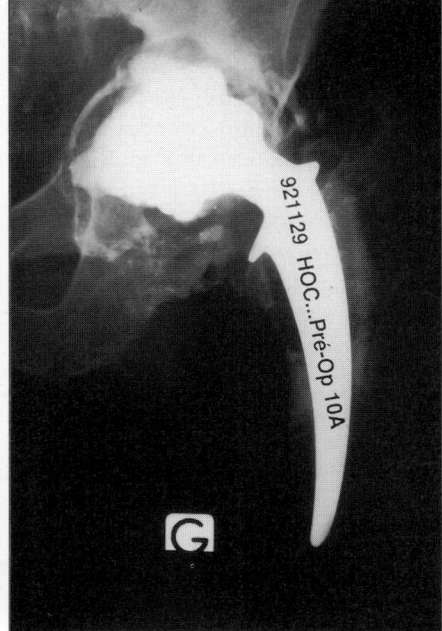

Figure 15.12 Femoral and acetabular loosening of a 12-year-old total hip prosthesis.

Figure 15.13 provides examples of aggressive granulomas around femoral prostheses which could be determined as aggressive granulomas (Figure 15.13a), medium osteolytic reactions (Figure 15.13b), and extensive osteolysis associated with stem sinking (Figure 15.13c) or not (Figure 15.13d). The topography of these osteolytic areas is determined according to the radiographic Gruen's areas (Gruen et al, 1979), which are described in the schematic presentation given in Figure 15.14.

In 1977, Willert and Semlitsch showed that osteolysis can be traced back to the accumulation of particles. Particulate products from the implanted components and from bone cement were directly transported into the capsular tissue by phagocytosis or indirectly transferred via the organisation of fibrin and necrotic cell masses. In the tissue they were stored in mononuclear histiocytes or multinucleated histiocytes (giant cells) and carried away via the perivascular lymph spaces. In cases of large amounts of particulate debris, the interfacial membranes became involved in particle storage, leading to bone resorption. More recently, it has been shown that the production of potentially osteolytic mediators (prostaglandin E_2, interleukin-1, etc.) and metabolic products by histiocytes is stimulated by the phagocytosis of particulate debris. All biomaterials (metals, polymethylmethacrylate, polyethylene, etc.) have been implicated in this process (Amstutz et al., 1992; Doorn et al., 1996).

15.5.1.4 Polyethylene Wear Particles

At present, polyethylene appears to be the most significant particle in wear-induced bone resorption. Particles arise from the wear of articulating surfaces. The size of the polyethylene particles varies from 0.5 to 300 μm according to different wear processes. For 0.5 μm particles, and for 30 mm^3 of wear of a 28 mm cup, the number of particles produced in a total hip replacement due to the abrasion between the bearing surfaces has been estimated at 500 billion particles per year (McKellop et al., 1995). Figure 15.15 shows an explanted acetabular implant with serious wear of the polyethylene insert.

According to their size, these particles are ingested by either mononuclear histiocytes or multinucleated foreign-body giant cells, leading in the case of accumulation to bone resorption.

15.5.1.5 Metal Wear Particles

In THR, the main sources of metal particles have been reported by Doorn et al. (1996), i.e. the bone–metal interface, bone–cement interface, impingement of the neck or collar and acetabular rim, inside of a modular cup, junction of the femoral head and Morse taper, porous coatings moving against the bone and intercoating movement. The renewed interest in metal-on-metal bearing surfaces as a means of avoiding the production of polyethylene wear particles could be a new source of metal wear particle that should be evaluated.

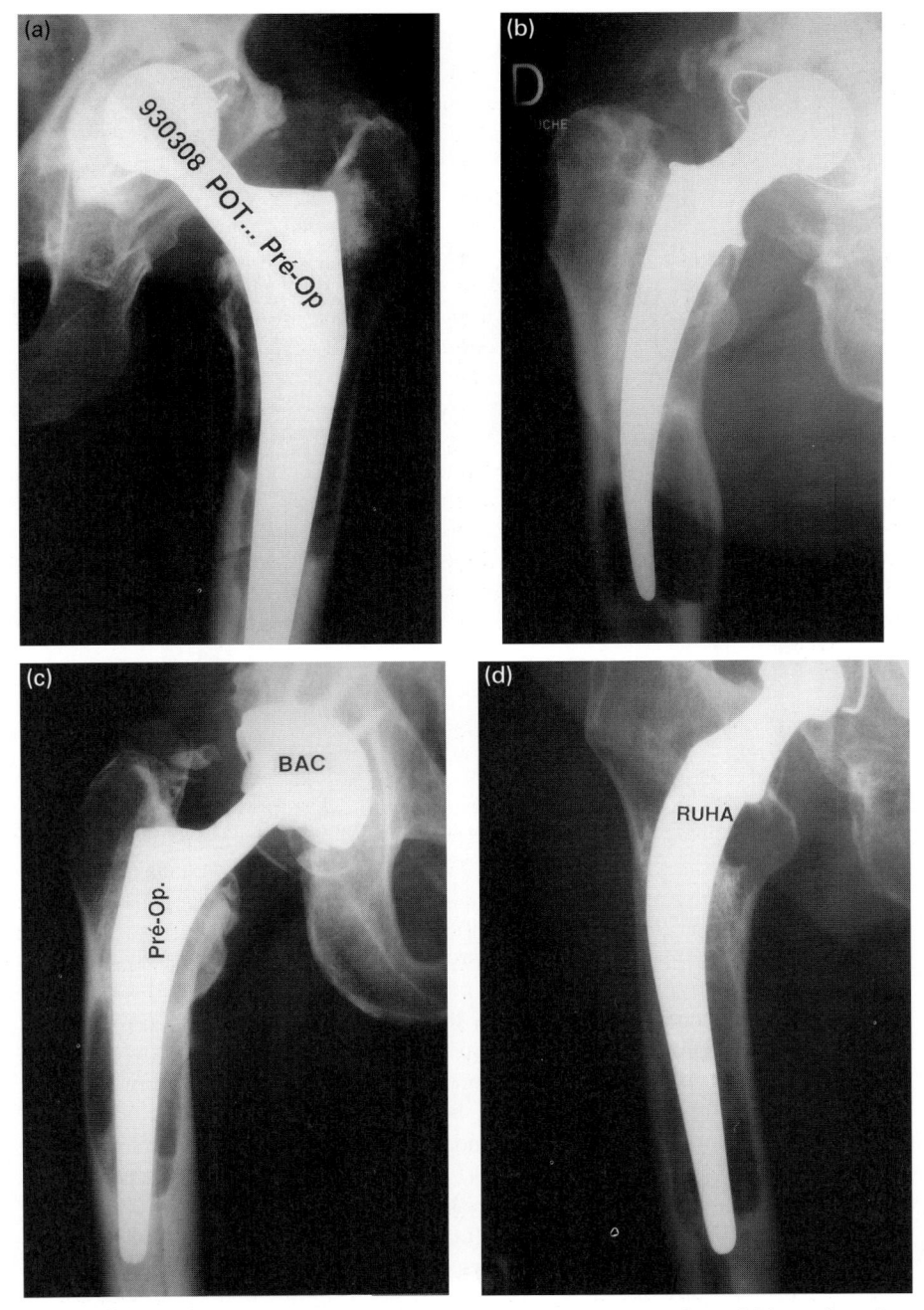

Figure 15.13 Osteolytic reactions around femoral stems of total hip arthroplasties. (a) Aggressive granuloma in zones 3 and 5; (b) osteolytic reaction in zones 2, 3, 5 and 6; (c) extensive osteolysis (zones 1, 2, 3, 5 and 6) associated with stem sinking; (d) extensive osteolysis (zones 1, 2, 3, 5, 6 and 7).

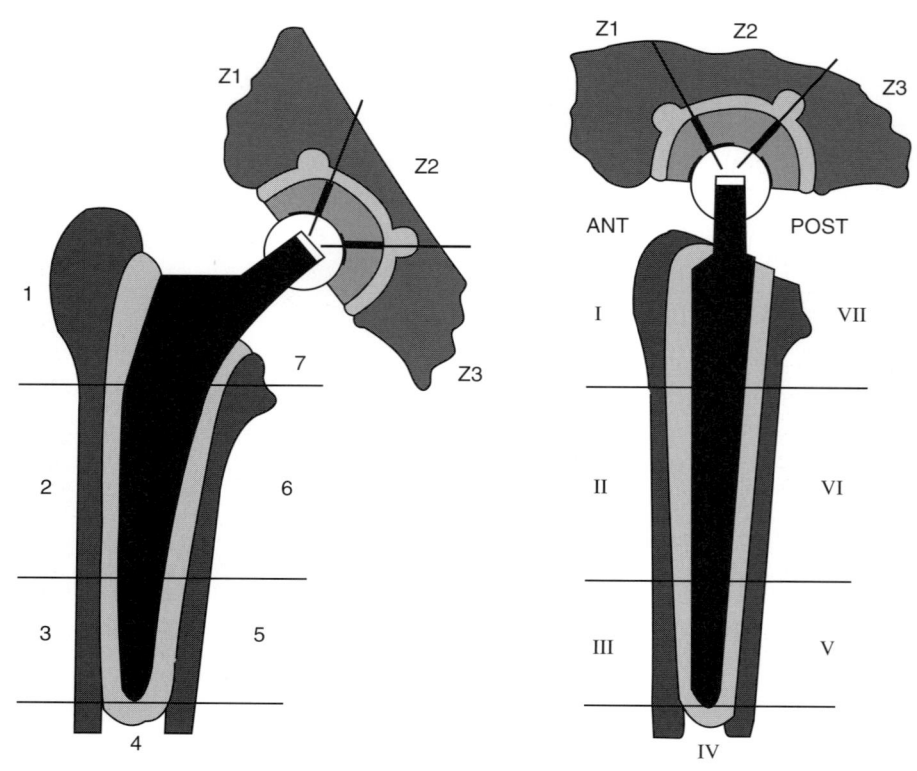

Figure 15.14 Gruen's zones allowing a topographic localisation of the osteolytic reactions.

Figure 15.16 shows different explanted prostheses. One THR presents severe metal wear due to the fretting of the stem in the cement mantle (Figure 15.16a). On another arthroplasty metal wear was provoked by the impingement of a ceramic head on the acetabular rim (Figure 15.16b). The third case presents a broken ceramic femoral head, the fragments of which liberated small ceramic particles that in turn produced very fast metal head wear of the metallic head (Figure 15.16c).

Titanium implants seem to produce more particles than CoCr implants (Howie, 1990). The size of particles varies from 0.1 to 400 µm according to the type of wear. Most studies indicate a size smaller than 3 µm and rarely larger than 100 µm. The number and type of metal particles in THR cannot be estimated precisely as these factors depend on the type of alloy, the forces exercised, the duration of abrasion, etc.

Metal particles provoke a macrophage tissue reaction, with phagocytosis by mononuclear histiocytes. Immunological reactions have also been reported, but their clinical implications remain unclear. The accumulation of metal wear particles in periprosthetic tissue leads to metallosis and osteolysis.

RETRIEVAL ANALYSIS

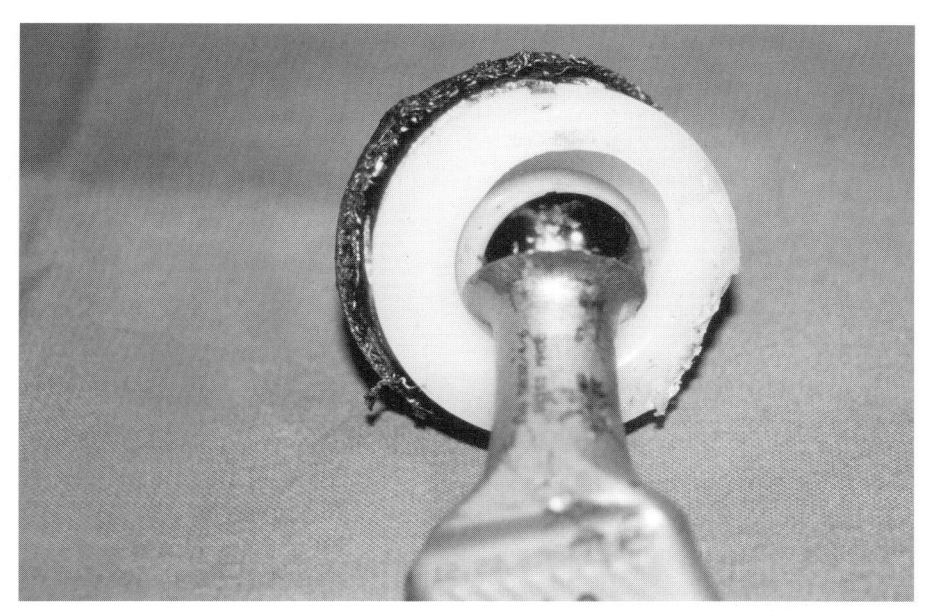

Figure 15.15 Wear of the polyethylene insert of a metal-backed acetabular implant (explanted).

Figure 15.17 shows a macroscopic feature of periprosthetic tissue around a total hip prosthesis with osteolysis and metallosis. Figure 15.18 illustrates a case of metallosis around a total knee prosthesis, induced by the impingement between the patella of the metal-back implant and the femoral implant. Radiographic investigation reveals osteolysis and loosening with important mobilisation of the femoral implant (Figure 15.18a, b). The perioperative picture shows the black appearance of the tissue, corresponding to metallosis, i.e. invasion of metallic wear particles (Figure 15.18c). The polyethylene insert (patellar and tibial) contained carbon. On the explanted femoral component there appears a deep track, which has been dug into the prosthetic trochlea, by the metallic part of the prosthetic patella (Figure 15.18d, e).

15.5.2 OSTEOSYNTHESIS MATERIALS

Any implant introduced into the human organism is exposed to at least two degradation phenomena: one is of physicomechanical origin due to the environment of the site of implantation, while the other concerns the electrochemical behaviour of implants due to the presence of chloride ions in the biological medium. In this way, an interaction between the implant and the tissue leads to a tissue response, especially in the vicinity of the implanted material. This reaction can be modified by

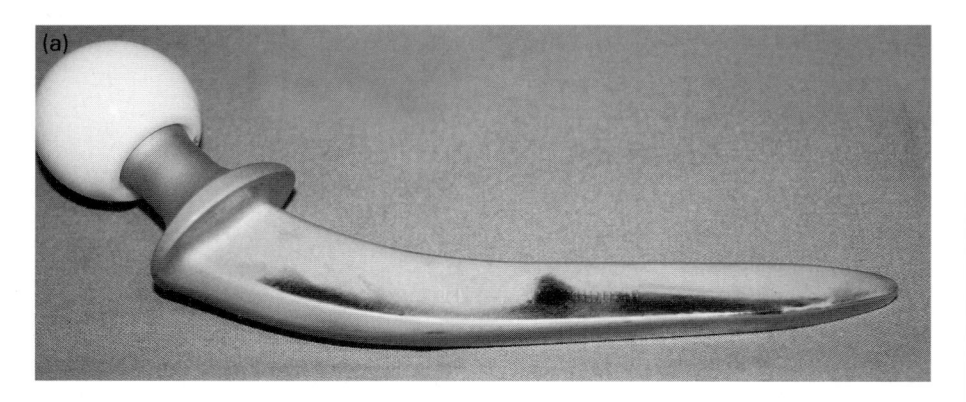

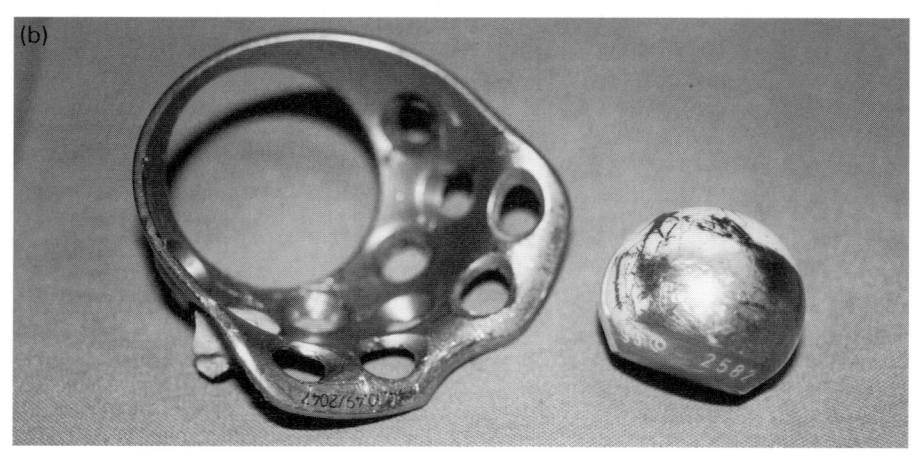

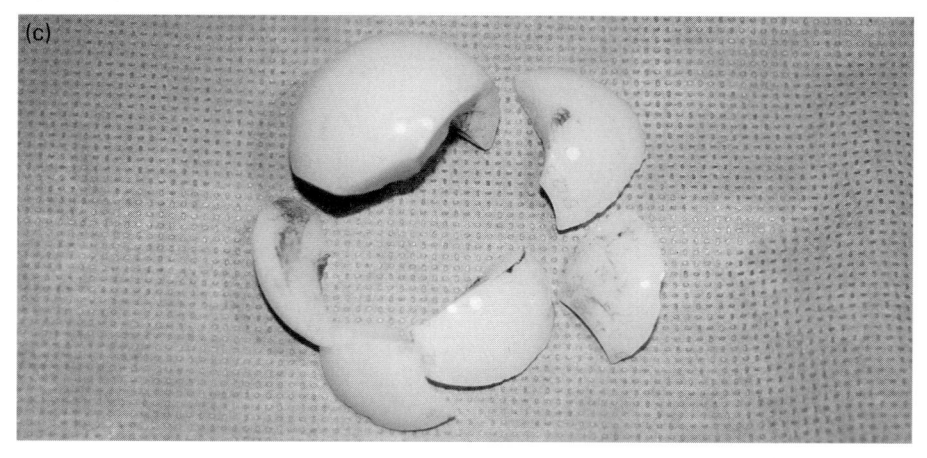

Figure 15.16 Explanted implants of total hip arthroplasties. (a) Explanted femoral prosthesis with fretting areas; (b) impingement of a ceramic femoral head on the acetabular rim; (c) broken ceramic femoral head.

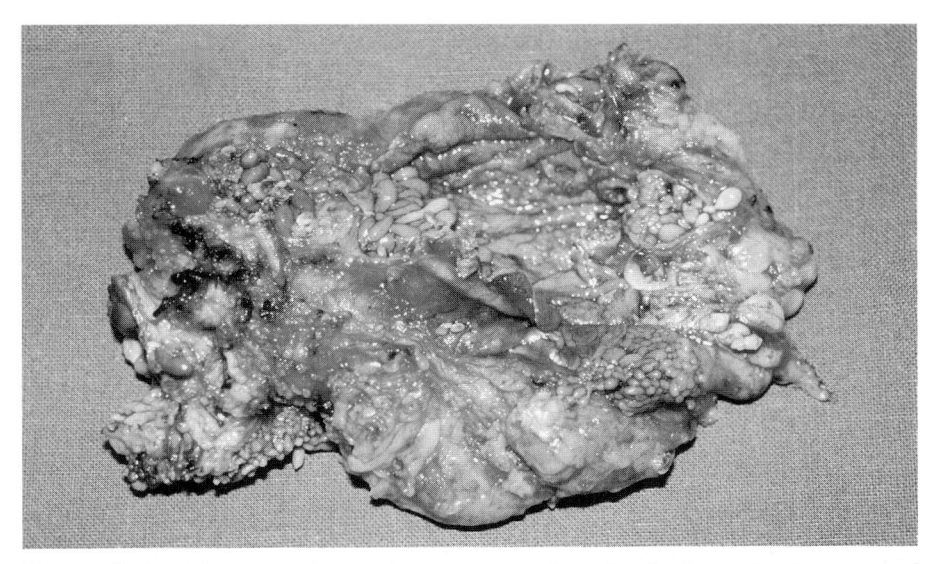

Figure 15.17 Macroscopic appearance of periprosthetic tissue in the case of granuloma in contact with a total hip prosthesis with metallosis.

various other factors, such as a local infection, pre-existing evolutionary pathology, local tissular trauma from the surgical intervention and movement of the implant acting as a static foreign body. Thus, inflammatory granulomas appear, mobilising phagocytic cells, which is a fundamental mechanism of non-specific defence. These cells are able to phagocytose and convey mineral or organic particles derived from either mechanical degradation or electrochemical corrosion. In addition, histological observations reveal an increased number of lymphocytes in the vicinity of the implants, which suggests an immunological process. Indeed, clinical and scientific research has emphasised a relationship between the use of these alloys and the increase in sensitisation to the metals contained therein, e.g. nickel, cobalt and chromium.

In 1988, Hildebrand *et al.* reported a study on the metabolism of the diffusing metal ions in patients after the removal of metal implants (osteosynthesis plates, nail-plates and centromedullary nails). In total blood, nickel and cobalt levels were significantly higher than the upper normal level. All orthopaedic implants displayed corrosion areas (pittings, crevices and galvanic corrosion areas). Some morphological changes to the tissue in the vicinity of the implant were observed, such as granulomas, the dark colour of which indicated the presence of metallic precipitates or wear particles. Connective tissue displayed an increase in cell density and high amounts of metallic intracellular and extracellular precipitates. Intracellular deposits were generally observed in macrophages, fibroblasts and histiocytes. Granulomous tissue was characterised by multinuclear giant cells (MGC) and also contained many electron-dense particles. Ultrastructural examination revealed quite different aspects of these structures, varying among patients, implant types and

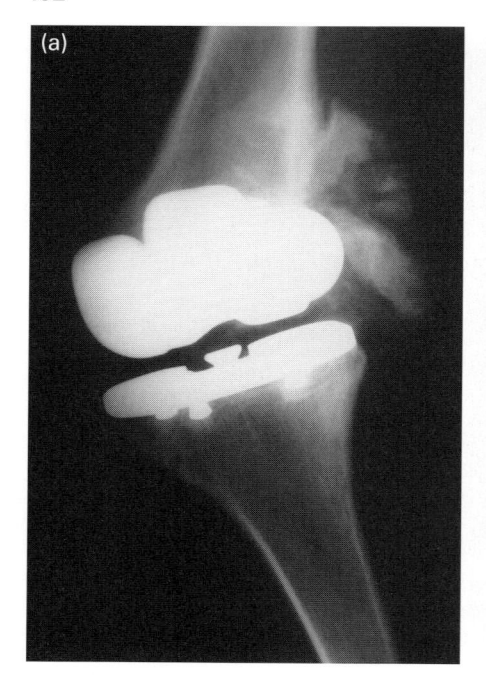

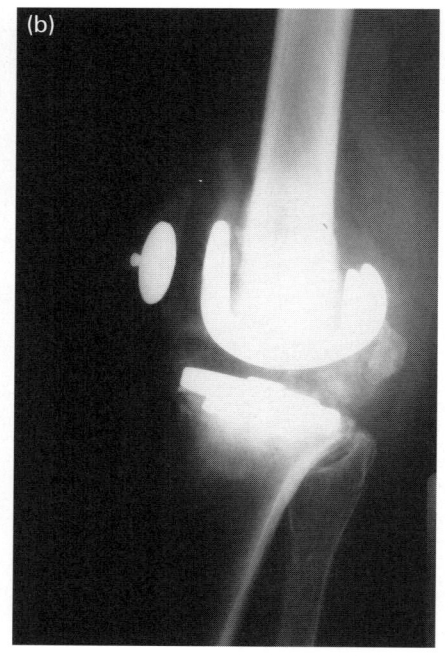

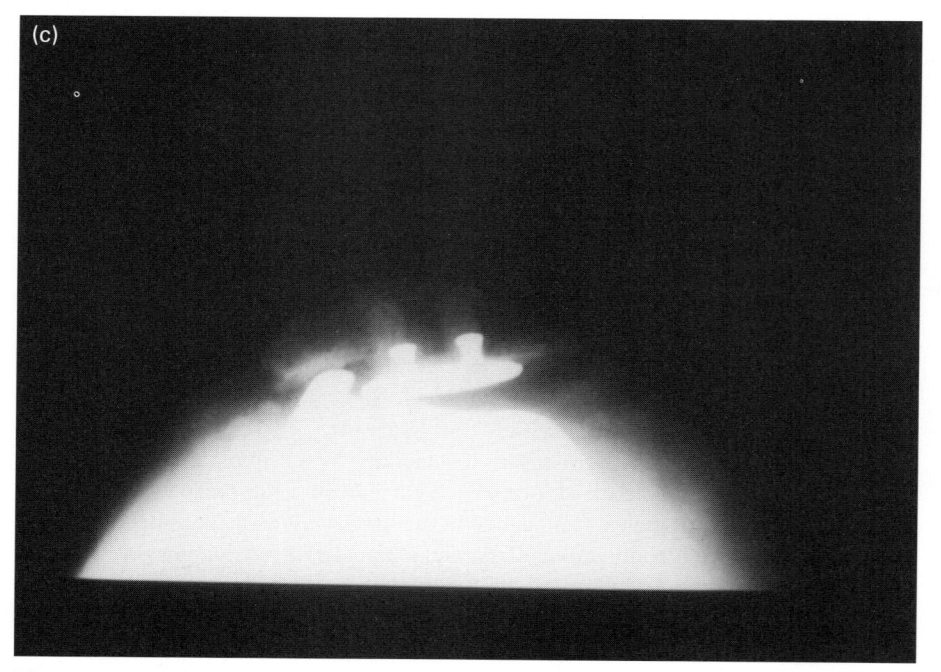

Figure 15.18 (a)–(c).

RETRIEVAL ANALYSIS

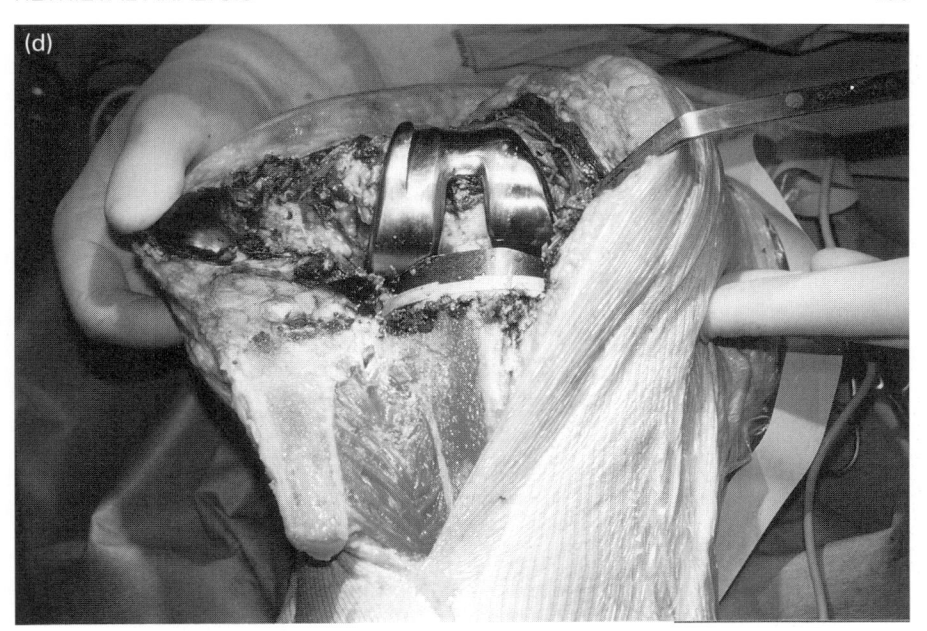

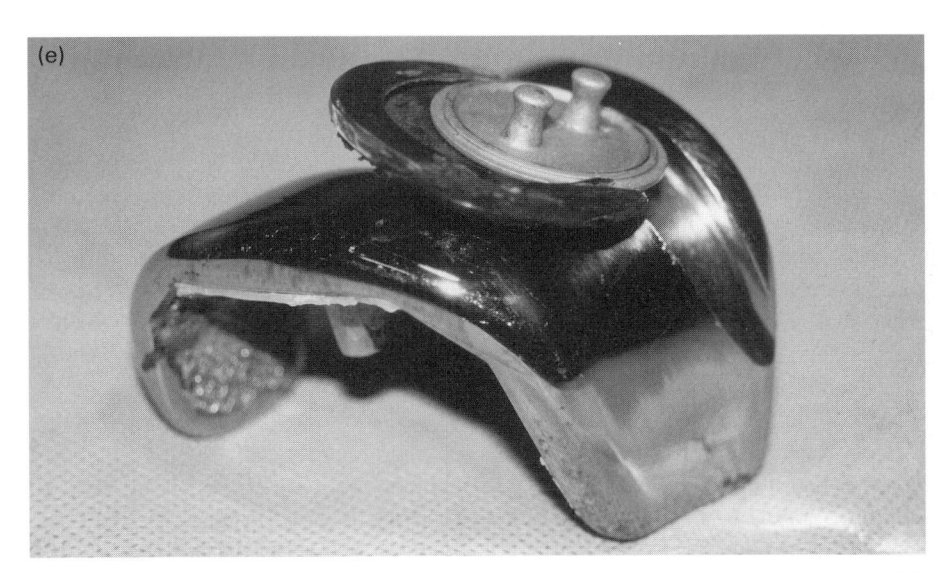

Figure 15.18 (a) Osteolysis and metallosis around a total knee prosthesis with serious wear; (b) anteroposterior and lateral radiographs of loosened total knee prosthesis with metallosis: mobilisation of the femoral component; (c) femoropatellar view, showing inpingement between the titanium femoral component and the patellar metal backing (CrCo); (d) perioperative view: typical metallosis with dark appearance of the periprosthetic tissues; (e) explanted prosthesis: considerable wear of the femoral component.

examinated tissues. There were amorphous precipitates besides crystalline particles and granular organic deposits next to membranous structures. The elementary composition of the particles and precipitates varies as a function of both their morphological differences and the initial composition of the implant alloy. Tissue analysis showed a striking increase in the distribution of nickel, cobalt and chromium in connective tissue next to nails, depending on the duration of exposure. An elevated content of nickel, cobalt and chromium has also been observed in hair, fingernails and toenails. Total blood, plasma and (if properly collected) urine are the most significant indicators of excessive internal exposure.

The authors concluded that orthopaedic implants of CoCrNi alloys can corrode in biological fluids as well as in implant-surrounding tissue. The metabolism and clearance of these metal ions are different: nickel and especially chromium are observed in the form of extracellular and intracellular precipitates, whereas cobalt seems to be bound to whole tissue in an unprecipitated form. The presence of other elements such as sulfur, chlorine, calcium and especially phosphorous suggests the metabolisation of the corrosion products and the existence of metallo-organic metabolites. In contrast to occupational exposure, orthopaedic implants are an internal source of contamination by allergenic and toxic elements. Alarmingly high concentrations of these elements are sometimes recovered in tissues and body fluids, so that more intensive monitoring of patients with such implants must be recommended.

15.5.2.1 Metal Carcinogenesis and Orthopaedic Implants: Case Report of Malignant Fibrous Histiocytoma

In 1971, a 26-year-old male suffered a motorcycle traffic accident. He sustained a fracture of the low extremity of his left femur. This fracture was treated by open reduction and internal fixation with a plate and screws of stainless steel. The functional recovery was complete.

In December 1990 pain arose in the lower part of his left thigh. At the time, the pain was related to a conflict between the iliotibial tract and the femoral plate. Gradually increasing pain and radiographic analysis (Figure 15.19a, b) indicated a surgical revision in January 1991 to remove the metallic implants. The surgeon discovered a large necrotic bone area in the posterior and lateral part of the femur. He removed the screws and the plate, took a biopsy and performed a curettage. Bacteriological findings were negative. Histopathological examinations suggested areas of necrotic bone and a very typical cellular proliferation appearing as bone sarcoma, but the biopsy was not sufficient for a positive diagnosis.

One month later, the patient suffered a pathological fracture on the same site and was referred to the Department of Orthopaedic Surgery in March 1991. Examination revealed a painful, large and firm swelling over the distal part of the thigh. Radiography revealed a large osteolystic area in the lower part of the left femur and a sub-condylar fracture (Figure 15.19d).

Computed axial tomography (CAT) and nuclear magnetic resonance (NMR) imaging scans showed a tumoural mass involving the lower third of the thigh, with osteolysis of the posterior and lateral cortices of the femur, invading the surrounding soft tissues. Another biopsy was performed on 7 March 1991, and histological study revealed a malignant fibrous histiocytoma (MFH) of the bone and the presence of numerous metallic foreign bodies in the tumour (Figure 15.20a, b).

A hip disarticulation was immediately performed. Histological findings and immunolabelling reconfirmed the diagnosis. The patient was released to a rehabilitation centre and resumed walking with an artificial limb. In June 1991, X-ray examinations revealed two metastatic pulmonary nodules. Chemotherapy with vindesine (3.5 mg m^{-2} on day 1), ifosfamide (2.5 g m^{-2} on days 1 and 2), doxorubicin (27.5 mg m^{-2} on days 1 and 2) and cisplatin (88.5 mg m^{-2} on day 3) was administered for 3 successive months. In August 1991, a right hemiplegia revealed cerebral metastasis which was resected in a neurosurgical department. Two additional periods of chemotherapy were then administered.

After 4 months of stabilisation, spreading of the disease and general metastatic diffusion were noticed. The patient died 21 years after the internal fixation of the fracture and 12 months after the diagnosis of MFH of the bone.

In conclusion, MFH of the bone may occur in normal bone but also as a late complication of pre-existing bone abnormalities (Mirra *et al.*, 1974; Capanna *et al.*, 1984; Boland and Huvos, 1986; Little and McCarthy, 1993). According to various authors, it represents from 1 to 5% of malignant bone tumours and occurs mainly from the second to the sixth decade of life. In young humans, it occurs more often in normal bone. It can also be observed on pre-existing abnormalities, mainly after the age of 60 years, such as bone infarct, Paget's disease, enchondroma, fibrous dysplasia, radiotherapy, dedifferentiated chondrosarcoma, multiple osteochendromas and chronic osteomyelitis.

Some cases have reported the occurrence of bone MFH at the site of metallic implants, plate and screws, hip prostheses and metallic foreign bodies from shrapnel fragments (Table 15.1). The causal relationship between this kind of tumour and metal implants in humans is difficult to establish (Lee *et al.*, 1984; Sunderman, 1988; Tait *et al.*, 1988; Haag and Adler, 1989; Nelson and Phillips, 1990; Goodfellow, 1992; Jacobs *et al.*, 1992).

In the case described here, the possible relationship between a malignant fibrous bone histiocytoma and the presence of the metallic implants (plate and screws) could be established (Laffargue *et al.*, 1998). This does not preclude a concomitant role of the repair process or bone necroses in the appearance of malignant transformation. In the last few years, reports on other associated tumours have been increasingly published and the interpretation of a simple coincidence should no longer be the only consideration (Mirra *et al.*, 1974; Troop *et al.*, 1990; Solomon and Sekel, 1992; Khurana *et al.*, 1994; Gillespie *et al.*, 1996; Lewis and Sunderman, 1996; Visuri *et al.*, 1996).

In spite of the small number of cases of malignant tumours arising with respect to the large number of metal implants used in humans, these arguments deserve serious consideration. As proposed earlier by Aspley (1989) and Jacobs *et al.* (1992), the establishment of an international or world-wide register of such cases would facilitate future knowledge.

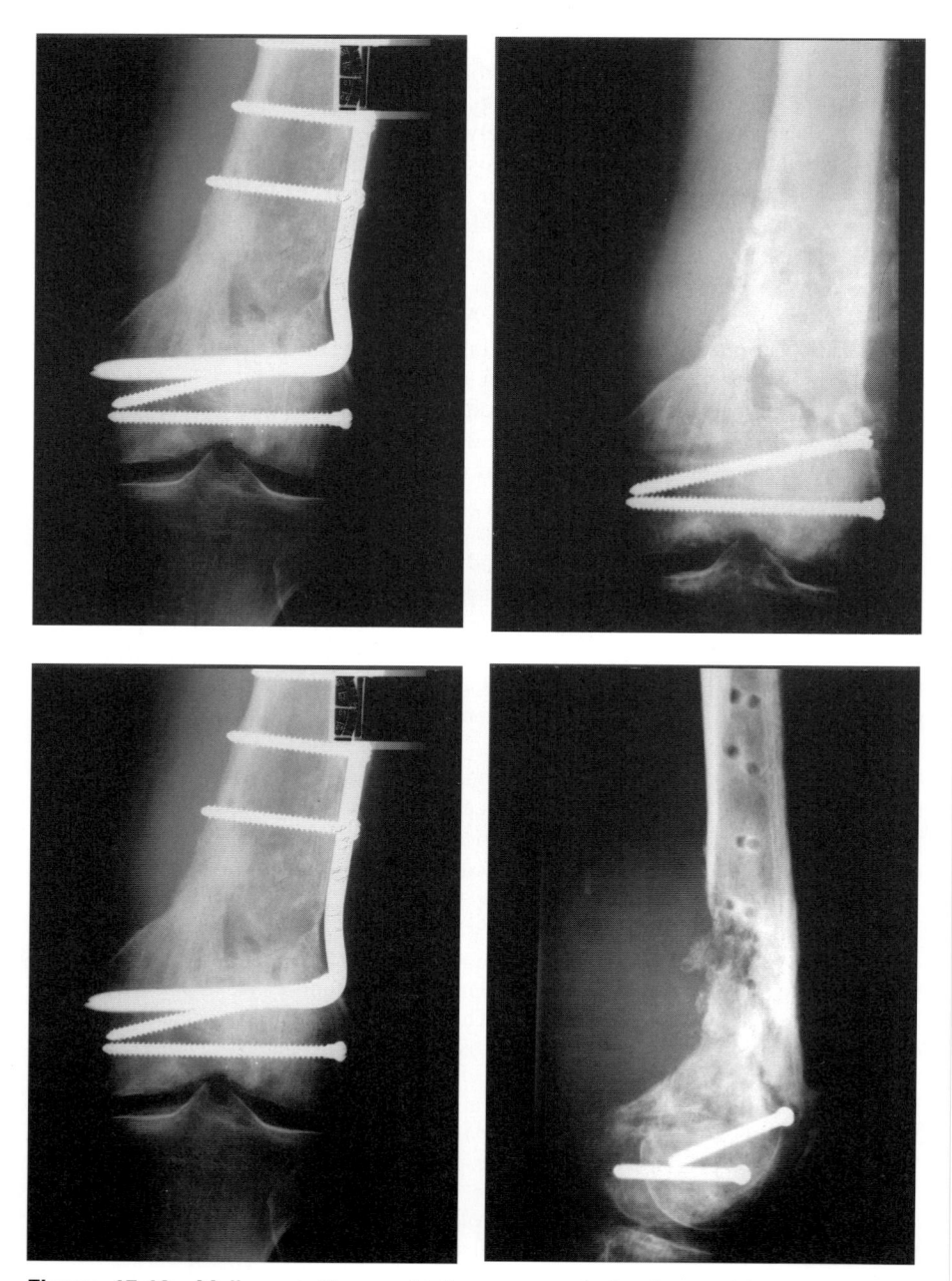

Figure 15.19 Malignant fibrous histiocytoma of the bone, 20 years after a femoral fracture.

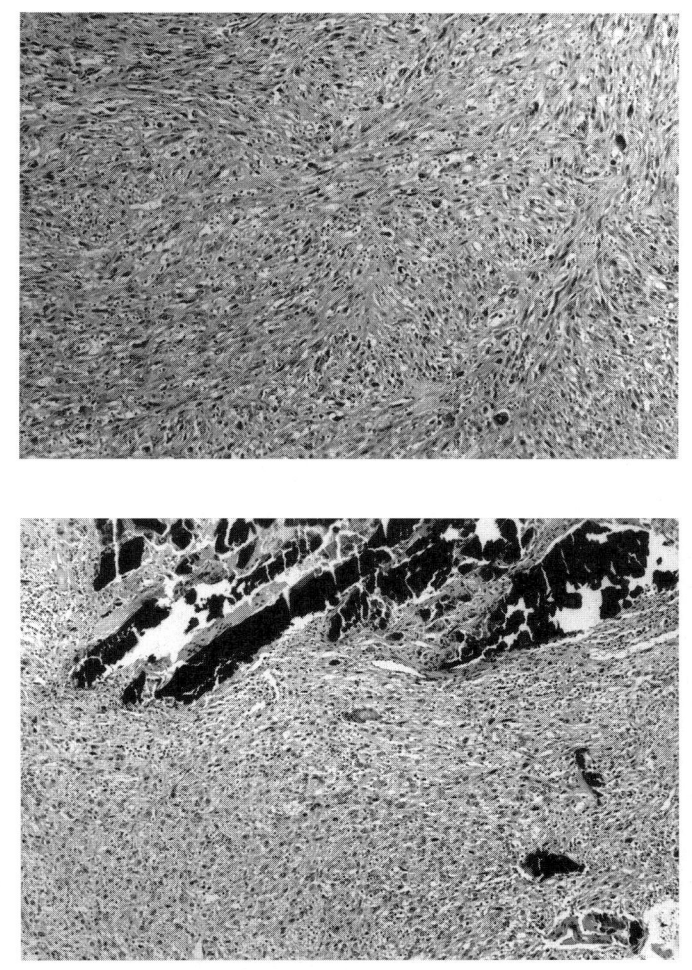

Figure 15.20 Malignant fibrous histiocytoma of the bone, 20 years after a femoral fracture.

15.6 CONCLUSION

Beside this analysis of failure and adverse effects of metallic implants in orthopaedic and traumatic surgery, the great improvements in the implants usually applied in the treatment of polytraumatism and osteoarticular diseases must be emphasised, as numerous patients have recovered satisfactory function and mobility.

However, the knowledge of these adverse phenomena should encourage the removal of metallic osteosynthesis materials as soon as they are no longer necessary, as well as the institutional organisation of registers allowing the periodic surveying of all patients with osteoarticular prostheses.

REFERENCES

Amstutz, H.C., Campbell, P., Kossovsky, N. and Clarke, J. (1992) Mechanism and clinical significance of wear debris-induced osteolysis, *Clin. Orthop.* **276**, 7–17.

Anke, M., Kronemann, H., Groppel, B., Henning, A., Meissner, D. and Schneider, H.J. (1980) The influence of nickel deficiency on growth, reproduction, longevity and different biochemical parameters of goats, in 3-*Spurenelement Symposium, Nickel*, Vol. 3 (eds M. Anke, H.J. Schneider and C. Brückner), Wiss. Beitr. Karl-Marx-Univ. Leipzig and Friedr-Shiller-Univ. Jena, pp. 3–10.

Aspley, A.G. (1989) Editorial: Malignancy and joint replacement: the tip of an iceberg? *J. Bone Joint Surg.* 71B, 1.

Barbosa, M.A. (1991) Corrosion mechanisms of metallic biomaterials, in *Biomaterials Degradation* (ed. M.A. Barbosa), North-Holland, Amsterdam, pp. 227–57.

Barrière, H., Boiteau, H.L., Geraut, C. and Metayer, C. (1979) Allergie aux détergents et allergie au nickel, *Ann. Der. Vener.* **106**, 33–7.

Bauer, T.W., Stulberg, B. N., Ming, J. and Geesink, R.G.T. (1993) Uncemented acetabular components, *J. Arthroplasty* **8**, 167–77.

Black, J. (1988) *In vivo* corrosion of a cobalt–base alloy and its biological consequences, in *Biocompatibility of Co–Cr–Ni Alloys* (eds H.F. Hildebrand and M. Champy), NATO-ASI Series A, Vol. 158, Plenum, pp. 83–100.

Black, J., Sherk, H., Bonini, J., Rostoker, W.R., Schajowicz, F. and Galante, J.O. (1990) Metallosis associated with a stable titanium alloy femoral component in total hip replacement, *J. Bone Joint Surg.* **72**, 126–30.

Bloebaum, R.D., Merrell, M., Gustke, K. and Simmons, M. (1991) Retrieval analysis of a hydroxyapatite-coated hip prosthesis, *Clin. Orthop. Rel. Res.* **267**, 97–102.

Boland, P.J. and Huvos, A.G. (1986) Malignant fibrous histiocytoma of bone, *Clin. Orthop.* **204**, 130–4.

Boss, J.H., Shajrawi, I. and Mendes, D.G. (1994) The nature of the bone–implant interface, *Med. Prog. Technol.* **20**, 119–42.

Buma, P. and Gardeniers, J.W.M. (1995) Tissue reactions around a hydroxyapatite-coated hip prosthesis, *J. Arthroplasty* **10**, 389–95.

Capanna, R., Bertoni, F., Bacchini, P., Bacci, G., Guerra, A. and Campanacci, M. (1984) Malignant fibrous histiocytoma of bone. The experience at the Rizzoli Institute: report of 90 cases, *Cancer*, **54**, 177–87.

Cheng, S.L., Davey, J.R., Inman, R.D., Binnington, A.G., Guelph, D.V.M. and Smith, T.J. (1995) The effect of the medial collar in total hip arthroplasty with porous-coated components inserted without cement, *J. Bone Joint Surg.* **77A**, 118–23.

Coleman, R.F., Herrington, J. and Scales, J.T. (1972) The concentration of wear products in the body following total joint replacement, *Br. J. Med. Biol.* **17**, 744.

Coleman, R.F., Herrington, J. and Scales, J.T. (1973) Concentration of wear products in hair, blood and urine after total hip replacement, *Br. Med. J.* **i**, 527–9.

Collier, J.P., Bauer, T.W., Bloebaum, R.D., Bobyn, J.D., Cook, S.D., Galante, J.O., Harris, W.H., Head, W.C., Jasty, M.J., Mayor, M.B., Sumner, D.R. and Whiteside, L.A. (1992a) Results of implant retrieval from postmortem specimens in patients with well-functioning, long-term total hip replacement, *Clin. Orthop. Relat. Res.* **274**, 97–112.

Collier, J.P., Surprenant, V.A., Jensen, R.E., Mayor, M.B. and Surprenant, H.P. (1992b) Corrosion between the components of modular femoral hip prostheses, *J. Bone Joint Surg.* **74B**, 511–17.

Cook, S.D. and Thomas, K.A. (1991) Fatigue failure of noncemented porous-coated implants, *J. Bone Joint Surg.* **73B**, 20–4.

DeYoung, D.J., DeYoung B.A., Aberman, H.A., Kenna, R.V. and Hungerford, D.S. (1992) Implantation of an uncemented total hip prosthesis technique and initial results of 100 arthroplasties, *Vet. Surg.* **21**, 168–77.

Dhert, J.A. (1994) Retrieval studies on calcium phosphate-coated implants, *Med. Prog. Technol.* **20**, 143–54.

Dobbs, H.S. and Minski, M.J. (1980) Metal ion release after total hip replacement, *Biomaterials* **1**, 193–8.

Doorn, P.F., Campbell, P.A. and Amstutz, H.C. (1996) Metal versus polyethylene wear particles in total hip replacements, *Clin. Orthop.* **329S**, 206–16.

Dorr, L.D., Bloebaum, R., Emmanual, J. and Meldrum, R. (1990) Histologic, biochemical and ion analysis of tissue and fluids retrieved during total hip arthroplasty, *Clin. Orthop. Relat. Res.* **261**, 82–95.

Frazier, M.E. and Andrews, T.K. (1979) *In vitro* clonal growth assay for evaluating toxicity of metal salts, in *Trace Metals in Health and Disease* (ed. N. Kharasch), Raven Press, New York, pp. 71–81.

Gilbert, J.L., Buckley, C.A., Jacobs, J.J., Bertin, K.C. and Zernich, M.R. (1994) Intergranular corrosion-fatigue failure of cobalt-alloy femoral stems, *J. Bone Joint Surg.* **76A**, 110–15.

Gillespie, W.J., Henry, D.A., O'Connel, D.L., Kendrick, S., Juszezak, E., Mcinneny, K. and Derby, L. (1996) Development of hematopoietic cancers after implantation of total joint replacement, *Clin. Orthop.* **329S**, 290–6.

Goodfellow, J. (1992) Editorial: Malignancy and joint replacement, *J. Bone Joint Surg.* **74B**, 645.

Griffith, H.J., Burke, J. and Bonfiglio, T.A. (1987) Granulomatous pseudotumors in total joint replacement, *Skel. Radiol.* **16**, 146–52.

Gruen, T.A., McNeige, G.M. and Amstutz, H.C. (1979) Modes of failure of cemented-stem-type femoral components: a radiographic analysis of loosening, *Clin. Orthop.* **141**, 17–27.

Haag, M. and Adler, C.P. (1989) Malignant fibrous histiocytoma in association with hip replacement, *J. Bone Joint Surg.* **71B**, 701.

Harris, W.H., McCarthy, J.C. and O'Neill, D.A. (1982) Femoral component loosening using contemporary techniques of femoral fixation, *J. Bone Joint Surg.* **64-A**, 1063.

Helsen, J.A., Jaecques, S.V.N. and Simon, J.-P. (1997) Measurement of mass eroded from a THR stem, in *13th European Conference on Biomaterials* 4–7 September, Göteborg, Abstracts, Paper no. 56, European Society for Biomaterials, Göteborg.

Hildebrand, H.F., Laffargue, P., Decoulx, J., Duquennoy, A. and Mestdagh, H. (1996) Retrieval analyses of total hip replacements, *Int. J. Risk Safety Med.* **8**, 125–34.

Hildebrand, H.F., Ostapczuk, P., Mercier, J.F., Stoeppler, M., Roumazeille, B. and Decoulx, J. (1988) in *Biocompatibility of Co–Cr–Ni alloys* (eds H.F. Hildebrand and M. Champy), NATO-ASI Series A, Vol. 158, Plenum, New York, 133–53.

Hofmann, J., Wiehl, N., Michel, R., Loer, F. and Zilkens, J. (1982) Neutron activation studies of the in-body corrosion of hip-joint prostheses made of Co–Cr-alloys, *J. Radioanal. Chem.* **70**, 85–107.

Howie, D.W. (1990) Tissue response in relation to type of wear particles around failed hip arthroplasties, *J. Arthroplasty* **5**, 337–48.

Hughes, S.S., Furia, J.P., Smith, P., Pellegrini, V.D. and Rochester, J. R. (1995) Atrophy of the proximal part of the femur after total hip arthroplasty without cement, *J. Bone Joint Surg.* **77A**, 231–8.

Jacobs, J.J., Rosenbaum, D.H., Hay, R.M., Gitelis, S. and Black, J. (1992) Early sarcomatous degeneration near a cementless hip replacement. A case report and review, *J. Bone Joint Surg.* **74B**, 740–4.

Khurana, J.S., Rosenberg, A.E., Kattapuram, S.V., Fernandez, O.S. and Shigeru, E. (1994) Malignancy supervening on an intramedullary nail, *Clin. Orthop.* **267**, 251–4.

Laffargue, P., Hildebrand, H.F., Lecomte-Houcke, M., Biehl, V., Breme, J. and Decoulx, J. (1998) Malignant fibrous histiocytoma in association with a metal implant. Analysis of corrosion products and their possible role in malignancy, *Int. J. Risk Safety Med.* in press.

Lee, Y.S., Pho, R.W.H. and Nather, A. (1984) Malignant fibrous histiocytoma at site of metal implant, *Cancer* **54**, 2286–9.

Lewis, C.G. and Sunderman, F.W., Jr (1996) Metal carcinogenesis in total joint arthroplasty, *Clin. Orthop.* **329S**, 264–8.

Little, D.G. and McCarthy, S.W. (1993) Malignant fibrous histiocytoma of bone: the experience of the New South Wales Bone Tumour Registry, *Aust. NZ J. Surg.* **63**, 346–51,

Lombardi, A.V., Mallory, T.H., Eberle, R.W., Mitchell, M.B., Lefkowitz, M.S. and Williams, J.R. (1995) Failure of intraoperatively customized non-porous femoral components inserted without cement in total hip arthroplasty, *J. Bone Joint Surg.* **77A**, 1836–43.

Mathiesen, E.B., Lindgren, J.U., Blomgren, G.G.A. and Reinholt, F.P. (1991) Corrosion of modular hip prostheses, *J. Bone Joint Surg.* **73B**, 569–75.

Matsuda, Y. and Yamamuro, T. (1994) Metallosis due to abnormal abrasion of the femoral head in bipolar hip prosthesis, *Med. Prog. Technol.* **20**, 185–9.

McCaskie, A.W., Roberts, M. and Gregg, P.J. (1995) Human tissue retrieval at post-mortem for musculoskeletal research, *Brit. J. Biomed. Sci.* **52**, 222–4.

McKellop, H.A., Campbell, P. and Park, S.H. (1995) The origin of submicron polyethylene wear debris in total hip arthroplasty, *Clin. Orthop.* **311**, 3–20.

McKellop, H.A., Sarmiento, A., Schwinn, C.P. and Ebramzadeh, E. (1990) *In vivo* wear of titanium-alloy hip prostheses, *J. Bone Joint Surg.* **72A**, 512–17.

Michel, R. and Zilkens, J. (1978) Untersuchungen zum Verhalten von Metallspuren im umgebenden Gewebe von AO-Winkelplatten mit Hilfe der Neutronen-aktivierungsanalyse, *Z. Orthop.* **116**, 666.

Mirra, J.M., Bullough, P.G., Marcove, R.C., Jacobs, B. and Huvos, A.G. (1974) Malignant fibrous histiocytoma and osteosarcoma in association with bone infarcts. Report of four cases, two in caisson workers, *J. Bone Joint Surg.* **56-A**, 932–40.

Nasser, S., Campbell, P.A., Kilgus, D., Kossovsky, N. and Amstutz, H.C. (1990) Cementless total joint arthroplasty prostheses with titanium-alloy articular surfaces: a human retrieval analysis, *Clin. Orthop. Rel. Res.* **261**, 171–85.

Nelson, J.P. and Phillips, P.H. (1990) Malignant fibrous histiocytoma in association with hip replacement, *Orthop. Rev.* **12**, 1078–80.

Pidhorz, L.E., Urban, R.M., Jacobs, J.J., Sumner, D.R. and Galante, J.O. (1993) A quantitative study of bone and soft tissues in cementless porous-coated acetabular components retrieved at autopsy, *J. Arthroplasty* **8**, 213–25.

Röckelein, G., Breme, J. and von der Emde, J. (1989) Lethal blockage of a Bjørk–Shiles artificial heart valve caused by strut fracture – the metallurgical aspect, *Thorac. cardiovasc. Surgeon* **37**, 47–51.

Sarmiento, A. and Gruen, T.A. (1985) Radiographic analysis of a low-modulus titanium-alloy femoral total hip component. Two to six year follow up, *J. Bone Joint Surg.* **67A**, 48–56.

Schmidt, H., Beck, H. and Zwicker, K. (1980) Untersuchungen über die Ursachen von Schaftbrüchen bei Hüftgelenkimplantaten 1. *Vortragsreihe des Arbeitskreises Implantate*, DVM, 169–180.

Schmalzried, T.P., Maloney, W.J., Jasty, M., Kwong, L.M. and Harris, W.H. (1993) Autopsy studies of the bone–cement interface in well-fixed cemented total hip arthroplasties, *J. Arthroplasty* **8**, 179–88.

Semlitsch, M. and Wintsch, W. (1972) Gefügeveränderungen am CoCrMoC-Implantatpräzisionsguss PROTASUL durch Hochtemperatur-Glühungen zur Erziehung optimaler Eigenschaften, *Beitr. elektronenmikroskop. directabb. Oberfl.* **5**, 701–21.

Solomon, M.I. and Sekel, R. (1992) Total hip arthroplasty complicated by a malignant fibrous histiocytoma. A case report, *J. Arthroplasty* **7**, 549–50.

Sunderman, F.W., Jr (1988) Carcinogenic risks of metal implants and prostheses, in *Biocompatibility of Co–Cr–Ni Alloys* (eds H.F. Hildebrand and M. Champy), NATO-ASI Series A, Vol. 158, Plenum, New York, pp. 11–19.

Sunderman, F.W., Jr (1989a) Mechanisms of nickel carcinogenesis, *Scand. J. Work Environ. Health* **15**, 1–2.

Sunderman, F.W., Jr (1989b) Carcinogenicity of metal alloys in orthopedic prostheses: clinical and experimental studies, *Fund. Appl. Toxicol.* **13**, 205–16.

Süry, P. (1974) Korrosionsgegossener und geschmiedeteter Implantatwerkstoffe unter Berücksichtigung von Verbundkonstruktionen bei Gelenkendoprothesen, Sonderdruck aus der Technische Rundschau SULZER, Forshungsheft, 1–12.

Tait, N.P., Hacking, P.M. and Malcolm, A.J. (1988) Case reports: malignant fibrous histiocytoma occurring at the site of a previous total hip replacement, *Br. J. Radiol.* **61**, 73–6.

Torgersen, S., Gjerdet, N.R., Erichsen, E.S. and Bang, G. (1995) Metal particles and tissue changes adjacent to miniplates, *Acta. Odontol. Scand.* **53**, 65–71.

Troop, J.K., Mallory, T.H., Fisher, D.A. and Vaughn, B.K. (1990) Malignant fibrous histiocytoma after total hip arthroplasty: a case report, *Clin. Orthop.* **253**, 297–300.

Visuri, T., Pukkala, E., Paavolainen, P., Pulkkinen, P. and Riska, E.B. (1996) Cancer risk after metal on metal and polyethylene on metal total hip arthroplasty, *Clin. Orthop.* **329S**, 280–9.

Wall, L. and Calcan, C.D. (1980) Occupational nickel dermatitis in the electroforming industry, *Contact Derm.* **6**, 414–20.

Weissman, B.N., Scott, R.D., Bridge, G.W. and Corson, J.M. (1991) Radiographic detection of metal-induced synovitis as a complication of arthroplasty of the knee, *J. Bone Joint Surg.* **73A**, 1002–7.

Willert, H.G. and Semlitsch, M. (1977) Reactions of the articular capsule to wear products of artificial joint prostheses, *J. Biomed. Mater. Res.* **11**, 157–64.

Index

actuation devices 81
adhesion 212, 213–15, 219–58, 293–6,
  see also cell adhesion, tissue adhesion
AFM, *see* atomic force microscopy
AISI 316L 257, 222, 414, 452
alkaline phosphatase 319
allergenic potency 265
allergies 277, 332, *see also* immunological reactions
alloys 266–7, 273 *see also* aluminium alloys, CoCr alloys, dental alloys, gallium-based alloys, NiTi alloys, shape memory alloys, titanium alloys
alumina 444, 446, 447, 449, 451, 458, 474
aluminium 127, 140, 268, 433, 440
  alloys 111
amalgams 40, 63–4, 134, 136
amino acids
  α 178–9
  proteinogenic 179
  single, adsorption of 189–90
anatase 138
anodic partial reactions 104, 105, 107, 124
artificial saliva 131
aseptic loosening 484, 485
atomic force microscopy 191, 359–400
Auger effect 346

bandwidth 83
beam-deflection scheme 367–70
beryllium 268
binding energy 345
biocompatibility 1, 7, 28, 97, 103, 112, 131, 138, 309–12, 429, 433, 440, 452, 461
biofunctionality 7, 24, 25
bioploymers 178–85
blasting
  abrasives 142
  treatment 142

Bode plot 119, 120–1, 122, 124, 410, 411, 423–5, 444–9, 461, 462, 463
body fluids, metal distribution in 478–81
bone
  decalcification 155
  formation 23
  healing process 193
  ingrowth 154–5, 160–1, 164
  properties of 43
  resorption 23, 91, 484, 485, 486
  structural modification 275
  see also osseointegration, osteoinduction, osteolysis 276
bovine serum 129, 131
brazing 47, 53, 58, 62, 219, 221–9
Butler–Volmer equation 307

cadmium 268–9
calcium 23
capacitative impedance 298–9
carbides 111, 112, 472
carbon 112, 137, 432, 433
carcinogenic
  agents 265
  features of metals 279, 331–2, 494–7
casting 154
catheters 88, 194
cathodic partial reaction 102, 104, 105, 107, 110, 124, 128
cell
  adhesion 293
  attachment 324–6, 327
  culture variability 323–4
  density 321
  lines 131, 132
  plating 320–1
  role of metals in 317–32
  viability 280–3
cellular interaction 324, 326–7
cementless implantation 3
ceramics 14, 15, 26, 219–58, 331

chain repulsion 203
chemical vapour deposition 172
chromium 111, 112, 137, 269, 433, 434, 439, 472, 474, 478, 479, 481, 494
clamping devices 79, 81
coated biomaterials 3, 4, 141–2, 143
coating, effect of 452–60
cobalt 269, 274
CoCr alloys 8, 9, 19, 37, 49–53, 103, 110, 132, 134, 137, 142, 154, 155, 156, 158, 172, 187, 188, 253, 266, 274, 279, 470, 471, 481
cold deformation 16, 17, 18, 19
collagen 183, 184–5, 191–3
compression stress 162–3
conformational relaxation 203
conformations 198
CoNiCr alloy 18, 27, 451
constant phase element 121, 408
contact angle 294
contact-mode operation in microscopy 375–8, 383
cooling restrictions 83
copolymers 202
copper 269–70
corrosion
   localised 104, 105, 108, 109, 144, 414
   processes 104–12, 306–9, 423–63, 471–2
   resistance 18, 19, 26, 27, 40, 103, 136, 137, 418, 427, 429, 442, 446, 449, 451, 452, 472, 478
creep 3, 15, 23, 27, 45
crevice
   corrosion 110
   width 125
crystallisable polymers 202
crystallisation process of glass ceramics 222
current–potential curves 105–6, 107, 115
CVD, *see* chemical vapour deposition
cytotoxicity 280–2
cytotronic effects 31

damping
   applications 79
   capacity 77

degradation 27, 83, 101–51, 460, 468, 469, 489
degree of deformation 45
density 47
density–potential curves 134–5
dental
   alloys 136, 266, 274, 278–9
   implants 160, 162–3, 166, 231
   restoration, materials for 40, 58–64, 127, 142
   see also orthodontics
depletion 110, 112, 140
deprotonation 31
dielectric
   constant 29, 31, 412, 420–2, 429
   properties of films 411–23
diffusion bonding 229–5
dispersion hardening 9
disulfide bridges 180
disuse atrophy 155
Dulbecco's modified Eagle's medium 131
Dupré equation 223

electric double layer (EDL) 213–14, 407, 420
electrical field strength 299
electrochemical
   impedance 120, 122
      data 441
      measurements 444
      spectrometry (EIS) 118, 405–63
   noise measurements 123–5
   reaction 104, 106–8
electrode 104
   counter 298–9, 405–9
   –myocardium interface 247
   potential 105
   reaction 409
   reference 114
   –tissue interface 246
   working 114, 298–9, 405–9
electron conductivity 188
electron mean free path 341
electronic properties of films 411–23
electrostatic
   bonding 222
   interaction 180

elongation at fracture 15, 47
energy efficiency 82
enthalpy 181, 183, 199
equilibrium potential 104
essential elements 265
European standards 127, 137
examination stages 113
experimental methods of examining degradation 112–33
extracellular fluid 414

fatigue 83
  corrosion 109, 112, 469
  failure 470–1
  strength 14, 15–16, 24, 25, 45–6, 48, 57, 160, 471
FCS, see foetal calf serum
Fermi energy 305, 345
fibre proteins 184, see also collagen
fibre-interferometric force microscope 367
fibroblasts 166–70
fibronectin 324–6
Fickian diffusion 204
films 411–52
Flory–Huggins theory 202
foetal calf serum 319–20
force
  curves 392–5
  sensors 364–70
forging 9–10
fracture
  energy 234
  toughness 15, 48, 49, 56
free recovery applications 79
frequency modulation 387
fretting corrosion 27, 109, 112, 138, 139, 439, 488
friction 9, 81, 113, 379–81, 474
fusion welding 235, 476

gallium-based alloys 136, 141
galvanic corrosion 102, 110, 111, 127, 143, 144
galvinostatic methods 115
genomic code, human 178
Gibb's adsorption isotherm 295
Gibb's enthalpy 185, 223, 224, 225

glass
  bondings 221–223
  transition temperature 199
gold 103, 136, 273, see also precious metals
grain
  boundary attack 110, 111, 471
  growth 19, 21
  size 14, 116, 121
granulated tissue 31
granulomas 275
gripper 92
growth factors 193
Gruen's zones 486, 488

H_2O_2 29, 31, 420, 421, 423, 427, 429, 440
Haber–Luggin capillary 114
Hall–Petch relation 21
Hanks solution 130, 140, 142, 444, 447, 448, 451, 452, 453
hard tissue 66
hardening time 64
hardness 49
HDH, see hydrogenisation–dehydrogenisation
heart valve, blockage of an artificial 476–8
heat of formation 29, 30, 223
Hellman–Feynman theorem 378 378
Helmholtz
  free energy 202
  layer 299
  potential 300–2
hingeless instruments 92
histiocytoma 494, 495
humidity 238
hydrogen
  adsorption 292
  bonds 180
  evolution 11, 105, 116
  peroxide 27
hydrogenisation–dehydrogenisation 158
hydrophobic interactions 186
hydroxyapatite 1, 3, 141, 142, 185, 193, 235, 236, 237, 238, 239, 240–5, 318–19, 452, 453, 454, 456, 458, 460, 469, 484
hydroxyl groups 27, 29, 31, 138, 139, 292
hysteresis 379

imflammatory reactions 28, 31, 272, 274, 276, 280, 282, 284, 484
immunological reactions 276, 309–12, 488
impedance
  measurements 121, 429, 444, 451
  modulii 458–60
  spectrometry 118–23, 405, 458
implant construction
  evaluation of 1
implant/body system, interactions causing injuries 29–31
implants
  comparison of materials 161–3
  electrodes 460–2
  environment 1, 177
  failed 481–84
  retrieval 467–98
  successful 481–84
  surface cavities 154–5
  surgical 266, 274, 277–8
implant–bone interface 155
in vivo degradation 132–3
inflammatory reactions 276, 322
inorganic media 130
insulators 300–1
intergrins 326–7
international standards 38, 49, 53, 280
interphases 197, 200
ion
  profiling 353
  release 142, 273, 479
iridium coatings 252, 461, 462
iron 270
isoelectric
  behaviour 24, 156, 159
  point 138, 302
isotropic molecular weight distribution 200
interstitial atoms 16

jaw, artificial 161, 162

kidney cells 28
knee sledge failure 474–6

L_{50} 280–3
Lewis acid–base interaction 214

limit of toxicity 28
locking 85, 90, 91
London forces 213
loosening of a hip prosthesis 484
lymphatic vessels 31

machining 10
  parameters for
    stainless steels 47
    CoCr alloys 52
macromolecules 197–200
malignant fibrous histiocytoma 494–7
manganese 233, 239, 240, 241, 266, 270, 433
martensitic transformation 73–5
matrix attachment force 327
mechanical loading, effect on biomaterials 14–15
medical instruments 92–6
membrane
  potential 329–31
  proteins 183
memory effect 76, 77, 79
metal
  allergies 332
  distribution of
    in fluid 27, 29, 478, 479
    in tissue 478, 479, 494
  ions
    classification of 141
    pharmacological effects of 327–8
  oncogenic effects of 331–2
  responsive elements 331
  roles in cells 317–32
  surfaces, protein adsorption on 188
  wear particles 486–9, 490–3
metallic biomaterial 14, 15, 16, 25, 27, 28, 29, 101, 102, 103, 104, 105, 110, 113, 127, 129, 130, 133, 137, 141, 220, 253, 265, 278, 337, 342, 345, 354, 355
  classification of 134
  combinations of 143–4
  strength, improvement of 16
  use of X-ray photoelectron spectroscopy for studying 337–55
metallosis 276, 270, 271, 470, 488, 489

INDEX

metal–polymer interaction 206
microscopy, background of 359–60
minimal invasive surgery 92
miniplates 31
modified Eagle's medium 131
molecular surface processes 185, 186
molybdenum 137, 233, 266, 270–1, 488, 489
moment of inertia 23, 24
Mott–Schottky analysis 303–4, 305–6, 411, 415–19
Mulliken electronegativity 305
multiphase alloys 18, 21

nanotechnology 395–9
Nerst equation 104–5
nickel 228, 229, 266, 271, 274, 278, 279, 286, 332, 433, 478, 479, 481, 483, 491, 494
NiCr alloys 62, 63, 221, 267, 283
niobium 40, 223, 231, 233, 234, 256, 266, 273, 291, 313
NiTi alloys 75, 85, 87, 92, 97
nitride layers on CoCr-based alloys 142
nitrogen implantation 9, 254
NMR, *see* nuclear magnetic resonance
noble metals 134, 136
non-contact–mode operation in microscopy 381–9
nuclear magnetic resonance 2, 201
nucleation 222
Nyquist plot 119, 120–1, 122, 406, 444–9, 451, 452, 454
Nyquist spectra 407–8, 444–9

on/off applications 81
open circuit potential 104, 105, 107, 108, 124, 418, 434–9, 440–2
organ cultures 131
organic
 coatings 177–94
 testing media 131
orthodontics 85–7
orthopaedics 90–1
osmotic pressure 322–3
osseointegration 11, 31, 153, 173, 355
osteoinduction 193

osteolysis 276, 485, 486
 periprosthetic 485–6, 487
osteonecrosis 276
osteosynthesis 90, 112, 470, 481, 484, 489–94
overpotential 106, 107, 128, 141
oxide films 411–52
oxygen 127, 128, 215, 227, 234, 270, 302, 305, 308, 309, 313, 323, 441, 474
 reduction 106, 309

PAA, *see* polyacrylic acid
pacemakers 235
palladium 136, 144
partial reactions 105
passive films 27, 107, 108, 109, 112, 134, 137, 138, 139, 140, 407, 411–52
Pauling electronegativity 305
Pauling–Corey peptide bond 179
peptides 178
pH 178, 189
photoelectric effect 338–9
photoelectron-spectroscopy 189
photoionisation cross-section 341
PHS, *see* photoelectron-spectroscopy
physical vapour deposition 172, 461, 474
piezoelectric effect 361
pin-on-disc method 129, 136
pK values 30, 138
pitting
 corrosion 109–10, 130, 136, 137
 potential 110, 111
plasma spraying 142, 451, 456, 458
plastic deformation 229
plating efficiency 321
platinum group elements 271
PMMA, *see* polymethylmetacrylate
pneumatic testing apparatus 160
point of zero charge 302–6
polarisation resistance 27, 28, 409, 429, 432–6, 439, 440, 442
polyacrylic acid 215
polycondensation 179, 181
polyethylene 23, 27, 133
 wear particles 486

polymer 197–218
  adsorption 206–7
  chain
    conformations 200
    dynamics 199
    metallisation of 206
    segment depletion 205–6
  polymer–polymer interfaces 197, 202–5
  polymethylmetacrylate 8, 15, 201, 214
  polypeptides 178, 179, 180
  polystyrene–PMMA 203
porosity 25, 26, 142, 158, 422, 427, 429, 460
porous sintering 25, 160–1, 247, 248
post-mortem retrieval 468–9
potentiodynamic polarisation 136
potentiostatic polarisation 115
power density spectra 125, 126
power/volume ratio 81–2
power/weight ratio 81–2
precious metals 40, 60–2, 134
precipitation hardening 16, 19, 20
probe–sample interactions 372–5, 390, 395–6
processing recommendations for stainless steel 46–8
properties of biomaterials
  biological 27–31
  chemical 26–7, 37–40, 47–50, 53, 59–60, 63, 64
  material-specific 1, 2
  mechanical 14–26, 42–6, 51, 61, 63, 65
  product-specific 1, 3
  physical 41, 50, 60, 63, 64
  surface 26–7
prostheses
  all-metal 7–13
  cemented 469
  hip 1, 3–5, 7–9, 12–13, 154, 158, 255–8, 468, 469, 472–4, 484
  hydroxyapatite-coated 469
  retrieved 9, 468, 471
proteins
  adsorption 185, 187–8
  fibre 184
  globular 191–3
  membrane 183

morphogenic 177, 193–4
  structure 180, 182
  surface binding of 319–20
  synthesis of 179–80
protonation 31
pseudoelasticity 75, 79
PVD see physical vapour deposition

reactive wetting 224, 226
recovery stresses 76, 77, 79
redox processes 423–63
refractory metals 40, 64–5, 291, 310, 311, see also titanium
reptation 204, 205
retrieval of implants 467–98
rigid materials 207
Ringer's solution 110, 130, 139, 141, 411, 432, 433, 441–4
Rouse relaxation 204

satellites 346–51
scanning
  force microcopy 364–95
  Kelvin microprobe 125–7, 128
  probe technology 360–4
  tunnelling microscope 359–60
self-diffusion coefficient 200
semi-conductors 134, 301–2, 415, 422
sensitisation 277
serum albumin
shape factor 170
shape-memory alloy 73–98
shear force microscopy 389–92
silver 136, 188, 206, 272, 278, 282
Simon Nitinol filter 95
slope detection 386–7
SMA, see shape-memory alloy
sol–gel 172–3, 241, 244, 245
solid–liquid interface 374
spatial adhesion maps 395
specific electrical resistance 49
specific heat capacity 60
stainless steel 17–18, 19, 27, 31, 32, 37, 38–48, 85, 103, 110, 111, 137, 266, 414, 416, 429, 439, 440, 441, 442, 449, 450, 452, 454, 456, 461, 462, 470, 478, 479, 481, 494
standard heat of formation of coatings 253

INDEX

stem machining 10
stents 87–9
strain point 222
stress corrosion cracking 112
superelastic
  applications 84
  deployable umbrellas 96
  effect 73–4, 76, 78, 84
  needles 94
  wires 95
surface
  binding of proteins 319–20
  characterisation techniques 140
  charge 297–8, 299–303
  chemical properties 14, 26
  coating 235–55
  composition 169–73
  elasticity 395
  electrified 396
  finishing 141–2
  metal 188
  modification 312–13
  polymer 200–2
  properties 14, 15, 26, 293–6
  structuring 153–8
  tension 293–6
  titanium oxide 191–3
synovial liquid 8, 129

Tafel constants 116–17
Tafel equation 306–7
Teflon 8
TEM, see transmission electron microscopy
temperature-activated applications 81–4
temperature-induced transformation 73, 75
tensile strength 15, 23, 66, 153, 154
tensile yield strength 60
thermal
  conductivity 66
  expansion behaviour 220, 221, 222
  expansion coefficient 66, 220, 221, 223, 231–3
  neutron-capture cross-section 66
  nitriding 251
  residual stress 219, 220
TiN-Thornton layers 247
tissue
  adhesion 153, 293

–implant interactions 291
  metal distribution in 478–81
  reactions 102, 103, 272, 275–6, 291
  soft 90, 468, 495
titanium 9, 11, 31, 32, 40, 53–8, 111, 133,
  137–41, 154, 155, 156, 157, 158, 161,
  172, 187, 188, 190, 193, 206, 223,
  266, 272, 291, 293, 295, 302, 312,
  313, 319, 321, 327, 338–9, 343, 355,
  411, 412, 418, 421, 422, 423, 424, 427,
  429, 434, 439, 452–6, 468, 470, 471,
  481
  alloys 10, 15, 17, 20–3, 40, 53–8, 134,
  137–41, 142, 153, 158, 160–1, 169,
  170, 172, 188, 193, 223, 225, 231, 232,
  233, 236–9, 240, 241, 245, 246, 249,
  251–4, 256, 275, 411, 412, 414, 416,
  418, 423–32, 439, 440, 454, 455, 458,
  460, 461, 470, 471, 474
  –ceramic coatings 246–53
  –hydroxyapatite composites 236–46
  oxide surfaces 189, 191–3, 222
tools, medical 92–6
toxicity 21, 28, 29, 141, 265, 267–73,
  280–4, 317, 331, 332, 467
trace elements 265
trans-configuration 179, 181
transfer
  function 118, 120, 122, 123, 468
  model 120
transmission electron microscopy 191
tungsten, see refractory metals

UHMWPE, see ultra high molecular weight
  polyethene
ultimate tensile strength 66
ultra high molecular weight polyethene 8–9,
  15, 25, 27, 254–5

vacuum plasma spraying 158
valence bands 351, 417
valve metals 134
van der Waals forces 360, 374, 375
van der Waals interaction 213, 381
vanadium 171, 172, 272–3, 275, 286, 433,
  439
Volta potential difference 126
VPS, see vacuum plasma spraying

Warburg impedance 122, 123
wear 470
   behaviour 101, 113, 129, 140
   debris 28, 470, 484, 485
   particles 8, 274–5, 470, 479, 484, 486, 488, 489
   rates 9, 27
   resistance 104, 119, 129, 134
wear-resistant ceramic coatings 253–5
welding 143, 219, 229–35, 476, 477
Wolff's law 24

X-ray photoelectron spectroscopy 337–55
X-ray satellites 347
XPS, *see* X-ray photoelectron spectroscopy

Young's modulus 4, 22, 23, 26, 66, 158–9, 160, 162–3, 166, 219, 233, 469
   vs density chart 6

zeta potential 297–8
zinc 273
   regulatory factor 331
zirconia 14, 27